Textbook of ORAL PATHOLOGY

Dr Mrinalini Sant MD
Former Head of the Department of Pathology
NSCB Medical College, Jabalpur, Madhya Pradesh

New Central Book Agency (P) Ltd
LONDON
DELHI KOLKATA PUNE HYDERABAD ERNAKULAM

REGD OFFICE

8/1 Chintamoni Das Lane, Kolkata 700 009, India
email: ncbapvtltd@eth.net

OVERSEAS

NCBA (UK) Ltd, 149 Park Avenue North, Northampton, NN3 2HY, UK

EXPORT

NCBA Exports Pvt. Ltd, 212 Shahpur Jat, New Delhi 110 049
email: ncbaexp@ncbapvtltd.com

BRANCHES

208B Peacock Lane, Shahpur Jat
New Delhi 110 049
email: ncbadel@ncbapvtltd.com

Shop Nos. 3 & 4, Vinayak Towers
681/B Budhwar Peth, Appa Balwant Chowk
Pune 411 002
email: ncbapune@ncbapvtltd.com

House No. 3-1-315, 1st Floor
Nimboliadda, Kachiguda, **Hyderabad** 500 027
email: ncbahydb@ncbapvtltd.com

GSS Shopping Complex, 1st Floor
Opposite College Post Office, Convent Road
Ernakulam 682 035
email: ncbaernk@ncbapvtltd.com

TEXTBOOK OF ORAL PATHOLOGY

First Published: January 2011

PUBLISHER AND TYPESETTER

New Central Book Agency (P) Ltd
8/1 Chintamoni Das Lane, Kolkata 700 009

PRINTER

New Central Book Agency (P) Ltd
Web-Offset Division, Dhulagarh, Sankrail, Howrah

COVER DESIGNER

Soumen Paul

COVER PRINTER

Liba Graphics, Kolkata

TECHNICAL EDITOR

Dr Mita Sen, MBBS

PROOF CHECKING

Subas Maitra and Kakali Banerjee

PROJECT TEAM

Prabhat Jas and Suman Dutta

ISBN: 978-81-7381-645-1

Price: ₹ 325.00

Dedicated
To My mother
Mrs Shanta Hamine
and
Loving memory of my father
Late Moreshwar Hamine

CONTENTS

Foreword vii

Preface ix

Acknowledgement xi

Chapter 1. Introduction 1-7

Chapter 2. Advanced Techniques in Pathology 8-15

Chapter 3. Developmental Disturbances of Oral and Paraoral Structures 16-47

Chapter 4. Healing of Oral Wounds 48-56

Chapter 5. Dental Caries 57-65

Chapter 6. Diseases of Pulp and Periapical Tissues 66-72

Chapter 7. Diseases of Periodontium 73-85

Chapter 8. Physical and Chemical Injury 86-100

Chapter 9. Bacterial, Viral, Fungal, and Parasitic Infections of Oral Cavity 101-137

Chapter 10. Osteomyelitis 138-146

Chapter 11. Diseases of Blood and Blood Forming Organs 147-175

Chapter 12. Skin Diseases Manifested in Oral Mucosa 176-198

Chapter 13. Oral Aspects of Metabolic Diseases 199-211

Chapter 14. Diseases of Bones and Joints with Oral Manifestations 212-223

Chapter 15. Oral Manifestations of Immunological Disorders 224-239

Chapter 16. Nutrition and Oral Cavity 240-258

Chapter 17. Diseases Affecting Nerves and Muscles 259-275

Chapter 18. Cystic Lesions of Oral Cavity 276-290

Chapter 19. Benign Tumours of Oral Cavity 291-310

Chapter 20. Premalignant Lesions and Conditions 311-324

Chapter 21. Malignant Tumours of Oral Cavity 325-355

Chapter 22. Salivary Gland 356-377

Chapter 23. Odontogenic Tumours 378-390

Chapter 24. Cytology 391-396

Chapter 25. Spread of Oral Infection 397-406

Index 407-415

FOREWORD

I am delighted that my colleague has chosen to write a book on Oral Pathology. It is a matter of great pride for me to write this foreword for her book. The author has long been a front line teacher and consultant to medical fraternity in the field of Pathology.

I have had my association with the author's earlier book *Textbook of Pathology*, which has been acclaimed and accepted as an informative textbook. The knack of presenting the subject in the classroom has helped her presentation look more original and insightful. It is an invaluable contribution, to say the least. It includes 116 subject-oriented photographs, 36 tables and 14 illustrations.

The author has, as the readers will understand, started from the fundamentals and later on proceeded towards advanced analysis casting conceptual light on various topics in relevant chapters.

Indeed, the book has aptly fulfilled the need of a good textbook for the dental courses in the medical field.

I have no doubt that the simplicity of the text and its exceptional clarity will be much appreciated by the readers. Special care has been taken to include literature from the latest references.

I would, in the end, exclaim what an effort by the author after retirement ! I wish happy reading for everybody and best wishes for the success of this book.

Dr J L Vegad
Former Professor and Head,
Department of Pathology and
Dean, College of Veterinary Science
and Animal Husbandry
Jabalpur 482001, India

Jabalpur
22.09.2010

PREFACE

In Pathology, knowledge regarding Etiology and Pathogenesis is increasing by leaps and bounds, more and more disease subunits are coming to the fore. Innovations in the field of Oral Pathology, naturally, continue to hold great promise. Advances in technology, and diagnostic and surgical techniques, and the development of new medications are providing doctors and scientists with even more powerful tools for diagnosing and treating diseases.

A brief overview of applied basic sciences have been given at the beginning of chapters to enhance understanding of clinical problems. This book includes 25 chapters. In each system, normal structure functions and the symptom signs that arise from pathological changes are discussed first in each chapter. Knowledge is essential for the Bachelor of Dentistry students.

This book is based on recent Medical Council of India syllabus, covering the modules of didactic teaching for the Bachelor of Dentistry students as per Medical Council of India and Indian Association of Dentistry recommendation.

Histology is an essential component of Pathology teaching in all dental courses; nevertheless, the scope, content and emphasis on microscopy vary considerably between different centres. This book is designed to meet as closely as possible the requirements of all these varied and differing courses.

The salient feature of this book is to make learning easy. Well-labelled diagrams and tables have been furnished at appropriate places all through the text. Latest state-of-the-art developments and new concepts are included in great detail.

Every effort has been made to keep the volume comprehensive, profusely illustrated and still handy—maintaining the emphasis on the needs of BDS students. A good number of coloured plates (116), tables (36) and illustrations (14) are provided to enhance the utility of the volume.

I hope my efforts would meet the expectations of the students. I would greatly welcome and appreciate suggestions, comments, criticisms from the interested students and erudite teachers to help me improve the quality of this book further.

The present volume is sure to prove highly beneficial to the students of oral pathology and oral medicine, as well as practising dentists.

22.09.2010 — Dr (Mrs) Mrinalini Sant

PREFACE

ACKNOWLEDGEMENT

At the outset I want to thank Almighty God who encourages each of us to discover the work we should do and is pleased when we perform that work with integrity.

I am grateful to Dr J L Vegad (former Professor of Veterinary Pathology) for his timely suggestions during the preparation of the text.

A handful of people deserve special mention. Dr Rajesh Dhirawani, Director, Jabalpur Hospital and Research Centre was instrumental in providing library facilities and continuous encouragement during the preparation of the manuscript. Dr Ashwin Deshmukh also contributed by providing valuable guidance. I am equally thankful to him for permitting me to use some relevant photographs provided by him.

I am thankful to Dr Manish Mishra and Dr Shyamji Rawat for providing valuable photographs.

I must express my thanks to Mr Arun Pillai, Librarian, NSCB Medical College, Jabalpur for full academic support.

My special thanks to Mrs Kiran Dubey for initiating me in the field of computers.

All the patients deserve special mention for their contribution. I am immensely indebted to them.

I still wish my father was alive. He taught me to work hard and believe in myself. My mother, brother and sisters must know that their love for me has kept me going for writing the second book. To each of the family members I offer my admiration, my appreciation and my heart-felt thanks.

Lastly, I must not forget my family members–notably my husband Dr S K Sant, retired Principal, Government Engineering College, Jabalpur, my son Ashish (BE, MTech), my daughter-in-law Kavitha (MCA), my daughter Ashwini (MSc, Applied Physics) and son-in-law Prassanna (BSc, MBA). Without their continuous wholehearted support it would not have been possible for me to complete the long-drawn job of the preparation of the manuscript.

I could not have worked with a better publishing house than New Central Book Agency (P) Ltd whose professional staff made the process of publishing my second book a wonderful experience for me. Success of the book should be equally attributed to effort and enthusiasm of the people we don't see, who ponder over the layout until it is just right, tirelessly promote the book in the market so that the book succeeds. I appreciate the effort of every single person in the Company. I have been blessed with marvellous publishing team of NCBA who minutely reviewed every word with devoted attention. Incidentally the same team was assigned for publishing my first book.

I express special gratitude to Mr Amitabha Sen, Director, NCBA for his earnest endeavour—in multifarious ways—in publishing this book. I would like to offer my special thanks to Mr Soumen Paul for expediting the work from time to time.

There is every possibility, that some names that should appear here have been inadvertently left out, if so, please accept my apology and know that your contribution has made a difference.

Vancouver, Canada

22.09.2010

Dr (Mrs) Mrinalini Sant

CHAPTER 1

INTRODUCTION

INTRODUCTION

Oral pathology deals with the nature of oral diseases, their causes, processes and effects. It relates the clinical manifestation of oral diseases to physiologic and anatomical changes associated with these diseases. It deals with commonly occurring premalignancies and malignancies and serves commonly with the scientifically based information. It also deals with dental science to administrative of law and furtherance of justice.

NORMAL STRUCTURE

Jaw consists of an upper maxilla, and a lower mandible, the bony part with a covering of skin and other soft tissues. The inner borders have teeth arranged all around and are covered by gingival.

MANDIBLE

Development

Mandible is developed from the first pharyngeal arch. The mandible is a flat bone with two layers of compact bone separated by a layer of cancellous bone.

The mandible is a U-shaped bone forming the lower jaw; it has alveolar processes for the mandibular teeth. It consists of a horizontal part—the body, and a vertical part, the ramus. The meeting point of the posterior border of the ramus with the lower margin of the body is known as the angle of mandible, where the stylomandibular ligament is attached.

Body of mandible

Inferior to the second premolar teeth is mental foramina. Forming the prominence of the chin is the mental protuberance, a triangular elevation of bone inferior to the mandibular symphysis—the region where the halves of the infantile mandible fuse.

Oblique line

Oblique line is the lower and forward continuation of the anterior border of the ramus. It runs towards the mental tubercle. It gives origin to the buccinator muscle. The inferior border of the body of the mandible presents the digastric fossa in the midline.

Ramus of the mandible

It is quadrilateral and has the anterior, posterior, superior, and inferior borders and the inner and the outer surfaces. The oblique line runs downwards from the anterior border of the ramus of the mandible. It gives origin to buccinator muscles. The mandibular foramen, lingual of the mandible and the mylohyoid groove are seen on the medial surface of the ramus.

Lingula is the tongue like process projecting from the anterior border of the mandibular foramen. It is directed upwards. Mandibular foramen is meant for the inferior dental nerve, and the vessels which run further in the mandibular canal. They supply the lower teeth of each half.

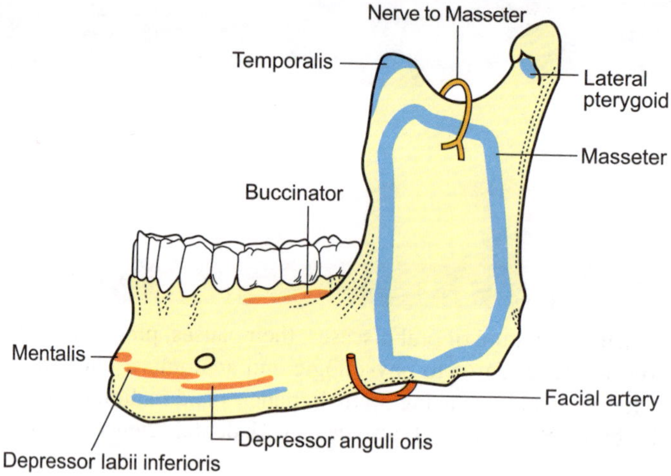

Fig.1.1: Showing mandible external surface

Sphenomandibular ligament runs from spine of the sphenoid to the lingual of the mandible below. The mylohyoid nerve and the vessels pierce it.

Superior border of the ramus of the mandible presents the notch bounded in front by the coronoid and behind by the condyloid processes. The notch gives the passage to the nerve to the masseter.

Condyloid process has the head. It is expanded transversely and is covered with the fibrocartilage. The head of the mandible articulates with the mandibular fossa of the temporal bone to form the temporomandibular joint.

Coronoid process provides insertion to the temporalis muscle along its medial surface and the neck of the mandible.

Posterosuperior part of the lateral surface of the ramus of the mandible is related to the parotid gland. Medial surface of the ramus of the mandible between the angle and the lingula gives origin to the medial pterygoid muscle.

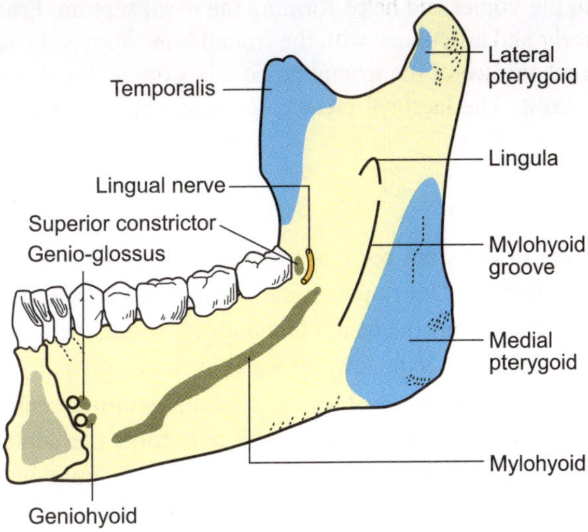

Fig.1.2: Showing mandible internal surface

MAXILLA

The maxillae form the upper jaw and are united at the inter-maxillary suture in the median plane. Their alveolar processes include the tooth sockets (alveoli) and constitute the supporting bone for maxillary teeth. The maxillae surround most of the pyriform aperture and form the infraorbital margins medially. They have a broad connection with the zygomatic bones laterally and have an infraorbital foramen inferior to each orbit.

Maxilla contributes to the formation of the face. Together they form the skeleton of the face, part of the nose, part of the orbit and anterior wall of the infratemporal and pterygopalatine fossae.

Face is divided into three equal parts—upper, middle, and the lower.

Frontal bone occupies the upper mandible and the lower, and the maxilla the middle.

Maxilla presents the body and four processes—namely the frontal zygomatic alveolar base directed medially towards the lateral wall of the nose. The apex is directed towards the zygoma. It has the base, apex, superior, inferior, posterior and anterior surfaces.

Superior surface forms the orbital floor and the inferior surface forms the roof of the oral cavity. Anterior surface points towards the face and the posterior surface forms the anterior wall of the infratemporal fossa.

Zygomatic process of the maxilla forms the anterior wall of the infratemporal fossa. Medial margin of the anterior surface of the maxilla forms the nasal notch, which forms the boundary of the anterior nasal aperture. Superior surface of the body of the maxilla has the groove meant for the infraorbital nerve, which enters the infraorbital canal and opens anteriorly 4 mm below the infraorbital margin on the face.

Anteromedial part of the orbital surface has a small notch which forms the limit of the canal for the nasolacrimal duct.

Orbital surface of the maxilla articulates with the zygomatic, ethmoidal and lacrimal above. Posterior surface of the maxilla forms the inferior limit of the infraorbital fissure. The zygomatic process is strong and thick and it forms the partition between the infratemporal fossa and the orbit. Palatine process forms the hard palate. It articulates posteriorly with the horizontal plate of the palatine. Nasal crest of the maxillae fits into the vomer and helps forming the nasal septum. Frontal process of the maxilla projects posterosuperiorly and articulates with the frontal bone above, the nasal bone in front, and the lacrimal behind. External surface of the frontal process has the lacrimal crest which continues, as the inferior margin of the orbit. The lacrimal crest gives attachment to the medial palpebral ligament.

TOOTH

Development

Teeth start developing in the sixth week of embryonic life due to proliferation of oral ectoderm along the whole length of the jaw. Development into an outer process leads to formation of the cheeks and lips and the inner process forms the dental lamina from which the teeth develop. A bud develops from the dental lamina, which descends down in the ecto-mesenchymal arches—the future mandible and maxilla—and forms a cap. The inside of the cap contains ecto-mesenchymal cells called the dental papilla. Surrounding the cap, the ecto-mesenchymal cells form the dental sac. This bud gradually grows to a bell-shaped structure, which is the future enamel, the pulp and dentin, while cells in the dental sac form the cementum and the periodontal ligament.

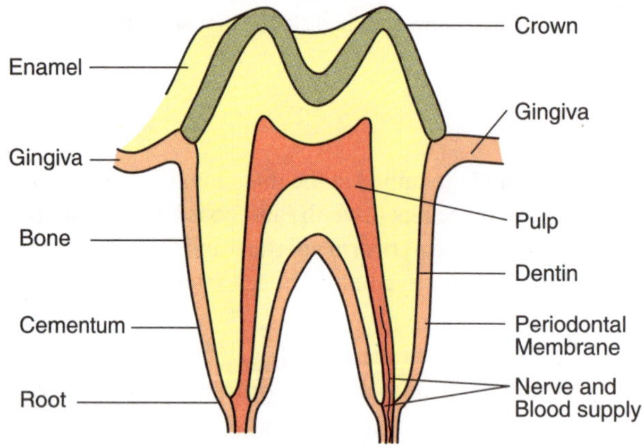

Fig.1.3: Parts of tooth

The tooth has two prominent parts—crown and root. Crown is visible in the oral cavity and root is embedded in the jaw bone. Teeth are named incisors, canines, premolar and molars commencing from the midline.

Structurally, each tooth consists of several parts:

Neck is the region of the tooth that is at the gum line, between the root and the crown.

Enamel, the outermost covering of tooth, is the hardest structure in the body with inorganic components, mainly with calcium salts. Enamel protects the tooth besides giving colour and lustre. Mature enamel is not considered to be a living tissue.

Dentin is also a calcified structure forming bulk of the tooth and it consists of collagen fibres. The dentin is composed of millions of tiny cells arranged in a tubular shape; it is sensitive to temperature and touch.

Cementin is another calcified structure covering the root portion.

Pulp, the central part of the tooth, viewed in a sagittal section, contains nerves carrying sensation and blood vessels serving nutrition to the tooth.

Root canal: Extension of pulp within the root of the tooth is called the root canal. The root canal connects with the surrounding tissue via the opening at the tip of the root. This is an opening in the cementum through which the tooth's nerve supply and blood supply enter the pulp from the surrounding tissue.

Periodontal ligament, a band of connective tissue, attaches the tooth to the alveolar bone. It carries pain and pressure sensations, and allows movement of tooth within physiological limits.

TONGUE

Structure of tongue

Tongue is the inverted shoe-shaped muscular organ covered with stratified squamous epithelium situated in the floor of the mouth with its tip directed anteriorly and base posteriorly.

Tongue is composed entirely of muscle and connective tissue covered with two types of mucosa.

The ventral surface is smooth and not involved in tasting food. Deep irregular veins can be seen as bluish structures running towards the tip.

The dorsal surface is on top and is covered with a thin, pink velvet carpet. The velvet is composed of tiny hair-like projections called filiform papillae.

The dorsal aspects of the tongue may be thought of as divided into thirds. The anterior two-third is known as oral tongue, and it is this portion that is mobile. A pharyngeal part (posterior one-third of the tongue) faces backward to the oropharynx.

The upper side of the posterior tongue (pharyngeal part) has no visible taste buds, but it is bumpy because of lymphatic nodules lying underneath.

Nerve supply

Mucous membrane of anterior two-third of the tongue is supplied by the lingual nerve and the chorda tympani. Posterior one-third of the tongue including the circumvallate papillae is supplied by the glossopharyngeal nerve.

The internal laryngeal nerve supplies posterior most part of the pharyngeal surface of tongue.

Blood supply

The lingual artery—the branch of the external carotid artery is the chief artery supplying the tongue through dorsal and the deep branches. Inferior alveolar artery—the branch of first part of the maxillary—also supplies the tongue.

Lymphatic drainage

Numerous lymph vessels from the tip of the tongue drain bilaterally in the submental lymph nodes. However, some reach jugulo-digastric nodes.

Central lymph vessels from the midline pass downwards through the core of the tongue and end in the jugulo-digastric group of both the sides.

Lymphatics from the lateral part of the anterior two-third of the tongue go to the submandibular nodes.

Lymphatics from the posterior one-third of the tongue go to the jugulo-digastric and to the jugulo-omohyoid nodes. Some of the lymphatic channels from the posterior one-third of the tongue may go to the retropharyngeal nodes.

WALDEYER'S RING

It is the name given to the collection of lymphoid tissues. They are the palatine, lingual, tubal and the adenoids found around the pharynx inside. The outer ring of the Waldeyer's consists of the group of lymph nodes outside the pharynx such as submental, submandibular, preauricular and postauricular and the occipital.

LIPS

Lips are thick muscular folds covered with the mucous membrane from inside and skin from outside. The meeting point of the skin and mucous membrane is known as the edge of the lip. The orbicularis muscle and other small muscles form the core of the lip. Lips meet laterally at the angle of the mouth. Frenulum—a thick mucous fold connects the lip to the gums in the midline.

CHEEK

It is made up of the skin, fatty tissue, buccopharyngeal fascia, buccinator muscle, submucous coat and the mucous membrane—arranged from lateral to the medial side.

GUMS

They form the dense fibrous structure along the margin of both the jaws, and fit the teeth like a collar. Fixed part is firmly attached to the jaws at the alveolar processes. Nerve supply of the lower gums comes from the inferior alveolar, lingual, and the buccal. Buccal nerve supplies the outer part of the lower gums up to the mental foramen.

Soft palate

Soft palate is the structure composed of mucous membranes, muscular fibres, and mucous glands—suspended from the posterior border of the hard palate forming the roof of oral cavity.

Hard palate

It is a semilunar area located between the upper alveolar bridge and the mucous membrane covering the palatine process of maxillary bones.

Floor of the mouth

It is a U-shaped area bounded by the lower gingival and the oval tongue.

SALIVARY GLANDS

ANATOMY

There are three major salivary glands in the mouth. The largest pair of—salivary glands—called the parotid glands—lies just behind the angle of the jaw, below and in front of the ears. Two smaller pairs—the sublingual glands and submandibular glands—lie deep in the floor of the mouth.

MINOR SALIVARY GLANDS

There are over 600 minor salivary glands located throughout the oral cavity within the lamina propria of the oral mucosa. They are 1-2 mm in diameter and, unlike the other glands, they are not encapsulated by connective tissue.

The minor salivary glands are scattered in the mucosa of nasal cavity, paranasal sinuses, oral cavity, oropharynx, hypopharynx, larynx and trachea.

The gland consists of number of acini connected in a tiny lobule. A minor salivary gland may have a common excretory duct with another gland, or may have its own excretory duct. All the glands produce saliva and aids in breaking down food as part of the digestive process. Their secretion is mainly mucous in nature.

Development

Both the major and minor salivary glands develop from the oral ectoderm as solid epithelial buds appearing between sixth to tenth week of embryonic life. The ingrowing epithelial buds enlarge and form branching structures and, subsequently they become hollow to form ducts. The distal end of these ductal structures differentiates to form secretory acini.

Histology

Acini: Salivary gland unit consists of numerous acini from which narrow intercalated ducts arise. The parotid gland acini are composed of large plump serous cells packed with basophilic zymogen granules.

Ducts: The ducts are lined by flattened to cuboidal cells. Intercalated ducts converge and unite to form intralobular ducts with tall columnar lining. Cytoplasm of these cells is acidophilic and reveals longitudinal radial striations. These intralobular ducts are also known as striated ducts.

Interlobular ducts: Intralobular ducts further combine forming interlobular ducts.

Secretory ducts: The interlobular ducts finally join together to form the secretory duct.

Myoepithelial cells: Salivary acini and ducts are lined by epithelial and myoepithelial cells, also known as basket cells. Myoepithelial cells lie directly on the basement membrane underneath the epithelial cells. Myoepithelial cells play an important role in salivary gland tumours.

Bibliography

Kadanse DK: *Kadanse's Textbook of Anatomy*, 2009, 2nd edition, Jaypee Brothers Medical Publishers (P) Ltd.

CHAPTER

2

ADVANCED TECHNIQUES IN PATHOLOGY

MICROSCOPY

A microscope is used to produce enlarged and well-defined images of objects too small to be observed with naked eyes. There are two main types of microscopy:

1. Light microscopy (0.2 μ resolution)

   Visible light—Routine microscopy

   Ultraviolet light—Fluorescent microscopy

2. Electron microscopy (0.2 nm resolution): Beam of electrons in an electromagnetic field are used to visualise the specimen.

There are two types of microscopes:

1. Simple microscope: This is a simple hand-magnifying lens. The magnification power of hand lens is from 2x to 30x.
2. Compound microscope can be uniocular or binocular.

DARK GROUND MICROSCOPE

In the dark ground microscope, reflected light is used instead of the transmitted light. The essential part of the dark field microscope is the dark field condenser with a central circular stop, which illuminates the object with cone of light.

Certain very slender bacteria, such as the spirochetes, are so freely retractile that they cannot be seen by ordinary microscopic method; and dark ground illumination is necessary for their demonstration.

Dark field microscope is also used to demonstrate trypanosomes, other microorganisms, body fluids, cell suspensions, flow cell techniques, parasites and auto-radiographic grain counting.

FLUORESCENCE MICROSCOPY

The technique involves conversion of invisible ultraviolet light into visible light by use of appropriate filters to visualise the reaction of antigen and antibody complex in histological section. Fluorescence microscopy can be utilised:

(i) For detection of tubercle bacilli; if a smear is stained with Rhodamine, or Auramine.

(ii) In the diagnosis of skin diseases e.g., pemphigus.

(iii) It can demonstrate, with the help of fluorochrome dyes (Thioflavin T for amyloid, and Acridine orange for malignant cells in exfoliative cytology).

(iv) For demonstration of antinuclear antibody and other tissue antibodies in SLE and other autoimmune diseases.

(v) It is used for detection of viral antigens in frozen tissue sections, acetone fixed cell smears, cells from virus infected cultures or vesicle fluid by direct or indirect fluorescent antibody technique.

(vi) Fluorescence microscopy of brain biopsy can be used for diagnosis of herpes simplex encephalitis and subacute sclerosing pancephalitis.

(vii) It is used for verification of rabies in the brain of animals suspected to be rabid.

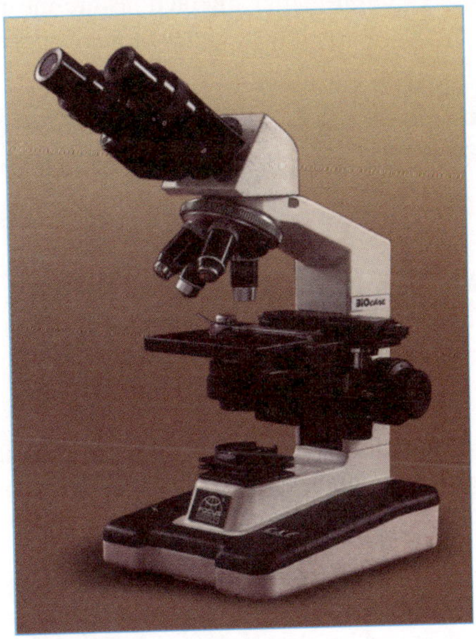

Fig.2.1: Showing compound binocular microscope

ELECTRON MICROSCOPY (EM)

In electron microscopy stream of electrons in magnetic fields are used. This stream of electrons has a very short wavelength (a 50 kv electron beam produces light of 0.0055 nm).

Uses of electron microscope

1. Renal pathology: E.M. aids are used for classification of kidney diseases; reveals all structural details of glomerulus. In renal pathology, E.M. is used in conjunction with immunofluorescence.
2. It is used to study pathology of liver diseases.

3. To study ultra-structure of tumours of uncertain histogenesis. E.M. plays an important but selective role in diagnostic study of tumours.
4. Electron microscopic study of skin, brain, rectum, muscles, and nerves in storage diseases.
5. Other tissues and cells studied by E.M. are liver, heart, nerves, macrophages, and respiratory epithelium.

Types of electron microscope

1. *Transmission electron microscope*: The transmission electron microscope is similar to the light microscope in that it uses lenses to form magnified image. The condenser lenses concentrate the incident beam upon the specimen. This beam passes through the specimen to the projector lens and forms an enlarged image on to a fluorescent screen.
2. *Scanning electron microscope*: It scans the surface of the objects. Advantages of SEM are:
   (i) Provides three-dimensional image.
   (ii) Specimens of large size or thickness can be studied.
   (iii) Differentiate B and T-lymphocytes on the basis of their surface morphology.
   (iv) For viewing of podocytes in renal epithelium.
3. Analytical electron microscope is an essential tool for microstructural investigations of non-structured material. Since electron-matter interactions are mostly elastic, high electron doses are necessary for all methods of analytical electron microscope.

ELECTROPHORESIS

The term electrophoresis describes the migration of a charged particle under the influence of an electric field.

Paper electrophoresis

In paper electrophoresis, Whatman 1, 2, 3 type of paper is used. A direct current of 0.5 to 7 mA is applied. The process is conducted for 16 hours. For proteins, bromophenol blue, amide black, azocarmine B are used for various types of staining. For lipoproteins, oil red O, Sudan III are used.

Gel electrophoresis

Gels of agar, starch, and polyacramide coated on microscopic glass slides could be used. In column electrophoresis, gel can be placed in column, in which various fractions like pre-albumin, post-albumin and hepatoglobin can be separated.

Immunoelectrophoresis

Principle: Immunoelectrophoresis is one of the elegant techniques in gel diffusion in which the antigenic mixture is primarily separated by electrophoresis and, subsequently, subjected to antibody in immunodiffusion. The resulting immunoprecipitates (arcs) assume different shapes and exhibit varying motilities.

Uses of immunoelectrophoresis

(i) To determine if two proteins in a mixture are antigenetically similar or different.
(ii) It is most suitable for the recognition of abnormal immunoglobulins and, hence, has an utmost utility in the diagnosis of multiple myeloma.
(iii) It is an important research tool for the assessment of purity of the protein component and monospecificity of the locally raised antibody.
(iv) In separation of various proteins like albumin, globulin, pre-albumin.
(v) In separation of various haemoglobins like HbA, HbS, HbC, and HBF.

(vi) In separation of complement components Clq, Clr, Cls, C3, C4, C5.

(vii) Identification of C reactive protein.

(viii) Separation of lipids like HDL, VLDL, and LDL.

Countercurrent immunoelectrophoresis

Principle: Under the influence of electric current, antigen (Ag) and its corresponding antibody (Ab) are driven in opposite direction (Ab moves from cathode to anode) and, when they meet in an optimum proportion, immunoprecipitate develops at the junction of the two wells.

Uses

The CIEP is perhaps the only technique used in the diagnostic immunology:

(i) It has a versatile utility for the rapid identification of microbial antigens, e.g., pneumococcal antigen, salmonella antigen.

(ii) It is used for demonstration of alpha-fetoprotein, complement, anti-DNA antibody and fibrin degradation products in human serum.

(iii) Detection of antigen HbsAg and antibody (Anti Hbs).

(iv) Detection of diphtheria toxin.

HAEMOGLOBIN ELECTROPHORESIS

Haemoglobin electrophoresis was done on cellulose acetate strip at alkaline pH 8.6, because it is the best method of separating abnormal haemoglobins as a routine procedure. This method is simple, rapid, and sensitive, and is satisfactory for distinguishing common haemoglobin variants.

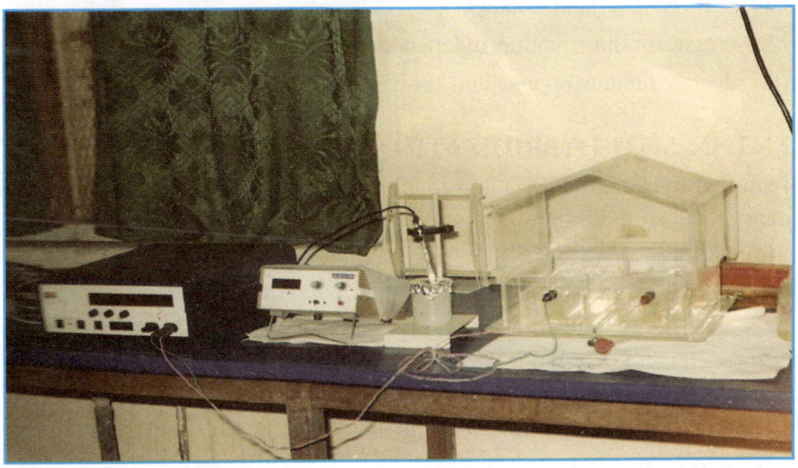

Fig.2.2: Electrophoretic tank, pH meter and power source used in the haemoglobin electrophoresis

At alkaline pH 8.6, hemoglobin is negatively charged protein and, in an electric field will migrate towards the anode. Most structural variants of haemoglobin will separate due to surface charge differences and, thus, allow identification of abnormal forms.

Haemoglobin H is the fast moving haemoglobin present in cases of alpha thalassaemia. The haemoglobin, which crosses HBA are HbH, Hb Bart, I, J, K, HbA2 and HbD migrate near anode. HbA2 is increased in thalassaemia minor and HbF in thalassaemia major. HbH and Hb Bart are present in alpha homozygous thalassaemia.

MOLECULAR PATHOLOGY

FLOW CYTOMETRY

Flow cytometry (FCM) is a rapidly expanding technology. It is a method for the separation, classification and quantification of blood cells and antibodies which affects blood cells. Complex computer operated instruments are used to pass a monocellular stream of cell, platelets, or other microscopic particulate elements—through a beam of laser light. The structural parameters measured by FCM are cell size, cytoplasmic granularity, surface antigens, DNA content, RNA content, chromatin structure, and enzyme content of the cells.

Applications of flow cytometry

Applications of flow cytometry are in the areas of immunology, oncology, and haematology:

1. Immunotyping of leukaemia, lymphoma, and plasmacytic neoplasm.
2. Detection of minimal disease in acute leukaemia below the detection limit.
3. Identification of reversal of T4 and T8 ratio in diagnosis and prognosis of AIDS.
4. To diagnose the cause of allograft rejection.
5. Diagnosis of autoantibodies in ITP and autoimmune neutropaenia.
6. DNA aneuploidy analysis in various types of cancer.
7. Enumeration of visible cells.
8. Oncogene protein detection.
9. Reticulate count.
10. Measurement of nucleic acid content.
11. It provides prognostic information independent of stage and grade of the tumour.
12. It helps to identify tumour relapse and tissue of origin of tumours.

FLUORESCENT IN SITU HYBRIDIZATION

Fluorescent in situ hybridization (FISH) is a highly refined technique for identifying numerical or structural changes in the chromosomes.

Tissue in situ hybridization (TISH) is the tissue equivalent of FISH. This is extensively used to identify activation of cell growth factors, proliferation potential markers and oncogenes.

FISH involves specific hybridization of a single strand labelled nucleic acid probe to a single strand complementary target DNA and RNA in the tissues. DNA probes are labelled with fluorescent dyes and spreads or interphase nuclei. The end product of hybridization is visualised by radioactive labelled probe (32P, 125I) or non-radioactive labelled probe biotin digoxigenin.

Applications of FISH technique

A. *Application of infectious diseases*

1. Viral diseases
   a. DNA probes have been employed to detect hepatitis B virus DNA in liver and serum of chronic hepatitis in carriers.
   b. Cytomegalovirus pneumonitis, detection of HPV 16 and 18 sequence of human papilloma virus in Pap smear and biopsy section.
2. Non-viral infectious agents: Tuberculosis, Neisseria gonorrhoea, *E. coli*.
3. Bacteria–like agents: Chlamydia, rickettsia.

4. Protozoa: Plasmodium, Leishmania.
5. Helminths: Schistosoma species.

B. *Applications in cancers*

In situ hybridization using oncogene probes in surgical pathology. In situ hybridization techniques are used to detect oncogene alteration in:

1. Chronic myeloid leukaemia
2. Neuroblastoma
3. Breast cancers or MYCN
4. Applications in human genetics
5. Human lymphoid tumours
6. FISH has been used for detection of numeric abnormalities of chromosomes:
   (i) Demonstration of subtle micro-deletions
   (ii) Analysis of gene application e.g., ERBB2, HER2/NEW.

Analysis can be performed on prenatal samples:

1. Cells obtained by amniocentesis
2. Chorionic villus biopsy
3. Umbilical cord blood
4. Peripheral blood lymphocytes
5. Tissue section.

Filter Hybridisation

1. Dot and blots: DNA dot blot hybridization is a rapid method of choice for the detection of a specific DNA sequence in a specimen. The main application of this method is in infectious disease diagnosis and forensic analysis. Dots or spots of the DNA containing samples are placed on to a nitrocellulose membrane—or nylon membrane—and fixed. This membrane is then hybridized to a radioactively labelled DNA segment of known sequence, specific for pathogenic DNA being tested for.

If the pathogenic DNA is present in the specimen, complementary DNA sequences present on the membrane will hybridize, or anneal producing a double stranded DNA segment with radioactive label incorporated into the molecule. The presence of radioactivity is detected by autoradiography; Non-isotopic signalling methods can also be used.

Northern blot is a similar procedure in which RNA is utilized as the test nucleic acid.

Southern blot: Southern blot technique was termed Southern blotting after its pioneer, EM Southern. Southern blot technique involves fractionation of DNA by electrophoresis and then transfer of separated patterns of nucleic acid to a solid support such as nitrosocellulose sheet with subsequent hybridization for identification of the separated fraction.

Western blot: In western blotting, protein antigens are separated according to their electrophoretic mobility and molecular weight by polyacramide gel electrophoresis, and then blotted on to nitrocellulose paper by standard blotting procedure. The patient's serum is allowed to react with blot. Antibodies attached to separated viral antigens on the nitrocellulose paper are detected by enzyme tagged-antihuman gamma globulin. Enzyme substrate changes colour in the presence of enzyme and permanently stain the nitrocellulose paper. The position of the band on the paper indicates the antigen with which the antibody has reacted.

Applications of blotting techniques can be used for the detection and determination of hormones, enzymes, viral antigens receptors, autoantibodies, DNA binding proteins, apolipoproteins, glycoproteins and oncogenes.

POLYMERASE CHAIN REACTION

The idea of polymerase chain reaction was conceived by Dr Kary Mullis in 1983 while working at the Citreus Corporation in Emeryville, CA. However, some pioneering work was done by Hargovind Khurana in 1971, who described the basic principle of replicating a piece of DNA using two primers.

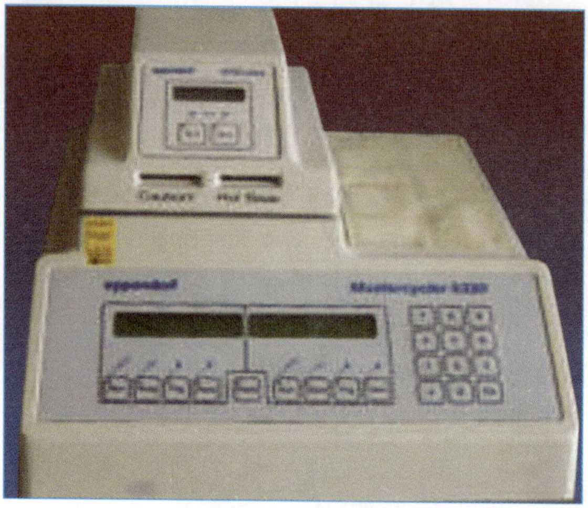

Fig.2.3: Showing photograph of thermocycler used for PCR

Uses of PCR

Polymerase chain reaction can be used for a broad variety of experiments and analysis:

1. PCR can identify organisms that can cause bacterial, viral, and fungal infections.
2. To identify parasitic infections (Leishmaniasis).
3. Tissue biopsy specimens can be analysed by PCR for gene mutations that signify the early development of cancer.
4. The DNA viruses (oncogenic viruses) associated with specific cancers can also be identified by PCR, e.g., cervical scrapings tested to see if they contact DNA from human papilloma virus—a causative agent for human cervical cancer.
5. PCR can also detect genetic mutation in atherosclerosis.
6. Detection of gene mutations by PCR in preneoplastic disorders such as inflammatory bowel disease may be helpful in early detection of colonic cancer.
7. In case of breast cancers early detection of mutated gene can be detected by PCR.
8. Insulin dependent diabetes mellitus has also been associated with gene mutation.
9. Mitochondria DNA extracted from hair, bone, platelets, leukocytes and saliva has been useful in both diagnostic and forensic pathology.
10. Finger printing, paternity testing can be done by PCR.
11. PCR can be used in detection of hereditary diseases, e.g., sickle cell anaemia, haemophilia, and Gaucher's disease.
12. It is also used in cloning genes, analysis of ancient DNA, genotyping of specific mutations comparison of gene expression.
13. mRNA can be tested to see if they contact DNA from human papilloma virus—a causative agent for carcinoma cervix.

The polymerase chain reaction (PCR) is used to multiply copies of specific nucleic acid regions quickly and exponentially. Each cycle in the exponential reaction consists of three steps:

1. **Heat denaturation,** typically at 90ºC, to dissociate double stranded DNA.
2. **Annealing:** The temperature is then reduced to 55ºC, promoting the primers to attach them to either end of target strip.
3. **Primer extension:** Polymerase enzymes then triggers the formation of new DNA strand from nucleotides. Extension of primers is done by a thermostable Taq polymerase.

These three steps are repeated again and again by manipulating the temperature, a process that is automated by the PCR machine. A cycle takes 3 to 5 minutes and, after 30 cycles taking about 2 hours, a single copy of DNA can be increased up to 1,000,000 copies.

Amplified sequences of the target DNA is present, it can be visualised by:

1. Gel electrophoresis and ethidium bromide staining
2. Southern blot and dot blot analysis with either radioactive or non-radioactive probes
3. Oligomer restriction
4. Oligomer hybridization
5. Reverse dot blot.

There are various modifications of this technique:

1. Reverse transcription PCP (RT-PCR) is a method used to amplify, isolate or identify a known sequence from RNA.
2. Touchdown PCR
3. Nested, hemi-nested and pit-stop PCR: It is used to increase the specificity of DNA amplification. It is often more successful in specifically long DNA products than conventional PCR, but it requires more detailed knowledge of the sequence of the target.
4. Solid phase PCR
5. Multiplex PCR
6. Quantitative PCR is used to measure the quantity of a PCR products.

Bibliography

Burns JC: Immunological methods and their application in the routine laboratory. Recent advances in Histopathology (10). Edited by Anthony PP and Wolff N. Churchill Livingstone, Edinburgh, London, and New York.

Coding BW: Audit, quality control, assurance and quality control. Recent advances in Histopathology (16) Anthony PP et al (Eds). London, Churchill Livingstone. PP 193. 1994.

Erlich HA, Geifand D, Snirsky JB: Recent advances in Polymerase chain reaction. Science. 252 1643-1651. 1991.

Erilch HA: 1989 PCR technology, principle, and applications of DNA amplification. Stockton Press, New York.

Quike P and Dyson JED: 1986 Flow cytometry, methodology and application in Pathology, J Path 149, 79-87.

CHAPTER 3

DEVELOPMENTAL DISTURBANCES OF ORAL AND PARAORAL STRUCTURES

DEVELOPMENTAL DEFORMITIES OF JAW

AGNATHIA

It is also called ***'hypognathous'* or *'agnathy'***.

Agnathia is a developmental defect characterised by total or partial absence of the lower jaw. It is a lethal anomaly characterized by hypoplasia or absence of the mandible with abnormally positioned ears, and also any form of holoprosencephaly.

Cause

It may be due to autosomal recessive inheritance. There is failure of migration of neural crest mesenchyme into the maxillary prominence at the fourth to fifth week of gestation.

Clinical features

Agnathia is associated with cephalocele, dysgenesis of corpus callosum, cerebellar hypoplasia, atresia of third ventricle, middle proboscis, hypoplastic tongue, cleft palate, microstomia, cardiac anomalies and adrenal hypoplasia. Hyoid bone is sometimes absent, despite the presence of a rudimentary tongue. In the place of buccal orifice, there may be vertical slit.

MICROGNATHIA

It is also sometimes called ***'mandibular hypoplasia'***

Definition: Micrognathia is defined as a smallness of the jaws, especially of the lower jaw.

Micrognathia is of three types—congenital, developmental, and acquired.

True micrognathia: In true micrognathia, the jaw is small enough to interfere with the infant's feeding. Infants with micrognathia need special nipples in order to feed properly.

It is further divided into:

Congenital—Abnormality present since birth.

Acquired—It is acquired later in life.

Causes

It can present as a birth defect in multiple syndromes including fetal alcohol syndrome, congenital rubella, DiGeorge's syndrome, Pierre-Robinson's syndrome, Hallermann Streiff syndrome, Trisomy 13 (Patau syndrome,) Trisomy 18 (Edward's syndrome), X0 syndrome (Turner's syndrome), Seckel syndrome, Progeria, Treacher's Collin's syndrome, Smith-Lemi- Opitz's syndrome, juvenile idiopathic arthritis, Cri-du-chat syndrome and Marfan's syndrome.

Micrognathia is believed to result from hypoplasia of the neural crest cell population in the first branchial arch.

Teratogenic factors also have been suggested to play a role in the etiology of micrognathia. Observations in fetuses of mothers who received radiotherapy during pregnancy showed an increased incidence of mandibular hypoplasia.

Clinical features

The clinical features comprises:

- It is common in infants, but is usually self-corrected during growth, due to the jaws increasing in size.
- There is abnormal alignment of teeth as there is not enough room for teeth to grow. If the upper jaw is short, then occlusion may also be abnormal.
- Symmetrical underdevelopment of the chin.
- Breathing difficulty.
- Cleft of the soft palate (seen in 45% of cases).
- The child has a characteristic bird facies. The most important complication of this condition is respiratory difficulty. This is thought to occur due to the failure of support of tongue musculature because of micrognathia.
- The tongue falls down, and backwards, which partially obstructs the epiglottis.

Treatment

Surgical treatment is necessary to restore facial form and the centric relationships of the dento-alveolar processes in order to reestablish the masticatory function.

Corrective and surgical procedures include selective sectioning of the body of the mandible or the ramus for purpose of elongating the bone, and bone grafting for restoration of adequate size and contour of the mandible.

MACROGNATHIA

It is also called ***'prognathic mandible'*** or ***'megnathia'***.

Macrognathia refers to the condition of abnormally large jaws. It could affect either mandible or the maxilla, or both the jaws together. Normally, there is symmetrical overgrowth of the jaw bones—it is termed as prognathism. Prognathism is a term used to describe the positional relationship of the mandible and/or maxilla to the skeletal base where either of the jaws protrudes beyond a predetermined imaginary line in sagittal plane.

Causes

It can be associated with systemic conditions like Acromegaly, Paget's disease of bone, fibrous dysplasia and Leontiasis ossea.

Clinical features

Characteristics of macrognathia

(i) There is abnormal forward projection of the affected jaw bone giving the patient ape-like appearance.

(ii) *'Gummy smile'* when maxilla is elongated. This is due to the upper jaw being too large.

(iii) Occasionally, there is prognathism which produces a severe facial deformity, and malocclusion of the teeth. It is caused by condylar growth.

(iv) Mandibular protrusion when mandible is affected and chins appears prominent.

Treatment

Treatment is surgical. Mandibular macrognathia is generally managed by resection of a portion of the mandible followed by orthodontic treatment.

FACIAL HEMIHYPERTROPHY

It is also called ***'Friedreich's'*** disease.

Definition: When one side of the face progressively enlarges over the other, the condition is known as facial hemihypertrophy.

Causes

The etiology of hemihypertrophy is not known (idiopathic). It is possibly related to neural, vascular, lymphatic, endocrine, or chromosomal abnormalities. It is associated with certain syndromes e.g., Curtius, Klippel–Trenaunay, Maffucci's syndrome, Ollier's syndrome and Silver-Russsel syndrome.

There can be an increased incidence of certain visceral tumours, particularly Wilm's tumour of kidney, hepatoblastoma, and haemangioma of skin.

Clinical features

It is more common in males than females. Onset of lesion in childhood. The disease is unilateral, with enlargement of both osseous and soft tissues. The opposite side of face is normal where–as affected side shows enlargement of facial bones and mandible. The skin is often thicker on the involved side and there may be more hair on the corresponding side of the head. A compensatory scoliosis may also develop as a result of pelvic obliquity associated with the discrepancy between the lengths of lower limbs. Associated other abnormalities are mental deficiency, hyperplasia of cerebral hemisphere, ventricular dilatation, and displacement of eye to lateral side.

Oral manifestations

The bone of the maxilla and mandible is also enlarged, being wider and thicker, sometimes with an altered trabecular pattern.

There is enlargement in the size of crown and roots of teeth. Primary teeth shed easily. Teeth on the affected sides are larger than those on the normal side.

The buccal mucosa on the affected side appears pendulous and velvety.

Tongue is commonly involved and bizarre patterns of enlargement of papilla, in addition to general unilateral enlargement of tongue.

The soft and hard tissues—such as lips and uvula, are also unilaterally involved.

The palate is asymmetric, and the permanent teeth, with the exception of the third molars, are enlarged on the involved side.

Treatment

There is no specific treatment.

FACIAL HEMIATROPHY

It is also known as ***'Romberg disease'*** or ***'Parry-Romberg syndrome'*** or ***'Progressive facial hemiatrophy'***. It was first described by Parry in 1825 and then expanded by Romberg in 1846.

Definition: The syndrome is characterised by slowly progressive unilateral atrophy of facial subcutaneous fat, muscle tissue, skin, cartilage, and bone. The condition typically progresses over a period of 2-10 years and then stabilises.

Etiology

Exact cause is not known. There are various causes, which include trigeminal neuritis, a chronic autoimmune neurovasculitis, sympathetic denervation, trauma, vascular malformations, immunologic abnormality, hereditary disease, infection by a slow virus and increased sympathetic nerve activity triggering facial atrophy.

Clinical features

The symptoms of Parry-Romberg's syndrome may begin at any age. In rare cases, the disorder is present at birth. The syndrome usually starts during the first two decades of life and completes progression within 2 to 15 years. Facial atrophy is more common in adolescent girls.

Usually left side is affected rather than the right. In some rare cases the atrophy may be bilateral.

The major features of this syndrome, which have been reported previously, are atrophy of the soft tissues on one side of the face with hyperpigmentation of the overlying skin and various neurologic findings, including migraine type headache, trigeminal neuralgia, and focal epilepsy.

Eye: There is ptosis of eyelids, ophthalmoplegia, convergence nystagmus, and papillary dilatation.

Neurological complications include seizures, facial neuralgia, hemiplegia, hemianopia, aphasia, migraine, headache, impairment of sweating, and ventricular dilatation.

CT and MR findings included unilateral focal infarctions in the corpus callosum, diffuse deep and subcortical white matter signal changes, mild cortical thickening, and leptomeningeal enhancement with dense mineral deposition.

Skin: The skin features in Parry-Romberg's syndrome include hypo-or hyperpigmentation of the forehead, cheek, or jaw. The cutaneous changes are characterised by dry, atrophic, and sometimes adherent skin with progressive atrophy of the underlying subcutaneous tissue, muscle and bone. The changes lead to a sunken-appearing hyperpigmented, hemiatrophic face.

Hair: There is greying of hair as well as abnormal bald patches on the scalp.

Ear: There is aplasia or hypoplasia of external ear and missing of ear canal.

Oral manifestations

In the individuals with this disorder, initial facial changes usually involve the tissues above the upper jaw (maxilla) or between the upper corners of the lip (nasolabial fold) and progress to involve the angle of the mouth, the areas around the eye, the eyebrows, the ear/or the neck.

Many individuals experience atrophy of half of the upper lip and tongue as well as abnormal exposure, delayed eruption and wasting of the roots of certain teeth on affected side. The symmetry of the face is lost, nose and chin is deformed. There is malformation of teeth on affected side with deformed palate.

Treatment

Treatments have included silicone injections, alloplastic implants, microfat injections, and microvascular free tissue transfer.

CONGENITAL LIPS AND COMMISSURAL PITS AND FISTULA

Commissural lip pits are by far the most common, occurring in 1-2% of newborns. They usually represent a rare developmental malformation that may occur alone or in combination with cleft lip, or cleft palate.

Commissural lip pits are small mucosal invaginations that occur at the corners of the mouth on vermilion border. Their location suggests that they may represent a failure of normal fusion of the embryonal maxillary and mandibular processes.

Clinical features

Age and Sex: Commissural lip pits appear to be common in adults, where they have been reported in 12% to 20% of the population. Their prevalence in children is considered lower, ranging from 0.2% to 0.7%. Commissural pits are seen more often in males than in females.

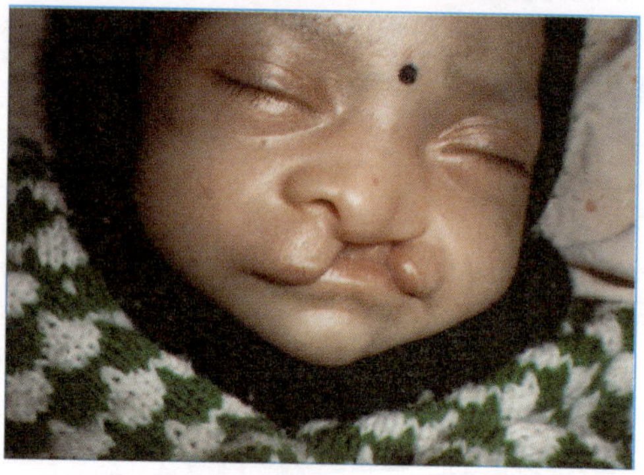

Fig.3.1: 2 months' female showing cleft upper lip

On examination: These occur at the corners of the mouth. They are frequently of pencil-lead size, from 1 to 4 mm deep, and may be filled with cellular debris. Lip pits, the congenital depressions, are usually bilateral and symmetrically placed on the vermilion portion of the lower lip. These pits may be circular or may be present as transverse slit. They often produce viscid saliva on pressure. The lip may be enlarged and swollen.

Microscopically: Microscopic examination reveals a narrow invagination lined by stratified squamous epithelium. Ducts from minor salivary glands may drain into this invagination. Small amount of mucinous secretion may accumulate at the depth of the pit.

Congenital lip pits may occur either as an isolated finding or they may be associated with cleft lip, and cleft palate.

CONGENITAL ANOMALIES OF LIPS AND PALATE

CLEFT LIP AND CLEFT PALATE

Cleft lip (cheiloschisis) and Cleft palate (palatoschisis)—which can also occur together as cleft lip and palate—are variations of a type of clefting congenital deformity caused by abnormal facial development during gestation.

The incidence of cleft lip and cleft palate is 1:600 live births and of isolated cleft palate is 1:1000 live births.

The incidence increases in Oriental groups (1:500) and decreases in the blacks. The highest incidence reported for cleft palate and lip occurs in the Red Indian tribes of Montana, USA (1: 276).

CLEFT PALATE

Cleft palate is a result of lack of fusion of the two palatal processes with each other or with the frontonasal process (primitive palate), varying in severity from the so-called bifid uvula (cleft of uvula to a cleft that involves uvula, soft palate, alveolar bridge, and upper lip).

Isolated cleft palate is more common in females.

CLEFT LIP

It results from abnormal development of the median nasal and maxillary process. Cleft lip is formed in the lip as either a small gap or an indentation in the lip.

Cleft lip can occur as one-sided (unilateral) or two-sided (bilateral). When unilateral, the cleft is more common on left.

Etiology

Etiology of cleft palate and cleft lip is as follows:

According to medical research, there has been no way to prevent the causes of cleft palate and cleft lip: however, from statistics, the cause may include hereditary or environmental factors.

1. Hereditary

Polygenic inheritance: The main possible mode of transmission is by number of genes producing small effects, which create this condition.

Monogenic inheritance: When clefting is influenced by only single gene it is called monogenic defect. A few cases are associated with chromosomal abnormality (e.g., Trisomy 13 and 18, Down's syndrome and Pierre-Robin's syndrome).

2. Environmental factors

Early pregnancy is prone to environmental influences affecting cleft lip and cleft palate:

(a) **Nutritional:** Folic acid and other nutrient deficiency cause cleft palate and cleft lip. Protective influence in the prevention of clefting with folic acid supplementation before and during the first trimester is now being postulated.

(b) **Defective vascular supply:** Defective vascular supply to the area may lead to ischaemia which in turn may lead to cleft formation.

(c) **Mechanical disturbances:** The size of the tongue may prevent the union of parts due to mechanical disturbances of the embryo.

(d) **Infection:** Infection from bacteria and virus (rubella) causes cleft palate.

(e) **Miscellaneous**

Other environmental factors include overdose of X-ray, maternal smoking, alcoholism, caffeine abuse, corticosteroid during pregnancy.

CLEFT LIP

Types of cleft lip

The types of cleft include central, lateral, complete or incomplete and single or compound.

I. **Central:** It is very rare and occurs due to failure of two median nasal processes.

II. **Lateral:** It is commonest variety where there is a cleft between frenum and the lateral part of the upper lip. This is due to imperfect fusion of maxillary process with median nasal process. Lateral variety can be unilateral or bilateral.

III. **Complete or incomplete:** In cases of incomplete variety, cleft lip extends to the floor of the nose. In cases of incomplete variety, the cleft does not extend up to the nostril.

IV. **Simple or compound:** Compound refers to cleft lip associated with a cleft in alveolus.

Clinical features

1. In 80% of the cases, cleft lip is unilateral and in about 60% of the cases it is associated with cleft palate.
2. In many cases nostril is widened.
3. Mal-development or mal-alignment in relation to cleft is common.

Functional effects

1. Presence of cleft lip does not interfere with sucking.
2. However there may be some difficulty in speech.

Cleft palate

Development of palate is as follows:

Palate is developed around 6-8 weeks of life from three components:

1. The premaxilla, which is developed from the median nasal process.

2 and 3: Maxillary process, which contributes one palatine process on each side. The line of fusion of these processes is in the form of the letter Y.

Imperfect fusion or developmental anomalies results in cleft palate.

Types of cleft palate

1. *Complete*: Failure of fusion of palatine processes and premaxilla results in complete cleft palate. In such situations, the nasal cavity and mouth are interconnected. When the premaxilla is not fused with both palatine processes, it hangs down from the septum of the nose.
2. *Incomplete*: When the fusion of three components of palate takes place, it starts from uvula and then backwards. Thus various types of incomplete fusion results:
   a. Bifid uvula.
   b. The whole length of soft palate is bifid.
   c. The whole length of soft palate and the anterior part of palate is normally developed. In about 25% of cases, the cleft palate alone and in 50% of cases, both cleft palate and cleft lip encountered.

Effects of cleft palate

1. Presence of cleft palate interferes with swallowing.
2. They are unable to utter consonant sounds like B, K, D, P, T.
3. **Teeth:** Upper lateral incisors may be small or even absent. The maxilla tends to be smaller. Teeth are crowded.
4. **Problems with respiration:** Due to underdevelopment of nasal bone, oral organisms contaminate the upper respiratory mucous membrane through cleft palate and leads to upper respiratory infection.
5. **Hearing:** Even with repair, acute and chronic otitis media and hearing problems can occur.
6. **Problem of articulation:** The cleft palate may cause malocclusion of loss of hearing followed by defects in articulation.
7. **Psychological problem:** The cleft-lip and cleft palate children may cause psychological problems to parents beside themselves.

MACROCHEILIA

It is a condition of permanent swelling of the lip that results from greatly distended lymphatic spaces. This causes an abnormal largeness of the lips.

DOUBLE LIP

Double lip is an oral anomaly which may be either congenital or acquired.

Congenital double lip may present either as an isolated anomaly in random association with other oral anomalies, or as a component of Ascher's syndrome.

It is also known as *'Ascher's syndrome'*. Double lip is an uncommon oral anomaly, which occurs mostly in the upper lip.

It may be congenital or acquired and occurs as an isolated case or in association with other lesions.

A triad of double lip, blepharochalasis and nontoxic thyroid enlargement characterises Ascher's syndrome.

Microscopically, double lip shows essentially normal structures; often there is an abundance of minor salivary glands. The blepharochalasis of Ascher's syndrome usually shows hyperplasia of the lacrimal glands and prolapse of orbital fat.

Treatment

Treatment consists of W-plasty or elliptical excision of hypertrophic mucosa and wound closure by primary sutures. Good functional and cosmetic results are usually obtained.

LABIAL AND ORAL MELANOTIC MACULE

Synonyms: The melanotic macules have been variously termed ephelis, melanosis, lentigo, solitary labial lentigo, labial melanotic macule, and oral melanotic macule.

Common solitary melanotic lesion of the oral cavity, and in large series, comprised 86% of all pigmented lesions.

Non-cancerous dark spots that are found in the lips or inside the mouth are known as oral melanotic macule.

An oral melanotic macule, which appears on the lips, is known as labial melanotic macule.

Causes

Regarding etiology, melanotic macules may result from racial pigmentation, endocrine disturbances, antimalarial therapy, trauma, haemochromatosis, or chronic pulmonary disease, or they may be idiopathic.

Some inherited diseases show brown pigmentation of the oral mucus membrane, e.g., Peutz-Jegher's syndrome, Laugier-Hunziker syndrome.

The congenital melanotic macule of the tongue has been reported in the literature.

Labial melanotic macule is provoked by sun exposure, and it is common in fair-skinned people.

Clinical features

- Usually solitary, a labial melanotic macule is most commonly seen in adult women but it also occurs in males and young people. Almost a fifth of the lesions are multiple.
- Labial melanotic macules are present in about 20-30% of children and adolescent. The intraoral lesions usually occur in patients older than 40.
- Labial melanotic macule is a well-defined, oval, brown to black, flat patch on the central third of the lower lip.
- Occasionally, the lesion can be on the upper lip.
- Size ranges from 1 to 8 mm. Most of the lesions are less than 1 cm in diameter, although occasional cases may be larger in size.

Intraorally, it may be found on the gingival, buccal mucosa, palate and termed as the oral melanotic macule.

Microscopically

The dark colour of the lesion is due to increase of melanin pigment of the basal cell layer, not from an increased number of melanocytes. Melanin may also be found in lamina propria. Deposits may also be seen within subepithelial stroma.

Treatment

No treatment is required for oral melanotic macule except for aesthetic considerations.

DEVELOPMENTAL DISTURBANCES OF ORAL MUCOSA

FORDYCE'S GRANULES

It is a developmental anomaly characterised by heterotopic collections of sebaceous glands at various sites in the oral cavity. Sebaceous glands are normal adenexal structure of the dermis but may also be found within the mouth, where they are referred to as Fordyce's granules or ectopic sebaceous glands.

Clinical features

They are not observed in children; rather, they appear only in the second or third decade of life. Men usually exhibit more Fordyce's granules than women. The granules tend to appear during puberty and increase in number with age.

They appear as rice-like white or yellowish white spots, either discretely separated or forming relatively large plaques often projecting slightly above the surface of tissue. They are 1-3 mm in greatest diameter.

Sites: Fordyce's granules occur at any site in oral cavity, but commonly, these granules occur at mucosa of the cheek, opposite the molar teeth. It is also found on the inner surface of lips, in retromolar area lateral to anterior faucial pillar and, occasionally, on the tongue, gingival, frenum and palate. Neoplastic transformation is rare but has been reported.

They don't appear to have any function in the oral cavity.

Microscopically

The glands are superficial and may consist of many lobules, all grouped around one or more ducts, which open on the surface of the mucosa. These ducts show keratin plugging. The surrounding connective tissue may contain occasional chronic inflammatory cells because of trauma with adjacent teeth. The peripheral cells of the Fordyce's granules are flat and darkly stained; whereas inner cells are rich in lipid and pale in appearance.

Treatment

No treatment is required for Fordyce's granules, except for cosmetic removal of labial lesions. Inflamed glands treated locally with clindamycin. When surgically excised, recurrence does not occur.

FOCAL EPITHELIAL HYPERPLASIA (HECK'S DISEASE)

Focal epithelial hyperplasia, also called '*Heck's disease*' is a benign disorder of the oral mucosa. This disorder is very common in natives of Central and South America, Eskimos, Swedish, Norwegians, Caucasians and Europeans.

Causes

Multiple more or less papillomatous lesions, possibly caused by a virus of papilloma virus, (HPV-13 and possibly HPV-32) characterise the condition.

The factors that determine disease susceptibility are unclear, but genetics—and having the human lymphocytic (B1-404) allele in particular—are thought to play a major role in disease vulnerability. The condition usually occurs in children and has familial predilection. Multiple papillary lesions similar to focal epithelial hyperplasia arise within with increased frequency in AIDS patients.

Clinical features

- Heck's disease primarily occurs in children, but lesions may occur in young and middle-aged adults. The lesions are quite prominent after 25 years of age.
- There is no gender predilection.
- **Sites:** Occur often on the lower lip. Other areas involved are buccal mucosa, upper lip, tongue, gingival, and anterior pillar of the fauces.
- The lesion measure several millimeters (1-4 mm) and have a papillomatous or fibroma-like appearance. The lesions may be multiple and clustered to present a 'cobble stone' appearance.
- Heck's disease presents clinically as a well-circumscribed, sessile pale elevation of the buccal mucosa.

Microscopically: It is characterised by hyperplastic mucosa with thin parakeratotic stratum corneum acanthosis and blunting. The most prominent feature is the presence of balloon cells in the malpighian layers. Due to hyperplasia of epithelium, the rete ridges become wide, elongated and sometimes anastomised (Bronze Age battle axe appearance) or club-shaped. Some superficial keratocytes show koilocytes. Other keratocytes show koilocytes within the spinous layer and demonstrate altered nuclei that somewhat resemble mitotic figures. These altered cells are called mitosid figures.

Electron microscopically there is clear cytoplasm with scattered ribosomes, a peripheral condensation of tonofilaments, a central aggregation of chromatin clumps with loss of nuclear membrane and an accumulation of desmosome fragments.

Treatment

Several treatment modalities such as surgical excision, laser ablation, cryotherapy, elecrocauterisation, topical intralesional, systemic interferon, and systemic retinoic acid have been used with inconsistent results and many side-effects. Yasar Sirin et al, 2009, reported three children of Turkish origin with focal epithelial hyperplasia successfully treated with imiquimod 5% cream. No serious side-effects were observed and recurrence did not occur during one-year follow-up period.

DEVELOPMENTAL DISTURBANCES OF GINGIVA

Fibromatous gingivae

It is also called ***'elephantiasis gingivae'***, ***'idiopathic fibrous hyperplasia'***, and ***'congenital microgingiva'***.

Exact cause is not known. It is due to some genetic defect, which causes developmental enlargement of gingival tissue. This condition may manifest as an autosomal recessive mode of inheritance.

Clinical features

This hyperplasia may be present at birth and at an early age. The gingival enlargement may delay the eruption of teeth and make cleaning of the teeth virtually impossible.

Idiopathic gingival fibromatosis is a slowly progressive benign enlargement that affects the marginal gingival, attached gingival, and interdental papilla. The fibromatosis may potentially cover the exposed tooth surfaces, causing aesthetic defect and, in extreme cases, may distort the jaws. The gingival tissues are usually pink and non-haemorrhagic, and have a firm, fibrotic consistency.

Microscopically

The underlying stroma mainly consists of thick, avascular bundles of mature and immature fibroblasts. The covering epithelium is hyperplastic with mild hyperkeratosis and elongated rete ridges. There is sparse collection of chronic inflammatory cell. Unusual findings include the presence of small calcified particles, amyloid deposits, islands of odontogenic epithelium, and osseous metaplasia.

Management

Idiopathic gingival fibromatosis is removed by gingivectomy, with recurrences being treated in the same fashion or by conservative removal of local areas of hyperplasia.

Retrocuspid papilla

The retrocuspid papilla (RCP) is a circumscribed nodule that lies lingual to the mandibular cuspid on the gingival tissue.

They probably represent developmental anomalies. This papilla is evidently a normal entity because its presence occurs in over 99% of a group of more than one children.

Clinical features

It is present in most children, but has decreasing incidence with increasing age. Retrocuspid papillae are common, having been reported in 25 to 99% of children and young adults.

It consists of a round epithelial papule on the attached gingival lingual to the mandibular cuspid. It is usually bilateral. Retrocuspid papillae are 2 to 4 mm in size. They are soft, of normal colour, and not associated with any causative factor.

Microscopically it is composed of loosely arranged delicate fibrous tissue with stellate multinucleated fibroblasts. Elongation of rete ridges and /or increased vascularity is also present in significant number of cases.

Retrocuspid papilla is a normal anatomical structure, which regresses with age and requires no treatment.

DEVELOPMENTAL DEFECTS OF TONGUE

Macroglossia

Macroglossia may be congenital or acquired:

TABLE 3.1
CAUSES OF MACROGLOSSIA

I. Congenital causes	
• Idiopathic muscle hypertrophy	• Down's syndrome
• Beckwith-Widemann syndrome	• Trisomy 22
II. Acquired causes	
a. Metabolic/Endocrine	
• Hypothyroidism	• Cretinism
• Diabetes	• Acromegaly
b. Inflammatory	
• Ludwig angina	• Syphilis
• Candidiasis	
c. Nutritional	
• Pellagra	• Scurvy

Contd.

d. Systemic
- Uremia
- Iatrogenic

e. Neoplastic
- Lymphangioma
- Carcinoma
- Lingual thyroid
- Haemangioma
- Plasmacytoma

f. Traumatic
- Surgery
- Radiation therapy
- Haemorrhage

Macroglossia is a congenital disorder characterised by an abnormally large tongue, often seen in cases of Down's syndrome.

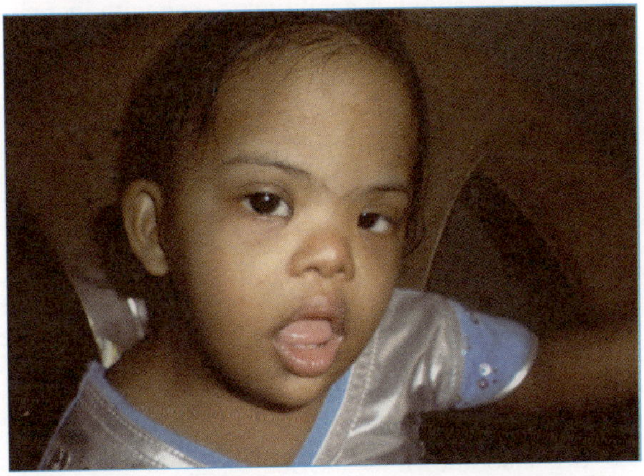

Fig.3.2: Shows macroglossia in a 1 year Mongolian child

Clinical features

- If large enough, the tongue may obstruct the airway and lead to sleep apnea.
- Mechanical obstruction of oral cavity can directly occlude the airway.
- Speech and swallowing may be affected.
- Shape of the oral cavity may be affected. Reduced pressure on the palate may lead to adenoid facies.
- Upper incisors can be pushed horizontally, inducing forward maxillary growth. If the tongue protrudes beyond the lips and is exposed to the air, drying of the tongue with resultant glossitis and bleeding is common.
- There is crenation or scalloping on the lateral border of the tongue.

Beckwith's-Wiedemann syndrome (BWS) is an overgrowth disorder present at birth characterised by an increased risk of childhood cancer and certain features. Common features of BWS are: Macroglossia (large tongue), macrosomia (birth weight and length >90th percentile), midline abdominal wall defects), (omphalocele, umbilical hernia, diastasis rectii), ear creases or ear pits, and neonatal hypoglycemia (low blood sugar at birth).

Other findings include: Naevus flammeus, prominent occipit, mid-face hypoplasia, hemiatrophy, genitourinary anomalies, cardiac anomalies, musculo-skeletal abnormalities, and hearing loss.

Microglossia

Microglossia refers to a small tongue, and aglossia refers to absence of the tongue. Although these conditions are sometimes seen in malformed fetuses, they are rarely seen in live born infants. Cases of complete absence of the tongue have been reported. Tiny tongue will pose many difficulties related to speech and swallowing.

Accessory tongue

Accessory tongue is a rare anomaly.

Cause

Tongue develops during the fourth week of intrauterine life, originating from a median swelling (tuberculum impar) on the floor of the pharynx and two lateral lingual swellings joining the central structure. These structures grow rapidly to cover the tuberculum impar to form the anterior two-thirds of tongue.

Fissured tongue (Scrotal tongue)

Etiology

The cause of fissured tongue is not clearly defined but it may occur with certain underlying syndromes or may be an inherited condition. It is sometimes seen in Melkersson-Rosenthal's syndrome and Down's syndrome. Although a specific etiology has not been elicited, a polygenic or autosomal dominant mode of inheritance is suspected because this condition is seen with increased frequency in families with an affected proband.

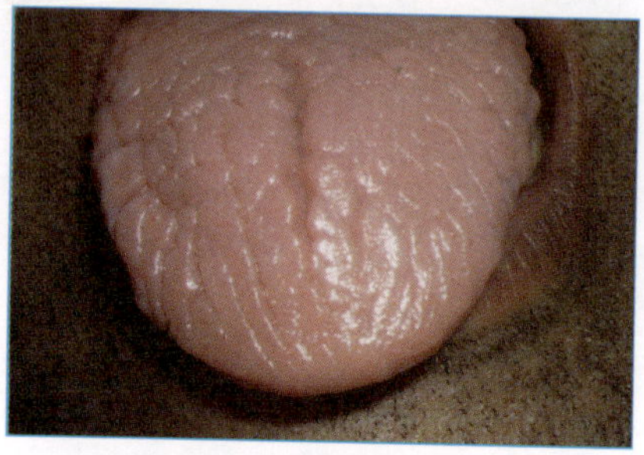

Fig.3.3: Fissured tongue

Clinical features

Fissured tongue is also known as 'lingua plicata'. Fissured tongue may be seen in 2 to 5% of the overall population. It becomes more noticeable with age and affects males more often than females. Fissured tongue affects the top surface of the tongue and often extends out to the edges of the tongue. The size and depth of the fissures vary and when particularly large and deep the fissures or grooves may be interconnected, separating the top surface of the tongue into what may look like several lobules. It is often associated with mild glossitis.

Tongue-tie

It is also known as ankyloglossia.

Cause

It is a developmental malformation in which the tongue is abnormally fixed to the floor of the mouth or lingual aspect of the gingival due to a short or malpositioned lingual frenulum. It occurs when the lingual frenulum is quite short, or when the frenulum is attached near the tongue tip.

Occurrence: It is rare, approximately one per 1,000 birth.

The lingual frenulum is short, thick, or thin and fibrous. The malformation may cause partial or complete immobility of the tongue.

Treatment

Treatment is surgical.

Cleft tongue

Partial failure of fusion of the left and right halves of the tongue causes a deep groove running in the midline of the dorsum of the tongue. Rarely, complete failure of fusion causes a bifid tongue.

Treatment

Treatment is surgical.

MEDIAN RHOMBOID GLOSSITIS

Median rhomboid glossitis is also known as ***"central papillary atrophy"*** and ***"posterior midline atrophic candidiasis"***.

Median rhomboid glossitis is an uncommon condition; the estimated prevalence in adults is less than 1%.

Cause

It is a rare developmental anomaly. It is a failure of developmental apparatus during the organogenesis of the fetus. A structure called "tuberculum impar" is supposed to withdraw when the two halves of the tongue come close to each other during development. When this does not happen, creating an area, which looks like a bald patch on it, traps the structure in-between the two halves of the tongue.

Median rhomboid glossitis has been strongly linked with the fungal infection caused by Candida albicans, where the tongue has an ovoid patch just before the entry into the oesophagus.

Clinical features

The condition is reportedly thrice as common in men as in women.

A reddish white patch is found in the midline just in front of the circumvallate papillae due to inadequate covering of the tuberculum impar.

Two clinical varieties are recognised

1. A smooth well-circumscribed red plaque that is devoid of normal papillae, slightly below the level of normal papillae.
2. Slightly below the level of the surrounding.

Microscopically

Median rhomboid glossitis shows a smooth nodular surface covered by atrophic stratified squamous epithelium overlying a moderately fibrosed stroma with somewhat dilated capillaries. Fungiform and filliform papillae are not seen. A mild chronic inflammatory cell infiltrate may be seen within subepithelial and deeper fibrovascular tissues.

Treatment

Treatment may include the use of antifungal drugs and surgical removal of the hyperplastic tissue.

Geographic tongue

It is also called benign migratory glossitis, glossitis migrans, wandering rash and glossitis areata exfoliativa and is a relatively common condition (affecting 1-2%) of population of unknown cause, which is usually asymptomatic. The colloquial names are due to the fact that the affected tongues sometimes resemble a map.

Etiology

Its cause is uncertain, though it tends to run in families and is associated with several different genes. Etiological factors include immunological reaction, allergic, emotional and hereditary factors, infections and nutritional deficiencies. A polygenic mode of inheritance has been suggested because it is seen clustering in families. Association with human leukocyte antigen (HLA-DR5, HLA DR-6, and HLA-Cw6) have been reported.

Clinically

Most patients are adults, but it is also seen in children. It often occurs in association with fissured tongue. Females have been reported to be affected twice as often as males. Patients with geographic tongue may present a burning sensation or an irritation of the tongue noted with hot or spicy food.

On examination it appears as an erythematous flat zone on the dorsum of the tongue resulting from loss of the filiform papillae and overcrowded in the greyish white borders. There is map-like or geographic appearance of tongue.

Microscopically

There is acanthosis, hyperkeratosis with migration of neutrophils throughout the epithelium to form microabscesses near the surface (Monro's abscess) accompanied by a mild inflammatory infiltrate in the lamina propria. Rete ridges are typically thin and considerably elongated with only a thin layer of epithelium overlying the connective tissue papillae.

Hairy tongue

Synonyms: Lingua nigra, lingua villosa, lingua villosa nigra, black hairy tongue.

Hairy tongue is a commonly observed condition of defective desquamation of the filiform papillae that results from a variety of precipitating factors.

Precipitating factors for hairy tongue include poor oral hygiene, the use of medications (especially broad-spectrum antibiotics), and therapeutic radiation of the head and neck. Hairy tongue has also been reported with greater frequency in males, those who use tobacco, those who heavily drink coffee and tea, patients infected with HIV, and those who are HIV negative and use intravenous drugs.

Symptoms: There is hypertrophy of filiform papillae. Normal filiform papillae are approximately 1mm in length; whereas filiform papillae in hairy tongue are more than 15 mm in length.

Microscopically: Section shows elongated filiform papillae with mild hyperkeratosis and inflammatory cells. External colonisation of the papillae by basophilic microbial colonies is a prominent feature.

LINGUAL VARICES

It is also called phlebectasis.

Varicose veins, whether in the mouth or elsewhere, represent an abnormal dilatation of veins.

The ventral surface of the tongue is a common location for varicose veins, it is also known as sublingual varices.

Dilated tortuous veins may be seen along the ventral surface of the tongue and tend to become more prominent with age. Isolated varices are also common on the lips and buccal mucosa.

Sublingual varices occur in up to 60% of individuals over the age of 60. They are common, but usually asymptomatic and harmless. They have been associated with portal hypertension and are known to bleed and lead to haemoptysis.

Microscopically

They are frequently composed of dilated and tortuous veins with thrombosis.

Treatment

No treatment is indicated for lingual varices. Isolated varices of the lip and buccal mucosa are surgically removed.

LINGUAL THYROID

In the first trimester of embryonic development, the thyroid gland originates in the back of the tongue and migrates to the front of the neck. If it fails to migrate properly, it can remain high in the neck or even in back of the tongue.

Lingual thyroid is ectopic tissue at the base or in the substance of the tongue, in the presence of a normally situated cervical thyroid gland.

Clinically

Lingual thyroid is four times more common in females than in males. The age of onset ranges from birth to the sixth decade.

Larger lesions can interfere with swallowing and breathing, but most patients are unaware of the mass at the time of diagnosis. There may be haemorrhage with pain and feeling of tightness or fullness in the throat.

Up to 70% of patients with lingual thyroid have hypothyroidism and 10% suffer from cretinism.

Macroscopically

The lesion appears as a nodule or mass in the foramen cecum area, reaching a size of a few centimetres. The overlying mucosa may show an increased vascularity.

Microscopically

Sections from lingual thyroid reveal a non-capsulated collection of embryonic or mature thyroid follicles that may extend between muscle bundles. Parathyroid tissue may be seen with lingual thyroid.

DEVELOPMENTAL DISTURBANCES OF ORAL LYMPHOID TISSUE

LYMPHOID PATCHES

Reactive lymphoid aggregates

Lymphoid patches are to be regarded as physiologic rather than pathologic and can be seen in almost every individual.

Lymphoid patches are localised, solitary or multiple lymph follicles occurring in the oropharynx, including the base of the tongue. In the tongue these patches are known as lingual tonsils.

Lymphoid patches are found in the posterior pharyngeal wall, appearing as single or multiple, slightly elevated projections of the mucosa. Their size may vary from a few millimetres up to 1cm. The colour is usually yellowish or greyish. During a cold the lymphoid patches may cause slight irritation but are otherwise asymptomatic.

Enlargement of the lingual tonsils may occur after tonsillectomy, probably because of a compensatory mechanism. In rare instances lingual tonsillitis and even abscess formation may occur.

Occasionally single or multiple lymphoid patches are encountered in the oral cavity, especially in the floor of the mouth. These are sometimes called oral tonsils. The diagnosis is usually based on clinical examination.

A few cases have been described of benign lymphoid hyperplasia of the hard palate, which may simulate malignant non-Hodgkin's lymphoma.

LYMPHOID HAMARTOMA

Synonyms: Angiofollicular lymph node hyperplasia, Angiomatous lymphoid, Castleman tumour, Giant benign lymphoma, Hamartoma of the lymphatics, and Giant lymph node hyperplasia.

Castleman's disease is a very rare disorder characterised by non-cancerous growths (tumour that may develop in the lymph node tissue at a single site or throughout body. It is named after Benzamin Castleman.

Cause: Castleman's disease is likely due to hypersecretion of cytokines IL-6. In tumour that is positive for Kaposi's sarcoma-associated herpes virus (KSHV), also called Human Herpes virus 8 (HHV-8), this is most likely due to expression of the virus-encoded cytokine vIL-6.

Classification

I. Based on clinical and radiological findings: (i) Unicentric Castleman's disease; (ii) Multicentric Castleman's disease.

II. Based on histopathology: (i) Hyaline vascular; (ii) Plasmacytic; (iii) Mixed cellularity.

III. Angiolymphoid hyperplasia

Unicentric Castleman disease: Nearly always plasma cell type. It represents with generalised lymphadenopathy, and hepatosplenomegaly. It may be associated with POEMS syndrome, which includes polyneuropathy, organopathy, endocrinopathy, M-protein, and skin change. There is associaton with Kaposi's sarcoma, large cell lymphoma of immunoblastic type.

Clinical features

Castleman's disease affects both males and females, and may occur at any age—but, typically it affect children.

Plasma cell type: 10% of cases are of plasma cell type. Individuals have fever, weight loss, fatigue, and skin rash. This type of Castleman's disease affects blood cells, leading to low numbers of red blood cells in the body (haemolytic anaemia) or abnormally high amounts of immune factors in blood (called hypergammaglobulinaemia).

Microscopically it shows that the lymph node germinal centres are poorly formed with dysplastic/ atrophic CD21 + follicular dendritic cell networks surrounded by an expanded mantle zone consisting of rim of small CD20+ lymphocytes arranged in an onion skin manner.

Mixed cellularity type: Mix cellular form of Castleman's disease has features of both hyaline vascular, and plasmatic types of Castleman's disease.

ORAL LYMPHOEPITHELIAL CYST

Causes

The pathogenesis of lymphoepithelial cysts is not understood; possible causes that have been suggested are local trauma and obstructed tonsillary crypts.

Clinical features

Oral lymphoepithelial cysts may develop in people of almost any age, but they are most common in young adults.

Oral lymphoepithelial cysts are most commonly located on the floor of the mouth (65.3%); about 13.7% of cases are located on posterolateral portion of the tongue.

Oral lymphoepithelial cysts presents a soft, fluctuant, movable painless submucosal nodule with a yellow white discolouration. Occasional cysts are transparent. Almost all cases are less than 0.6 cm in diameter. But cases up to 2 cm are reported in medical literature. The oral lymphoepithelial cyst develops within a benign lymphoid aggregate or accessory tonsil of the oral or pharyngeal mucosa.

Microscopically

Cystic cavity is lined by stratified squamous epithelium without rete ridges. This epithelium is typically parakeratinised, with desquamated epithelial cells seen filling the cyst lumen. In rare instances the epithelial lining also may contain mucous cells. The most striking feature is the presence of lymphoid tissue in the cyst wall with formation of germinal centers.

Treatment

The treatment of oral lymphoepithelial cysts consists of conservative surgical removal; recurrences are rare.

TREACHER COLLIN'S SYNDROME

This is also termed as ***'mandibulofacial dysostosis'***. The condition is hereditary and is thought to occur due to the retardation or failure of differentiation of the maxillary mesoderm. It is representative of

Tessier's clefts 6, 7, and 8. Their pattern of inheritance is autosomal dominant with an incidence of 1 in 10,000 births.

Clinical features

Clinical features vary from the typical to the atypical.

Features of this syndrome are:

- Antimongoloid palpebral fissures (downward slanting eyes)
- Coloboma of the outer portion of the lower lids
- Hypoplasia of the facial bones, especially the mandible
- Malformation of external ear
- Macrostomia
- Facial clefts
- Mental retardation
- Absence of eyelashes in the medial third of lower lid.

The face gives a bird–like or fish–like appearance. The prognosis of these patients is good, and most have a normal lifespan.

Treatment

Facial defects can be corrected by surgery to a reasonable extent.

DEVELOPMENTAL DISTURBANCES OF TEETH

Developmental dental disorders may be due to:

1. Abnormalities in the differentiation of dental lamina and tooth germs (anomalies in number, size, shape).
2. Abnormalities in the formation of the dental hard tissues (abnormalities in structure).

Variation in tooth number

Decrease in number

Anodontia

In dentistry, anodontia is also called ododontia vera, is a rare genetic disorder characterised by the congenital absence of all primary or permanent teeth.

Causes

Anodontia is usually part of a syndrome and seldom occurs as an isolated entity. Complete absence of teeth is rare; it is often associated with the uncommon condition hereditary ectodermal dysplasia, cleidocranial dysplasia, craniofacial dystosis, cleft lip and cleft palate. The tooth germs may fail to initiate, or initiation may occur but further development of the tooth germ will be aborted. It may be due to radiation injury to the developing tooth germ.

Types of anodontia

True total anodontia (oligodontia) is the agenesis of six or more permanent teeth without associated systemic disorders. It involves both deciduous as well as permanent teeth.

Partial (hypodontia): Partial onodontia is known as hypodontia. It is congenital absence of one or more teeth. Congenital absence of all wisdom teeth or third molars, maxillary lateral incisors, maxillary or mandibular second premolar is relatively common. Absence of less than six teeth is referred to as hypodontia. Syndromes associated with hypodontia are ectodermal dysplasia, achondrodysplasia, Reiger's syndrome, Down's syndrome, and cleft palate and cleft lip.

False anodontia: It is due to extraction of teeth.

Pseudoanodontia

Increase in number

Hyperdontia: ("supernumerary" teeth)

Hyperdontia is the condition of having supernumerary teeth, or teeth which appear in addition to the regular number of teeth. Hyperdontia occurs in primary and permanent dentition.

Supernumerary tooth can occur in both males as well as females. These are far more common in maxilla (90%) as compared to mandible.

Types: Most common supernumerary teeth are:

Mesiodens: The most common supernumerary tooth is a mesiodens, which is a mal formed peg-like tooth that occurs between the maxillary central incisors. It may occur singly or paired, erupted or impacted or even inverted.

Distomolar: An accessory tooth distal to the third molar is a distomolar.

Paramolar: Supernumerary molar located buccally or lingually to the maxillary molars or inter-proximally between 1st 2nd and 3rd maxillary molars.

Hyperdontia can be seen due to inheritance conditions or environmental factors. It is inherited as an autosomal dominant trait, is associated with syndromes. Multiple supernumerary teeth can occur in association with number of disorders including Gardner's syndrome, cleidocranial dystosis, Down's syndrome, craniofacial dystosis and Sturge-Weber angiomatosis.

Clinical features

Supernumerary teeth may sometimes produce crowding or malocclusion and they cause cosmetic problems.

Dentigerous cysts may sometimes develop from an impacted supernumerary tooth.

Treatment

Supernumerary teeth are mostly nonfunctional and they should be extracted.

DISTURBANCES OF ERUPTION OF TEETH

Premature eruption

For the past two hundred years many reports of infants born with teeth or teeth erupting immediately after birth have appeared in medical and dental literature. These teeth have been referred as *'Natal teeth' 'congenital teeth'* and *'precocious dentition'*. Natal teeth indicates teeth in the oral cavity in birth and neonatal teeth those which erupt during the neonatal period; from birth to the thirtieth day of life. Neonatal teeth often present in hypoplastic enamel, adrenogenital syndrome, and underdeveloped roots.

Delayed eruption

Eruption of deciduous teeth starts about 6 months after birth, usually with the appearance of lower incisors, and is complete by two years. Mass failure of eruption is very rare.

Delayed development and eruption of all the permanent molars is a rare phenomenon, which can cause disturbance in the developing occlusion.

Causes of delayed tooth eruption include impacted teeth, cytotoxic therapy, radiotherapy, Down's syndrome, cleidocranial dysplasia, congenital hypopituitarism, congenital hypothyroidism, Gaucher's disease, and osteopetriosis.

Impacted and embedded teeth

An impacted tooth fails to fully pass through the gums. An impacted tooth remains embedded in soft gingival tissue or bone beyond the normal eruption time. The cause may be overcrowding, often because the jaw is too small to fit the third set of molars. Teeth may also become twisted, tilted, or displaced as they try to emerge—resulting in impacted teeth.

Symptoms of impacted tooth are

- Pain or tenderness of the gum or jaw bone.
- Unpleasant taste when biting down on or near the area.
- Visible gap where a tooth did not emerge.
- Bad breath.
- Redness and swelling of the gums around the impacted tooth.
- Swollen lymph nodes of the neck.
- Difficulty in opening the mouth.
- Prolonged headache or jaw ache.

Impacted wisdom teeth

Impacted wisdom teeth are very common. A dentigerous cyst may develop around the coronal portion of the tooth. Furthermore, cases of ameloblastoma have been reported to develop in the wall of such a cyst.

Impacted mandibular third molars

The third molars generally erupt between the ages 18 and 24 years, although there is wide variation.

Approximately one or more third molars are absent in approximately 25% of adults, but they may be still present in adults.

Types of impaction

Mesioangular impaction is the most common form (44%), and means the tooth is angled forward, towards the front of the mouth.

Vertical impaction (38%) occurs when the formed tooth does not erupt fully through the gum line.

Distoangular impactions (6%) mean the tooth as angled backward, towards the rear of the mouth. Typically, distoangular impactions are easier to extract in maxilla and most difficult to extract in the mandible.

Horizontal impaction (3%) is the least common form, which occurs when the tooth is angled fully ninety degrees forward, growing into the roots of the second molar.

Impact wisdom teeth may also be categorised on whether they are still completely encased in the jaw bone.

Bony impaction: If it is completely encased in the jaw bone, it is a bony impaction.

Soft tissue impaction: If the wisdom tooth has erupted out of the jaw bone but not through the gum line, it is called soft tissue impaction.

Operculum: Sometimes the wisdom tooth fails to erupt completely through the gum bed and the gum at the back of the wisdom tooth extends over the biting surface, forming a soft tissue flap or lid around the tooth called operculum.

Management

The extraction of impacted third molar teeth is one of the most frequent surgical procedures carried out by National Health Services.

Surgical procedures for extraction of unerupted third molar teeth are associated with significant morbidity including pain, and swelling, together with the possibility of temporary or permanent nerve damage, resulting in altered sensation of lip or tongue.

ANKYLOSIS

Ankylosis is a dental situation in which the roots of primary teeth lose their normal attachment to the bone and become fused directly to the bone.

Prevalence rate of ankylosed deciduous teeth vary from 1.3% to 14.3% of the population.

Tooth ankylosis is the fusion of the tooth to the bone, preventing the tooth from erupting. This can happen in both primary (baby) teeth and permanent teeth, and may occur at any stage during development of eruption.

Causes

Causes of ankylosis are:

- Inflammation and infection
- Problems with metabolism or normal bone growth
- Congenital tenderness
- Gaps in the membranes around the tooth
- Abnormal pressure from the tongue
- Crushing or other damage.

Clinical features

Ankylosis may occur at any age; however, clinically, the condition is most obvious if the fusion develops during the first two decades of life. An ankylosed tooth has a higher pitched sound or dulled sound as opposed to the more cushioned sound of a normal tooth.

Deciduous mandibular molars are affected with more than ten times the frequency of deciduous maxillary molars. It is quite common for primary molars to become ankylosed. If this occurs before eruption the teeth will fail to appear in the mouth, if it occurs post-eruption, the tooth will appear to submerge into the alveolus.

Problems can occur when ankylosed deciduous molars become submerged or significantly intra-occluded and these include tipping of adjacent teeth, space loss, over-eruption of antagonists and ectopic or failure of eruption of permanent teeth.

ALTERATION IN SIZE

Microdontia

As the term microdontia suggests, this condition is recognised by presence of teeth that are significantly smaller than normal.

Three types of microdontia are recognised

1. **True generalised microdontia:** When all the teeth in both arches are uniformly smaller than normal the condition is known as true generalised microdontia. True microdontia can be associated with systemic diseases such as hypopituitarism in the child dwarfism, Down's syndrome and congenital heart disease.
2. **Relative generalised microdontia:** Normal or slightly smaller teeth present in jaws that are larger than normal. Relative microdontia often exhibits spacing in between the teeth.
3. **Localised microdontia:** Usually only one tooth is involved. Affects maxillary lateral incisors and third molar. When maxillary lateral incisors are involved the teeth often appear cone or peg shaped and are often designated as peg laterals. These peg laterals carry an autosomal dominant type of inheritance pattern. It occurs with congenital heart diseases, Down's syndrome and progeria (Hutchinsons-Gliford syndrome characterized by dwarfism and premature senility). These are also the common missing teeth.

Macrodontia

Abnormally large tooth is an uncommon condition. Macrodontia is a condition in which the teeth appear larger than normal.

A. Generalised macrodontia

1. **True generalised macrodontia:** It is commonly associated with pituitary gigantism, pineal hyperplasia, angioma of face and facial hemi-hypertrophy.
2. **Relative generalised macrodontia:** Teeth are normal or slightly larger than normal, but present in a smaller jaw.

B. Localised macrodontia

Localized macrodontia is occasionally seen on the affected side of the mouth with hemi-facial hypertrophy.

ALTERATION IN SHAPE

Germination

It manifests as a twinning of teeth, usually incisors. It is assumed that a single tooth germ attempts to divide producing a **'double crown or double root'**. A notch in the incisor edge of the affected tooth often recognises doubling of the crown. Tooth counting reveals a normal number of teeth.

Fusion

It is also called synodontia. It is transmitted as autosomal dominant trait with reduced penetration. Fusion is the joining of two tooth germs, resulting in a single large tooth. Fusion may involve the entire length of the teeth, or only the roots, depending on the stage of development of the teeth at the time of union. Majority appcars as large bifid crown with pulp chamber. Few teeth have two pulp chambers.

Dental caries is common in fused teeth.

Dilaceration

It is a developmental disturbance in shape of teeth. It refers to angulations, or a sharp band or curve, in the root or crown of a formed tooth.

Etiology: The condition is thought to be due to developmental disturbances and trauma during the period in which tooth is forming. The result is that the position of the calcified portion of the tooth is changed and the remainder of the tooth is formed at an angle.

Clinical features

Dilaceration can be seen in both the permanent and deciduous dentition and it is more commonly found in posterior teeth and in the maxillary incisors.

Concrescence

It is also called false germination. In concrescence, the roots of two adjacent teeth are joined by cementum.

It most commonly affects maxillary molar teeth.

Types

- True concrescence: This situation occurs during tooth development.
- Acquired concrescence

ACCESSORY CUSPS

Talons cusps

These occur more commonly on maxillary permanent lateral incisors (55%) or in central incisors.

Dens invaginatous, Dens in dente—***'Tooth within a tooth'***.

It is also called dilated composite odontome, or gestant odontome.

Dens invaginatous is a malformation of dental papilla during the tooth development. Affected teeth show a deep infolding of enamel and dentin starting from the foramen coecum or even the tip of the cusps and which may extend deep into the root. Teeth most commonly affected are maxillary lateral incisors and bilateral occurrence is not uncommon.

There are coronal and a reticular form, with the coronal form being more common.

Reticular form: These teeth often contain pulp necrosis and apical lesions. It is lined by cementum.

Coronal form: No sexual predilection:

Mild type

Moderate type

Severe type

Dens evaginatous: It is also called Leong's premolar, evaginated odontome, or occlusal enamel pearl. This defect is found predominantly in individuals of Mongoloid origin including Chinese, Japanese, Philippines and American Indians.

C. Taurodontism

Taurodontism is a condition in which tooth roots have a thick 'bull like appearance'. Such teeth have been found in fossils of Native Americans and Insuits. Taurodontism is a condition found in teeth where the body of the tooth and pulp chamber is enlarged. As a result, the floor of the pulp and the furcation of the tooth are moved apically down the root. Third molars are most severely affected and first molars are least affected. Conditions with taurodontism include Klinefelter's syndrome, Orofacial-digital syndrome type II, Amelogenesis imperfecta, and Down's syndrome.

D. Enamel pearls, enamel drops

An enamel pearl is a condition of teeth where enamel is found on locations where enamel is not supposed to be, such as on a root surface. They are found usually in the area between roots, which are called a furcation of molars. Enamel pearls are not common in teeth with single root enamel defects. Enamel pearls do not exhibit periodontal attachment.

Cause

This anomaly appears to be caused by the localised failure of Hertwig's epithelial root sheet to separate from the dentin. Prolonged contact with the dentin presumably induces this odontogenic epithelium to secrete enamel, albert in limited quantity, while preventing the normal deposition of cementum by adjacent cementoblasts.

Microscopically, the pearl is a flat enamel patch located on dentin and surrounded by otherwise normal cementum. It is located just apical to the cemento-enamel junction. The enamel pearl is lined with reduced enamel epithelium. Epithelial cell rests can be seen close to the normally formed adjacent cementum.

Amelogenesis imperfecta

The prevalence varies from 1:700 to 1:40,000—according to the population studied.

Amelogenesis imperfecta is a genetic disorder of teeth development. This condition causes teeth to be usually small, discoloured, pitted or grooved and prone to rapid wear and breakage.

Amelogenous imperfecta presents with abnormal formation of the enamel or external layer of teeth. Enamel is composed mostly of mineral, which is formed and regulated by the proteins in it. Amelogenesis imperfecta is due to the malfunction of proteins in the enamel ameloblastin, tufflin and amelogenin.

Up to date, mutation in the AmELX, ENAM, MMP20, and KLK-4 genes have been found to cause amelogenesis imperfecta.

Clinical features

There are four types of amelogenesis imperfecta:

1. Hypoplastic type
2. Hypomineralised or hypocalcified type
3. Hypomaturation type
4. Hypomaturation/Hypoplasia/Taurodontinsm

1. Hypoplastic type shows the typical pattern of X-linked inheritance—heterozygous females can pass mutant gene to children of either sex with chance of being 50%. It may show autosomal dominant pattern of inheritance. The condition affects males and females in strikingly different ways. Males show the trait fully. They may have only a thin layer of enamel of normal colour and translucency. The enamel is of normal hardness but does not develop to normal thickness. The enamel may be smooth, pitted or locally rough or it may have alternating vertical bands of normal and abnormal enamel. Lack of normal depth of the enamel layer is frequently observed in the yellowish to brownish, and, generally, both primary and permanent teeth are affected.

2. Hypomineralised form or hypocalcified type: This is most common type of amelogenous imperfecta. The enamel may be stained by exogenous agents and tends to be brown or black. In hypocalcified amelogenous imperfecta, the enamel surface is pitted, and chips off, thereby exposing the dentin. The teeth are sensitive to changes in temperature. In hypomineralised form the enamel is rough, soft and discoloured. The enamel is of normal thickness but opaque or yellowish white luster on newly erupted teeth. It is so soft that it is lost after eruption.

3. Hypomaturation form: In hypomaturation form the enamel is of normal thickness and hardness but with a whitish-yellow surface. A dental exposure may penetrate the surface enamel in the X-linked recessive type. In the autosomal recessive type, the enamel tends to chip way.

Microscopically

In hypoplastic type there is thin lamellar or somewhat thicker amorphous enamel on a proximal surface with no rods or incremental lines visible. In cases of hypocalcified amelogenesis imperfecta the affected enamel is porous and appear opaque. In hypomaturation type, enamel cannot be distinguished from dentin on roentgenogram.

Radiologically

Enamel is radiodense and, therefore, poorly mineralised compared with normal enamel. In hypocalcified type the enamel is of normal thickness but has a moth-eaten appearance.

Management

Treatment depends on the severity of the problem. Full crowns will improve the appearance of the teeth, and protect them from damage.

ENAMEL HYPOPLASIA

Enamel hypoplasia is a defect in tooth enamel that results in less quantity of enamel than normal. The defect is usually localised, which can be a small pit or dent in the tooth or can be so widespread that the entire tooth is small or misshaped.

This makes the tooth's surface very rough, and the defects often stand out because they are brown or yellow in colour. In severe cases, the tooth enamel is missing entirely, causing the affected tooth to be misshapen or abnormally small.

TABLE 3.2
CAUSES OF ENAMEL HYPOPLASIA

A. Hereditary

B. Acquired

- Nutritional deficiency
  Poor pre-natal or post-natal nutrition
- Exanthematous diseases
  (i) Measles
  (ii) Scarlet fever
  (iii) Chicken pox
- Congenital syphilis
- Hypocalcaemia
- Birth injury due to haemolytic disease of newborn
  Injury due to incubation of premature infants
- Local infection or trauma
- Fluoride toxicity
- Idiopathic

Many conditions can produce defects in enamel production. Most are acquired, not inherited. Among them are inflammation, vitamin deficiencies, microbial infections, trauma, and excessive fluoride ingestion.

Enamel hyperplasia due to local infection or trauma

Sometimes enamel hypoplasia shows up as distinct white spot on the tooth. This is often referred to as ***'Turner's tooth'*** or ***'Turner's hypoplasia'***, and is typically caused by a trauma to the tooth during its mineralisation phase. It is most commonly observed in (permanent) bicuspid teeth secondary to infected primary molars and permanent central incisors (secondary to injury to the primary incisors).

Vitamin deficiency: Another possible explanation for pitted irregular hypoplastic tooth enamel is irregular vitamin D metabolism, which prevents proper absorption of calcium. This can occur due to nutritional deficiency of vitamin D, an X-linked dominant disorder known as vitamin-D rickets.

Hypocalcaemia is a specific cause of enamel hypoplasia. This type of defect may cause tooth sensitivity, may be unsightly or may be more susceptible to dental cavities.

DENTIN DEFECTS

DENTINOGENESIS IMPERFECTA

It is also known as hereditary opalescent dentin.

Dentinogenesis imperfecta is an autosomal dominant trait and was first reported by Talbot. Roberts and Schour proposed dentinogenesis imperfecta in 1939.

Types of dentinogenesis imperfecta are:

Type I: Dentinogenesis imperfecta combines with osteogenesis imperfecta.

Type II: It is an isolated trait of dentinogenesis imperfecta. It occurs in people without other inherited disorders, e.g., osteogenesis imperfecta. A few families have progressive hearing loss in addition to dental abnormalities.

Type III: Dentinogenesis imperfecta was first identified in a population from Bradywine, Maryland. There is Bandywine opalescent dentin. It is a rare variety characterised by shell teeth, with very little dentin and multiple pulp exposures in the primary teeth.

Researchers now believe that type II and type III may be the same disorder.

Dentinogenesis imperfecta is a disorder of tooth development which results from an inherited structural deficiency of collagen formation. This condition causes the teeth to be discoloured (most often a blue-grey or yellow brown colour) and translucent.

Cause

Mutations in the DSPP gene cause dentinogenesis imperfecta.

Clinical features

Teeth are also weaker than normal, making them prone to rapid wear, breakage, and loss. These problems can affect both primary and permanent teeth. Patients affected with dentinogenesis imperfecta show a peculiar colour deviation from the natural dentition that ranges from grey to brown-violet or yellowish-brown, with a characteristic unusual translucent or opalescent hue. This is attributable to the dentinal disturbance, with enamel being normal. These teeth are prone to excessive wear and fracture due to primary abnormality in the structure and composition of dentin-enamel junction that lacks normal scalloping.

Radiographs show that the roots are short and conical, and that the pulp chambers are wide in the early stages but narrowed or completely obliterated later, giving typical 'tulip' appearance.

Microscopically: The remainder of the dentin shows reduction of tubules, cellular inclusion, and numerous resting lines giving the appearance of stratification. The tubules may be irregular in shape, size, number and course.

Dentin dysplasia

In 1920, Balchsmiede first reported 8 cases as ***'root less teeth'***. Later Rushton, in 1939, described it as ***'dentinal dysplasia'***.

Dentin dysplasia is a genetic disorder of teeth, commonly exhibiting an autosomal dominant inheritance. It is characterised by presence of normal enamel but atypical dentin with abnormal pulpal morphology.

There are two types:

Type 1 is the reticular type, and type 2 is the coronal type.

Reticular type

Synonyms: Opalescent dentin, type 1 dentin dysplasia, reticular dentin dysplasia, rootless teeth, pulpless teeth, Thistle tube teeth.

Reticular type is characterised by the presence of primary and permanent teeth with normal appearance of the crown but no or only rudimentary root development, incomplete or total obliteration of the pulp chamber and periapical radiolucent areas or cysts. The pulp chamber is described as having a **'crescent shaped'** appearance.

Coronal type

Synonyms: Anomalous dysplasia of dentin, pulp stones, pulpal dysplasia and type II dentin dysplasia.

Coronal dentin dysplasia is transmitted by autosomal dominant trait.

It is characterised by abnormal development of the hard tissue (dentin) that is beneath the enamel, surrounds the pulp and forms major part of the teeth. In those with coronal dysplasias, the baby teeth (primary and deciduous teeth) are brownish-blue with a translucent opalescence. However, permanent teeth appear normal in colour. The pulps are enlarged and are described as having ***'thistle tube appearance'***. Pulp stones may be found.

Radiographs

In type I: Show short pointed roots, periapical radiolucencies and obliteration pulp chambers and root canals.

In type II: The pulp-containing canals within the roots of the teeth (root canal) are smaller than normal.

Management

Successful oral rehabilitation with complete denture after extraction of all teeth and curettage of cysts has been described.

DEFECTS IN ENAMEL AND DENTIN

Odontodysplasia: It is a condition in which there is localised arrest in tooth development due to regional vascular anomaly. There is ghost-like appearance with short roots and shell-like crowns. There is large diffusely calcified pulp chamber.

Microscopically: There is distortion of enamel matrix, absence of enamel rods and focal calcifications in the connective tissue around the crown.

REGRESSIVE ALTERATION OF TEETH

ATTRITION

Attrition is the mechanical wearing down of the biting and surfaces of teeth. The tooth-to-tooth contact during chewing grinds down the surfaces. This type of tooth wear takes place in all mouths, and may be physiological and occurs as a natural consequence of ageing. Interproximal attrition occurs at proximal surfaces of adjacent teeth when they move against one another on occlusal loading. Movement of teeth is in the vertical direction. Amelogenesis imperfecta may create unaesthetic appearance, dental sensitivity and attrition. In cases of dentinogenesis imperfecta the exposed dentin may undergo severe and rapid attrition.

Clinical features

The back teeth become flatter, and the front teeth become shorter. Characteristic feature is development of facet (flat surface with circumscribed and well-defined border).

Signs of attrition include flattening of biting surfaces, wearing away of enamel, and exposure of underlying dentin. Dentin may be yellow or stained from food or tobacco. Severe attrition of the front of teeth will have a disfiguring effect on the face. It may infrequently cause sensitivity to sweet, hot and cold food and drinks. Severely worn teeth as a result of long term habit of grinding and clenching teeth results in **'gummy'** appearance. It results not from too much gum tissue but from having short teeth.

Management

Bruxism should be investigated as it can cause severe damage to teeth, fillings, and crowns. If bruxism exists, then either a soft or hard nightguard should be made depending on the clinical situation.

If damage to teeth should be repaired carefully by using composite white fillings, onlays or crowns to restore the patient bite, stop the tooth sensitivity and improve the aesthetics of the teeth.

ABRASION

Abrasion is the loss of tooth structure by mechanical forces from a foreign element. If this force begins at the cementoenamel junction, then progression of tooth loss is rapid since enamel is very thin in this region of the tooth. Once past the enamel, abrasion quickly destroys the dentin and cementum structures.

Friction between a tooth and exogenous agent causes wear called abrasion. If teeth are worn on their occlusional surfaces, incisional surfaces, or both, by friction from the food bolus, this wear is termed **'mastication abrasion'**. Masticatory abrasion also can occur on the facial and lingual aspects of teeth as coarse food is forced against these surfaces by the tongue, lips and cheeks during mastication.

Causes

Abrasion can occur as a result of overzealous tooth brushing, improper use of dental floss and tooth-picks, or detrimental oral habits such as chewing tobacco, biting hard objects such as pens, pencils, or pipe stems, opening hair pins with teeth, and biting finger nails. The clamps of partial dentures can produce abrasion. Occupational abrasion may occur among tailors, steam stresses who server thread with teeth, teamstresses, shoemakers and upholsterers who hold nails between their teeth, glassblowers, and musicians who play wind instruments.

Clinical features

The teeth of abrasion causes V shaped or wedge shaped notches in the lower third of the teeth near gum line. Notches made by the toothpicks may occur between the teeth. The teeth most commonly affected are premolars and canines. Traditionally, cervical lesions caused by abrasion have sharply defined margins and a smooth hard surface. Symptoms of tooth abrasion include erosion of tooth enamel, increased tooth and sensitivity to heat and cold.

Complications of tooth abrasion are tooth infection, tooth loss and tooth decay.

Treatment of abrasion

The patient's toothbrushing technique should be assessed and modified where necessary. Switching to a soft brush or an electric toothbrush can also help to reduce abrasion.

Where the root surface is exposed and sensitive to air, it should be covered by composite resin fillings to stop the dentin sensitivity.

EROSION

Erosion is defined as loss of tooth structure by chemical reaction, not that associated with bacteria.

It is secondary to presence of acid or chelating agent. Source can be dietary (e.g., vinegar, lemons).

Types

I. **Internal:** Erosion that occurs due to intrinsic causes, e.g., gastric secretions, perimolysis.
   - Acid reflux or heart burn
   - Anorexia or bulimia
   - Hiatus hernia
   - Excessive consumption of alcohol
   - Morning sickness in early pregnancy
   - Over-eating.

II. **External**

   A. **Foods with high acid contents are**
   - Soft drinks, citrus fruits, oranges, lemons and grape fruits
   - Fruit juices
   - Vinegar and pickles
   - Yoghurt
   - Acids.

B. Industrial, atmosphere

- Electroplating
- Galvanising acid pickling
- Battery manufacture
- Sanitary cleanser manufacture
- Sulphuric acid and hydrochloric acid manufacturer
- Copper smelter
- Chemical dye and petroleum industry
- Fertiliser company

Foods, which have a high acid content, can cause the enamel and dentin to be eroded. The acids dissolve the calcium in the tooth.

Dental erosion appears as a smooth silky-shining, glazed, enamel surface. Further progression may lead to the development of shallow concavities or to rounding and grooving of the edges or the cusps of the tooth surfaces. In patients with severe dental erosion, the enamel is often totally removed, leaving a vulnerable dentin surface which is often associated with a painful sensitivity and is prone to further erosion and mechanical wear daily.

It commonly affects facial surface of maxillary anterior and appears as shallow spoon shaped depressions in cervical portions of the crown. Posterior teeth exhibit loss of occlusal surface, where dentin is destroyed more rapidly than enamel, resulting in concave depression of dentin surrounded by elevated rim of enamel.

Erosion limited to facial surfaces of maxillary anterior dentition is usually associated with dietary acid.

Consequences of erosion

- Sensitivity
- Weakening of the teeth
- Reduced lifetime.

Management

The patient's diet and medical history should be analysed so that the cause of the erosion can be identified. Where dietary factors are causing the erosion, medical advice should be sought.

Saliva production should be encouraged to neutralise the acids that cause erosion. Saliva production is increased by the use of sugar gum.

Composite resin fillings or crowns should repair deep erosion cavities. Root canal treatment may become necessary if the erosion cavities have exposed the pulp of the tooth. Use fluoride paste daily.

ABNORMALITIES OF DENTAL PULP

Pulp calcification

Synonyms: Dental pulp calcification, pulp calculus, pulp nodule, and pulp stone.

Definition: A calcified body found in the pulp chamber of a tooth may be composed of irregular denticles (true dentin) or due to ectopic calcification of pulp tissue (false denture).

Causes

Conditions initiating pulp stones—for instance aging, circulatory disturbances, caries, and pulp pathos, and arteriosclerosis.

Three types of pulpal calcification are:

1. Denticles; 2. Pulp stones; 3. Diffuse linear calcifications.

Diffuse linear calcifications exhibit areas of fine, fibrillar, irregular calcification that often parallel the vasculature. These calcifications may be present in the pulp chamber or canals and the frequency with age.

X-ray

Pulpal calcifications are identified on dental radiographs and may be located either within the pulp chamber appearing as focal intrapulpal radioopacities, or within the root canals, as diffuse radioopacities giving the appearance of calcific obliteration.

Pulp stones are also frequently encountered in certain forms of osteogenesis imperfecta.

The root resorption is the breakdown or destruction, and subsequent loss of the root surface of the tooth. This is caused by living body cells attaching part of the tooth. When damage extends to the whole tooth, it is called tooth resorption.

Root resorption occurs as a result of differentiation of macrophages into osteoclasts in surrounding tissue, which, if in close proximity to the root surface will resorb the root surface, cementum and underlying root dentin. This can vary in severity from evidence of microscopic pits in the root surface to complete devastation of the root surface.

Deciduous root resorption is a natural processes which allows exfoliation of the primary teeth to make way for the secondary teeth. Deciduous root resorption is caused by osteoclast differentiation due to pressure exerted by the erupting permanent tooth.

Root resorption of secondary teeth can occur as a result of pressure on the root surface. This can be in the path of the root, inflammation, excessive loading, aggressive tumours and growths.

TABLE 3.3
CAUSES OF RESORPTION

A. External resorption
- a. Conditions which causes resorption of teeth
  - i. Periapical inflammation
- b. Excessive mechanical or occlusal forces
- c. Cysts and tumours
- d. Reimplantation of teeth
- e. Impacted teeth
- f. Idiopathic

B. Internal resorption
- a. Idiopathic

Types include internal resorption and external resorption.

Internal resorption

Internal resorption is an unusual condition of a tooth when the dentin and pulpal walls begin to reabsorb centrally within the root canal.

Clinical features

The first evidence of this lesion may be the appearance of a pink-hued area on the crown of the root; this condition is referred to **'pink tooth of Mummery'**, after the 19th century anatomist James Howard Mummery, and represents the hyperplastic, vascular pulp tissue filling-in the resorbed areas.

Microscopically

Carious destruction of dental hard tissues frequently produces pulpitis, an inflammatory lesion of the pulp, which may be acute or chronic. The lesion may be non-infective, as a result of trauma or very marked changes in temperature, but more often eosinophilic acellular dentin, the characteristic uniform layer of vascular connective tissue and large numbers of chronic inflammatory cells. The connective tissue appears to be extending into the dentin and eroding it extensively. Most of the chronic inflammatory cells are plasma cells, and among them are Russel bodies, large plasma cells with much intensely eosinophilic cytoplasm. Resorption of dentin continues until both dentin and enamel of the crown of the tooth are absorbed.

Radiologically

Radiological findings include an increase in diameter of the pulp chamber.

Treatment

If the condition is discovered prior to perforation of the crown or root, endodontic therapy (root canal therapy) may be carried out with the expectation of a fairly high success rate. Severe tooth resorption is very difficult to treat and often requires extraction of teeth.

External resorption

External resorption is an inflammatory process in which tooth is dissolved away from the root surface inward, towards the pulp. As the tooth resorps, the space previously occupied is replaced with bone.

Inflammatory resorption

In addition to apical root resorption caused by apical root, periodontitis as a consequence of pulpal necrosis.

There are two main forms of external resorption associated with inflammation in the periodontal tissues, namely:

- Periapical inflammatory root resorption (PARR)
- External inflammatory root resorption.

Both forms are triggered by destruction of cementoblasts.

In PIRR, the osteoclast activating factors, which perpetuate the resorptive process, does an inflammatory lesion in the adjacent periodontal tissues provided.

Peripheral inflammatory root resorption: A damaged cervical root resorption, e.g., due to excessive scaling or other trauma, is usually covered by functional epithelium. Sometimes this does not occur, instead, the damaged area will be repopulated by connective tissue. In the presence of a periodontal lesion the onset of a resorptive process is triggered. It is conceivable that the inflammatory cells in the lesion recognised osteoclast-activating factors of the denuded root surface and thus initiate and maintain clastic activity. This type of resorption is found immediately apical to the marginal tissues and pocket depth and may, thus, not always be cervical in position.

Ankylosis replacement resorption

In replacement resorption the tooth structure is resorbed and replaced by bone resulting in ankylosis in which bone fuses directly to the root surface. The characteristics of ankylosis are lack of physiologic mobility, failure of the tooth to erupt along with adjacent teeth.

HYPERCEMENTOSIS

Some teeth in some individuals display massive over-production of cementum—known as hypercementosis.

Hypercementosis is the thickening of increased deposit of cementum on the root surface. It may involve the entire root surface, but, more commonly, it appears as a bulbous mass involving the root end.

The cause is unknown, but it also occurs in unerupted teeth.

Causes of hypercementosis

- A broken or fractured teeth
- An abscess or low-grade inflammation at the tip of the root
- Osteitis deformans
- Hyperocclusion of teeth
- Reports are available where hypercementosis is associated with Paget's disease of jaw
- The extension of a tooth from its normal position due to the loss of the opposing tooth from the opposite arch
- Acromegaly, rheumatic fever.

It refers to abnormally large cellular cementum deposits on the apical third of one or more teeth. Such deposits form bulbous enlargements on the roots that may interfere with dental extractions.

It may be diffuse or circumscribed, e.g., it may affect all the teeth or only certain parts of one tooth.

Clinical features

Hypercementosis occurs predominantly in adulthood, and the frequency increases with age. Mandibular molars are affected most frequently, followed by the mandibular and maxillary second molars and mandibular first molars.

Microscopically

The periphery of the root exhibits deposition of an excessive amount of cementum over the original layer of primary cementum.

Radiologically

X-ray shows thickening of the cementum layer as well as blunting or rounding of the root's tip. There is increased deposition of cementum immediately beneath the periodontal membrane and the bulging of the peridental membrane and lifting of the lamina dura from the surface of the root.

CEMENTICLES

Cementicles are small, spherical, discrete globular mass of cementum that may lie free in the periodontal ligament adjacent to the cementum surface. These are classified as free cementicles. They can also attach to cementum surface (attached or sessile cementicles) or incorporated into cementum layer (imbedded cementicles).

Cementical tears have been reported in the periodontal literature associated with localised, rapid periodontal breakdown. Common causative factors are aging and traumatic occlusion but the exact etiology is not known.

Cementicles are spherical in shape and varies in size. They are seldom larger than 0.2 to 0.3 cm.

Structure: Cementicles may be composed of fibrillar or afibrillar cementum, or a mixture of two. True cementicles consist of collagenous matrix intermingled with a non-collagenous ground substance.

Bibliography

AB Neville, BWD Damm, C Allen, J Bouquot: *Oral and Maxillofacial Pathology* 2nd edition 2002 page 20.

Bennet Lindsey, Hinshaw Molley: Heck's disease: *Diagnosis and Susceptibility*: *Pediatric Dermatology*, Volume 26, Number 1, January 2009 PP 8-89 (3)

Robert J Gorlin, Henry M Goldman: Thomas *Oral Pathology*. Volume 1. 6th edition. CV Mosby: 1970.

Stewart ML and McClanahan SB: *Cemental tear*: *A case report* (2009) International Endodontic Journal. Vol 39(1) p 81-89

Yasar Sirin, Ayse Tulin, Serdar Zehra Asiran, Goktav Fatih, Aslan Canan: *Paediatric Dermatology*, Volume 26, August 2009. PP 465-468.

CHAPTER

4

HEALING OF ORAL WOUNDS

WOUND HEALING

Definition: Wound healing or wound repair is the body's natural process of regenerating dermal or epidermal tissue. Wound healing is a complex phenomenon, involving a number of well-orchestrated processes including regeneration of parenchymal cells, migration and proliferation of both parenchymal and connective tissue cells, synthesis of extracellular matrix proteins, remodeling of connective tissue and parenchymatous components, and collagenisation and acquisition of wound strength.

Wound healing may be defined as the process whereby an injured tissue is repaired, resulting in regeneration of the cell lining of the tissue with the reorganisation of deeper tissue components into the scar.

FACTORS WHICH AFFECT WOUND HEALING

1. Growth factors

These include:

A. **Epidermal growth factors (EGF)** were the first cytokine described and is potent mitogen for epithelial cells, endothelial cells, and fibroblasts. Epidermal growth factor stimulates fibronectin synthesis, angiogenesis, fibroplasias, and collagenase activity.

B. **Platelet derived growth factor (PDGF)** is released from the alpha granules of platelet and is responsible for the stimulation of neutrophils and macrophages and for the production of transforming growth beta factor. PDGF is a mitogen and chemotactic agent for fibroblasts and smooth muscle cells and stimulates angiogenesis, and collagenase.

C. **Fibroblastic growth factor** is a mitogen for mesenchymal cells and an important stimulus for angiogenesis. Fibroblast growth factor is a mitogen for endothelial cells, fibroblasts, keratocytes, and myoblasts. This factor also stimulates wound concentration and epithelisation and production of collagen, fibronectin and proteoglycans.

D. **Keratinocyte growth factor (KGF)**, a member of the fibroblast growth factor family of mitogen (FGF-7), is a secreted protein, which is predominantly produced by various types of mesenchymal, but not the epithelial cells. However, most types of epithelial cells express the only known high affinity receptors for KGF, transmembrane protein tyrosine kinase.

E. **Transforming growth factors** are of two types—alpha and beta. Transforming growth factor beta is released from the alpha granules of platelets and has been shown to regulate its own production in an autocrine manner. This factor is an important stimulant for fibroblast proliferation and the production of proteoglycans, collagen and fibrin. The factor also promotes accumulation of extracellular matrix and fibrosis. Transforming growth factor- beta has been demonstrated to reduce scarring and to reverse the inhibition of wound healing by glucocorticosteroids.

F. **Vascular endothelial growth factor (VEGF):** It promotes blood vessel formation in early development (vasculogenesis) and has a central role in the growth of new blood vessels (angiogenesis) in cancers, chronic inflammatory states and healing wounds. VGEF is a specific stimulator of lymphatic formation.

2. Extracellular matrix and cell matrix interaction

These basically include:

A. **Collagen** from a major portion of connective tissue in healing wound.

B. **Adhesive glycoprotein**

(i) **Fibronectin** binds to number of other extracellular matrix components (including collagen, fibrin, heparin) and is involved in attachment, spreading, and migration of cells.

(ii) **Laminin** is a glycoprotein, mediates cell attachments to connective tissues substances; in culture, it alters the growth, survival, morphology, differentiation and motility of various cell types. It also causes capillary tube formation in angiogenesis.

3. Proteoglycans glycosaminoglycans (GAGS)

Glycosaminoglycans are negatively charged, extended molecules that occupy large volumes. The most abundant are hyaluronic acid, chondroitin sulphate, heparan sulphate and keratin sulphate.

Factors affecting the healing of oral wounds

There are different factors that affect wound healing in the oral cavity.

Wound healing is an intricate process in which a selection of cellular and matrix components act together to restore the integrity of the injured dental tissue:

1. **Location of dental wounds:** The location of the dental wound is important in the fast healing of the dental wound. It is faster to heal a dental wound in which there is a good vascular bed than dental wounds in an area which is moderately avascular as observed in dental surgical microscope.

2. **Local factors**

   i. **Immobilisation** of dental wound is important in dental wound healing. Early motion, particularly before tensile strength, has been established, subjects a wound to persistent trauma, thereby preventing or retarding healing.

   ii. **Circulatory factors:** Healing wound needs good blood supply. Diminished blood supply due to arterial disease and poor circulation from any cause (varicose vein) delays healing. Anaemia is reported to be responsible for causing delay in wound healing.

iii. **Infection:** Wound infection is likely the most common reason for poor wound healing. Infection of wound, which is necessarily of secondary type, delays healing. Infection leads to formation of more scar tissues. Infected granulation tissues may overgrow and impede regeneration of epithelium.

3. **Physical factors**
   a. **Trauma:** Severe trauma to tissue delays wound healing and mild traumatic injury favours wound healing.
   b. **Local temperature:** Wounds heal slowly in cold weather. In environmental hyperthermia, wound healing is accelerated.
   c. **Radiation injury:** Prior irradiation leaves vascular lesions that interfere with blood supply and result in slow wound healing. Acute irradiation of a wound blocks cell proliferation and inhibits contraction of granulation tissue.
4. **Nutritional factors**
   a. **Protein:** Low protein levels in the diet have an adverse effect on healing. Of special importance are two sulphur containing amino acids—methionine and cystine. Malnutrition causes a decreased rate of fibroblastic proliferation and neovascularisation and impairs both cellular and humoral immunity.
   b. **Vitamins:** Vitamin C increases the conversion of proline to hydroxylysine. Scurvy caused by deficiency of vitamin C is a classic cause of defective wound healing. Vitamin A deficiency retards healing. Riboflavin and pyridoxine deficiency also results in a delay of the healing process.
   c. **Zinc and iron** are needed for wound healing, and there is evidence that increasing the content of zinc in a patient's diet may help wound healing.
5. **Presence of foreign body or necrotic tissue or blood** in the wound impairs healing.
6. **Age** is often identified as an important factor in wound healing. It has been suggested that wound complication in the elderly may have more to do with cardiovascular and respiratory problems than the effects of aging itself.
7. **Tobacco** affects postoperative wound healing following surgical and non-surgical tooth extractions, routine maxillofacial surgeries, implants, and periodontal therapies. In an experimental study, bone regeneration after distraction osteogenesis was found to be negatively affected by smoking. Thus, tobacco, a peripheral vasoconstrictor along with its products like nicotine increases platelet adhesiveness, raises the risk of microvascular occlusion, and causes tissue ischemia. Smoking tobacco is also associated with catecholamines release resulting in vasoconstriction and decreased tissue perfusion. Smoking is believed to suppress the innate and host immune responses, affecting the function of neutrophils—the prime line of defence against infection.
8. **Hormones:** Steroids hinder the formation of granulation tissue, and their immunosuppressive effects may predispose to local infection. These agents also inhibit collagen synthesis.
9. **Underlying systemic disease** in a patient with a wound can dramatically diminish wound healing. Diabetes mellitus is a classic example. Healing is also delayed in cases of neutropaenia, renal failure, and tumour cachexia.
10. **Miscellaneous**

    Wound sutured with non-absorbable sutures are weaker than those sutured with absorbable ones.

Cynoacrylate adhesions: It permits uncomplicated healing and also hastens the healing process.

Healing process

Healing process can be categorised into primary, secondary and third intention.

Healing by first intention (primary union)

Healing of clean, uninfected surgical incision approximated by surgical suture is referred as primary union or healing by first intention.

There are five major interrelated and overlapping phases to the healing process.

1. Immediately

The capillaries on either side of wound are thrombosed. The gap is filled up with blood, which coagulates and seals the defect. If clot reaches the surface, it dries to form a crust or a scab.

2. Inflammatory phase

Day one: Neutrophils appear at margins of incision and there is an acute inflammatory response on each side of the narrow incisional space leading to swelling, redness, and pain at the wound site. Epithelial cells at edge of wound undergo mitosis and begin to migrate across the wound.

3. Proliferative phase

Cellular proliferation (Day 2): Cellular proliferation involves three key processes angiogenesis, fibroblast proliferation, and epithelial cell proliferation.

Angiogenesis: The wound surface or edge is relatively ischaemic and healing cannot effectively proceed until sufficient blood flow is restored to allow delivery of nutrients. Angiogenesis is also known as neovascularisation. This involves formation of new blood vessels by the proliferation and migration of endothelial cells from preexisting blood vessels.

Angiogenesis takes place under the influence of vascular endothelial growth factor (VEGF). The receptors for VEGF are expressed only on endothelial cells. Fibroblast proliferation collagen fibres are now present in the margins of the incision.

Epithelial cell proliferation: The epidermis at its cut edges thickens as a result of mitotic activity of basal cells, within 24 to 48 hours spurs of epithelial cells from both edges migrate and grow along cut margins of dermis, depositing basement membrane components as they move. They fuse in the midline, beneath the scab, thus producing continuous but thin epithelial layers.

Day 3: Macrophages largely replace neutrophils. Granulation tissue gradually fills the incision, but in the beginning these are vertically oriented and do not bridge the incision. Epithelial cell proliferation continues, thickening the epidermal covering layer yields mature epidermal architecture with surface keratinisation.

Connective tissue formation: (Day 5). Incisional space is filled with granulation tissue. Neovascularisation is minimal. Abundant collagen fibrils now begin to bridge the incision. Epidermis recovers its normal thickness and differentiation of surface cells occurs.

Day 7: Interstitial matrix production.

Day 10. Wound contracture phase begins about **10th day**.

Wound remodeling

Day 30, the scar comprises of a cellular tissue largely devoid of inflammatory cells and covered by an essentially normal epidermis.

3 months: There is devascularisation of tissues, remodeling of collagen by enzyme action. Scar is now minimal and merges with surrounding tissues.

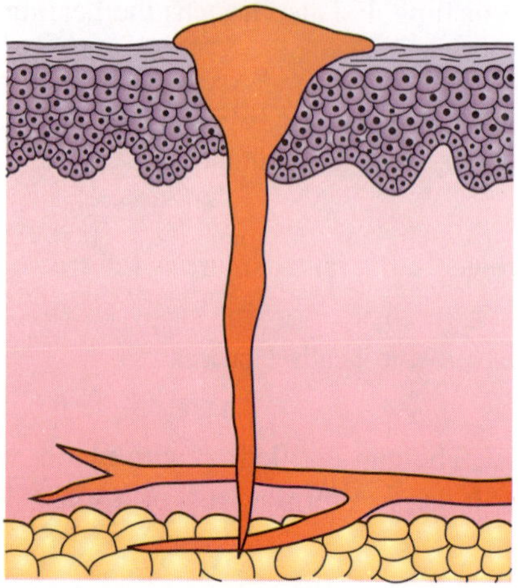

Fig.4.1: Clean incision

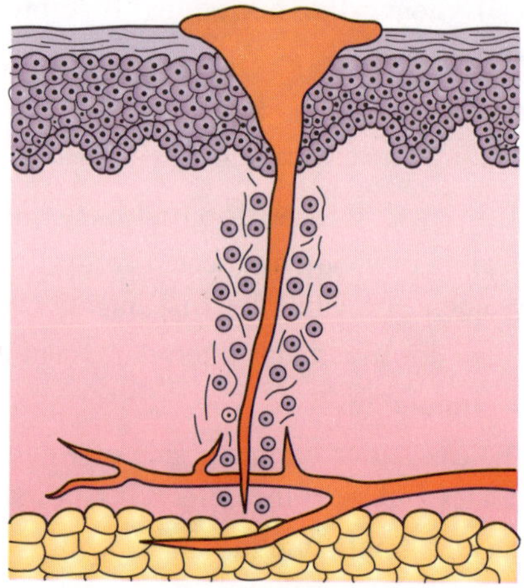

Fig.4.2: Blood clot, fibrin fill up the gap

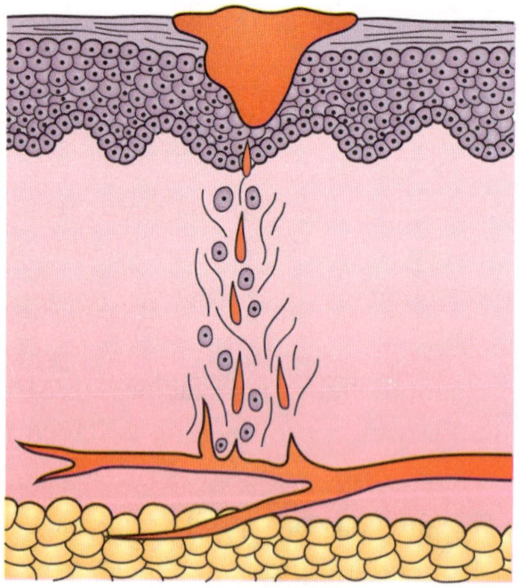

Fig.4.3: Macrophage activity removing clot

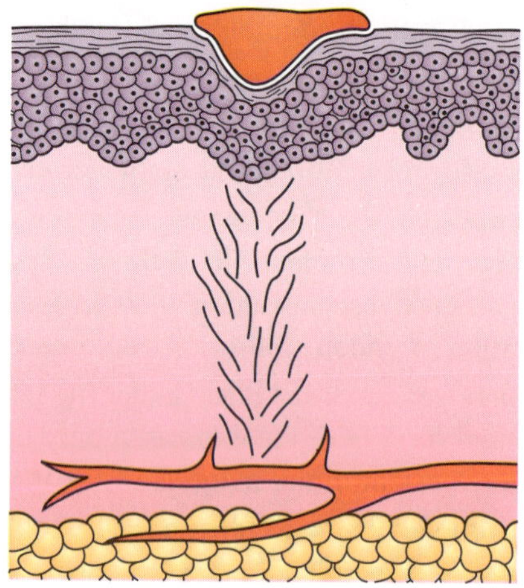

Fig.4.4: Scab loose and epithelial covering complete

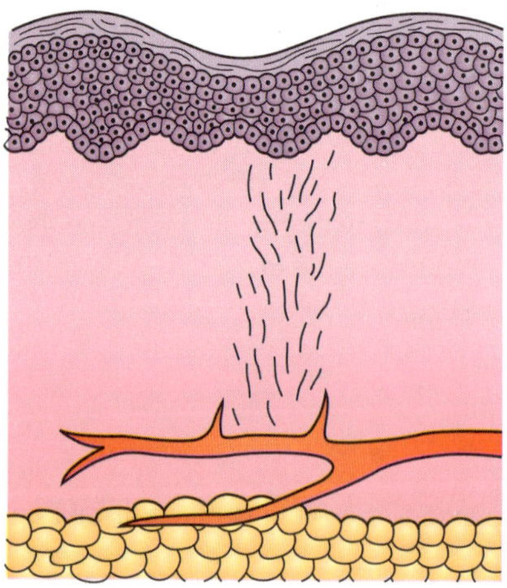

Fig.4.5: Fibroblast close gap, epithelium grows over

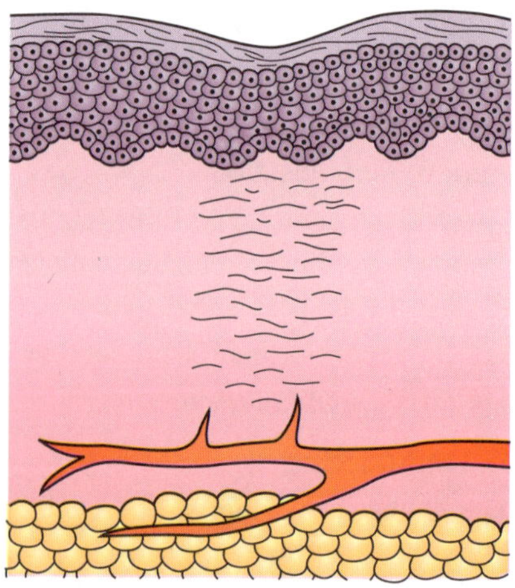

Fig.4.6: Healed

Healing by second intention (secondary union)

Healing by secondary intention occurs in an open wound, because of the presence of infection, excessive trauma or skin loss, and the wound edges come close together naturally by means of granulation tissue and contraction are not brought together by sutures.

The basic process of healing by second intention is approximately same as healing by first intention. The major differences are that wounds healing by second intention are more open and are more prone to infection and that much more granulation tissue is necessary to close the wound.

Early phase: The edges of a wound cannot be brought together and a defect remains. The base of the wound may become covered with plasma. The plasma oozes out from the damaged blood vessels in the base of the wound. Wounds are filled with the blood from the cut ends of capillaries, fibrin threads, and platelets.

One week approximately: The fibrovascular granulation tissue gradually fills the wound space and the epithelium grows over its surface. The exudative inflammatory changes and the migration of neutrophils also subside. There is formation of loose connective tissue by the fibroblasts. Macrophages come to clear the debris, and granulation tissue grows into the wound from its base.

Second week onwards: During the second week, there is continuous accumulation of collagen and proliferation of fibroblasts. The leukocytic infiltration, edema, and increased vascularity are greatly reduced. There is increasing collagen deposition within the incisional scar and disappearances of vascular channels.

Months: The contraction of wound is brought about by microfibroblasts present in granulation tissues. Wound contraction occurs at the time when active granulation tissue is being formed. Wound contraction is probably caused by shrinkage of granulation tissue that develops in the wound. Both the fibrocytes and the endothelial cells in granulation tissue are contractile and pull the edges of wound together.

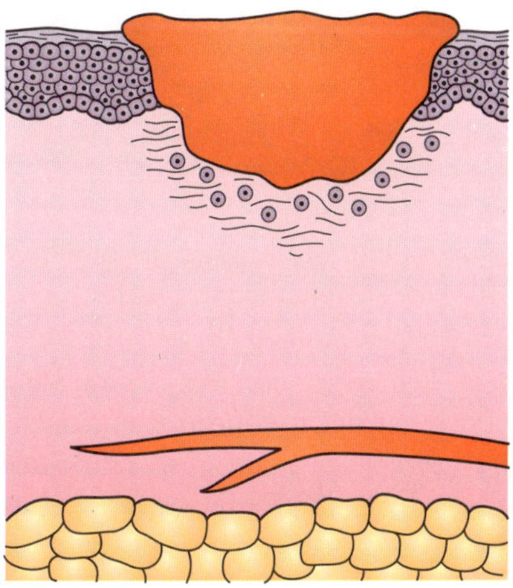

Fig.4.7: Cavity fills with blood and fibrin clot at the junction of living tissue

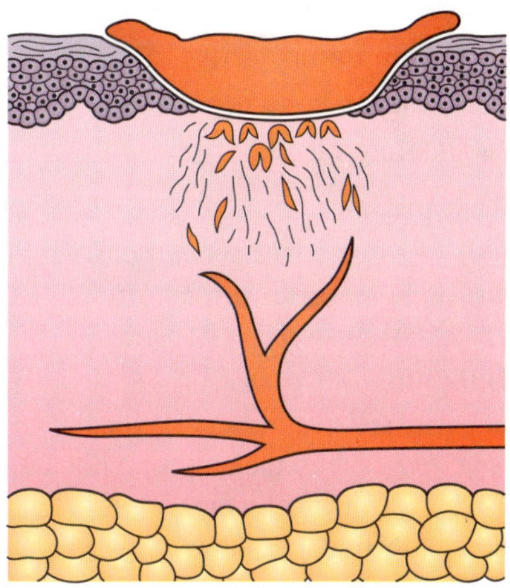

Fig.4.8: Contraction of wound size, mitotic activity in epithelium, new capillary loops macrophages, neutrophils, and fibroblasts.

Healing by third intention (delayed primary closure)

A primary closure technique is used where temporarily left open wound to be closed on later day (4-7 days).

Complications of wound healing

1. **Contracture:** This is permanent; or crippling deformity due to severe contraction of the scar and a common occurrence following extensive burns.

2. **Occasional complications**

   A. **Exuberant granulation:** Pyogenic granuloma is an overgrowth of granulation tissue extending through a breach in the overlying epithelium and forming a little mass, usually a centimetre or less in diameter.

   B. **Keloid:** Synthesis of excessive amounts of collagen in wound healing results in formation of abnormal nodular masses of collagen (keloids) at the site of skin injury. Keloids are most common in wounds of the neck, deltoid region and upper part of chest.

   Microscopic examination shows excessive collagen as thick hyalinised bands.

C. **Fibrosis**

   1. In case of hollow viscera, cicatrisation leads to formation of stricture, e.g., stenosis of oesophagus.
   2. Healing of valves in rheumatic valvulitis by fibrous tissue may produce harmful effects.
   3. Healing by fibrosis gives rise to stricture of urethra.
   4. **Neoplasia:** Rarely scar may be the site for the development of carcinoma later, e.g., squamous cell carcinoma in marjolin ulcer.

HEALING OF FRACTURE

Events following a fracture are:

There are three major phases of fracture healing and five histologic stages of fracture healing.

1. Reactive phase:
   i. Fracture and inflammatory phase
   ii. Granulation tissue formation.
2. Reparative phase
   i. Callus formation
   ii. Lamellar bone deposition.
3. Remodeling phase.

1. Reactive phase

Stage I. (A) Fracture: When bone gets fractured there is rupture of intraosseous blood vessels. Endosteum and preosteum striped off with laceration of soft tissue surrounding it. Fusiform haematoma comes to surround ends of fragments.

(B) Inflammatory phase: There is aseptic inflammation. Secondary necrosis is possible due to tearing of periosteal vessels and Haversian vessels. There is swelling due to collection of exudates and haematoma. Invaded by the polymorphonuclear leukocytes, macrophages, (also responding to cytokines), which phagocytise debris, blood clot, cells, and damaged matrix. There is decalcification of bone adjacent to fracture, along with enzymatic digestion of soft tissues.

Stage II. Granulation tissue formation: Within 24-48 hours proliferating fibroblasts and capillary sprouts grow into blood clot in injured area, forming granulation tissue, in response to cytokines released by tissue damage.

2. Reparative stage

Stage III. Callus formation: The term callus (derived from Latin *callus* for hardskin) is most appropriately applied to the hard-calcified granulation tissue uniting the fractured bone. A provisional callus is fully formed within 2 to 3 weeks and consists of three parts. Granulation tissue becomes denser and cartilage is formed from primitive mesenchymal cells or demodulation of other cells. Callus temporarily binds and stabilises bone.

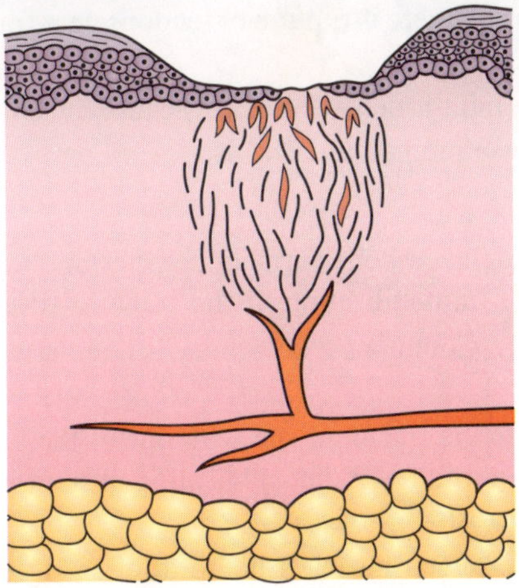

1 week approximately   Surface debris has been shed

Fig.4.9: Loose connective tissue formed by fibroblast
Granulation tissue at the base of the wound

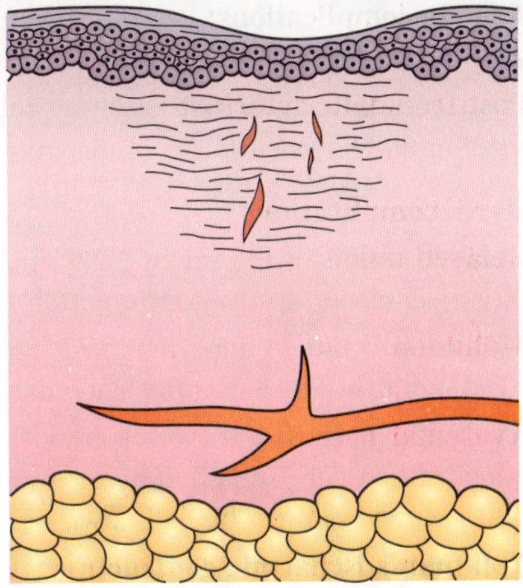

Fig.4.10: Collagen arranged transverly.
Capillaries less prominent

Stage IV. Lamellar bone formation: Provisional callus is transformed into fully formed bone. Structure of newly formed bone is remoulded to suit mechanical stresses and strains and pressure.

Stage V. Remodeling phase: Uneven or protruding surfaces are gradually removed and heal bone; especially in young individuals assume its normal contour remodeling (months to years).

COMPLICATION OF FRACTURE HEALING

General complications

1. Fat embolism may occur in fractures of long bones due to entry of fat from the marrow cavity into the torn ends of veins.
2. Shock
3. Venous thrombosis
4. Tetanus.

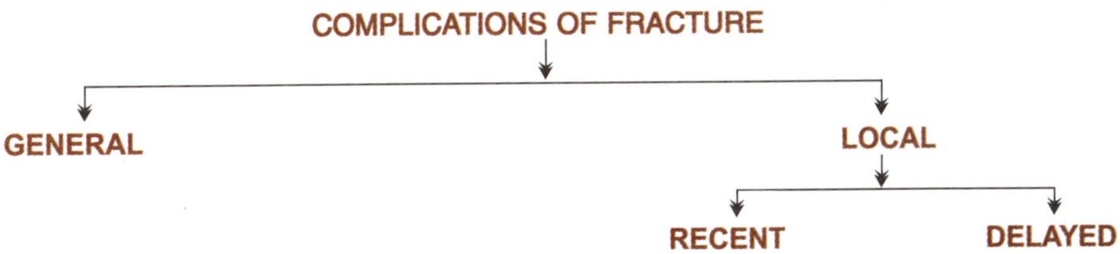

LOCAL COMPLICATIONS

I. Recent complications

1. **Infection:** If underlying skin is breached in any way, i.e., the fracture is compound; the risk of infection is greatly increased.
2. **Neurovascular injuries:** Injury to neighbouring joint causes joint stiffness. Gangrene and ischaemic contracture of muscles is due to injury to blood vessels by fractured bone.
3. **Muscle complications:** Torn muscles may adhere to other sites, leading to stiffness of joints. There is diffuse atrophy of muscles.

4. **Tendon complications:** Patients develop tendinitis and there is rupture of tendons near fracture site.
5. **Post-traumatic arthritis:** Fractures into the joints (intra-articular fractures) cause the bones to meet at an abnormal angle in the joints. It can cause premature arthritis.

II. Delayed complications

1. **Delayed union** of the fracture site may be due to delayed bone formation either due to poor blood supply or suspended infection or inadequate immobilisation of the fracture site.
2. **Malunion** is due to imperfect position of bone ends. Commonest deformity is angulation and overlapping with shortening and malunion.
3. **Avascular necrosis:** If there is poor blood supply to the fractured site with one of the broken bones not properly supplied by the blood, the bony portion will die and healing of the fracture will not take place. This is known as avascular necrosis of bone.
4. **Volkman's ischaemic contracture:** Ischaemia of skeletal muscle (due to arterial or venous obstruction) leads to Volkman's ischemic contractures.
5. **Post-traumatic ossification:** In children and young adults in whom periosteum is loosely attached to bone.

Pathological fracture: When the break occurs at the site of preexisting disease of bone, the term *'pathological fracture'* is applied.

CHAPTER

5

DENTAL CARIES

INTRODUCTION

'Caries' is Latin for ***'rot'*** or ***'rotten'***. Dental caries is the term used to describe rotten teeth or tooth decay, which results in cavities or holes in the teeth.

Definition: Dental caries is defined as chronic, irreversible disease of the hard structures of teeth characterised by demineralisation of inorganic components of teeth and dissolution of organic substance of microbial etiology.

Epidemiology

Worldwide, most children and an estimated ninety percent of adults have experienced caries, with the disease most prevalent in Asian and Latin American countries and least prevalent in African countries. In United States, dental caries is the most common childhood disease.

Dental caries is an important dental public health problem and it is the most prevalent oral disease in the world. The prevalence of dental caries is of great interest for long and is a principal subject of many epidemiological researches carried out in our country and abroad. In India, prevalence of dental caries is reported to be 50% to 60%.

This disease not only causes damage to the teeth, but is also responsible for several morbid conditions of the oral cavity and other systems of the body.

Caries is a result of bacterial growth in unhygienic oral cavity, leading to acid production. Acids eat away the enamel and cavities are formed.

Plaque formation: Microorganisms breed in the oral cavity in the food debris and produce acids by fermentation. The acids thus produced are lactic acid, propionic acid, and acetic acid. The bacteria and acids they form become part of the sticky deposit – called dental plaque—that clings to the surface of the teeth.

In addition to the bacteria, plaque is composed of saliva and food particles. The texture of the plaque is slightly rough and particularly noticeable on the surfaces of back teeth. Plaque adheres most strongly in pits and grooves (fissures) of the molars and premolars, in the areas just above the gum line, between teeth and at the margins of fillings.

Stages of tooth decay

Stage I. Pellicle: A pellicle or coating on the teeth starts to form as soon as you put down your toothbrush. The coating contains proteins from the saliva and 'hosts' bacteria, which attach to the pellicle. This is the beginning of the plaque.

Stage II. Plaque formation: Plaque is also known as biofilm. Plaque appears as soft, gooey substance that sticks to the teeth. It is, in fact colonies of bacteria, protozoa, mycoplasma, yeasts and viruses—clumping together in a gel-like organic material. Also in the mix are bacteria byproducts, white blood cells, food debris, and body tissue.

Stage III. Demineralization: The first indication of tooth decay is white spot on the enamel caused by the loss of calcium. Acids bring about demineralisation of the enamel. Caries appears as black spot or cavity in the tooth. The destruction of the enamel begins as bacteria proliferate in the food and debris are trapped in one of the pits or fissures in the enamel or in a plaque in which the bacteria are attached to the smooth surface by a glycoprotein matrix. At this stage the tooth can remineralise and fix the weakened area itself with the help of minerals in saliva and fluoride.

Stage IV. Enamel involvement: If the demineralisation process outruns the natural mineralisation process, the lesion grows. Over time, the tooth enamel begins to break down beneath the surface while the surface remains intact. Once the decay continues and breaks through the surface of the enamel, the damage is permanent.

Stage V. Dentin involvement: Once the enamel is penetrated, the underlying softer dentin becomes vulnerable. The dentin contains tiny canals leading to the pulp at the core of the tooth. When enough of the sub-surface enamel is eaten away, the surface collapses, forming a cavity. The decay must be cleaned out and the cavity filled by a dentist.

Stage VI. Pulp involvement: If bacteria reach the sensitive pulp, the pulp becomes inflamed. Blood vessels within the pulp swell and, because there's no room within the rigid tooth to expand, patient experiences the pain.

Stage VII. Abscess formation: White blood cells collect at the site to counteract bacterial invasion from the tooth into the surrounding tissues. This kind of bacterial infection may result in a tooth abscess. The tooth pain is consistent, especially during night.

Caries is most frequent in the molars, then the bicuspids then upper incisors but rarely involves the lower incisors.

Causes of dental caries

Dental caries is outcome of a multiple complex process involving factors like diet, microorganisms, trace elements, saliva, genetic predisposition, and tooth morphology. Apart from these, many related factors like individual, social, environmental and cultural factors are also responsible.

Tooth decay is the result of three interacting factors: Bacteria growth, dietary sugars, and vulnerable tooth surface:

1. Tooth surface
2. Caries causing bacteria
3. Fermentable carbohydrate.

The process by which the three factors interact is described:

1. **Tooth surface:** There are certain diseases and disorders affecting teeth, which may leave an individual at a greater risk for caries.

   Amelogenesis imperfecta is a disease in which the enamel does not fully form or forms in insufficient amounts and can fall off a tooth.

2. **Caries causing bacteria:** Streptococcus mutans, Lactobacillus acidophilus, Actinomyces viscosus, and Nocardia are most closely associated with caries, particularly root caries. Streptococcus mutants and lactobacillus are acidogenic and aciduric—meaning that they can produce acids, which can dissolve the tooth substance, and that they survive and produce acids in a low pH environment. Compared to other oral flora, Streptococcus mutans and lactobacillus are cariogenic and have enzymes with greater resistance to acids.

3. **Fermentable carbohydrate:** Carbohydrates (sugar and starches) increases the risk of tooth decay. Sticky foods are more harmful then non-sticky foods because they remain on the surface of the teeth. Sugars such as glucose, fructose, maltose and lactose are found in all carbohydrate foods—these sugars are more destructive than maltose.

Acidic pH: After having a meal, snack or drink, the bacteria of the dental plaque start to convert sugar and carbohydrates of food into acids. The normal pH of 6.2 to 7.0 starts to drop to acidic values.

If the mouth environment becomes too acidic (pH below 5.5-6) the acids start to dissolve the minerals (calcium and phosphates) of the tooth's surface creating microscopic lesions or tooth enamel (demineralisation), which weakens its structures.

Risk factors

1. Poor dental hygiene
2. Low fluoride exposure: Fluoride works primarily via topical mechanisms, which include:
   a. Inhibition of demineralisation at the crystal surfaces inside the tooth.
   b. Enhancement of remineralisation at the crystal surfaces.
   c. Inhibition of bacterial enzymes.

Fluorides in drinking water and in fluoride containing products reduce tooth decay via these mechanisms.

3. Acidic food and drinks
4. Defects of the tooth.

4. **Reduced saliva production:** Reduced saliva is associated with increased caries since the buffering capability of saliva is not present to counter-balance the acidic environment created by certain foods. As a result, medical conditions that reduce the amount of saliva produced by salivary glands—particularly submandibular gland and parotid gland—are likely to lead to widespread tooth decay. Examples include Sjogren's syndrome, diabetes insipidus, and sarcoidosis.
5. **Recession of the gums:** Gum recession occurs because of periodontal disease and lack of good oral hygiene. In addition, the periodontal conditions result in layers of plaque composed of food particles, bacteria and saliva. Plaque gives rise to inflammation, swelling, pain, and bleeding. This further progresses to tooth decay.
6. **Excessive dental fillings:** Fractured or weakend fillings may allow for bacterial infiltration.
7. **Pregnancy:** Excessive intake of carbohydrates in pregnant women causes dental caries.
8. **Psychological stress:** Recently, it has been suggested by several authors that psychologic stress might be a factor in cariogenesis.

Clinical features

Dental caries shows some relation to the arches regarding prevalence pattern and the mandibular arch is affected more often than the maxillary arch. On comparing caries in relation to right and left side of the oral cavity it is evident that dental caries occurs predominantly as a bilateral phenomenon:

(i) Initially caries remains asymptomatic.

(ii) Lodging of food particles between teeth is often a common complaint and, if oral hygiene is not maintained, may lead to cavity formation.

(iii) When caries/cavity reaches the dentin, the individual would complain of sensitiveness to hot and cold food substances resulting in pain.

(iv) Toothache: Painful and tender tooth is a late symptom of an untreated tooth cavity. Toothache may also be caused by an infection, injury, or the absence of a tooth.

(v) Jaw pain may also occur as a result of dental cavity as the nerve supply of a tooth follows a path around or near the jaw.

(vi) Tenderness upon pressure and air entering through mouth breathing.

(vii) Halitosis.

(viii) Bleeding.

Classification of dental caries

Generally there are three types of caries when separated by location:

1. Smooth-surface caries
   - i. Proximal
   - ii. Buccal or lingual surface.
2. Pit and fissure caries
   - i. Occlusal
   - ii. Buccal and lingual caries.
3. Root caries.

G. V. Black classification

1. Pit and fissure caries (Class I caries).
2. Smooth surface caries – Class II, Class III, Class IV, Class V and Class VI.

Dental caries are classified depending on the onset of the process:

1. Acute dental caries
2. Chronic dental caries.

Primary caries

Secondary caries

Acute dental caries

Nursing bottle caries

It is also called baby bottle decay, baby bottle syndrome, and bottle mouth syndrome.

Baby bottle decay is a dental problem that frequently develops in infants that are put to bed with a bottle containing a sweet liquid. Bottles containing such liquids as milk, fruit juices, sweetened drink mixes, and sugar water continuously bathe the infant's mouth with sugar during naps or at night. The bacteria in the mouth use this sugar to produce acid that destroys the child's teeth.

It usually affects children between the ages of 1 and 2 years. Breastfed infants who fall asleep while breastfeeding are also at risk. The upper front teeth (primary maxillary incisors) are typically the ones most severely damaged. The primary first molars are second in frequency. The most remarkable finding is that the mandibular incisors are seldom involved. This is thought to be related to the protective effect of the tongue during sucking.

Symptoms of nursing caries include

- White spots on the teeth
- Early development of cavities (brown areas on the tooth that lead to tooth destruction).

I. Pit and fissure caries

Pit and fissures are anatomic landmarks on a tooth where the enamel folds inward. The occlusal surfaces of teeth forms 12.5% of all tooth surfaces but are the location of all dental caries.

Among children, pit and fissure caries represent 90% of all dental caries.

Fissures are mostly located on the occlusal (chewing) surfaces of posterior teeth and palatal surfaces of maxillary teeth. Pit and fissure caries appears as a conical-lesion, with the base of the cone at the dentinoenamel junction. Pit and fissure caries infects more dentin than smooth surface. As the decay progresses, caries in enamel nearest the surface of the tooth spreads gradually deeper. Once the caries reaches the dentin at the dentinoenamel junction, the decay quickly spreads laterally. Within the dentin, the decay follows a triangle pattern that points to the tooth's pulp.

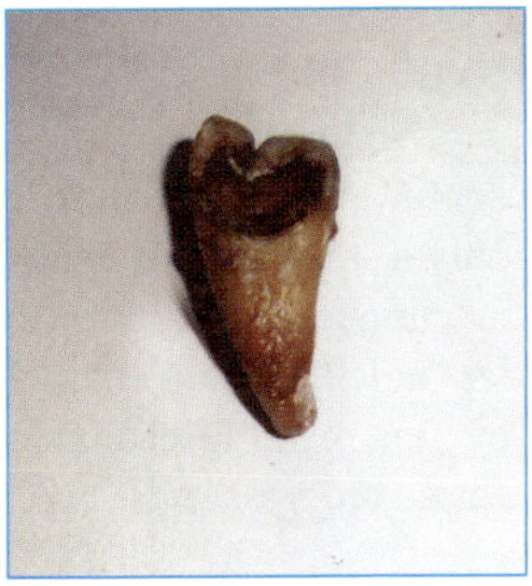

Fig.5.1: Caries tooth

II. Occlusal caries

Occlusal caries is observed radiographically only after the decay process has penetrated the enamel fissures to the dentoenamel junction. Here the caries spreads and, on a radiograph, shows a radiolucent line at the dentinoenamel junction.

III. Recurrent caries is that which recurs in a previously treated restored tooth. The caries may occur under a restoration or along its margins. As the recurrent caries progresses closer to the pulp, a layer of secondary dentin may sometimes form to protect the pulp from the carious lesion.

Radiographically, recurrent caries produces a diffuse radiolucency.

IV. Smooth-surface caries

There are three types of smooth-surface caries:

Type I: Proximal caries, also called interproximal caries, form on the smooth surfaces between adjacent teeth.

Type II: Root caries form on the root surfaces of teeth.

Type III: The third type of smooth surface caries occurs on any other smooth tooth surface. Smooth surface caries appears as a conical–lesion, with the base of the cone at the dentinoenamel junction.

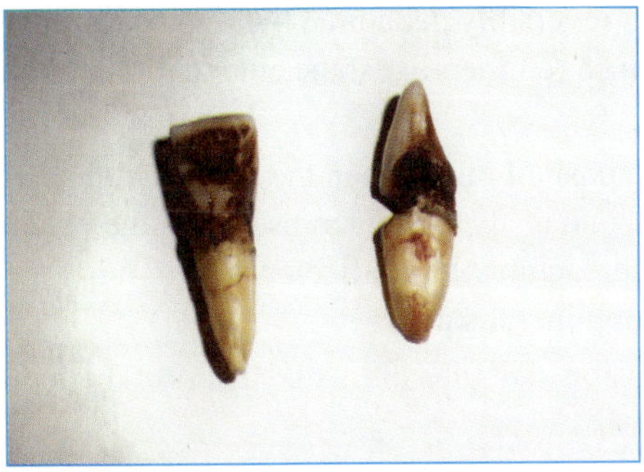

Fig.5.2: Showing caries teeth

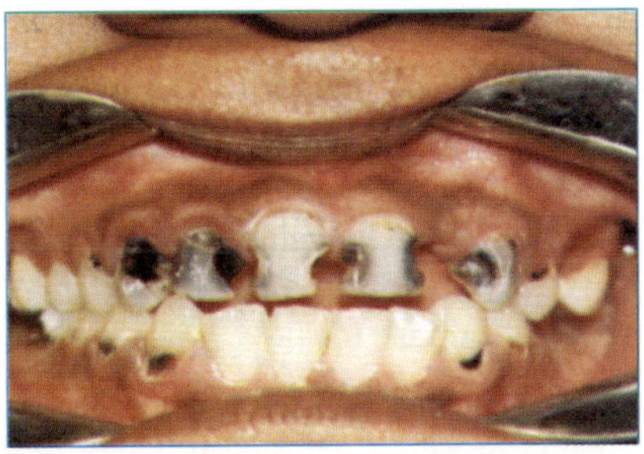

Fig.5.3: A set of teeth showing dental caries. The cavity is formed in between the upper incisors and on the teeth close to the gum as well as near the lower end of the crown.

Caries on tooth's surface that are nearest the cheeks or lips are called ***'facial caries'***.

Caries on surfaces facing the tongue are called ***'lingual caries'***.

Facial and lingual palatal caries originate in pits and grooves on the facial and lingual surfaces. Its shape is round, oval or semilunar, and depends on its location and degree of extension.

The lesions of smooth surface caries are cone-shaped. On smooth surfaces, enamel of decalcification produces cone-shaped lesions, the tip pointing at the dentinoenamel junction and the wide end facing the external surface. Since most of enamel rods are oriented perpendicular to the external surface and destruction of the rods follow them, the lesion's long axis is also perpendicular to the tooth surface.

Histopathology of dental caries

Depending on which hard tissues are affected, it is possible to describe caries as involving enamel, dentin, and cementum. Thus, caries are classified histologically into enamel caries, dentin caries, and cementum caries.

Dentin caries

Eventually the cone shaped lesion contacts dentin along the dentin enamel junction. At first only a small spot of dentin is exposed to the action of carious microorganisms. Because the dentin is less calcified than enamel (70%) and is perforated by innumerable channels (dentin tubules) dentin caries progress more rapidly than enamel caries.

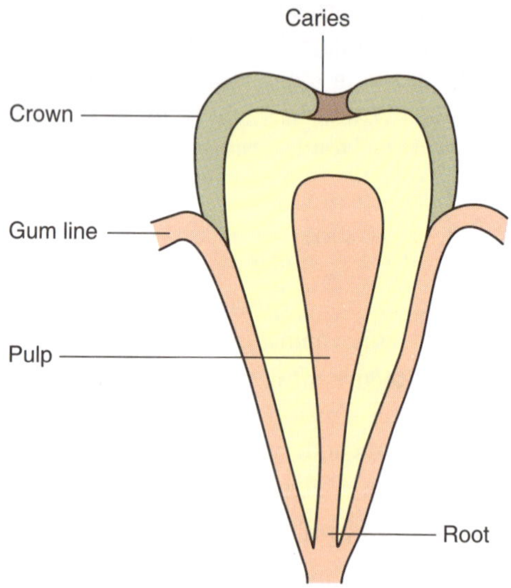

Fig.5.4: Diagrammatic representation of Enamel caries

Microscopically

While enamel is still intact, the lesion is darker than the surrounding unaffected enamel. The lines of Retzius are much more conspicuous than in surrounding enamel. Increased lines on individual enamel rods are also affected, a change indicating that rod dissolution is not far away.

Zones of dentin caries

Zone 1. Sub-transparent dentin: Inner carious dentin is characterised by increasing levels of minerals, as compared to outer carious dentin. Bacterial acids have dissolved minerals and collagen to some extent. The acid affects the dentin prior to bacterial invasion and bacteria are much less frequent in this layer. The dentinal structures with odontoblasts in tubules and the narrowing of the tubules prevent bacterial invasion. The collagen has been partly and reversibly denatured but retains its cross-banded structure. In the inner carious dentin the collagen can be remineralise if the outer carious dentin is removed.

Zone 2. Transparent dentin: The odontoblasts have deposited minerals in the lumen of the denticles tubules and a transparent zone is often present. This zone is also demineralised to some extent. It this zone, mineral content and hardness increases when approaching the unaffected dentin. It is softer than normal dentin. No bacteria present. In is capable of remineralisation.

Zone 3. Turbid zone: This is the zone of bacterial invasion. Tubules are with bacteria. The tooth is non-capable of remineralisation. Tooth must be removed.

Zone 4. Outer carious dentin: Decomposed dentin filled with bacteria. It is the most superficial part of the caries lesion facing the oral cavity. Bacterial acids have completely demineralised the tissue and the collagen is necrotic. This is soft decalcified and intensive and contains bacteria. The border to the layers—the inner carious dentin—is often irregular.

Enamel caries

Zones of enamel caries

Zone 1. Translucent zone: It is not always present. It is more porous than the normal enamel. These pores are larger than the normal enamel. Pore volume is 1% as compared with 0.1% in normal enamel. Chemical analysis shows that there is fall in the magnesium and carbonate content as compared to the normal enamel.

Zone 2. Dark zone: This zone contains pores 2-4% by volume. Some pores are large and some are smaller than the translucent zone suggesting that some mineralisation has occurred. In rapidly advancing lesion the dark zone is narrow. It is also known as positive zone because it is always present.

Zone 3. Body of lesion: This zone has pore volume of 5 to 25%. It contains appatite crystals larger than the normal enamel. This is more of an effort for the remineralisation but by further dissolution of the mineral. Thus this is the zone of maximum demineralisation.

Zone 4. Surface zone: This is about 40 micrometer thick. This part is relatively normal because in this area there is maximum remineralization from the inorganic component of both the plaque and saliva.

Cementum caries (root caries)

Root caries are the third most common type of caries and usually occur when the root surfaces have been exposed due to gingival recession. Root caries are most likely to be found on facial surfaces, then the interproximal sufaces, then the lingual surfaces. Mandibular molars are the most common location to find root caries, followed by mandibular premolars, maxillary posteriors, and mandibular anteriors.

The term cementum caries may be used to describe the decay on roots of teeth, very rarely does caries affect the cementum alone. Roots have a very thin layer of cementum over a large layer of dentin, and, thus, most caries affecting cementum also affect dentin.

Cementum caries progresses along Sharpey's fibres, the laminated appearance begins to disappear, and the surface of the cementum gets destroyed.

The on-going, caries process can eventually lead to a breakdown of the intact layer and then bacterial invasion occurs through the dentinal tubules. In such carious teeth several layers can be distinguished.

First layer: The layer containing bacteria is soft and contains little mineral.

Second layer: Second layer in pulpal direction still has an intact collagen structure but in a state of demineralisation.

Third layer: The third layer is that of sclerotic dentin—characterised by higher mineral content and a greater hardness than the original sound dentin.

Root caries or cemental caries on radiograph produces a saucer shaped (scooped out) appearance.

Rampant caries

Rampant caries may be seen in individuals with xerostomia, poor oral hygiene, stimulant use and large sugar intake.

Rampant caries signifies advanced or severe decay on multiple surfaces of many teeth.

If rampant caries is a result of previous radiation to the head and neck, it may be described as radiation-induced caries.

Complications of dental caries

1. **Pulpitis:** Inflammation of dental pulp is known as pulpitis. It results from invasion by the oral bacteria involved in dental caries. Acute or chronic pulpitis—if untreated—results in complete necrosis of the dental enamel.
2. **Periapical abscess:** A cavity filled with pus forms at the apex of the tooth and is surrounded by acute inflammation. Occasionally a peripheral abscess causes osteomyelitis, sinusitis, or fistula leading to the gingival mucosa.
3. Open pulpitis.
4. Closed pulpitis.
5. Apical periodontal infection.
6. Chronic peri-apical odontitis.
7. **Periapical granuloma:** The bone at the apex of the tooth is slowly reabsorbed and replaced by granulation tissue, forming a spheroidal lesion 2 to 5 mm across. Alpha-1 antitrypsin, alpha-2 macroglobulin, C reactive protein, complement concentrations and oxidase activity of cerulosplasmin are elevated in chronic periapical granuloma.

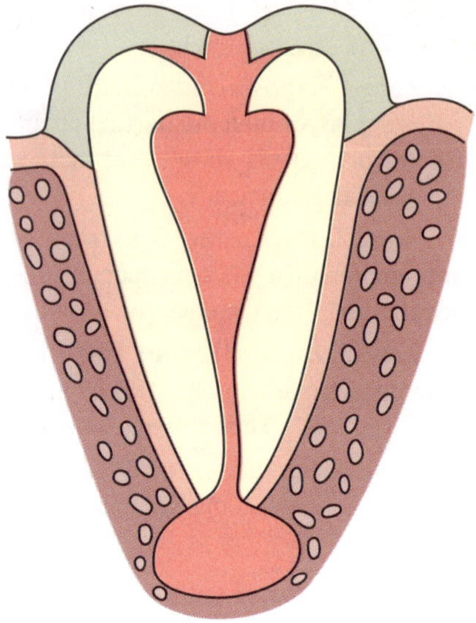

Fig.5.5: A tooth abscess occurs when Bacteria enter through a decayed area and spread inward. Infecting the pulp, root and even the bone surrounding the tooth

Microscopically: Periapical granuloma consists of proliferating mass of chronic inflammatory tissue within a fibrous capsule that is an extension of the periodontal ligament. Granuloma shows heavy infiltration by monocyte/macrophages, lymphocytes and plasma cells.

4. Fractured tooth.

Prevention

Caries remains a major public health problem. Extensive damage from caries can lead to major problems for the individual affecting quality of life—both functionally and esthetically. Hence, preventing caries is an important element in public health:

1. **Oral hygiene:** Oral hygiene is necessary to prevent cavities. This consists of regular professional cleaning (every six months), brushing at least twice a day, and flossing at least daily. The primary focus of brushing and flossing is to remove and prevent the formation of plaque.
2. **Fluoride:** Fluoride is often recommended to protect against dental caries. Topical fluoride is also recommended to protect the surface of the teeth. This may include fluoride toothpaste or mouthwash.
3. **Fissure sealant:** Fissure sealants are used on occlusal surfaces of the teeth. Occlusal surface have fissures that make tooth cleaning difficult and allow caries to start. The method involves applying a thin, very fluid, plastic material directly to the fissures. To retain the material to the tooth, its surface is pretreated with an acid that creates small pores in the enamel. The material fills the pores and, thereby, mechanically bonds to the tooth surface, creating a smooth and even surface.

Diet: Avoid chewy, sticky, sugary foods, particularly as snacks. Foods such as candy-coated nuts, dry cereal, doughy bread, raisins and dry fruit clinging to the teeth. When person eats them advise to brush teeth within 20 minutes afterwards. Acid production by the bacteria that promote tooth decay is most active after this time.

Bibliography

Dental caries: *Mayo Clinic Family Health Book* Scott C Litin, Editor in chief. 3rd edition. 2003

Pandit Kusuk, Kannan AT, Sarna A, and Agrawal K: *Prevalence of Dental Caries and Associated Teeth Cleaning Habits Among Children in Four Primary Schools*. 1986 International Journal of Epidemiology Volume 15(4) page 581-583

Saravanan, S Mandivanan I, Subashini B, Felix JW, *Prevalence Pattern of Dental Caries in Primary Dentition Among School Children*. Indian, Journal Dental Search (2005) Volume 16 (4) page 140-6.

CHAPTER

6

DISEASES OF PULP AND PERIAPICAL TISSUES

PULPITIS

Definition: Inflammation of dental pulp, known as pulpitis, result from invasion by the oral bacteria involved in dental caries trauma, or multiple restoration.

Classification

There are two forms of pulpitis: Acute and chronic.

It may be partial or total, open or closed, and exudative or suppurative.

Pulpitis can also be classified as reversible or irreversible.

Reversible pulpitis is caused by caries encroaching on the pulp and manifests itself as mild inflammation of the pulp. It does not have to be treated, as it will heal on its own over time.

Generalised pulpitis: If most of the pulp is diseased than the term total or generalised pulpitis has been used.

Focal reversible pulpitis: It is also known as pulp hyperaemia. Caries, cracks, restorative procedures or trauma may cause a pulp to become inflamed. The patient's chief complaint is usually of an exaggerated response to thermal stimulus but once the stimulus is removed, the discomfort does not linger.

Irreversible pulpitis is caused by the progression of reversible pulpitis and manifests itself as severe inflammation of the pulp. The available treatment for irreversible pulpitis is either endodontic (root canal) treatment or tooth extraction.

Causes of pulpitis

- **Dental caries:** The bacterial action can increase pressure within the tissues of tooth decay that has penetrated through the enamel and dentin layers of the tooth. This rise in tissue pressure causes pain.
- **Traumatic exposure:** Trauma to the tooth caused by forces from grinding, clenching, and/or injury to the tooth cause pulpitis. Trauma resulting in crown fracture and pulp exposure creates an avenue

for bacterial pulpal death. Concussive force from blunt trauma can result in pulpal inflammation and death of the pulp tissue without the bacterial influx seen with pulp exposure

- Marginal leakage
- Cracked tooth
- Coronal fracture
- Attrition
- Abrasion
- **Traumatic restoration procedure:** Effects of cavity preparation and restorative materials may further complicate pulpitis caused by caries or other causes. Cavity preparations, speed, and coolant may cause pulp irritation.
- Invaginated odontome
- Advanced periodontitis (advanced periodontal-endodontic lesion)
- **Barotrauma:** Flying at high altitude in unpressurised aircraft, or rapid decompression of divers cause pulpitis. Pulpitis is attributed to formation of nitrogen bubbles in pulp tissue or vessels.

ACUTE PULPITIS

A common condition affecting a tooth accompanied by severe relentless pain and the acute inflammation associated with it invariably causes pulp death requiring pulp extirpation or tooth extraction.

Clinical features

Signs and symptoms

1. Bitter taste in the mouth
2. Breath odour
3. Persistent aching or throbbing pain in a tooth
4. Sensitivity to sweet, hot, or cold foods, or liquids
5. Pain when chewing: Pain in acute pulpitis, reflects increase in the pressure of the pulp chamber caused by edema, and exudates
6. Swollen lymph nodes in the neck
7. A swollen area of the mouth, face or neck
8. Fever and general malaise.

Complications

I. Infectious sequelae of pulpitis

Apical periodonitis: Acute inflammation of the periapical tissue usually represents an extension of acute pulpal inflammation. The periapical tissues become inflamed and the tooth is usually very tender when used in mastication.

a. Periapical abscess

It is an acute inflammation of the periapical tissue characterized by localized accumulation of pus at the apex of a tooth. Usually, the gum swells near the root of the tooth.

Often various strains of staphylococci and streptococci are causative microorganisms; however, a wide variety of other anerobe microorganisms such as bacteroides, peptococcus, peptostreptococcus, Actinomyces, Eubacterium, and Fusobacterium, are sometimes found.

The body attacks an infection with large number of white blood cells. Pus is the accumulation of these white blood cells, dead tissue and bacteria. Usually, pus from the tooth infection spreads from the root tip through the bone into the soft tissues.

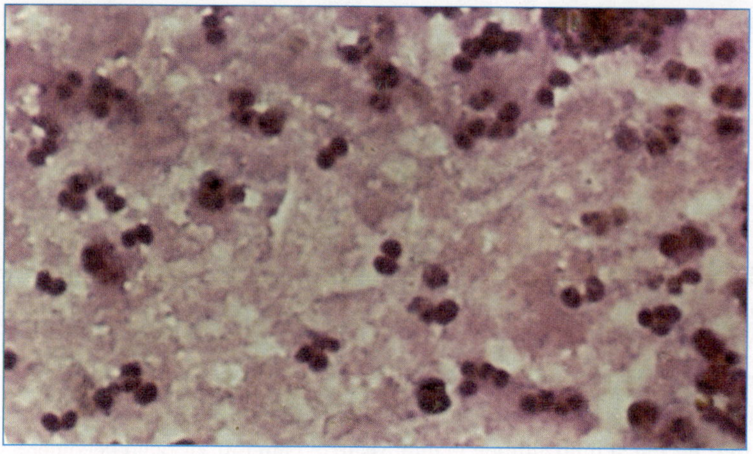

Fig.6.1: Shows necrotic debris, edema fluid and polymorphonuclear leukocytes

A tooth abscess is a complication of tooth decay. It may also result from trauma to the tooth, such as when a tooth is broken or chipped. Opening in the tooth enamel allow bacteria to infect the center of the tooth (pulp).

Clinical features

It is a painful condition that results from an advanced necrotic pulp. In advanced cases the pain is spontaneous, dull, throbbing and persistent; exacerbated by lying down. Tooth is extremely sensitive to percussion. There is horizontal or vertical mobility of tooth or, often, there is hyperocclusion. There is no response to heat. The abscess area is painful, and the surface of the skin over the abscess feels warm and rubbery to palpation and shows fluid-like feel. Aspiration usually produces yellowish pus.

Infection may spread out from the root of the tooth and to the bones supporting the tooth.

If treatment is delayed, the infection may spread directly through adjacent tissues, causing cellulitis, varying degrees of facial edema, and fever.

Management

To treat the periapical abscess we should perform the following in the treatment plan:

- Perform emergency treatment guidelines
- Expose a periapical radiograph of the affected tooth. The abscess will appear as a radiolucency around the apex of the tooth
- Drain the abscess
- If a carious lesion is present, gently excavate the cavity.

Periapical granuloma

Definition: A growing mass of granulation tissue surrounding the apex of a non-vital tooth and arising in response to necrosis of the tooth pulp. Also called apical granuloma, dental granuloma. Periapical granuloma is a common result of pulpitis.

Etiology

It is formed secondary to pulp necrosis of the associated tooth. It may develop following periapical abscess formation or may form as pulpal death which eventuates without abscess precursor.

The principal cause of apical granuloma is the persistence of microorganisms in the root canal system. The microorganisms found in these cases are predominantly Gram-positive (cocci, bacilli and filaments) such as Actinomyces, Enterococcus, and propionibacterium.

Alpha-1 antitrypsin, alpha-2 macroglobulin, C reactive protein, complement concentrations and oxidase activity of ceruloplasmin are elevated in chronic periapical granuloma.

Clinically

Usually it is asymptomatic. The involved tooth is sensitive to percussion and patient feels pain while chewing solid food. Hyperaemia, edema and inflammation of the apical periodontal ligament cause hypersensitivity of tooth. There is tenderness at root apex on palpation.

Microscopically

Periapical granuloma consists of proliferating mass of chronic inflammatory tissue within a fibrous capsule that is an extension of the periodontal ligament. Granuloma is composed of capillaries, inflammatory cells, fibroblasts, collagen and macrophages. Granuloma shows heavy infiltration by monocyte/macrophages, lymphocytes and plasma cells. The more numerous cells are plasma cells, usually in cellular region of granulation tissue where they are tightly pressed.

There is accumulation of cholesterol in the tissues. It appears as needle-like spaces or clefts. Cholesterol crystals may accumulate in periapical granulomas and are almost invariably associated with multinucleated giant cells of foreign body type. The incidence of cholesterol crystals in periapical lesions varies between 18 to 44% of all lesions. They are surrounded by macrophages, and multinucleated giant cells.

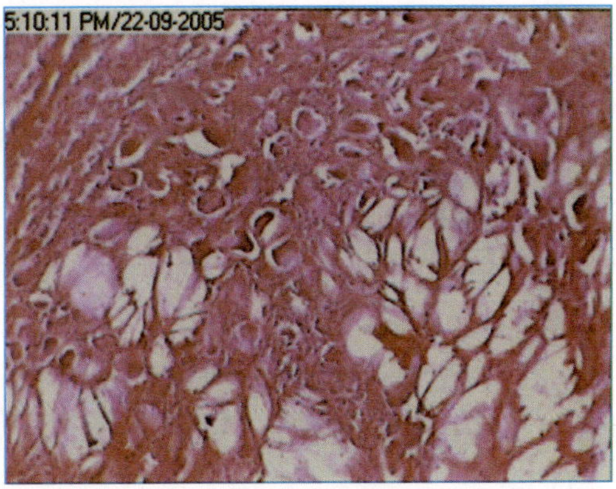

Fig.6.2: Showing cleft-like cholesterol crystals and multinucleated giant cells

In apical granulomas it is common to find nests of epithelium, formed from epithelial cell rests of Malassez, having a latent capacity to proliferate. Epithelial cells are normally arranged in layers forming small islands, strands, and trabecula of varying thickness.

Pulse granulomas: The essential histological features consist of a connective tissue stroma containing variable numbers of inflammatory cells and foreign body giant cells associated with hyaline rings and ovoid fibrillary or amorphous hyaline masses. Oral pulse granuloma is a histological diagnosis for a localised lesion resulting from implantation of food particles of plant origin. It often occurs in the posterior regions of an edentulous mandible in association with a full lower denture but it may also be found in periapical areas of grossly decayed teeth or retained roots and teeth with a history of endodontic therapy, where the root canal has been left open at some stage, associated with impacted lower third molar teeth with a history of pericoronitis or as part of a cyst wall where there has been a communication with oral cavity.

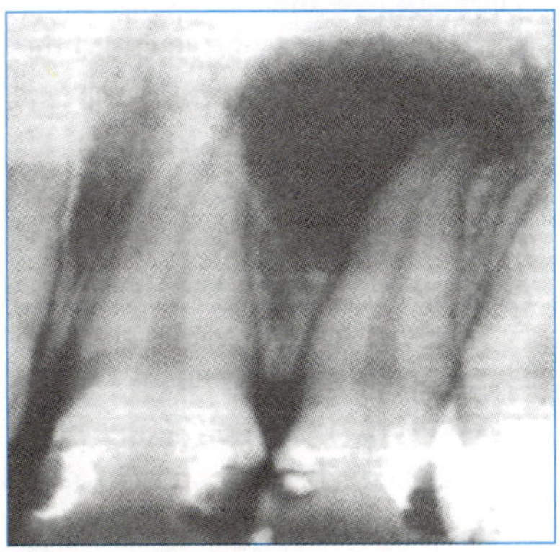

Fig.6.3: Radiograph of upper anterior teeth with large restorations. The upper lateral incisor is non-vital and a radiolucency is present in the bone around the apex of the tooth

More than half of the plasma cells are IgG positive, about 20% IgA positive; up to 10% are IgM, rarely IgE and, sporadically, IgD positive cells. In the vascular walls and their surroundings as well as in the phagocytes fine granular to granular positivities of C3 and C4 components of complement are present. The majority of lymphocytes bleared markers of T lymphocytes of which T suppressor cells are most frequent.

Radiologically

The associated radiolucencies are variable, ranging from small, barely perceptible lesions of the apical lamina. The lesion may be circumscribed or ill-defined and may or may not demonstrate a surrounding radioopaque rim. Root resorption is not uncommon. There is thickening of periodontal ligament at the root apex.

Periapical cyst

Periapical cyst is the most common odontogenic cyst.

A periapical cyst often forms from proliferation of islands of odontogenic epithelium presents within a radicular granuloma. The cystic lesion consists of a fluid-filled cavity that is lined by epithelium. The cyst generally develops from a long-standing periapical granuloma.

Pathogenesis of cysts in three phases:

Phase I: Infection of tooth leads to necrosis of pulp. Toxins exit the apex of the tooth, lead to periapical inflammation. During the first phase, the epithelial cells rests of Malassez begin to proliferate as a direct result of inflammation, and influenced by bacterial antigens, the epidermal growth factors, metabolic and cellular mediators. This inflammation results in the formation of a periapical granuloma that may be infected or sterile. Eventually, this epithelium undergoes necrosis caused by lack of blood supply—the granuloma becomes a cyst.

Phase II: In the second phase, a cavity is formed, lined by the epithelium.

Phase III: The cyst grows, probably by osmosis.

Clinical features

It is common in all ages and most common in third and fourth decades. They are the most common cystic lesions affecting the jaws. They are most commonly found at the apices of the involved teeth, however, they may also be found on the lateral aspects of the roots in relation to lateral accessory root canal.

Clinically, most of the radicular cysts are symptomless. Patient often complains of slowly enlarging swelling. Occasionally, a sinus may lead from the cyst cavity to oral mucosa.

Macroscopically

Most radicular cysts appear as round or pear-shaped, unilocular lucent lesion in periapical region. They are less than 1 cm in diameter and are bordered by a thin rim of cortical bone. Yellow nodules of cholesterol may project into the cavity. The associated tooth usually has a deep restoration or large carious lesion. The cyst displaces adjacent teeth and cause mild root resorption.

Microscopically

The common histological findings are:

1. The cyst is lined by stratified squamous epithelium of an extremely variable thickness depending on the degree of inflammation. Ulceration of epithelium is common. It may show metaplasia, calcification and hyaline body.
2. Surrounding inflammatory granulation tissue shows typical features of periapical granuloma. It shows plump endothelial cells, foamy histiocytes, cholesterol clefts and the pathognomic 'Rushton bodies' composed of RBC surrounded by empty spaces. There are aggregates of cholesterol crystals surrounded by macrophages, multinucleated giant cells and plasma cells.

Cellulitis: The infection may break through cortical bone and spread in various tissue spaces of the head and neck causing cellulitis.

Osteomyelitis: A periapical abscess, if not treated, rapidly extends to the adjacent bone where it produces osteomyelitis. Osteomyelitis of the mandible or maxilla is an uncommon complication of odontogenic disease—usually of periapical infection. Similar to osteomyelitis of other bones, it may become localised or propagate within the jaw bones.

An untreated severe tooth abscess may become large enough to perforate bone and extend into the soft tissue. From there it follows the path of least resistance and may spread either internally or externally.

This may leave a sinus tract (a channel) between a persistent focus of infection and the skin or mouth, which can discharge from time to time.

II. Spread from maxillary teeth may cause

a. Purulent sinusitis spread of infection to the nearby sinus in the face bone

b. Meningitis

c. Brain abscess

d. Orbital cellulitis

e. Cavernous sinus thrombosis.

Once the pus tracks into the soft tissue, further spread is determined by:

(i) Site of bony penetration by pus, and (ii) whether the infection was in the upper or lower jaw.

III. Spread from mandibular teeth may cause

a. Ludwig angina

b. Parapharyngeal abscess

c. Mediastinitis

d. Pericarditis

e. Empyema

f. Jugular thrombophlebitis

CHRONIC PULPITIS

Chronic pulpitis may develop with or without episodes of acute pulpitis or it may occur as a chronic onset from the beginning. It may be the result of persistent mild to moderate irritation of the pulp or it may follow a period of acute pulpitis.

It has been classified as open form and closed form.

Open form of chronic pulpitis: In open form of chronic pulpitis the pulp is cariously exposed and is characterized by the formation of abscess at the point of exposure.

Closed form of chronic pulpitis: The closed form of chronic pulpitis may occur due to trauma, restorative procedure, orthodontic tooth movements or periodontal lesion, but carious lesion is absent.

A common condition affecting a tooth accompanied by dull bearable pain; the chronic inflammation associated with it usually causes pulp death requiring pulp extirpation or tooth extraction. Pain is less intense than acute. Affected teeth do not respond to pulp sensitivity tests. There is tenderness to biting. Chronic pulpitis may either resolve itself or continue with slow destruction of the entire pulp involving also the periapical tissues. Chronic pulpitis may also develop into an acute infection in presence of virulent organisms that have reached the pulp from the mouth.

Microscopically

There is presence of chronic inflammatory cells with multinucleated giant cells. There is increase in vascularity of tissues, proliferation of fibroblast and laying down of collagen fibres in the affected area.

Radiologically

There is widening of periodontal ligament space to a large area of destruction of periapical tissue.

Chronic hyperplastic pulpitis

It is also known as pulp polyp or proliferative pulpitis.

It is an uncommon and specific type of inflammatory hyperplasia that is associated with a non-vital tooth.

Causes

Clinical features

Chronic hyperplastic pulpitis is commonly seen in the teeth of children and young adults. The teeth commonly involved are the deciduous molars and the first permanent molars. The affected tooth exhibits a large carious lesion. The polyp is usually painless but may cause discomfort during mastication due to transmission of pressure to the apical region. The polypoid tissue may bleed easily because of rich vascular supply.

Physical findings

- A spongy, soft tissue nodule exudes from the cavitated or fractured surface of a tooth.
- The surface varies from pink and smooth to red and white and granular.
- Polyps typically enlarge to fill the entire cavitated area to pulp chamber of the tooth.
- Soft tissue may merge with the adjacent attached gingival.
- A pulp polyp is a single lesion but multiple teeth may be affected.
- Polyps usually develop in carious primary molars and first permanent molars because anatomically—in young persons—these teeth have large pulp.
- Teeth with open or incomplete apexification of the root apices are the most susceptible.

Microscopically

Histopathologically, a blood clot, fibrin and inflammatory cells may be present at the pulp surface immediately after traumatic or carious pulp exposure, due to tissue trauma and microbial irritation. If treatment is delayed, the pulp may develop a proliferative (hyperplastic) pulpitis. The surface of the pulp usually shows epithelisation, even parakeratisation, and depends on the age of the polyp. The tissue in the pulp chamber is often transformed into granulation tissue, which projects from the pulp into carious lesion. There may be fibrosis and calcific degeneration in some areas of coronal pulp, whilst the radicular pulp tissue may be healthy or contain few chronic inflammatory cells.

PULP NECROSIS

It is also called gangrenous necrosis of pulp.

Pulp necrosis may follow pulpitis, or trauma to apical blood vessels. There is coagulative necrosis after ischaemia. Liquefaction necrosis after pulpitis may become gangrenous with foul odour upon infection by putrefying bacteria from caries.

Gangrene of the pulp root infrequently is the result of acute inflammation; the over-supply of blood in arteries compresses the veins at the dental foramen, interrupting the circulation so as to cut of all nutrition from this territory, causing death to the pulp in a body. In dry gangrene the pulp becomes a dry and shrivelled mass, or mummified.

Symptoms of pulp necrosis include dull or throbbing pain, no response to heat or cold, and moderate to severe pain on biting.

Treatment

Treatment consists in the removal of all remnants of pulp and perfect disintegration of the root canals before filling.

CHAPTER

7

DISEASES OF PERIODONTIUM

INTRODUCTION

Periodontal diseases are classified into two general groups on the basis of the pathologic processes present:

1. Inflammation (gingivitis and periodontitis)
2. Juvenile periodontitis (gingivosis and periodontitis).

PELLICLE

Certain proteins in saliva (glycoproteins) are absorbed by the surface of the teeth, creating a microscopically thin, clear coating on the teeth called the 'acquired pellicle'. The pellicle starts forming immediately after brushing teeth; within few minutes, teeth feel slippery and moist. The pellicle helps shield the teeth against acid that can cause tooth decay. However, the pellicle also is a prime surface for bacteria and other organisms to collect and lead to the development of plaque.

DENTAL STAINS

Dental stains are classified according to source and location. Stains that develop according to location are either extrinsic or intrinsic.

Stains that develop from a source are known as exogenous and endogenous.

Extrinsic stains occur on the external surfaces of teeth and may be removed by mechanical means such as brushing, scaling, or polishing.

Intrinsic stains occur on the internal surfaces of teeth and may not be removed by mechanical means.

Exogenous tooth stain

Nathoo classification of system of extrinsic dental stain describes 3 categories as follows:

Nathoo type I (N1): N1 type coloured material chromogen binds to the tooth surface. The colour of the chromogen is similar to that of dental stains caused by tea, coffee, wine, chromogenic bacteria, and metals.

Nathoo type II (N2): N2-type coloured material changes colour after binding to the tooth. The stains actually are N1-type food stains that darken with time.

Nathoo type III (N3): N3 type coloured material changes colour after binding to the tooth and undergoes chemical reaction to cause a stain. N3-type stains are caused by carbohydrate-rich foods (apples, potatoes), stannous fluoride, and chlorhexidine.

Tobacco stains from cigarettes, cigars, pipes, and chewing tobacco cause tenacious dark brown and black stains that cover the cervical one-third to one-half of the tooth. Tobacco stains are commonly called **'nicotine stains'** results from combustion of coal tar present in tobacco and also due to penetration of tobacco juices and pigments into the substance of the teeth.

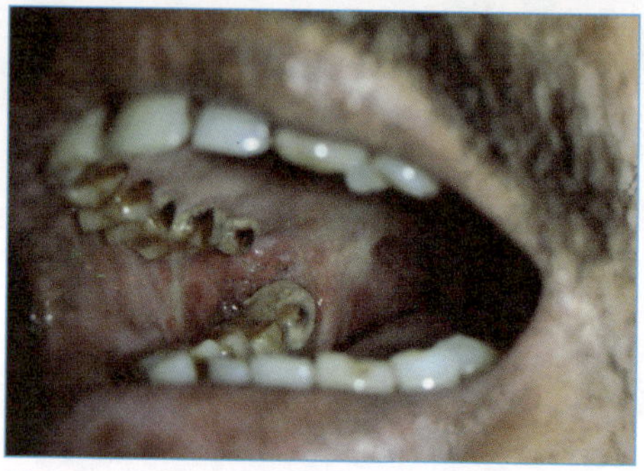

Fig.7.1: Showing black coloured pigment deposition due to betel leaves

Deposition of tannins found in tea, coffee, and their beverages cause brown stains on the outer surfaces of teeth.

Betel leaves (pan), common in Eastern countries discolours teeth dark brown to black colour.

Metallic compounds stains

Metallic compounds are also implicated in dental discolourations because of the metals with dental plaque to produce surface stains. Industrial exposure to iron, manganese, and silver may stain the teeth black. Mercury and lead dust can cause blue green stain. Copper and nickel green-to-blue-green stain.

Chromogenic bacteria produce exogenous stain.

The colour of the stain depends on the type of bacteria involved. Pigmentation in black, green, and orange have been described. These pigments are deposited in the cervical one-third of both the buccal and lingual teeth. The stain is generally observed in youngsters between the ages of 6 and 14 years. Black stain tends to develop only in children who are caries-free. Green and orange stains are associated with caries.

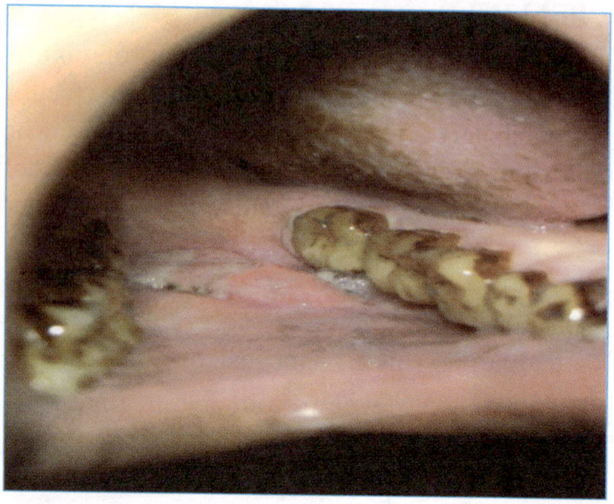

Fig.7.2: Showing orange coloured pigment deposition on teeth

Dental fillings can also be the cause of some types of tooth surface discolouration. Tooth coloured white fillings can change in colour and become darker as time passes. Metal fillings, like amalgam, even if not directly seen, can show through the translucent tooth enamel or even be the cause of staining.

Trauma: Falls and other injuries can produce sizable cracks in the teeth, which collect large amounts of stains and debris.

Fluorosis: In severe form it is characterised by black and brown stain.

CALCULUS

Definition: Tooth calculus or tartar is a hard, yellowish deposit on teeth. It is composed of mineral salts, food and other debris that has hardened over time.

Distribution of calculus

Calculus comes in two forms

1. Supragingival (above the gum line) calculus is the visible deposit that forms on the surface of the teeth.
2. Subgingival (below the gum line): Tartar forms in pockets between teeth and gums. Subgingival calculus is more harmful as it facilitates faster growth of plaque. Sometimes, calculus—normally the subgingival variety—forms from a fluid containing a greater or lesser amount of gingival fluid. This can lead to calculus containing the blood product haem and variety of its breakdown products. This leads to a brown or brown green calculus referred to as *'serumnal calculus'* in recognisation of its source.

Incidence of calculus deposition

Dental calculus is widespread in all groups from teenagers onwards throughout the world. However, the levels of calculus are dependent on the population studied and are affected by a number of factors. Oral hygiene habits, excess of professional care, diet, age, ethnic origin, time since last dental cleaning, systemic disease, and use of prescription medications.

Composition of calculus

There is no fixed composition of dental calculus because the type and amount of calcium phosphate salt which precipitate on to the tooth surface is affected by various factors such as the concentration of calcium and phosphate, the relative amounts of each ion present locally, the pH, the presence of other calcium phosphate mineral.

Calculus comprises a mixture of calcium phosphate minerals such as: brushite, octacalcium phosphate, tricalcium phosphate and biological apatite.

Clinical implications

Calculus forming at the gingival margin whether it is sub-or supragingival will cause inflammation of the gingival (gingivitis), which may progress to periodontal disease. The inflammation is the result of physical irritation of the gingival as well as the presence of bacterial toxic byproducts in the calculus.

GINGIVAL DISEASES

Definition: Gingivitis is an inflammatory process limited to the mucosal epithelial tissue surrounding the cervical portion of the teeth and the alveolar process.

TABLE 7.1
CLASSIFICATION OF GINGIVAL DISEASES

A. Dental plaque induced gingival diseases
1. Gingivitis associated with dental plaque only
2. Gingival diseases modified by systemic factors
   a. Associated with endocrine system
      1. Puberty associated gingivitis
      2. Menstrual cycle associated gingivitis
      3. Pregnancy associated gingivitis
      4. Diabetes mellitus associated gingivitis.

Contd.

Contd.

- b. Associated with blood dyscrasias
  - 1. Leukaemia associated gingivitis
  - 2. Others.
- 3. Gingival diseases modified by medications
  - a. Drug influenced gingival diseases
    - 1. Drug influenced gingival enlargement
    - 2. Drug influenced gingivitis
      - a. Oral contraceptive-associated gingivitis
      - b. Other.
- 4. Gingival diseases modified by malnutrition

B. Non-plaque induced gingival lesions

- 1. Gingival diseases of specific bacterial origin
- 2. Gingival diseases of viral origin
  - A. Herpes virus infections
    - 1. Primary herpetic gingivostomatitis
    - 2. Recurrent oral herpes
    - 3. Varicella zoster infections
    - 4. Other.
- 3. Gingival diseases of fungal origin
  - 1. Candida species infections
  - 2. Linear gingival erythema
  - 3. Histoplasmosis
  - 4. Others
- 4. Gingival lesions of genetic origin
  - 1. Hereditary gingival fibromatosis
  - 2. Other.
- 5. Gingival manifestations of systemic conditions
  - a. Mucocutaneous disorders
    - 1. Lichen planus
    - 2. Pemphigoid
    - 3. Pemphigus
    - 4. Erythema multiforme
    - 5. Lupus erythematosus
    - 6. Drug induced
    - 7. Others
  - b. Allergic reactions
    - 1. Dental restorative materials
    - 2. Reactive attributable to
      - a. Toothpastes/dentifrices
      - b. Mouth rinses/mouth washes
      - c. Chewing gum additives
      - d. Foods and additives
- 6. Traumatic lesions
  - a. Chemical injury
  - b. Physical injury
  - c. Thermal injury

Characteristics of plaque induced gingivitis

- Plaque present at gingival margin
- Disease begins at gingival margin
- Change in gingival colour—reddish or bluish in colour
- Change in gingival contour due to edema or fibrosis
- Sulcular temperature change

- Increased gingival exudates
- Bleeding upon provocation
- Absence of attachment loss
- Absence of bone loss
- Reversible with plaque removal
- Increase bleeding on probing and increased gingival bleeding.

Gingivitis associated with dental plaque only

Gingivitis is an irritation of gums. It is usually caused by bacterial plaque that accumulates in the small gaps between the gums and the teeth and by calculus that forms on the teeth. These accumulations may be tiny, even microscopic, but the bacteria in them produce foreign chemicals and toxins that cause inflammation of the gums around the teeth. This inflammation can, over the years, cause deep pockets between the teeth and gums and loss of bone around teeth—an effect otherwise known as periodontitis.

Gingivitis associated with endocrine system

Pregnancy associated gingivitis

Pregnancy gingivitis is a condition caused by increased hormone levels that can cause swollen red and tender gums. It is often accompanied with bleeding while brushing teeth.

Gingival diseases associated with blood dyscrasias

Leukaemia can cause gingivitis. In fact, gingivitis is the first sign of disease in about 25% of children with leukaemia. An infiltration of leukaemia cells into gums causes gingivitis, and a reduced ability to fight infections worsens it. The gums appear red and bleed easily. Often, the bleeding continues for several minutes and more because blood does not clot normally in people with leukaemia.

Gingival diseases modified by medications

Gingival bleeding may occur with use of anticoagulants and fibrinolytic agents. Phenytoin, oral contraceptive agents, and calcium channel blockers may cause gingival hyperplasia.

Gingivitis has been observed with use of protease inhibitors, vitamin A and analogues, danazol, pentamidine, misoprostol, methotrexate and gold compound. Gingivostomatitis has been observed in exposure to arsenic, gold, bismuth, mercury, nickel, sulphur dioxide, lead, thallium, zinc, methyl violet, and tropical chlorhexidine.

Gingival diseases modified by malnutrition

Plaque accumulation show increased effect in the condition known as scurvy (vitamin C deficiency)

Non-plaque induced gingival diseases

Gingivitis due to infections

Viral infections can cause gingivitis.

Herpetic gingivostomatitis is common, mild, and short-lived and requires no intervention in most adults. In immunocompromised persons, however, reactivation of herpes simplex virus infection is frequent and may be severe.

Acute herpetic gingivitis is a painful viral infection of the gums and other parts of the mouth caused by herpes virus. The infection turns the gums bright red and causes many small white or yellow sores to form inside the mouth.

Hereditary gingival fibromatosis

Gingival fibromatosis presents as a generalised but irregular enlargement of the facial and lingual aspects of the attached and marginal gingival.

Goddard and Gross under the descriptive term, 'fungus excrescence of the gingival' first reported the entity in 1858.

Incidence: Hereditary gingival fibromatosis is rare, affecting only in 750,000 people.

Histology shows mild epithelial hyperplasia and marked interwoven fascicles of dense fibrous tissues. Slender fibroblastic nuclei are scattered throughout the stroma. There is mild chronic inflammatory cell infiltration.

Causes: Hereditary gingival fibromatosis (HGF) is a rare condition that can occur in an isolated disease or as a part of a syndrome or chromosomal abnormality.

Generalised or localised diffuse fibrous overgrowth of the gingival tissue are usually transmitted as an autosomal dominant trait, but some cases are idiopathic and others produced by drugs.

Histological and cell culture studies have uncovered some of the molecular and cellular changes associated with hereditary gingival fibromatosis.

Recent studies about the genetic characteristics of hereditary gingival fibromatosis have provided novel clues about the potential pathogenic mechanisms. In particular, mutation in the son-of sevenless (SOS 1) gene has been associated with one form of disease.

Thus far, GINGF locus has been mapped on chromosome 2, at 2p21, and a second possible locus has mapped to 2p13.

Researchers identified a new locus, GINGF2, on chromosome 5q13-q22 with a maximum two-point lad score of 4.31 at D5S1721.

Traumatic injury

Misaligned teeth, rough edges of fittings, and ill-fitting or unclean mouth appliances (such as braces, dentures, bridges, and crowns) can irritate the gums and increase the risk of gingivitis.

Complications of Gingivitis

1. Recurrence of gingivitis
2. Periodontitis
3. Infection abscess of the gingival or the jaw bones
4. Trench mouth (bacterial infection and ulceration of the gums).

Periodontium consists of gum, and structure that supports the tooth (cement covering the root, fibers of the periodontal membrane and alveolar bone).

Periodontal disease is group of conditions in which inflammation and destruction of the attachment apparatus of the teeth.

GINGIVAL ENLARGEMENT

TABLE 7.2
CLASSIFICATION OF GINGIVAL ENLARGEMENT

- Inflammatory enlargement
- Drug induced enlargement
  - Anticonvulsants such as phenytoin and succinamides
  - Chemical channel blockers such as nifedipine and verapamil
  - Cyclosporin
- Enlargement associated with systemic factors
  - Conditioned enlargement
    - Pregnancy

Contd.

Contd.

- Puberty
- Vitamin C deficiency

- Systemic diseases causing enlargement
  - Leukaemia
  - Granulomatous diseases such as Wegner's granulomatosis
  - Sarcoidosis
  - Neoplasms
    - Benign neoplasms such as fibromas, papillomas, and giant cell granulomas
    - Malignant neoplasms as a carcinoma or malignant melanoma
- False gingival enlargement, such as when there is underlying bony or dental tissue lesion

DILANTIN INDUCED GINGIVAL HYPERPLASIA

Dilantin sodium has been used for the treatment of grandmal and psychomotor epilepsy.

It causes enlargement of gingival.

The incidence varies from 0% to 84.5% and occurs more frequently in young individuals. In most patients it develops 2 to 3 months after the starting of therapy and peaks in severity after 12 to 18 months.

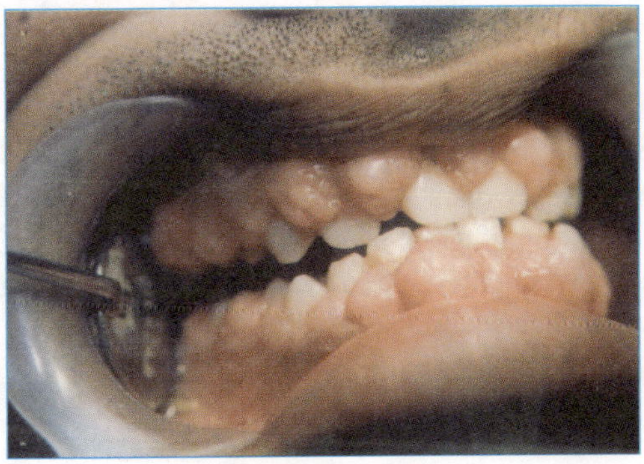

Fig.7.3: Shows enlargement of gum in case of dilantin sodium ingestion

Clinically

Uncomplicated cases of phenytoin induced gingival hyperplasia presents with a hard firm, resilient and intensive gingival with little tendency to bleed. The surface has a normal pink colour, is stippled and has a granular or smooth appearance. If secondary inflammation is present, the tissue may become dark red, odematous, spongy, friable, and ulcerated and bleed easily with gingival enlargement.

GINGIVAL ENLARGEMENT WITH LEUKAEMIA

Gingival hyperplasia is secondary to infiltration of the gingival tissue with leukaemia cells and is well-described in literature. In most extensive review of the topic, gingival hyperplasia was observed in acute myelogenous leukaemia with frequency of 0.5% to 5% among 1,076 patients.

Gingival hyperplasia is most commonly seen with the acute myeloid leukaemia subtypes acute monocytic leukaemia (M5), acute myelomonocytic leukaemia, and acute myelocytic leukaemia.

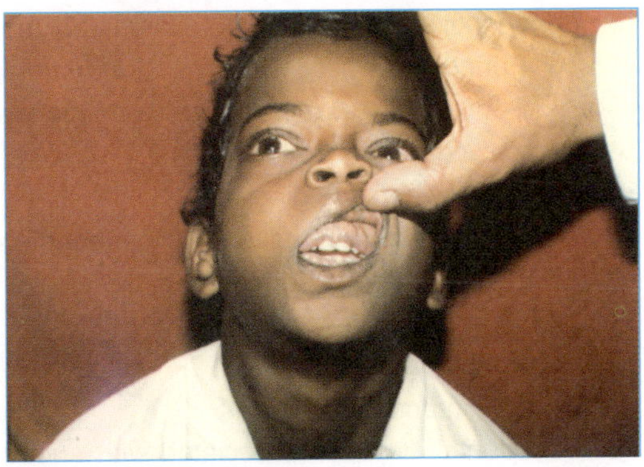

Fig.7.4: Gum hyperplasia in case of acute myeloid leukaemia

Clinically

Gingival enlargement is characterised by progressive enlargement of the interdental papillae as well as the marginal and attached gingival. In the condition's most pronounced form, the crowns of the teeth may be covered. Gingiva appear swollen, devoid of stippling and pale red to deep purple in colour. Mucosal haemorrhages, ulcerative gingivitis, infectious gingivitis and odontolgia may be observed. Pallor, spontaneous haemorrhage, petechiae and ulceration have been described to occur more frequently in acute than chronic leukaemia.

Microscopically

Typically, the lamina propria is densely packed with leukaemic cells extending from the basal layer of epithelium into the gingival. Regional blood vessels are compressed by the infiltrate.

GINGIVAL HYPERPLASIA DURING PREGNANCY (PREGNANCY GRANULOMA)

Pregnancy tumour is a primarily oral disease, which appears in the mouth as an overgrowth of tissue due to irritation, trauma, or hormonal factors.

A pregnancy granuloma is a growth on the gums that occurs in 2% to 10% of pregnant women. It is also known as pyogenic granuloma. They occurs in the 1st trimester of pregnancies, grow until delivery, and regress spontaneously without therapy, but may reappear with subsequent pregnancy.

They are red, purple, and pink nodules, typically found near the upper gum-line but can also be found elsewhere in the mouth. They can be smooth or lobulated. The growths bleed easily and can form an ulcer or crust over. Pregnancy granulomas are attached to the gum or mucus membrane by a stalk of tissue.

HYPERPLASIA ASSOCIATED WITH VITAMIN C DEFICIENCY

Gums are swollen, oedematous, soft, spongy; swelling of gums and gingival interdental papillae followed by gingival haemorrhage. Gums are red, tumid, very sensitive and retracted from the teeth, and subsequently ulcerated along their margins. Gum-line usually has a 'mushy' appearance. Haemorrhages are also seen in other parts of the body.

TABLE 7.3 CLASSIFICATION OF PERIODONTITIS According to American *Academy of Periodontology* (APP)
1. Chronic periodontitis ❖ Localised ❖ Generalised 2. Aggressive periodontitis ❖ Localised ❖ Generalised 3. Periodontitis associated with systemic diseases ❖ Periodontitis associated with haematological disorders ❖ Periodontitis associated with genetic disorders 4. Necrotizing periodontal diseases ❖ Acute ulcerative gingivitis ❖ Acute necrotising ulcerative periodontitis 5. Abscesses of the periodontium ❖ Gingival abscess ❖ Periodontal abscess ❖ Pericoronal abscess 6. Periodontal diseases associated with endodontic lesions

Contd.

Contd.

7. Developmental or acquired deformities and conditions
   - Localised tooth related factors
   - Mucogingival deformities
   - Conditions on edentulous ridges
   - Occlusal trauma
     a. Primary occlusal trauma
     b. Secondary occlusal trauma

Periodontitis associated with systemic diseases

There is increasing evidence that a number of complex diseases are related to opportunistic infections that have their source in periodontal disease. Subsequently, there has been increased interest in oral microbiology, oral mucus immunity and connection to systemic diseases such as preterm low birth weight, pulmonary diseases, cardiovascular diseases, diabetes, and osteoporosis.

Periodontitis severity and prevalence are increased in diabetics and worse in poorly controlled diabetics. Periodontitis may exaberate diabetes by decreasing glycaemic control. This indicates a degree of synergism between the two diseases. Impaired neutrophil function has been demonstrated in diabetic patients.

Periodontitis associated with haematological diseases

Langerhans cell histiocytosis

Langerhans cells histiocytosis presents with single or multiple site involvement. The skin, oral mucosa, bone, and lymph nodes are typical locations for single site involvement.

Clinically

Between 10% and 20% of patients present with infiltration of the oral cavity, usually the posterior mandible. The typical dental presentation of Langerhans cell histiocytosis is characterised by:

1. Eruption of the primary molars at or soon after birth.
2. Pain, ulceration, enlargement, inflammation, or recession of gingival and motility of teeth because of expansion of the alveolar bone.
3. Dental radiographs may show discrete, destructive bone lesions that make the teeth appear to be floating on air.
4. Periosteal new bone formation and single root resorption also may be present.
5. Cases may present as aggressive periodontitis lesions that do not respond to routine periodontal therapy.

Periodontitis associated with genetic disorders

1. Familial and cyclic neutropenia
2. Down's syndrome
3. Leucocyte adhesion deficiency syndrome
4. Papillon-Lefevre syndrome
5. Chediak-Higashi syndrome
6. Histiocytosis syndrome
7. Glycogen storage diseases
8. Infantile genetic agranulocytosis
9. Cohen syndrome

10. Ehler's -Danlos syndrome
11. Hypophosphatasia
12. Others.

Acute necrotising ulcerative gingivitis

Synonyms: It is also known as **'*Plaut Vincent angina*'**, Vincent stomatitis, acute ulcerative gingivitis or **'trench mouth'**.

The condition received its name because during World War I (1914-1918) it occurred in soldiers who were fighting in trenches under conditions of stress, poor hygiene and poor nutrition.

Acute necrotising ulcerative gingivitis is a polymicrobial infection of the gums leading to inflammation, bleeding, deep ulceration and necrotic gum tissues. Acute necrotising ulcerative gingivitis not only affects the gums but also may spread to adjacent tissues of the face, neck, and bone.

There is halitosis, fever, and bleeding from gums.

The teeth become loose, and lymph nodes of the neck are often swollen.

A grey pseudomembrane may be present.

Causes: Causative organisms include anaerobes, such as bacteroides, and Fusobacterium as well as Spirochetes.

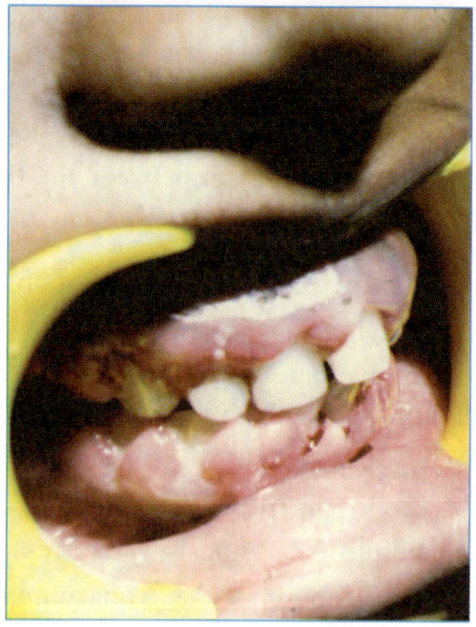

Fig.7.5: Photograph showing swollen gums with severe infection and ulcer formation (acute necrotising ulcerative gingivitis)

Risk factors

1. The condition is caused by an overpopulation of established oral bacteria due to a number of interacting factors such as poor hygiene, life-style and other infections. Other factors also contribute to periodontitis.
2. Conditions such as malformation of teeth, faulty dental restorations or ill-fitting appliances, root fractures, cervical root resorption and cemental tears all contribute to periodontal disease.
3. **Age:** This condition is commonly seen in the younger generation.
4. **Tobacco:** Cigarettes, cigars, pipe smoking and chewing tobacco all promote the growth of the bacteria in mouth and weaken immune system, making one more vulnerable to infection.
5. **Diabetes:** Elevated blood sugar can damage gums. Diabetes increases risk of cavities, gingivitis, tooth loss and variety of infection.
6. **Decreased immunity:** If person has a weakened immune system, he is susceptible to infections to all kinds including gum infection.
7. **Stress and heavy smoking** are probably the factors that most increases the risk of for necrotising ulcerative gingivitis.

Complications of gum disease

Advanced gum disease (periodontitis) does more than just damage to the gums. There is greater risk of:

1. **Heart disease and stroke:** Research suggests a link between oral bacteria and clogged arteries and blood clots, which can lead to heart attack and stroke. Some evidence shows that people with gum disease are more likely to have a heart attack or stroke than one those with healthy mouths. The more severe the gum disease the greater the risk of heart disease.

2. **Uncontrolled diabetes.**
3. **Pneumonia:** If patient has serious gum disease and lung problems, inhaling bacteria from mouth enter into lungs may result in pneumonia.
4. **Osteoporosis:** Researchers suspect a link between the loss of bone mineral density from osteoporosis and an increased susceptibility to oral bacteria. If osteoporosis also causes to lose density, that may increase risk of gum disease and tooth loss. Sometimes, gum disease or tooth loss may be an indication of osteoporosis.
5. **Adverse pregnancy outcomes:** New research suggests that women who have gum disease during pregnancy are at increased risk of giving birth to low weight, preterm babies.

PERIODONTAL DISEASE

Periodontal disease is the inflammation of gingival gum and periodontal ligament. Unhygienic oral cavity leads to deposition of inorganic salts on the teeth surface towards the gum and is commonly known as tartar. Tartar cannot be removed by brushing. It irritated the gingival, producing gingivitis. Gingivitis progresses to periodontitis, leading to abscess and loosening and exfoliation of teeth. Periodontal disease is more common amongst persons suffering from diabetes mellitus, nutritional deficiency, especially protein and vitamin C deficiency.

PERIODONTITIS

When an inflammatory process, whatever its cause, extends from the gingival into the underlying bone, the lesion is referred as periodontitis.

Periodontitis or pyorrhea is a more severe form of chronic gingivitis.

Clinically: Changes in gingival colour, loss of stippling, edema, hyperplasia, or recession, formation of clefts, presence of true pockets and tooth mobility characterise periodontitis.

Chronic periodontitis results from the consequences of chronic gingival inflammation in relation to the presence of calculus plaque between the gingival and the tooth. These are:

1. Destruction of the tooth in its pocket.
2. Progressive deepening of the pocket between teeth and gingival, which contains even-increasing amounts of the subgingival plaque.

Radiographs show evidence of bone destruction seen as a reduction in the height of the interdental and interradicular septa. Loss of the lamina dura on the alveolar crest gives the crest a concave or shaggy appearance.

Periodontal abscess formation: If the chronic inflammatory process becomes accelerated by acute bacterial infection this accelerates the destruction of the alveolar bone, and pus may extrude into the alveolar cavity or alongside the tooth in the gingival pocket.

JUVENILE PERIODONTITIS

Juvenile periodontitis occurs in children and can be classified into

1. Periodontitis, which occurs in otherwise healthy individuals
2. Periodontitis, which occurs in juveniles with systemic disease.

Two forms of juvenile periodontitis are recognised

1. Localised in which the destruction is limited to the incisors and first molar.
2. Generalised, involving all teeth. Generalised juvenile periodontitis includes early onset adult periodontosis, recurrent necrotising ulcerative and true generalised form.

Gottlieb described localised juvenile periodontitis as a chronic degenerative, non-inflammatory disease of periodontal tissues, which is referred as diffuse atrophy of alveolar bone. Localised juvenile periodontitis is not associated with plaque formation and inflammation. Localised juvenile periodontitis becomes apparent about the time of puberty, usually between the ages 10 and 15.

Juvenile periodontitis is connected to a defect in the immune system and has a genetic component. Recent evidence suggests that Actinobacillus actinomycetemcomitans, a gram-negative facultative anaerobic rod, plays a dominant role in the disease process.

Clinical features

As the disease progresses, the affected teeth may become increasingly mobile, with labial movements and spacing of incisors. Bleeding or probing of the periodontal pockets is also evident, reflecting ulceration of the cervicular epithelium.

Microscopically

There are numerous areas of chronic inflammation containing polymorphonuclear leukocytes, lymphocytes and large number of plasma cells. The covering epithelium is hyperplastic non-keratinising squamous, with pseudoepithelial hyperplasia.

AGGRESSIVE PERIODONTITIS

Aggressive periodontitis is considered as a multifactorial disease, comprising of a heterogenous group of infectious diseases characterised by the complex host-microbial interaction in the periodontium. Immune deficiencies and genetic link have been shown to be possible factors for all types of aggressive periodontitis. Recent study shows association of HLA-A9, and HLA-A10 with aggressive periodontitis in South India.

Clinical features

- A bacterial disease of the teeth and gingival that manifests before age 35, often in prepubescent children.
- **Swelling:** There is swelling of gum with little or no pain.
- **Discolouration:** When the periodontium begins to display patches of purple or red colour, this can be a sign of aggressive periodontitis.
- **Tenderness:** Gums may feel tender to the touch, especially in the closest teeth.
- **Gum recession:** Someone who is suffering from aggressive periodontitis may notice that their gums are appearing to pull from their teeth. This is called a recessive gum line.
- **Gapping:** During the recession of the gum line, new gaps will form between the teeth. This is because human teeth taper as they go down into the jaw, forming a root. As the gum line pulls away from the teeth, this tapering becomes apparent.

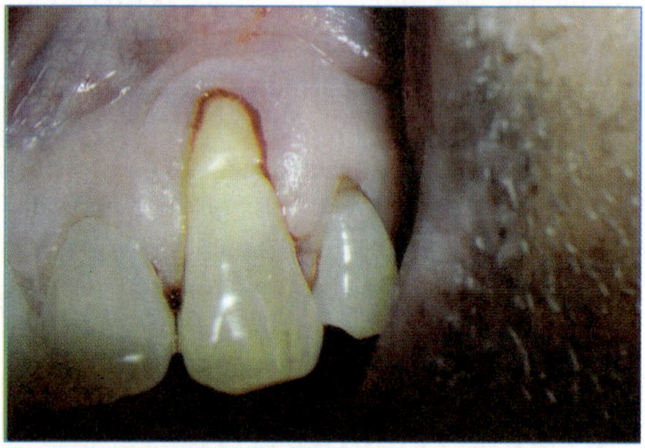

Fig.7.6: Showing recession of gum. Gums are pulled from the teeth and bleeding.

- **Infection and necrosis:** The later stages of aggressive periodontitis come with appearance of pus between the teeth nearest the gum lines. When pus is apparent, this is usually due to necrosis of the periodontium tissue. The gums experience discolouration, varying in hue from deep red to a greenish grey hint.
- **Tooth and bone loss:** Recession of gum tissues and necrotic infection will mostly result in the loss of many teeth in seemingly short period of time.

Papillon-Lefevre syndrome (PLS)

Papillon-Lefevre syndrome was first described by two French physicians Papillon and Lefevre in 1924. The prevalence is estimated to be 1 to 4 million persons in the general population with a carrier rate of 2 to 4 per 1,000.

Papillon-Lefevre syndrome is an autosomal recessive genetic disorder caused by a deficiency of cathepsin C. The gene responsible for PLS has recently been localised to chromosome 11q 14-21.

Males and females are equally affected and there is no racial predominance.

Papillon-Lefevre syndrome is characterised by periodontitis and palmo plantar keratoderma. The severe destruction of periodontium results in loss of most primary teeth by the age of 4, and most permanent teeth by age of 14.

Skin lesions

Often there is associated hyperkeratosis of the palms and soles resulting in a foul-smelling odour.

Microscopically, the skin lesions consist of hyperkeratosis, parakeratosis, acanthosis, and a slight perivascular inflammatory infiltrate.

Bibliography

Stephen J. Mcphee, Maxine A Papadakins: *Current medical diagnosis and treatment* 2008 Mcgraw Hill Lange 47th edition.

Xao S; Bu l; Yang m; Qian; M; Hu L; Liu J; Zhao G; Kong X. *Genomics*, volume, 74, number 2, June 2001. P P 180-185 (6).

CHAPTER

8

PHYSICAL AND CHEMICAL INJURY

INTRODUCTION

Trauma is the most common cause of ulceration of the oral mucous membranes. Traumatic ulceration may result from physical, chemical, or thermal injury to the tissue.

PHYSICAL AGENTS

Indirect trauma

FRACTURE TEETH

Fractures of the crown or root or both, luxation of the teeth, and indirect trauma to the pulp are all observed in automobile accidents, bicycle falls, professional sportsmen (boxers, baseball and football players, hunters, parachutists, and jockeys, etc), chewing hard objects and physical fighting.

Classification

Ellis classification

Ellis I: This level of injury includes crown fracture. Fractures involve only the enamel, these injuries may show minor chipping with rough edges.

Ellis II: Fractures involve enamel and dentin, patients complain of pain to touch and sensitivity to air. A pale yellow exposure of the dental processes, which communicate directly with the pulp, can occur.

Ellis III: Fractures involve enamel, dentin, and pulp layers. These teeth are tender and have visible areas of red, pink or even blood at the centre of the tooth.

Clinical features

Approximately 82% of traumatised teeth are maxillary teeth.

There are different types of tooth fractures and breaks, each of which require different treatment:

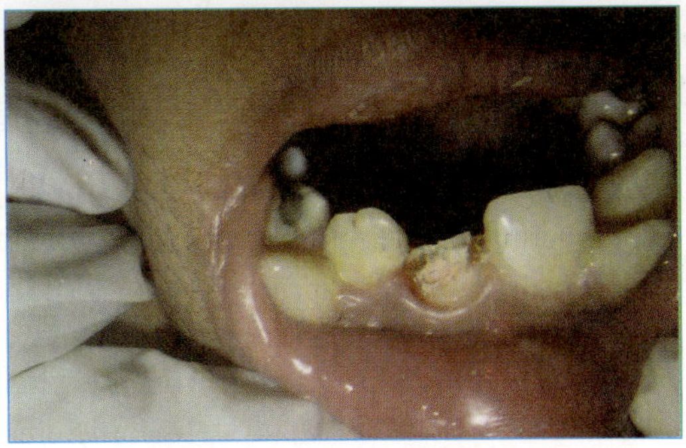

Fig.8.1: Showing fracture tooth

- **Minor cracks:** Crazed lines are tiny cracks that affect only the outer enamel of the tooth. They are common in all adult teeth and require no treatment. Dentist may sand the areas, but this generally does not need any treatment.
- **Cracked tooth:** This type of crack extends from the chewing surface of the tooth vertically towards the root and sometimes below the gum line.
- **Broken cusp:** When a cusp or pointed part of chewing surface of tooth becomes weakened, the cusp will fracture. These are rarely painful and may not affect the pulp of the teeth.
- **Chipped teeth:** Slight chip or fracture of tooth enamel only or with possible minimal dentin involvement. They are usually repaired using filling, especially if this occurred in front where it would require a tooth-coloured filling.
- **Serious breaks:** A serious fracture that exposes both the dentin and the pulp tissue should be treated promptly. The tooth may be displaced and loose and gums may bleed. In most serious injuries vertical, horizontal or diagonal fractures of the tooth roots.
- **Split tooth:** A split tooth is a cracked tooth in which the crack has progressed so there are two distinct segments that can be separated from one another.
- **Vertical breaks or split root:** It is the fracture of the root, which starts below the gum line and extend toward the chewing surface. These breaks are painful because the area around the root may be infected. It is the common complication of endodontic therapy. In most cases, the tooth will have to be removed.
- **Decay induced break:** In this case, the tooth has broken or crumbled because a cavity weakened it from the inside out.

Fracture of mandible and maxilla

Symptoms of fracture of the mandible and maxilla may include some of the following:

- Difficulty in breathing, talking, eating or swallowing
- Pain when mandible or maxilla is moved
- An inability to move the mandible or maxilla, bleeding from the gum and around the teeth
- Numbness of lower lip
- Abnormal occlusion
- Abnormal movement of maxilla and mandible.

Signs of mandibular fracture and maxilla

- Sublingual haematoma
- Edema
- Abrasion and lacerations

Nocturnal parafunctioning habits, such as bruxism (i.e., grinding of the teeth) and thumb sucking may be associated with the development of traumatic ulcers of the buccal mucosa, the labial mucosa, the lateral borders of the tongue, and the palate.

BRUXISM

Bruxism, or bruxomania, is the medical term for tooth grinding that is not a normal part of chewing movements.

Causes of bruxism

- As an effect of some drugs used for treating depression, like prozac, calexa and cocaine.
- Abnormal alignment of upper or lower teeth.
- Growth and development of the jaws and teeth in children.
- **Personality type:** Some studies show that persons with aggressive, overlying competitive, controlling or hyperactive personalities have an increased incidence of bruxism.
- **Central nervous system dysfunction:** Some theories link bruxism to the central nervous system disorders such as Huntington's disease or Parkinson's disease.

Predisposing factors

- **Age:** Bruxism is common in young children but usually goes away by adolescence.
- **Stress:** Increased anxiety or stress can lead to teeth grinding. So can anger and frustration.

Symptoms

Symptoms of bruxism are:

- An unexplained morning tension type headache.
- Regular contractions of the jaw muscles accompanied by facial pain.
- Damaged teeth, breaking of dental fillings, injured gums–this may be caused by the erosion of the outer most enamel layer by the teeth rubbing together. The exposure of the dentin causes tooth sensitivity.
- Grinding noise during sleep.
- Temporomandibular joint disorders.
- Other symptoms include anxiety, insomnia, eating disorders, and stress.

TRAUMATIC ULCER

Definition: Traumatic ulcer is a form of acute or chronic mechanical injury to the oral mucosa leading to loss of all epithelial layers.

Etiology

It can result from sharp or broken tooth, an ill-fitting amalgam restoration, orthodontic materials, accidental biting during mastication, sharp foreign bodies, and clumsy use of dental instruments.

Localisations: Tongue, buccal mucosa, lips, gingival, mucobuccal folds.

Clinical features

Traumatic ulcer usually presents as a single, ill-defined, painful ulceration, with smooth surface and erythematous or whitish borders. The size may range from a few millimetres to several centimetres. There is a close relationship between the ulcer and irritating cause.

The ulcer may persist for long time, but usually heals within 7-10 days after elimination of cause.

Treatment

Removal of etiological factors

Symptomatic.

Sublingual ulcerations (as in Riga-Fede disease) may occur as a result of chronic mucosal trauma due to adjacent anterior primary baby teeth. It may also occur in older infants after the eruption of primary lower incisors with repetitive tongue thrusting habits and in children with familial dysautonomia (insensitivity to pain).

Typically, the lesion begins as an ulcerated area on the ventral surface of the tongue with repeated trauma. It may progress to an enlarged fibrous mass with appearance of an ulcerated granuloma. It may interfere with proper suckling, feeding, and put the infant on nutritional deficiencies.

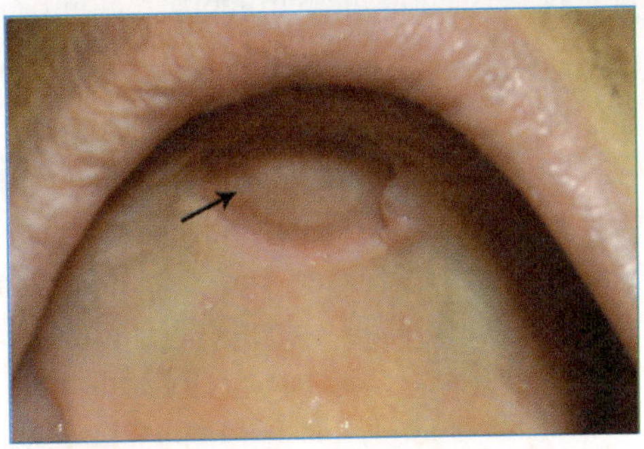

Fig.8.2: Showing traumatic ulcer tongue due to ill-fitted denture

Microscopically

The individual lesions present as erythema surrounding a centrally removable, yellow fibrinopurulent membrane. Often the lesion develops a rolled white hyperkeratotic border immediately adjacent to the ulceration. Occasionally, however, the underlying proliferative granulation tissue results in a raised exophytic lesion similar to pyogenic granuloma. The pseudomembranous pattern, termed atypical histiocytic granuloma, may be clinically misdiagnosed as a malignancy.

Fractured or malposed teeth and ill-fitting dentures may cause mucosal ulcers of the buccal mucosa, lateral and ventral surfaces of the tongue, and the alveolar mucosa overlying the osseous structures.

NICOTINE STOMATITIS

Nicotine stomatitis (smoker's palate), a lesion of the palatal mucosa, has been described in the literature since 1926.

Smoker's palate or nicotine stomatitis is a common tobacco-related type of keratosis that exclusively occurs on the hard palate and is typically associated with pipe and cigar smoking.

Cause: It is the temperature, not the chemicals in the smoke that is responsible. Concentrated heat stream of smoke from tobacco products causes nicotine stomatitis.

Clinical features

Men and women who smoke tobacco products are affected equally. Women smoke pipes for less often than men.

Clinically, the palatal mucosa responds initially with redness. Later, it becomes wrinkled and takes on a diffuse whitish-grey colour with numerous micronodules of inflamed and dilated salivary glands.

FRICTIONAL KERATOSIS

Frictional keratosis is seen in teenagers and young adults of both genders. Many individuals have a thin, slightly raised white keratotic line along the occlusal plane of the buccal mucosa, often bilateral. This linea alba considered to be a variation of normal anatomy but is called frictional keratosis, chronic cheek bite keratosis or Morsicatio buccarum when it becomes pronounced. There is usually a clenching or bruxing habit and the most severe lesions are found in person with the habit of constantly pushing the cheeks between the teeth with a finger while gently biting on the buccal tissues.

The surface of frictional keratosis may be quite rough and irregular, and on the buccal mucosa may show a scalloped effect as the tissues take on the contours of adjacent teeth. Such focal areas of pink mucosa may be seen, representing in which the patient has peeled off the thick surface keratin with his or her teeth.

Linear line of excess keratin may be found along the lateral edges of the tongue, often with crenations from chronically pushing the tongue against the teeth. Rounded or irregularly shaped white plaques may be seen on the anterior dorsal surface of the tongue from a chronic tongue thrust habit, and may be seen in the retromolar region because of trauma from the maxillary dentition.

Histological features are

1. Acanthosis and hyperkeratosis
2. Keratin is ragged and delaminated
3. No bacterial colonies lodges in surface irregularities
4. Granular cell layer is often quite prominent
5. The cells of the spinous layer often demonstrate intraepithelial oedema
6. Occasional vacuolated cells with pyknotic nuclei resemble koilocytes
7. There is no dysplasia in epithelium and there is no increase in mitotic activity
8. There is a mild scattered chronic inflammatory cell infiltrate within underlying fibrovascular stroma.

Habitual lesions: Saw tooth irregularities and V-shaped or U-shaped notches are seen in seamstresses, tailors, and fishermen who cut thread with their incisors.

SEXUAL ABUSE

Several physical injuries are strong signs of sexual abuse. The oral cavity is a frequent site of sexual abuse in children. The presence of oral and perioral gonorrhea or syphilis in pre-pubescent children is a strong sign of sexual abuse. Gags applied to the mouth may leave bruises, scratching, or scarring at the corners of the mouth. Unexplained injury or petechiae of the palate, particularly at the junction of the hard and soft palate, may be evidence of forced oral sex.

HUMAN BITE

Human bite injuries are usually considered as those injuries that occur because of a person being bitten by another person. Commonly, human bites by an assailant occur extraorally but in few occasions they also occur intraorally. The size and severity of the injuries vary ranging from small lacerations, punctures, or cuts, to total avulsion and loss of relatively big chunks of tissue. Human bites may become infected with a wide variety of aerobic and anaerobic bacteria that are the parts of oral microflora.

TRAUMATIC BONE CYST

Pathogenesis of simple bone cyst is unknown. Evidence exists that venous obstruction and blockage of interstitial fluid drainage, in an area of rapidly growing and remodeling cancellous bone, play an important role in the formation of unicameral bone cyst.

Macroscopically: Simple bone cyst is a fluid filled cavity in the bone, lined by compressed fibrous tissue. Occasionally blood products may be found within the fluid if a previous fracture has occurred. A membrane of varying thickness lines the inner wall of the cyst. Fibrous septa may form after a fracture and create a multilocular appearance.

Microscopically: Mesothelial cells line simple bone cysts. The inner wall of bone adjacent to mesothelial membrane consists of well-vascularised new bone produced by the overlying periosteum. Multinucleated giant cells may be present within the cyst wall.

EOSINOPHILIC ULCERATION

Tongue ulceration with eosinophilia (eosinophilic ulcer, ulcerative eosinophilic granuloma, Riga-Fede disease).

The initiating event is presumably traumatic (crush injury to the tongue muscle), hence alternative designation as traumatic ulcerative granuloma.

Riga-Fede disease is a form of eosinophilic ulcer that develops in infants and usually occurs on the anterior ventral side of the tongue. Lip and buccal mucosa are sites of predilection. The distinctive, self-limiting ulcerations develop as a result of chronic mucosal trauma from adjacent anterior primary teeth and, usually, occur in association with breast-feeding.

Clinical features of eosinophilic ulcer

Eosinophilic ulcers develop in individuals of all ages, ranging from infants to those aged 92 years. Mean patient's age at onset is 46 years.

An ulcer develops that may not be painful in two-third of cases and persists for months. This benign self-healing lesion may be misdiagnosed and clinically confused with squamous cell carcinoma.

Eosinophilic ulcer typically presents as an irregular, solitary ulcer with a fibrinous membrane on the surface. A zone of erythema surrounds the ulcer.

They range from 0.5 cm to several centimetres in size.

Microscopically, it shows a polymorphic inflammatory infiltrate rich in eosinophils, extending into the submucosa, muscle, and minor salivary agents.

CERVICOFACIAL EMPHYSEMA

Cervicofacial emphysema is an infrequently reported sequela to dental surgery. Most cases result from the accidental introduction of air into the soft tissues during the use of air-driven high-speed hand-pieces or air/water syringes.

It is normally restricted to only moderate local swellings. However, spread of larger amounts of air into deeper spaces may sometimes cause serious complications including airway compromise due to accumulation of air in the retropharyngeal space, pneumomediastinum, and pneumopericardium.

Clinical features

Clinical presentation is characterised by a sudden onset of hemifacial swelling with sensation of fullness of the face and closure of the eyelids on the involved side. Crepitation is noted on palpation. Fatal air embolism and soft tissue infections through dissemination of oral flora microorganisms along the emphysematous tracts have also been described.

DENTURE STOMATITIS

Denture related stomatitis indicates an inflammatory process of the mucosa that bears a complete or partial removable denture appliances, typically a denture.

Etiology

It is caused by mechanical irritation from dentures, candida albicans, or a tissue response to microorganisms living beneath the denture.

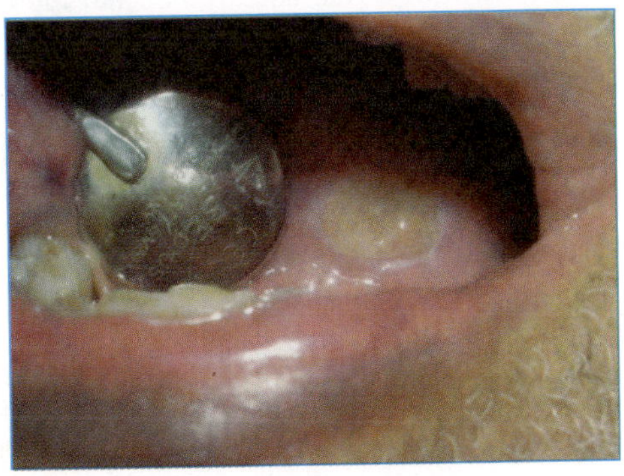

Fig.8.3: Shows features of denture stomatitis (Traumatic ulcer tongue)

Clinical features

Lesions are usually asymptomatic.

Patients may complain of halitosis, slight bleeding, and swelling of the involved area, or a burning sensation, xerostomia or taste alteration. Mucosa beneath the denture is red and edematous, with or without white spots. Papillary projections may develop in chronic cases. The mucosa below lower denture is rarely involved.

Complication

- Angular stomatitis
- Papillary hyperplasia in the vault of the palate
- Denture sore mouth

EPULIS FISSURATUM

It is also known as granuloma fissuratum, inflammatory fibrous dysplasia, denture epulis, and denture induced fibrous hyperplasia. It is an oral pathologic condition that appears in the mouth as an overgrowth of connective tissue.

Epulis fissuratum develops slowly over a prolonged period of time in patients with ill-fitting dentures.

Clinical features

Epulis fissuratum occurs in the fifth, sixth and seventh decades but it can be observed at almost any age.

More commonly found in women, it can appear in either the mandible or maxilla, but is more commonly found in anterior portions of the mouth rather than the posterior.

Epulis fissuratum appears as a single or multiple fold of tissue that grown in excess around the vestibule, which is the area where the gums meet the inner cheek.

The lesions made up of excess tissue are usually firm, fibrous and pink. The surface of the epulis fissuratum mass tends to be smooth, however occasionally, it is ulcerated or papillary. The size of the epulis fissuratum is variable.

Microscopically

Epithelial cells are usually hyperkeratotic, and irregular, hyperplastic rete ridges are often seen.

INFLAMMATORY PAPILLARY HYPERPLASIA

It is also known as papillary hyperplasia of the palate, palatal papillomatosis.

It is found in three out of every 1,000 adults.

Inflammatory papillary hyperplasia is an oral pathologic condition that appears in the mouth as an overgrowth of tissue usually beneath the denture.

Causes

It is associated with poor dental hygiene, denture overuse, and ill-fitting dentures. Other suspected contributing factors include denture-cleaning solutions, which may contain chemical irritants, putrefaction of food, decreased salivary flow, smoking and allergy.

Clinical features

Most patients with inflammatory papillary hyperplasia are in the third, fourth, and fifth decades of life and average is 40.2 years.

Majority of cases occur on the vault of the palate, but some may involve palatal shelves and even alveolar mucosa. The papillary projections are normally 3 mm in size, broad based, firm, and nontender, giving a 'cobble stone' appearance.

Microscopically

Histologically, the lesion shows numerous papillary projections that are covered by parakeratotic-stratified epithelium which quite frequently exhibits pseudoepitheliomatous hyperplasia as well as formation of keratin pearls and microcysts.

Small to moderate numbers of chronic inflammatory cells are present, perhaps occasional polymorphonuclear leukocytes.

CHEMICAL INJURIES

Chemical burn

This is an injury to the oral mucosa caused by topical application of caustic agents. Inappropriate or careless use of chemical agents in dental practice may cause oral lesions. Some of these agents may be introduced into the mouth by patient. The severity of lesion depends on the type of chemical agent utilised and the concentration and duration of contact of the noxious agent with the tissue.

DRUGS

Aspirin

Chemicals such as aspirin that are held or that come in contact with the oral mucosa may cause tissues to become necrotic and slough off creating an ulcerated surface. The healing of the painful 'aspirin burn' usually takes a week or more.

Dilantin causes stomatitis and gingival hyperplasia.

Tetracycline

Drugs such as tetracycline are well-known as agents that produce discolouration of the teeth. Generally, the colour changes from yellow to slightly brown or blue. Discolouration is usually bilateral, affecting multiple teeth in both arches. The teeth affected are those were mineralising while the drug was used. Tetracycline is incorporated with calcium and may be observed in dentin or enamel, which arc tooth structurcs. Greater the rate of mineralisation, the greater the amount of tetracycline finds its way into the tissues.

The mechanism for the characteristic dental defect produced by tetracycline is related to the potent chelating ability of the drug. Tetracycline forms a complex with calcium orthophosphate and becomes incorporated into bones and teeth undergoing calcification.

A clinical history of treatment with tetracycline and fluorescent teeth (yellow fluorescence) under ultraviolet light are criteria in making the diagnosis.

Management

Two approaches have been used to treat tetracycline discolouration:

(1) Bleaching the external enamel surface

(2) Intracoronal bleaching following intentional root-canal therapy.

Cancer therapy

Chemotherapeutic drugs affect hard palate, the lips, tongue, floor of the mouth, inside of cheeks, and soft palate.

Oral mucosal tissue injury is both a direct and indirect consequence of cancer therapy, with manifestations that include damage and a number of other potentially serious sequelae. Chemotherapy induced stomatitis is a common side effect of many of the antineoplastic drugs and may present as an excruciatingly painful mucositis involving any of the oral mucous membranes either in a localised or generalised fashion. Other manifestations include infections, pain and bleeding.

Chemicals used in cavity preparations

It is possible for the pulpal inflammation to be caused by chemicals used in cavity preparations. The cutting of dentin in routine cavity severs odontoblastic processes causing, in many cases, odontoblast death and subsequent inflammation.

Previously cavity preparation was performed without cooling water sprays. Such **'dry cutting'** elevated the temperature of dentin causing pulpal inflammation.

AMALGAM TATTOO

First formal investigation of the effects of dental amalgam on the periodontal structures was by Zander (1957).

Amalgam tattoo (focal argyrosis) is the most common exogenous pigment in the oral cavity. Amalgam is a combination of mercury, silver, tin, copper, and sometimes zinc.

Overall, amalgam tattoo is found in approximately 1 per 1,000 adults.

Causes

Amalgam dust can be introduced into the oral tissues through mucosal abrasion. The deposition occurs after a number of different dental procedures that include diffusion through soft tissues from root-end fillings, accidental deposition of fine metallic particles into the gingival by high speed-drills, accidental abrasion of the mucosa by high speed rotary instruments, or deposition of amalgam scrapes left behind during extraction.

The macules are present on the gingivae, the buccal and alveolar mucosae, the palate, and/or the tongue. Amalgam restoration produces a chronic inflammation of the adjacent gingival tissues. It has been documented in dental literature that electric currents are generated when amalgam fillings are placed in teeth.

Amalgam tattoos appear as macules and may be black, blue or grey in colour. The borders are well-defined, irregular or diffuse. It is usually less than 0.5 cm in greatest diameter, although rare examples have been more than 3.0 cm in size.

Microscopic examination reveals that amalgam is present in the tissues in two forms: as irregular dark, solid fragments of metal or as numerous discrete fine brown or black granules dispersed along collagen bundles, and blood vessels and nerves. In the lamina propria there is a finely granular black/brown pigment and within the cytoplasm of histiocytes. Larger fragments may elicit a foreign body giant cell response. Giant cells can surround or engulf the metallic particles, and, sometimes, huge pieces can be seen within their cytoplasm.

Treatment

Advances in laser technology now allow amalgam tattoos to be removed by the Q-switched ruby laser.

GUTTA-PERCHA

The word gutta-percha comes from the plant's name in Malay, *getah persa*, which translates as percha sap.

Gutta-percha is the predominant material used to obdurate or fill empty space of tooth after it has gone endodontic therapy. Gutta-percha cone is the most widely used material for root canal filling. It can cause chronic inflammation and irritation of pulp.

ZINC PHOSPHATE

Zinc phosphate cement has been, and still is, the most frequently used luting agent for crowns and bridges. Pulpal reactions initially occurring in deep cavities will subside over time.

ALCOHOL

Clinically affected area is covered by a whitish membrane (due to necrosis). The dead mucosa can be easily scrapped off, leaving a red bleeding surface. The lesion is painful.

Oral health care products

Toothpastes and mouthwashes contain a multitude of agents recognised as allergents. Additionally, ingredients such as pyrophosphates and zinc citrate and (tartar control) and sodium lauryl sulphate (surfactants) are contact irritants that have been implicated in mucosal sloughing and apthaeform ulcers, respectively.

PHENOL

Chemical burns can also be seen in patients who have used phenol for treating recurrent aphthous ulcers. Phenol is used in dentistry as an antiseptic or for local cautery. It is an extremely caustic chemical agent and careless application may cause necrosis. Clinically there is a whitish surface that later desquamates, exposing a painful erosion or ulcer that heals slowly.

TRICHLOROACETIC ACID

Trichloroacetic acid burns were frequent in the past because this agent was used in cautery of the gingival. It is an extremely caustic agent, and improper use may result in serious chemical burns.

Clinically, there is a white surface due to tissue necrosis. Underneath there is inflammation and erosion or ulceration. The lesion usually heals spontaneously.

SODIUM HYPOCHLORITE

Sodium hypochlorite, or dental bleach, is commonly used as a root canal irritant and may cause serious ulcerations due to accidental contact with oral soft tissues.

HYDROGEN PEROXIDE, alcohol, and chloroform are routinely used for washing out cavity preparations. Hydrogen peroxide may reaches the pulp and produce microemboli in the capillaries which will rupture, causing haemorrhages and tissue anoxaemia. It results in epithelial necrosis and sloughing of the epithelium.

EUGENOL BURN

Eugenol is used as an antiseptic and local anesthetic in dentistry. The noxious potential of the drug is limited but may on occasion cause a mucosal burn. A eugenol burn appears as a white-brownish surface with underlying erosion. The lesion heals spontaneously within a week.

ACRYLIC RESIN BURN: Autopolymerising acrylic resins are used in dentistry for the construction of temporary prostheses and may cause local burns due to heat evolving during polymerisation or to monomer excess. The mucosa is diffuse red with or without superficial erosions. In deeper cavities these resins causes inflammation of pulp and damage to the odontoblastic tissue.

IODINE BURN

Mild burn may occur after repeated application of concentrated alcoholic iodine solutions. The affected mucosa is whitish and red and has a rough surface.

STRONG ALKALI

Accidental ingestion of caustic agents may cause devastating injury in children. Strong alkalis are present in wide range of household and industrial cleaners and beauty products, often attractively packaged and easily accessible to children, both at home and low shelves in shops.

COCAINE

Ulcers may arise (e.g., on the palate) with the use of powdered cocaine or through smoking of crack cocaine. The effects of cocaine in the oral cavity vary depending on the form used and the route of administration. Rarely, sorting cocaine may cause necrosis, possibly associated with ischaemia of the floor of the nose, and, eventually, causing ulcers of the hard palate as well as fistula formation.

NON-ALLERGIC REACTIONS TO CHEMICALS USED SYSTEMICALLY

ARSENIC

Acute and chronic intoxication occurs from the ingestion of insecticides, or administration of organic arsenicals. Harmful effects of arsenic compounds (in pesticides, chemotherapy drugs, paints, etc.), most often from insecticide exposure. Industries that use inorganic arsenic and its compounds include wood preservation, glass production, non-ferrous metal alloys, and electronic semiconductor manufacturing.

Oral manifestations

The most prominent clinical findings associated with acute arsenic poisoning are related to gastrointestinal tract. Acute indigestion may lead to oral irritation and burning sensation in the mouth and throat. Oral lesions in arsenic poisoning consist of gingivitis and stomatitis, ulceration, purpura, and mobility of teeth. Arsenic stomatitis is an oral condition associated with arsenic poisoning characterised by dry, red, painful oral mucosa, ulceration, bleeding beneath the mucosa, and mobility of teeth.

LEAD (Plumbism)

Classically *'lead poisoning'* or *'lead intoxication'* has been defined as exposure to high levels of lead typically associated with severe health effects.

Occupational exposure is common cause of lead poisoning.

Neurological signs of acute poisoning, typically, are paraesthesia, pain, muscle weakness, encephalopathy with headache, convulsions, delirium and coma.

Possible complications of lead poisoning include behaviour or attention problems, hearing problems, kidney damage and slowed body growth.

Oral manifestations

Oral tissues are exposed to lead through direct contact with ingested lead, and through secretion of lead in the saliva.

Industrial dusts and fumes containing lead are deposited on the enamel. Prolonged exposure also results in intrinsic staining of the enamel, dentin, or cementum. Lead produces brown stain on teeth. The formation of a lead line (Halosaturninus or Burtonian's line) occurs in lead poisoning. Bruton's line is a blue purplish line on the gums seen in lead poisoning. It is caused by a reaction between circulating lead with sulphur ions released by oral bacterial activity, which deposits lead sulphide at the junction of the teeth and gums. Other oral manifestations include tremors of the tongue on thrusting, advanced periodontal disease, excessive salivation and metallic taste.

BISMUTH (BISMUTHISM)

Clinical features

Signs and symptoms in bismuth poisoning are vague gastrointestinal disturbances, nausea, vomiting, blood diarrhoea, *'bismuth grippe'* and *jaundice.*

An abnormal oral condition is caused by systemic use of bismuth compounds over prolonged periods. A blue-black line 'bismuth line' on the inner aspect of gingival sulcus or dark pigmentation of the buccal mucosa, sore tongue, metallic taste, burning sensation in mouth, ulcerative gingivostomatitis characterises it. Chronic use of bismuth can cause a black discolouration of normal filliform papillae and its appearance may resemble black hairy tongue. The papillae are not enlarged and stain is removable.

Microscopically

The granules of the sulphide are seen in tissue section as small irregular black collection of pigments, sometimes perivascular in location.

MERCURY

Mercury poisoning may be acute or chronic.

It is also known as mercurialism, or hydragyria, which is a disease caused by exposure to mercury or its compounds.

Mercury is still used in hospitals in thermometers and blood pressure instruments, and commercially in batteries, switches, and fluorescent light bulbs. Large quantities of metallic mercury are employed as electrodes in the electrolytic production of chlorine and sodium hydroxide from saline. These uses still give rise to accidental and occupational exposure.

Clinical features

Common symptoms include peripheral neuropathy (presenting as paresthesia or itching, burning or pain), skin discolouration (pink cheeks, fingertips and toes), edema (swelling and desquamation (dead skin peels off in layers).

Central nervous system disturbances in the form of tremors, headache, depression and insomnia.

Oral manifestations

Oral manifestations consist of increased salivation, stomatitis and glossitis, swelling of salivary glands, and, sometimes, a dark line on the gingival. The oral mucosa is prone to ulceration on the gingival, palate, and tongue. Salivary glands are enlarged and the tongue is also swollen and painful. Mercuric sulphide also causes significant destruction of the alveolar bone with resultant loosening of and exfoliation of the teeth.

Acrodynia

It is also known as Pink disease or Swift's disease. The term is derived from Greek roots meaning '*extremity*' and '*pain*'.

Chronic mercury exposure in infants and children is termed acrodynia.

Clinical features

It occurs most frequently in young infants before the age of two years although children can occasionally be affected up to age of 5 years or 6 years.

Children initially become listless, drowsy, and irritable, with a tendency to cry. Anorexia (loss of appetite) and subsequent weight loss can occur. More than 50% of patients demonstrate photophobia. Hypotonia (loss of muscle tone), the inability to hyperextend or overextend the limbs and atrophy of muscle is noted.

Oral manifestations

Oral signs include excessive salivation with dribbling, ulcerative gingivitis, bruxism, sore mouth, gingival hyperplasia, alveolar bone destruction and mobility of teeth and premature loss of teeth.

DENTAL FLUOROSIS

The magnitude of problem of fluorosis in India is roughly estimated to the tune of 66.62 million people at risk, of which an estimated 6 million are children below the age of 14 years. Fluorosis is an endemic health problem in 22 other nations around the globe.

Drinking water from sources having high fluoride is the cause of dental fluorosis. To cause mottling, fluorides must be present in concentration of several times of that found in controlled fluorinated water supplies. Fluoride in toothpaste, mouth rinses, varnish and sodium fluoride tablets—administered as prescription—can contribute to the fluoride burden of the body leading to dental fluorosis. Dental fluorosis is an aesthetic and social problem, besides being a health problem.

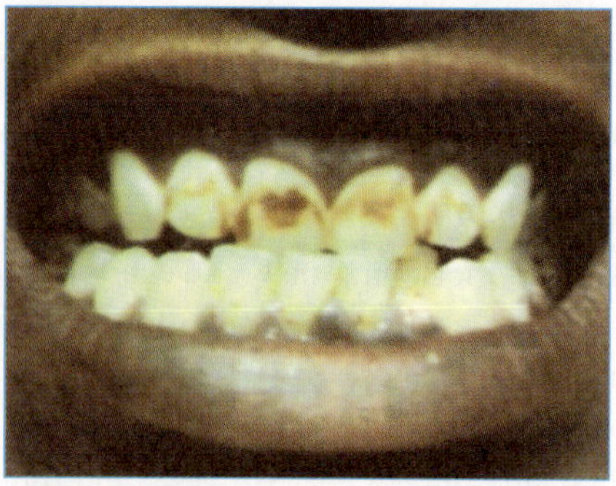

Fig.8.4: Brown colouring of teeth away from gums in dental fluorosis

The discolouration of the teeth may progress from white, yellow, brown to black. The discolouration may be in spots, or as streaks invariably horizontal in orientation, since new layers of the matrix are added on horizontally during tooth development.

Fluorosis is seen as (a) mild (b) moderate, and (c) severe, involving the whole or part of the crown.

In dental fluorosis, the discolouration will be away from the gums and on the enamel surfaces and it can never be removed, as it is an integral part of the tooth matrix. In dental fluorosis, the enamel will lose its lustre and shine.

Persons with discoloured teeth due to dental fluorosis develop inferiority complex, presenting psycho-sociological problems to self and the family.

Calcium-rich constituents of teeth, viz. enamel and dentin, have strong affinity for fluoride during the formation of teeth. Fluoride combines with calcium forming calcium fluoroapatite crystals during the mineralisation of teeth. Mottled enamel or dental fluorosis is a form of enamel hypocalcification, which results from the ingestion of excessive fluoride during the period of enamel formation.

THERMAL INJURY

Hot food and liquids: Hot food and liquids may cause oral ulcerations also. The classic example of this type of injury is the 'pizzas burn' from hot melted cheese contacting the palate.

Clinical features: The lesions commonly present as zones of erythema and ulceration—often exhibiting remnants of necrotic epithelium at the periphery.

Thermal and electrical burn

Electric burns of oral cavity are found to be more frequently in boys as compared to girls in a ratio of 2 : 1.

Sites: In children the major traumatic injuries in this group include electrical and/or thermal burns of the lips, perioral areas and commissure areas. Tongue, gingival, alveolar ridge, floor of mouth, and mucobuccal folds may also be less frequently affected.

Cause

Children tend to be curious about electrical cords and other items unknown to them, and as they explore these items, they tend to put them in their mouth.

Clinical features

Electric burns in oral mucosa present as a painless, white-grey, coagulated lesion with no bleeding and surrounded by a narrow rim of erythema. Extensive ulcerations with necrosis may develop. Progressively, the white grey surface evolves into brown-black charred tissues and, finally, sloughs, leaving a deep ulcer that may bleed.

The affected teeth may become non-vital.

Complications: The involvement of lips and angle of the mouth, if untreated, may lead to the development of deformities such as microstomia, mucosal-alveolar adhesions, alteration in shape of lips.

Treatment

It is supportive. Surgical reconstruction may be necessary in severe cases.

Ionising radiation

Miners, industrial workers, soldiers, and research scientists may become accidentally exposed to radiotherapy.

Radiation mucositis: Reactions that results from radiation therapy for malignancies in the oral cavity and oropharynx may be quite severe. Radiation mucositis is an early and acute reaction usually beginning during the second week of radiation. It usually presents as erythema followed by spotty mucositis. The spotty mucositis will coalesce to form areas of ulceration covered by a yellow white pseudomembrane with a bright erythematous border. The lips are often involved with a tenacious pseudomembrane and crusting being noted in the area of ulceration.

Radiation can cause a temporary sore throat, hoarseness, temporary partial or complete loss of taste, difficulty in swallowing, stiffness in jaw, bone pain and bone damage.

CHANGES IN THE SKIN

External beam of radiation may cause sunburn-like skin changes, nausea, vomiting and fatigue. The skin may become itchy and dry.

Acute effects in the skin usually manifest initially as a slight erythema. Epilation can also occur early in the course of treatment. As further radiation is given, reddening as well as inflammation of skin tends to increase. Desquamation, which can be dry in nature, show little more than surface flaking to the stratum corneum can also appear.

In some cases, it can progress such that a moist exudates begin to be released from portions of the irradicated skin.

EFFECTS ON SALIVARY GLANDS

Radiation therapy may be used as the main treatment in some cases of inoperable salivary gland cancers. Radiation therapy can be used after surgery as an additional treatment to try to kill any cancer cells that may have been missed by surgery.

Most common side-effect from radiation to the salivary gland is decreased production of saliva—which leads to dry mouth.

EFFECTS ON TEETH

Cervical caries and occasional internal or external resorption are seen. Ankylosis of teeth is sometimes noted.

EFFECTS ON BONE

Irradication of mature bone results in vascular and cellular changes best characterised as osteopenia. The incidence of osteopenia varies between 8% and 23%. Osteoblasts are sensitive to X-ray radiation. There is localised osteoporosis due to imbalance between bone formation and bone resorption. There is increase susceptibility of bone to infection.

Alveolar bone presents coarse trabeculae and osteolytic and osteosclerotic areas.

Fractures are common.

LASER RADIATION

Recent developments of laser dentistry have led to an increasing acceptance of this technology by both professionals and the general public. The potential hard-tissue applications are: Vaporise carious lesions, desensitise exposed root surfaces; endodontically, vaporize organic tissue, glaze canal plug wall surfaces and fuse an apical plug with the potential to resist fluid leakage; roughen tooth surfaces, in lieu of acid etching, in preparation for bonding procedures, preventively, to treat enamel, arrest demineralisation and promote remineralisation, and debond ceramic orthodontic brackets.

Effect on teeth

Laser with a wave length of 694 nm shows a crater-like morphology surrounded by a glass-like appearance at the irradicated zone, which seems to be caused by fusing, melting and recrystallisation of enamel crystallites.

Laser electron microscope shows a smooth area with concentric lines formed by melting with recrystallisation of dentin, areas of granulation, vitrified surface, numerous cracks, and irregular areas of descamative dentin.

Effect on pulp

In human beings: Studies revealed a severe irreversible damage to the pulp as a result of excessive heating. Laser irradiation of oral calcified structure can cause pulpal inflammation using a pulsed ruby laser.

In animals: Reports of effect of laser radiation on pulpal tissue in animals are available in literature. There is haemorrhagic necrosis, with acute and chronic inflammation, and coagulative necrosis of osteoblastic layer.

Effect on soft tissue

There is non-specific ulceration of epithelium with purulent inflammation after laser therapy on oral cavity.

CHAPTER 9

BACTERIAL VIRAL FUNGAL AND PARASITIC INFECTIONS OF ORAL CAVITY

IMPETIGO CONTAGIOSA

Impetigo is a contagious superficial skin infection caused by staphylococcus in most instances and perhaps by the haemolytic streptococcus in a few cases.

Predisposing factors

The predisposing factors, which lead to this disorder, include crowded living conditions, poor hygiene, preexisting eczema, and scabies and reduced resistance due to preceding influenza or herpes simplex infection.

Clinical features

1. Impetigo contagiosa most frequently affects primary school children. The face (especially around the mouth and nose) is commonly affected. As the name suggests, the disease is highly contagious and rapidly spreads in the family and among playmates.
2. The thin-walled blister rapidly ruptures to form an area of exudation and honey-coloured crusts. Yellowish-gold crust surrounds the lesions, which appear and spread within a few days. Removal of crust reveals erosion. Lesions are usually multiple. Regional lymphadenopathy is frequent.
3. Streptococcal impetigo may be followed by glomerulonephritis.

Microscopically

A submucous vesicle or bulla is produced as the initial or primary lesion. Neutrophils migrate through the living cellular portion of the epidermis and accumulate between it and the overlying cornified portion (the stratum corneum).

Laboratory diagnosis

Gram stain of the exudates shows polymorphs with intracellular and extracellular Gram-positive cocci in chains and cluster.

Pus culture helps to establish the diagnosis.

Management

Oral antibiotics are effective for treatment of impetigo as antistaphylococcal penicillins, amoxicillin, cephalosporins, and macrolides.

A topical skin cream such as mupirocin (bactroban) also may be prescribed.

ERYSIPELAS

Erysipelas is superficial spreading infection of skin caused by streptococcus pyogens. The organisms may gain entry through a superficial break in the skin.

Clinical features

1. Erysipelas appears as an acute erythematous, warm, indurated, rapidly spreading plaque with sharply defined advancing edge.
2. When it involves the face it can have a characteristic butterfly distribution on the cheeks and bridge of the nose.
3. Superficial vacuolation may occur on the plaque.
4. Patients typically develop symptoms including high fevers, shaking chills, fatigue, vomiting and general illness within 24 hours of the initial infection.
5. Associated constitutional symptoms are invariable and may antedate obvious cutaneous lesions.
6. Most severe infections can result in vesicles, bullae, and petechiae with possible skin necrosis.
7. Facial erysipelas, if untreated, may prove fatal. Recurrences may occur in the same area and eventuate into lymphedema.
8. Lymph nodes may be swollen, and lymphedema may occur.
9. Complications include bacteremia, infective endocarditis, septic shock, and necrotising fascitis.

Histological features

Section shows edema and dilatation of lymphatics and capillaries. There is infiltration of dermis by neutrophils.

Management

Depending on the severity, treatment involves either oral or intravenous antibiotics using penicillins, clindamycin, or erythromycin.

SCARLET FEVER

Scarlet fever is a complication of the streptococcal infection by strain of group A streptococci which produce the erythrogenic exotoxin.

Clinical features

Characteristic diffuse, bright scarlet to dusky red skin rash, which appears on the second or third day of illness.

Oral manifestations

It includes the involvement of pharynx, tonsils, soft palate and tongue.

Exudative tonsillitis preceding scarlet fever is often accompanied by erythematous oral mucous membrane, along with petechiae and punctate red macules on the hard and soft palate and uvula.

Strawberry tongue: On day 1 or 2, a white coating covers the dorsum of the tongue with reddened papillae projecting through, giving rise to the white strawberry tongue.

Raspberry tongue: On day 4-5 the white coating disappears showing fiery red tongue with prominent papillae.

Diagnosis

Diagnosis is confirmed by detection of antigens that are specific for group A, beta haemolytic streptococci.

Management of scarlet fever

Antibiotics: Penicillin or erythromycin is treatment of choice given for a full 10 days. A cephalosporin is an effective alternative to penicillin, but not if penicillin-allergic.

GONORRHOEA

Galen in 130 A.D was first employed the gonorrhoea (meaning, flow of seed).

The incubation period is 2-8 days.

The cocci penetrate through intercellular spaces and reach the sub-epithelial connective tissue by the third day of infection.

The surface of the organism is covered by hairy projections called pili. This helps the invasion of the mucosal surfaces by the gonococci.

Gonococci pili mediate the attachment of epithelial cells and prevent them from being washed away by normal vaginal discharges or by the strong flow of urine.

Clinical features

The ulceration in the urethra may heal by fibrosis and end in a structure, which may lead to hypertrophy and dilatation of bladder, ureter and renal pelvis.

Urethritis, pharyngitis, and proctitis are the most common syndromes, determined by the preferred route of sexual contact.

In female, the infection remains hidden for longer period, but produces more devastation. It causes cervicitis, and purulent inflammation of Bartholin glands. The most common consequence of gonorrhoea, however, is pelvic inflammatory disease, a potentially serious infection of the female pelvic organs.

Gonococcal infection may be transmitted to infants during passage through the birth canal. The affected neonate may develop purulent infection of the eyes (Ophthalmia neonatorum)—an important cause of blindness in the past.

Complications include bacteraemia, arthritis, and dermatitis, increased risk of tubal pregnancy and sterility in both sexes.

Oral manifestations

Pharyngeal gonorrhoea: When gonorrhoea is found in the throat, it is called 'pharyngeal gonorrhoea'. In a man, gonorrhoea can also be spread from a man's penis to the throat of his sex partner during oral sex (Gonorrhoea). People can transfer the bacteria from the genital area to the mouth with their fingers.

Most patients who have gonorrhea in the throat also have the infection in other parts of their body as well (penis, rectum, or vagina).

When symptoms are seen, they can include pharyngitis, a sore throat, and tonsillitis.

Gonococcal stomatitis: Isolated ulcers, gingivitis, and membranous gingivostomatitis may develop in gonococcal stomatitis.

Gonococcal arthritis: The joints involved in order of frequency are knee, wrist, elbow, shoulder, hip, ankle, and temporomandibular joint. The exudates may be serous or slightly turbid and, later on, it becomes purulent. In the later condition it may damage the articular surfaces followed by bony ankylosis.

Diagnosis

Demonstration of intracellular, Gram-negative diplococci in stained smears provides a presumptive evidence of gonorrhoea in the male.

Recently DNA amplification technique such as ligase chain reaction is used.

Management

Because a high proportion of men and women who have gonorrhoea also have chlamydia, the goal of treatment is to cure both infections. Partner should be treated at the same time.

Treatment of uncomplicated gonorrhoea consists of antibiotics, including ceftriaxone, cefixime, ciprofloxacin, or ofloxacin for gonorrhoea along with azithromycin, doxycycline or erythromycin for chlamydia.

DIPHTHERIA

It is a life-threatening disorder caused by a highly contagious bacterial infection caused by Gram-positive bacilli, Cornybacterium diphtheriae.

Pathogenesis

The organisms infect most commonly the mucus membrane of pharynx and adjoining structures and because of the liberation of powerful exotoxins they cause extensive mucosal necrosis as well as lead to damage to the heart, nerves, and brain cells.

Clinical features

Diphtheria pseudomembrane is elevated greyish green ('wash-leather') first appears on tonsils or posterior pharyngeal wall and causes fever, red sore throat, weakness and headache. It has well defined edge, is firm and adherent, and is surrounded by a zone of inflammation.

The toxin destroys the normal throat to swell. As the tissue dies the toxin form a thick greyish-white membrane that completely cover the throat. The membrane then spread either upward into nasal passages or downward into the larynx and trachea. In laryngeal diphtheria mechanical obstruction may cause suffocation unless the airway is restored by intubation or tracheostomy.

According to clinical severity diphtheria may be classified as

1. **Malignant or hypertoxic:** In which there is severe toxaemia, with marked cervical adenitis (bull neck). Death is due to myocarditis, palatal paralysis, and neurological complications. Neurological involvement occurs in 75% of cases. After tonsillar or pharyngeal diphtheria it usually starts after 10 days. Paralysis of accommodation often follows, manifest by difficulty in reading small print. Generalised polyneuritis with weakness and paraesthesia may follow the 10-14 days.
2. **Septic:** Which leads to ulceration, cellulitis, and even gangrene around the pseudomembrane.
3. **Haemorrhagic:** Which is characterised by bleeding from the edge of the membrane, epistaxis, conjunctival haemorrhage, purpura and gastrointestinal bleeding tendency.
4. **Laryngeal diphtheria:** With anterior nasal infection there is nasal discharge, frequently blood stained. In laryngeal diphtheria a husky voice and high pitched cough signal-potential respiratory obstruction requiring tracheotomy. If infection spreads to the uvula, fauces and nasopharynx, the patient is gravely ill.

Diagnosis

Laboratory diagnosis consists of isolation of diphtheria bacillus and demonstration of toxicity.

Smears prepared from throat swabs are stained by Loffler's methylene blue, Albert's stain, Neisser's stain and Ponder's stain.

Treatment

Three main areas of management are:

- Administration of antibiotics.
- Adminstration of diphtheria toxin
- Strict isolation procedure.

Penicillin 1200 mg 6-hourly I.V. or amoxicillin 500 mg 8-hourly should be administered for 2 weeks to eliminate C. diphtheriae.

Patient must be managed to strict isolation attended by staff—with diphtheria toxoid following recovery.

TUBERCULOSIS

Mycobacterium hominis, M. tuberculosis bovine and M. microti (human and bovine) causes tuberculosis. Mycobacterium Africanum is a rare pathogen causing tuberculosis in Africa. In addition there are **'opportunistic Mycobacterium'** that are responsible for the atypical forms of tuberculosis including the M. avium intracellulare which complicates the cases of AIDS.

Epidemiology

Tuberculosis poses a significant threat to global health, causing the second highest rate from an infectious disease worldwide, after human immunodeficiency virus. Currently, 30 percent of the world population is estimated to be with the disease. Till 2020, an estimated 1000 million will become newly infected, 150 million will contract disease, and 36 million will die.

India is the highest tuberculosis burden country in the world and accounts for nearly one-fifth (20%) of global burden of tuberculosis.

Mode of transmission

1. **Inhalation:** Inhaling infective droplets coughed or sneezed into air by patients with open case of tuberculosis infects humans with M. tuberculosis most frequently.
2. **Ingestion:** About 1% of infected cows develop lesions in the udder and bacilli are excreted in the milk, which can infect people who drink it raw.
3. **Inoculation:** The bacilli are directly inoculated on an abrasion or a minor cut in the skin of the hands. This mode of infection is seen in butchers, surgeons and pathologist.
4. **Transplacental:** The infection may occur through transplacental route as the placenta has been found to be infected with organisms.
5. **Prenatal:** Conceptional or germinative tuberculosis, as a result of infection of the spermatozoa, would surely destroy the ovum.

Tuberculosis is a chronic infectious granulomatous disease that is caused in human beings by mycobacterium tuberculosis and, less frequently, by mycobacterium bovis. Atypical mycobacteria have been recognised in some cases.

Oral manifestations

Oral tuberculous lesions may be either primary or secondary to occurrence.

Primary tuberculosis of the oral mucosal is very rare. It is associated with drinking raw milk of tuberculous cows. It usually develops when the deciduous tooth is being shed or extracted. Primary lesions are seen in younger patients and present as single painless ulcer with regional lymph node enlargement.

Predisposing factors for primary oral tuberculosis include poor oral dental hygiene, dental extraction, periodontitis, and leukoplakia. It is postulated that such infections are acquired by inhalation, with harboring of disease in Waldeyer's ring.

Secondary tuberculosis: Oral tuberculosis is usually post-primary and occurs in patients affected with advanced pulmonary tuberculosis. It is believed that the organisms enter the mucosa through a small break in the surface. Self-inoculation of patient usually results from infected sputum or by haematogenous or lymphatic dissemination. There is relation between oral tuberculosis and HIV infection.

Sites: The sites most frequently affected are tongue, hard palate, tonsils, pharynx, buccal mucosa and lips. Tongue is the commonest site for oral tuberculous lesion. Extra-pulmonary tuberculosis like tuberculosis of gingiva is an uncommon condition.

Oral tuberculous lesion may take the form of nodules, ulcers, or elevated fissures. Ulcers are irregular with undermined edges, are painful and increase slowly. Tuberculosis of tongue has also presented as macroglossia. It may also be present around the upper aerodigestive tract as parotitis, intraosseous lesions, pre-auricular swelling and trismus, tracheitis and laryngitis.

Microscopically

The biopsy from lesion consists of normal squamous epithelium overlying epitheloid granulomas with caseation, Langhan's giant cells, lymphocytes and fibrous tissue.

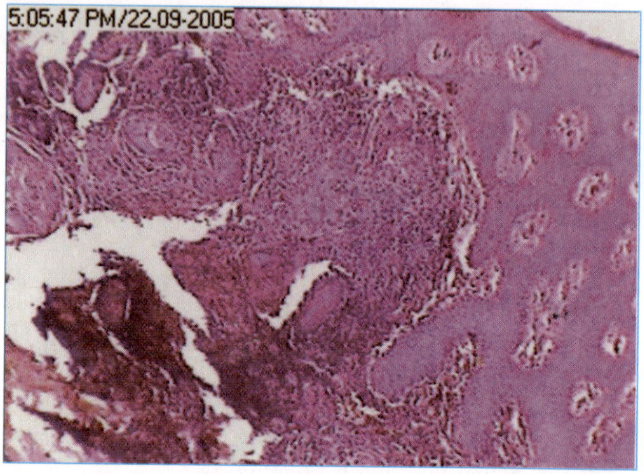

Fig.9.1: Showing epithelial hyperplasia, caseating granulomas with epithelioid cells, Langhan's giant cells and lymphocytes

Management

Antitubercular drugs employed are rifampicin, isoniazid, pyrazinamide, streptomycin, ethambutol, ethionamide, thiacetazone, Paraaminosalicylic acid, and cycloserine.

LEPROSY

Leprosy is a chronic granulomatous disease of man involving primarily the skin, peripheral nerves and nasal mucosa, but capable of affecting any tissue or organ. Mycobacterium leprae was discovered by Almauer Hansen Gerhard of Norway in 1883—leprosy is known as Hansen's disease. It was the first bacillus to be associated with human disease.

Epidemiology

The worldwide prevalence of leprosy is reported to be 5.5 million cases. Eighty percent of cases are formed in five countries—India, Myanmar, Indonesia, Brazil and Nigeria. The states of Chennai, Andhra Pradesh, Bihar, Orissa, West Bengal, Pondicherry and Assam are considered hyperendemic for leprosy, but no state in India is free from leprosy.

Morphology: Mycobacterium leprae is a straight or slightly curved rod, 1-8μ × 0.2-0.5μ in size. The organism is an acid-fast rod, decolourised by acid alcohol. It cannot be cultured, but can be grown in the footpad of mouse or in nine-banded armadillo.

Classification: Two extreme polar forms of disease are lepromatous and tuberculoid type.

Currently, leprosy is classified into following groups:

1. Lepromatous type
2. Borderline lepromatous
3. Indeterminate

4. Mild borderline
5. Borderline tuberculoid
6. Tuberculoid
7. Histoid type
8. Pure neural type.

Clinical features

Lepromatous leprosy

1. Lepromatous leprosy is the generalised form of the disease and is found in individuals where the host resistance is low.
2. Patients develop numerous nodular skin lesions (lepromata on face, earlobes, hands, and feet and, less commonly, trunk. The skin lesions are multiple, slightly hypopigmented, and erythematous macules, papules, or diffuse infiltration).
3. Bacilli invade the mucosa of the nose, mouth, and upper respiratory tract and are shed in large numbers in nasal and oral secretion.
4. Cooler parts of the body, such as ear lobes, are particularly affected.
5. The eyebrows are lost and classical lion (leonine) facies may develop. Eye involvement occurs, creating pain, photophobia, decreased visual acuity, glaucoma and blindness.
6. Nasal infiltration causes saddle nose deformity.
7. Aseptic necrosis and osteomyelitis can occur after repeated trauma.
8. Sensory loss is unusual.
9. Involvement of large peripheral nerves causes disturbances of sensations as well as trophic disturbances and neuroparalysis.
10. Claw-shaped hands, hammer toes, and pendulous ear lobes are common deformities.

Microscopic features

There is thinning of epidermis, atrophy of rete ridges and loss of melanin pigment. The dermal lesions show an extensive cellular infiltrate that is almost invariably separated from the flattened epidermis by a narrow zone of normal collagen. Macrophages with abundant foamy or vacuolated cytoplasm—so-called lepra cells or Virchow cells—predominate. Using Fite stain, innumerable acid-fast bacilli are seen within the lepra cells, where they often lie in bundles, like pack of cigars; if degenerated, in large clumps called globi. Bacilli layden Schwann cells infiltrate the dermal nerves and, eventually, the nerve undergoes fibrosis. It extends into the subcutaneous fat.

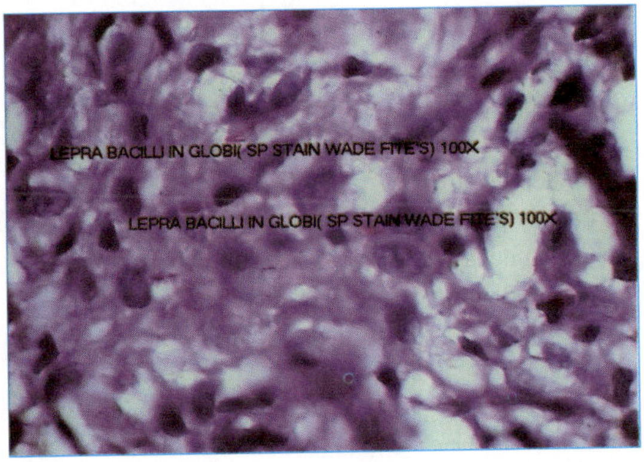

Fig.9.2: Tissue section stained by Wade Fite technique shows acid fast bacillus in a case of lepromatous leprosy

Tuberculoid leprosy

Clinical features of tuberculoid leprosy

1. Erythematous large hypoesthetic plaque with defined borders that are elevated and slope down into an atrophic centre.
2. There is a large asymmetric hypopigmented macule characterised by hypoesthesia and hypopigmentation.

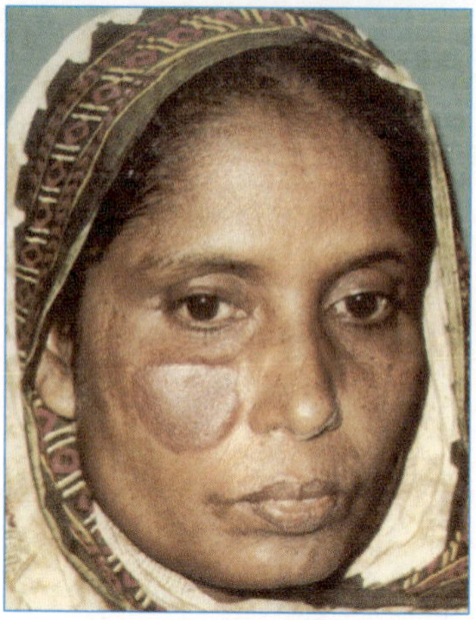

Fig.9.3: A case of Lepromatous leprosy shows depigmented patch over face

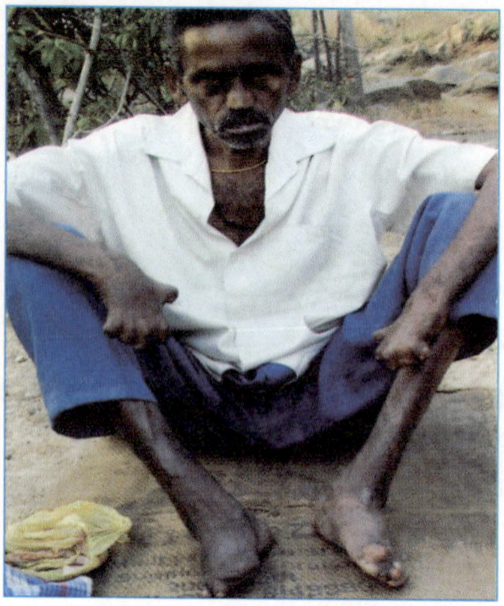

Fig.9.4: A case of tuberculoid leprosy showing destruction of toes and fingers

3. There is hair loss, impairment of sweating, and alopacia.
4. Neural involvement occurs early and may be pronounced leading to deformities, particularly hands and feet.
5. Superficial nerves in the vicinity of lesion may be palpable, e.g., median nerve at wrist and ulnar nerve at the elbow. In severe cases there is paralysis, claw hand, foot drop and anesthesia.
6. There are no systemic manifestations.

Microscopically

Lesions in tuberculoid leprosy consist of tubercle-like epitheloid granuloma which reaches up to epidermis. No clear zone at dermoepidermal junction. Non-caseating granulomas consists of Langhans giant cells, lymphocytes around skin appendages. The infiltration is focal and perivascular, perifollicular, perineural and periglandular. Nerves are infiltrated endoneurone; bacilli are few and more frequently encountered inside nerves.

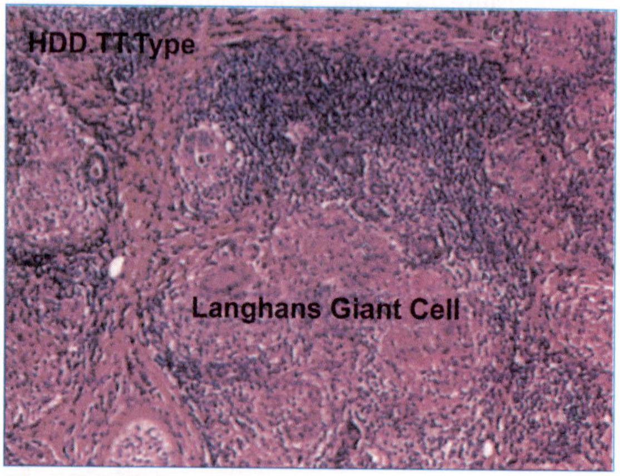

Fig.9.5: Showing non-caseating Granulomas with giant cells and lymphocytic infiltration in a case of tuberculoid leprosy

Oral lesions

Leprotic oral lesions are more common in lepromatous leprosy; indicate a late manifestation and have a great epidemiological importance as a source of infection. Oral lesions usually appear in lepromatous leprosy and occur in 20-60% of cases.

Morphologically, the lesions vary from exanthemas to ulcers, perforations and scars, passing through papules, nodules and superficial erosions. They can involve the following areas:

1. **Palate:** Lepromas formed on the soft palate result in ulceration, necrosis and fibrosis.
2. **Tongue:** The lesions are seen mostly on the top of tongue, which varies from superficial, silver erosions with loss of papilla to heavy nodular infiltration with characteristic paving-stone appearance.

3. **Uvula:** In extreme cases there is intense fibrosis with partial loss or even complete destruction of uvula.
4. **Lips:** Small tumour-like masses called lepromas develop on the lips. These nodules have a tendency to break down and ulcerate. There may be macrocheilia (caused by infiltration) or microstomia (caused by ulceration and subsequent repair with fibrosis of perioral or lip lepromas).
5. **Gums:** They are usually affected in the areas behind upper central incisors, often by contiguity, of lesions of the hard palate. Chronic gingivitis, periodontitis and periodontoclasia may occur. Gingival hyperplasia with loosening of teeth has been reported. In long-standing cases there is pulpal necrosis due to invasion of pulp by granulomatous tissue. This gives a pinkish-red discolouration to the teeth.

Maxilla: There may be destruction of the anterior maxilla and loss of teeth.

Laboratory diagnosis

Tissue smear: An incision is made in the skin and the scalpel blade is used to obtain fluid from a lesion. The fluid is placed on a glass slide and stained using the Ziehl-Neelsen acid-fast method to look for organisms.

Skin biopsy: This should be examined for morphology and for acid-fast bacilli. Biopsy is useful for histological typing of leprosy.

CERVICOFACIAL ACTINOMYCOSIS

Cervicofacial actinomycosis is a chronic infection of the head and neck occurring most often in adult males and caused by bacteria of the genus actinomyces.

Actinomyces supp are part of normal flora of the oropharynx. The most common pathogen is Actinomyces Israelii, Gram-positive anaerobes with a filamentous branching growth pattern.

Risk factors

Risk factors for cervicofacial actinomycosis include:

- Tooth decay
- Dental operations
- Maxillofacial trauma.

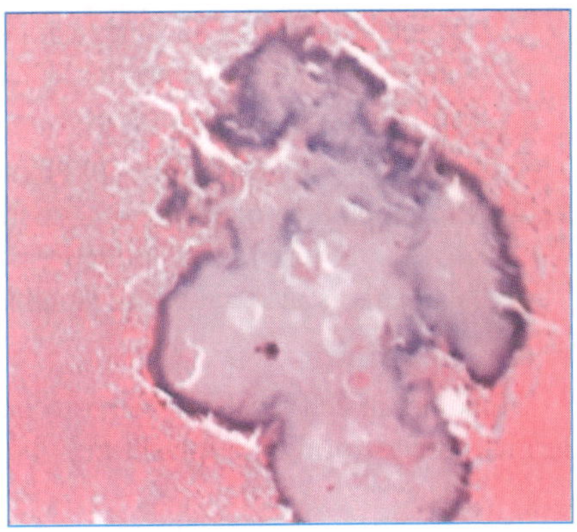

Fig.9.6: Fungal grain from a case of actinomycosis

Clinical features

1. Early signs include a small, flat hard swelling in the mouth or on the neck or jaw (subperiosteal).
2. Many small communicating abscesses then appears with surrounding granulation and sinuses that discharge sulphur-like granules containing the organism.
3. Actinomycosis of teeth usually presents as a painful local swelling.
4. Actinomycosis of tongue is very rare. It usually presents as a painful firm nodule involving the lateral portion of the mobile tongue and is often mistaken for malignancy.
4. The next most common involvement is the cheek. These probably arise from maxillary teeth or mucosal injury.
5. The body of maxilla itself, the pre-maxillary space, and the maxillary sinus may be involved.

Microscopically, there are varying numbers of granules present in periapical actinomycosis is reported usually in association with previous trauma to a tooth, or a dental procedure.

SYPHILITIC LESIONS

The lesion develops at the primary site of infection with Treponema pallidum.

Primary syphilis: The primary lesion develops in the skin or mucous membrane at the site of infection, 2-12 weeks after infection, and heals in 2-4 weeks. If patient have engaged in oral sex, then the chancre may occur in the oral cavity. Extragenital syphilis occurs commonly on the lips. The upper lip is affected more often than the lower lip, and the lesions are often in the middle of the lip. The chancres are occasionally seen on the tongue or tonsil, and rarely on the gum or in the pharynx. It produces a painful ulcer with large significant enlargement of regional lymph nodes.

It may be seen in the adult or in the child. Chancre of the tongue is more frequent in men than in women, and in middle-aged or elderly men gives rise to a suspicious of a malignant growth.

The chancre is usually an isolated ulcer, situated on the free edge of the lip. The ulcer is painful, slow-growing with increasing duration.

Microscopically

The section shows an ulcer with edema and dense infiltration by plasma cells, macrophages, and lymphocytes. The cells accumulate particularly around the small blood vessels. The vascular endothelial cells are enlarged and prominent and may proliferate, causing a reduction of the lumen (endarteritis and periarteritis).

Secondary syphilis: Secondary lesions appear at a variable interval, usually 2-3 months after infection.

Oral lesions are multiple greyish erosions on the mucus patches occurring anywhere on the oral mucosa; however, the tongue, lips, soft palate and tonsils are the most commonly affected sites.

The lesions of the mucosa in the secondary stage of syphilis are of several varieties

1. Among the earliest is a small red papule to be seen on the soft palate, lips, cheeks, tonsils, anterior pillar of the fauces and tongue surrounded by an area of bright erythema.
2. Typical mucous membrane lesions tend to be white, oval, serpiginous, raised erosions or ulcers with an erythematous border. There is an overlying grey or silver membrane. These ulcers are known as **'snail-track ulcers'**.
3. Sometimes these lesions can appear as leukokeratosis. Ulcers heal with fine tissue paper scar.
4. The moist area of the body—such as nasal cleft and angle of mouth—may show raised warty growths covered with sodden epithelium, greyish-white in appearance and called condyloma lata. This is also called as Hutchinson's wart.

Microscopically

Endothelial cell swelling, perivascular infiltrates with a preponderance of plasma cells, and epidermal psoriasiform hyperplasia may be observed.

Diagnosis

Laboratory diagnosis consists of demonstration of the spirochetes under microscope and antibodies in the serum.

In condyloma, and mucous patches or ulcers of the mouth, the secretions may be swarming with spirochaetes and are highly infectious. Spirochaetes can be demonstrated by dark ground illumination.

Tertiary syphilis: Tertiary lesions appear irregularly, especially in the internal organs, skin and mucous membranes.

There are two types of lesions in tertiary syphilis:

1. Gummas on the palate that produce palatal perforation
2. Chronic inflammation of the tongue associated with arteritis.

Gumma consists of parenchymal necrosis, surrounded by a layer of granulation and fibrous tissue showing usual infiltration by mononuclear cells.

Congenital syphilis

Congenital syphilis is acquired by transplacental infection and its severity depends mainly on the duration of maternal infection.

Oral lesions consist of Hutchinson's incisors, Pfluger and mulberry molars, gummas, glossitis, mucus patches, and fissuring and scarring of the corners of the mouth.

Hutchinson's incisors: These teeth may resemble a screwdriver, or may show notching of the incisor edges. There is also pitting of the first permanent molars.

Mulberry and Pfluger Molars: The occlusal surfaces are much narrower than normal and give the crown a pinched appearance.

Moon's teeth: Dome-shaped deformity of the first permanent molars called moon's teeth.

RHINOSCLEROMA

Hebra described it in 1870. It is an infective granuloma caused by Klebsiella rhinoscleromatis.

The disease is worldwide distributed and is endemic in South and Central America, and in central parts of Eastern Europe.

Sites: The disorder always begins in the nose. It may extend in the larynx, pharynx, trachea, bronchus, lacrimal glands, brain and occasionally skin of the upper lip.

Clinically

There is a hard, progressive nodular swelling of the nose accompanied by ulceration and foul discharge. There is impairment of sensation of taste anesthesia of soft palate, enlargement of uvula and upper lip. Nasal obstruction is common and laryngeal and oesophageal stenosis can occur. It occurs at any age and in both sexes.

Histopathology

The cellular infiltrate is very rich in plasma cells and lymphocytes. The characteristic cells are known as Mikulicz cells—called after a German surgeon. Mikulicz cell is a large histiocyte measuring up to 100 μ in diameter. They are filled by pale gelatinous material, giving the cytoplasm a foamy appearance and eccentric nucleus. One finds within the cytoplasm of Mikulicz cells many bacilli called Klebsiella Rhinoscleromatis Offrisch bacilli. They can be visualised with Giemsa's stain or a silver stain.

Russel bodies are round to ovoid formations, measuring from 20 to 40 μ in diameter. They have a homogeneous, bright red light refractile cytoplasm with no nucleus.

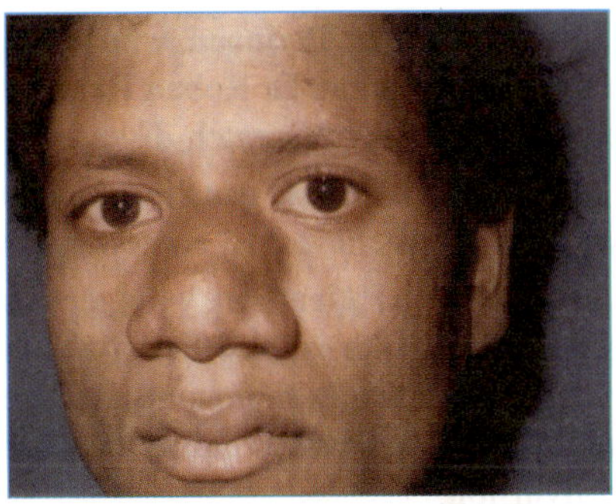

Fig.9.7: Showing swelling inside nasal cavity (Rhinoscleroma)

Management of rhinoscleroma

Surgery combined with antibiotic therapy is beneficial in patients with granulomatous disease and nasal or pharyngeal obstruction or nasal sinus involvement due to the proliferation of lesions.

NOMA

Noma (Cancrum oris or gangrenous stomatitis): It is a gangrenous condition occasionally seen in poorly nourished children and tends to complicate debilitating infections; it begins on the gum and spreads to the cheek.

(inguinal in males and pararectal in females) become inflamed and adherent to the overlying skin. The bacilli multiply in lymph nodes. The enlarged inguinal lymph nodes are known as bubos. Resolution is by rupture and discharge of pus or by involution without rupture.

Metastatic complications may sometimes occur involving joints, eyes, and meninges.

Oral lesions

Tongue is the most common site. Lesion consists of small, slightly painful superficial ulceration with non-indurated borders, which appear on lip.

Diagnosis

1. Smears from bubo (inguinal adenitis) or scrapping of urethra, cervix, or vagina are stained by Giemsa stain. Elementary bodies (Miyagawa's granulocorpuscles) may be detected in positive smears.
2. **Serological tests for detection of antibodies:**
   (i) **Microimmunofluoresence:** Staining of smears by fluorescent antibodies may also show elementary bodies.
   (ii) Complement fixation test becomes positive two weeks after infections.
3. **Culture:** Material is inoculated into the yolk sac of chick embryo, mice or tissue culture.
4. PCR for chlamydia trachomatis.
5. DNA probes can be used for antigen detection.
6. **Frei's test:** It is a skin test using LGV antigen and shows delayed type of hypersensitivity.

VIRAL INFECTIONS

Members of the human herpes virus and human papilloma virus (HPV) families are the most common causes of primary viral infections of oral cavity. Many other viral infections can affect the oral cavity in humans as either localised or systemic infections. Other viral conditions of the oral cavity are human immunodeficiency virus, Coxsackie virus infection, mumps, measles (rubeola), and rubella.

HERPES SIMPLEX VIRUS INFECTION

Cold sores are called fever blister or herpes simplex because they are caused by herpes simplex virus type I, which is very contagious and occur outside the mouth.

The most frequent viral infection of oral epithelium is caused by herpes simplex type I virus. This occurs in the primary form as acute herpetic gingivostomatitis characterised by extensive painful ulceration and occasionally generalised upset. Both keratinised and non-keratinized oral mucosa may be involved.

The herpetic infection is triggered by cold or sun exposure, stress, trauma, ultraviolet light, and respiratory tract infection, and weakened immune system.

Clinical features

Herpetic gingivostomatitis is transmitted by close contact. 90% of people develop antibodies in early childhood. Vesicles (2-3 mm diameter) followed by circular sharply define shallow ulcers (with yellowish or greyish floor and red margins) and affect any part of the oral mucosa. Gingivitis is characterised by red and swollen margins. Lymphadenopathy is associated with fever of variable severity. Lesions resolve within a week to 10 days.

Secondary or recurrent herpetic lesions are more frequent, especially at mucocutaneous junctions round the lips, nose, tongue, and cheeks. The initially vesicular phase is followed by ulceration and crusting.

Microscopically, the vesicles begin as an intraepithelial focus of intracellular and intercellular edema.

CONDYLOMA ACCUMINATA

Condyloma accuminatum—also known as venereal wart—is produced by infection with either Human Papilloma Virus (HPV-6, or HPV-11).

Site: They may develop in any oral mucosa including the gingival. They occur more commonly on non-keratinised mucosa than on keratinised mucosa.

Clinical features

These lesions are usually cribriform, pink, and sessile, and solitary or multiple.

Gingival lesions tend to be characterized by multiple, white finger-like projections, which are covered by keratin. These papillary lesions can be multiple or single and tend to develop on interdental papillae.

Diagnosis

1. Viral cultures of vesicular fluid.
2. Direct fluorescent antibody staining of scraped lesions remains the standard of diagnosis.
3. HSV can be identified using polymerase chain reaction (PCR).
4. The presence of intranuclear inclusion bodies and multi nucleated giant cells on a Tzanck preparation or Calcofluor stain is supportive of a diagnosis of herpetic viral infection.

HERPES ZOSTER

Shingles

Herpes zoster is a common, predominantly dermal, and neurologic disorder caused by the varicella-zoster virus (VZV)—a virus morphologically and antigenically identical to the virus causing varicella.

An increased incidence of herpes zoster occurs in Hodgkin's disease, leukaemias, and other malignancies, HIV infection, after administration of corticosteroids and other immunosuppressive drugs, and during radiation therapy.

Clinical features

Zoster most commonly manifests in one or posterior spinal ganglia or cranial sensory ganglia, presumably because viral particles have been preserved within these ganglia in a dormant state since the original episode of varicella. This results in pain and characteristic cutaneous findings along the corresponding sensory dermatoses of the involved ganglion.

Although thoracic dermatoses are most commonly involved, the ophthalmic division of the trigeminal nerve is frequently implicated; vesicles may appear on the cornea and lead to ulceration. Geniculate ganglion involvement causes the Ramsay Hunt syndrome of facial palsy, ipsilateral loss of taste and buccal ulceration, plus a rash in the external auditory canal.

Oral manifestations

Oral lesions are less common than cutaneous shingles, but do occur and are painful. An itching sensation and pain, which may simulate pulpitis, precede oral lesions. These begin in as unilateral clusters of vesicles, which rupture, in 2-3 days leaving ulcers surrounded by broad erythematous area. Rarely osteomyelitis, necrosis of jaw bone or loss of teeth may occur in immunocompromised patients.

Within the oral cavity the mucosa presents with numerous small papulovesicular lesions, which can appear on the palate to the midline. These lesions can involve the gingival, buccal mucosa, tongue, and the palate. The lesions are seen on the jaw tongue.

Microscopically

Varicella-zoster virus induces vesicles in the epidermis and mucus membranes. These vesicles show epithelial degeneration, necrosis, multinucleate giant cell formation, intranuclear eosinophilic inclusion bodies and haemorrhage. Secondary bacterial infection is rare, but does occur, and turns the haemorrrhagic vesicles into a pustule. When this occurs, the basal cell layer of the epidermis is destroyed, leading to long-term scars.

HERPANGINA

The term is derived from herp, an itching, and angina, a sore throat, literally 'choking'.

Etiology

It is uncommon infection of the oral mucosa by coxsackie virus A, occurs as vesicular lesion on the palate. It can be caused by coxsackie 1-5, echoviruses 3, 6, 9, 11, 16, 17, 22, 25, and 30, enterovirus 71.

Enteroviral infections occur worldwide.

Clinical features

It is most common in children and very contagious. It typically occurs during summer and spreads via the fecal-oral route. Fresh water sources, e.g., lakes may act as a reservoir for transmission.

All enteroviral infections may cause fever, which may be the first apparent symptom. Sore throat may develop.

Small number of lesions usually (2-6) forms in the back area of the mouth, uvula particularly the soft palate or tonsillar pillars.

In patients with herpangina, lesions characteristically appear as erythematous macules initially. These evolve into vesicles that ulcerate centrally creating an erythematous halo.

ACQUIRED IMMUNODEFICIENCY SYNDROME

Luc-Montagnier and Robert Gallo of the Pasteur Institute in Paris isolated the first HIV-1 virus in 1983 and labelled it lymphadenopathy associated virus or LAV. Gallo et al (1984) described numerous isolates of a retrovirus called HTLV-III from homosexuals, haemophiliacs with AIDS and AIDS related complex.

Epidemiology

AIDS has rapidly established itself throughout the world, and likely to endure and persist well into the 21st century. A total of 39.5 million (34.1-47.1 million estimated) people are living with HIV infection in 2006. Total numbers of adults died due to AIDS were 2.6 million and total numbers of children died due to AIDS were 390,000.

In sub-Saharan countries adults and children are acquiring HIV at a higher rate than ever before. In Botswana, a shocking 35.8% of adults are now infected with HIV, while in South Africa, 19.9 % are infected. With total of 4.71 million infected people, South Africa has the largest number of people living with HIV/AIDS in the world.

In India, as elsewhere, the epidemic continues to shift towards women and the young. As this is a disease of reproductive age group, newborn children are also becoming affected by vertical transmission from the mother. Maharashtra, Chennai, Andhra Pradesh, Manipur and Nagaland, HIV infection has crossed 1% or more in antenatal women.

Etiology

Acquired immunodeficiency syndrome (AIDS) is a widespread fatal disease that is caused by human immunodeficiency viruses 1 and 2 (HIV 1 and HIV 2). The recent edition of a new Cameron variant (HIV-M) has thrown open the possibility of finding more of these in the future. The fundamental lesion in AIDS is infection of CD4 + helper T lymphocytes by HIV, leading to the depletion of this cell population and consequent impaired immune function.

Morphology

HIV is a spherical virus, about 90-120 nm in diameter with a three-layer structure. In the centre are two identical copies of ssRNA associated with reverse transcriptase and surrounded by an icosahedral capsid, which, in turn, is surrounded by a matrix protein followed by a host cell membrane

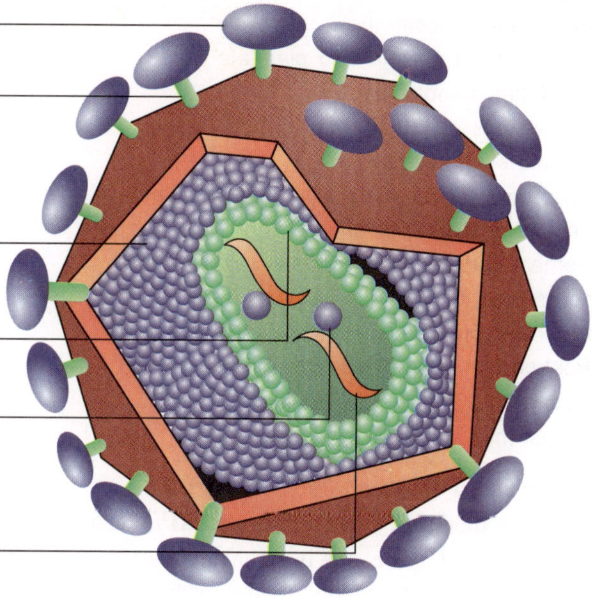

Fig.9.8: Structure of HIV virus

derived lipid bilayer envelop from which project 72 glycoprotein peplomeres. Encodes core or a capsid and matrix protein, the pol gene encodes the reverse transcriptase (polymerase) and the env gene encodes the virion envelope peplomer protein.

Acquired immunodeficiency syndrome (AIDS) is a widespread fatal disease that is caused by Human deficiency viruses 1 and 2(HIV-1 and HIV-2)

TABLE 9.1
MAJOR ANTIGENS OF HIV

Antigens	HIV-1	HIV-2
Spike antigen	gp 120	gp 140
Transmembrane Pedicle antigen	gp 41	gp 36
Matrix protein antigen	P17	P16
Capsid protein antigen	P24	P26

TABLE 9.2
COMMON MODES OF TRANSMISSION OF HIV

I. Sexual intercourse
- Anal, vaginal, oral

II. Blood and blood products
- Blood transfusion
- Factor VIII concentrate
- Recipients of plasma and platelets

III. Contaminated needles
- Intravenous drug abusers sharing needles
- Needle stick injuries
- Injections with unsterile syringes, needles

IV. Tissue and organ transplant
- Semen, cornea, bone marrow, kidney, liver

V. Mother to fetus
- Antenatal (in utero)
- Post-partum (at birth) Blood, amniotic fluid
- Post-natal
  Breast milk

Mode of transmission of virus

There are three modes of transmission of HIV: Sexual, parenteral, and perinatal.

1. **Sexual contact:** Homosexual, bisexual and heterosexuals are the spreaders of infection, while in contact with blood or lymph. In prostitutes, rates up to 25% have been reported. As with any venereal infection, the risk rises with the number of sexual partners. This is reflected in the association of infection with other sexually transmitted diseases. Anal intercourse facilitates transmission of the infection to blood stream. Heterosexual transmission is the major mode of transmission of HIV in many developed countries.

   Risk of transmission is 8 to 10 times higher in sexually transmitted diseased patients. If an STD, such as syphilis, chancroid or herpes, causes ulceration in the genital or perianal region it is of the infected partner, it becomes far easier for HIV to pass into his or her tissues.

2. **Blood transmission**

   a. HIV has been isolated from blood including lymphocytes, macrophages and plasma. Parental transmission may occur through blood transfusion. Transmission of HIV has been recorded in a few recipients of blood transfusion even when the blood transfused was found negative for HIV antibodies. This occurs when the blood is collected in the **'window period'** i.e., the interval between the time of exposure to the virus and development of detectable levels of antibodies.

      Blood component recipient who are non-haemophiliacs, but who received transfusion of components (platelet and plasma), composed 2.5% of the patients. It can also be transmitted from the donors of bone marrow, semen, and organs like cornea, kidney, and liver. Therefore, donors of various fluids and organs should be screened for AIDS before they donate them.

   b. **Intravenous drug abusers:** Sharing blood-contaminated syringes can also transmit AIDS. Therefore, HIV is more common in intravenous drug users who share syringes and needles. The incidence is 18.4%.

c. **Haemophiliacs, especially** those who received large quantity of factor VIII concentrate, made up 1% of all the cases.

d. **Contaminated needles and syringes** and inadequately sterilised medical equipments can trasmit HIV virus. Any skin piercing (including injections, ear piercing, tattooing, acupuncture or scarification) can transmit the virus.

e. **Transplacental spread**, ante-partum, during delivery, and via ingestion of HIV contaminated breast milk.

Mechanism of action

Stage 1. Attachment and entry

A. Entry of HIV into CD + cells occurs when the gp120 envelope proteins interact directly through conserved CD binding site, and other cell surface

B. The virus enters cells through chemokine receptors such as CCR5 and CXCR4.

C. Then by pinocytosis, the nucleocapsid of the virion enters into host cell. After entering into the cell, the nucleocapsid releases its RNA into the cytoplasm.

Stage 2. Reverse transcription and integration: After penetrating the cell and uncoating, NA copy is transcribed from the RNA genome by the reverse transcriptase (RT) enzyme that is carried by the infecting virion. This cDNA is transported into the nucleus and integrated randomly within the host cell genome via integrase enzyme.

Stage 3. Transcription, translation and replication: The provirus then either remains latent or is transcribed into messenger RNA (mRNA). These then migrate to the cell surface and are assembled using the host surface, incorporating the host cell membrane as their own lipid bilayer coat, and cell lysis occurs.

Stage 4. Maturation and viral dissemination: To complete the life cycle, nascent virus is assembled in the cytoplasm and disseminated to other target cells. This is accomplished either by fusion of an infected cell with an uninfected one or by the budding of virions from the plasma membrane of the infected cell.

Clinical features

Clinical features of HIV infection have been classified into four broad groups:

1. **Initial infection with the virus and development of antibodies:** Within 3-17 weeks after exposure to HIV, 30-50% cases develop an acute viral illness of 2 weeks resembling infectious mononucleosis, showing headache, high grade fever, joint pain, lymphomatosis, myalgia, skin rash, sore throat, aseptic meningitis and encephalitis. The development of detectable antibodies to HIV occurs approximately 8 to 12 weeks after initial infection.
2. **Asymptomatic carrier stage:** All persons with HIV, whether they develop seroconversion illness or not, pass through a long asymptomatic period of 1 to 12 years.
3. **AIDS related complex:** A person with AIDS related complex has illnesses caused by damage to the immune system, but without the opportunistic infections and cancer associated AIDS. The typical constitutional symptoms are fatigue, unexplained fever, persistent diarrhoea, and generalised lymphadenopathy, occasional night sweat and marked night sweat.
4. **Full blown AIDS:**
    1. Pulmonary diseases

       Bacterial pneumonia: Commonest pneumonias are pneumococcal lobar pneumonias, other include the klebseilla, staphylococcus aureus, haemophilus and pseudomonas.
    2. Pneumocystis carinii pneumonia is a common disorder of the late stages of AIDS with low CD4 + T cell counts in Europe and America.

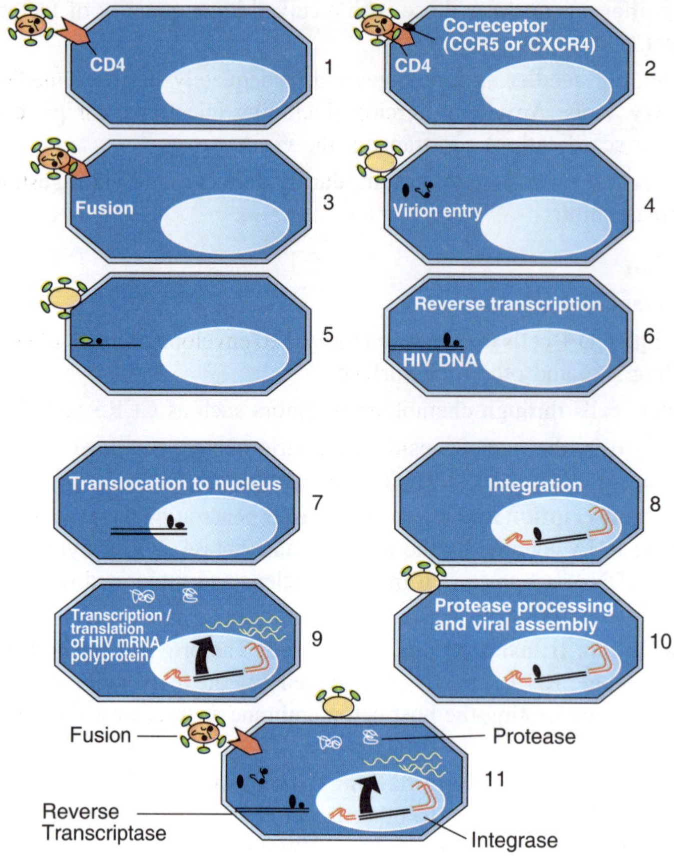

Fig.9.9: Life cycle of HIV virus

3. **Fungal infection:** Histoplasma capsulatum infection is relatively infrequent in patients with HIV disease. It may present with scattered pulmonary infiltrate. Other fungal infections include Cryptococcus neoformans, Aspergillous fumigatous and Coccidioidomycosis immitis can occur.
4. **Tuberculosis:** Mycobaterium avium intracellulare an opportunistic pathogen causes severe disseminated infection in AIDS patients. The organisms are resistant to antituberculous agents. Tuberculosis is widely recognised as the commonest opportunistic disease associated with HIV infection.

Heart: Cardiac valvular lesions are quiet common in AIDS. Other lesions include Marantic endocarditis, left ventricular dysfunctions dilated cardiomyopathy, and accelerated atherosclerosis.

Opportunistic infections like Trypanosoma cruzi, toxoplasmosis, infective endocarditis, fungal myocarditis are common in AIDS patients.

Generalised lymphadenopathy: This is largely due to HIV and occurs commonly in the posterior cervical lymph node chain. Lymphadenopathy in the HIV patients may occur as a result of tuberculosis, non-Hodgkin's lymphomas and toxoplasmosis. Three pattern of changes can be encountered, e.g., hyperplasia, partial depletion and complete depletion.

Neurological disease: Dementia, encephalopathy, myelopathy, peripheral neuropathy, diminished concentration and memory and motor disturbances such as tremors and loss of balance.

Renal abnormalities: A specific HIV-associated nephropathy presents as severe nephrotic syndrome as a consequence of glomerulosclerosis, which may progress to end stage renal failure.

Gastrointestinal tract: Between 50 to 90% of AIDS patients in USA have gastrointestinal symptoms. The underlying disorders include infections, tumours, and HIV related enteropathy; all of which present with intractable diarrhoea and malabsorption.

Eyes: Cytomegalovirus retinitis is one of the leading etiological agents. HIV retinopathy, a benign transient focal ischemia, seen as a cotton wool spot, is quite common.

Skin: Skin lesions include, pruritis, dermatitis, herpes lesions, xeroderma, seborrheic warts, psoriasis, dermatophytosis, folliculitis, and molluscum contagiosum.

HIV related malignancy: Kaposi's sarcoma is the most common malignancy associated with HIV-1 infection. Human herpes virus 8 has been proposed as a possible cause of Kaposi's sarcoma in AIDS patients.

Systemic non-Hodgkin's lymphoma and primary cerebral lymphoma usually complicates late stage of HIV.

Cervical carcinoma is also increased in patients with AIDS. This is attributable to a high prevalence of human papilloma-virus infection in patients with AIDS and AIDS related immunocompromise.

ORAL MANIFESTATIONS OF HIV

TABLE 9.3
COMMON HIV ASSOCIATED ORAL DISORDERS

INFECTION

Fungal

Candidiasis, cryptococcus, mucormycosis

Histoplasmosis, aspergillosis, cryptococcus neoformans, geotrichosis

Viral

Herpes simplex virus, varicella zoster, Epstein-Barr virus, human papilloma virus, cytomegalovirus, oral hairy leukoplakia

Bacterial

Bacillary angiomatosis, linear erythematous gingivitis, necrotising ulcerative periodontititis, syphilis, actinomycosis, tuberculosis

Mycoplasma avium intracellulare

Neoplasms

Fungal-Kaposi's sarcoma

Viral-Non-Hodgkin's lymphoma

Squamous cell carcinoma

Immune mediated

Fungal-Major aphthous ulcer

Viral-Necrotizing stomatitis

Waldeyer's ring lymphoid hyperplasia

Others

Salivary gland disorders, Xerostomia

Contd.

Contd.

Neurologic disorders: Paraesthesia, facial palsy, dysphagia

Bacterial: Nutritional

Miscellaneous: Xerostomia, Toxic epidermolysis, granuloma annulare, thrombocytopaenia, hyperpigmentation, exfoliative chelitis

Xerostomia

Xerostomia is a major contributing factor in dental decay in HIV infected individuals

Candidiasis

Oral candidiasis is commonly encountered among the following patients:

1. Those who wear dentures
2. Those who are debilitated
3. Those with diabetes mellitus
4. Those with anaemia
5. Those undergoing chemotherapy
6. Those receiving corticosteroids or broad-spectrum antibiotics.

Candidiasis and HIV: Candidiasis is often the first manifestation of HIV infection, and HIV testing should be considered in patients with no known predisposing cause for candida over-growth. The cause of candidiasis in known HIV infected patient correlates with the degree of immune suppression and overall disease progression, heralding the subsequent development of AIDS.

Based on clinical appearances, oral candidiasis can appear as one of the four distinct clinical entities:

1. Erythematous or atrophic candidiasis
2. Pseudomembranous candidiasis
3. Hyperplastic or chronic candidiasis
4. Angular cheilitis

Erythematous candidiasis: The condition presents as red flat subtle lesion on the dorsal surface of the tongue or on the hard or soft palates. It may present as **'kissing'** lesion if a lesion is present on the tongue, the palate should be examined for a matching lesion or vice versa.

Pseudomembranous candidiasis appears as creamy, white, curd like plaques on the buccal mucosa, tongue and other mucosal surfaces. The mucosa may appear red when plaque is removed.

Hyperplastic candidiasis: This type of candidiasis is unusual in persons with HIV infection. The lesion appears white and hyperplastic. The white areas are due to hyperkeratosis and, unlike the plaques of pseudomembranous candidiasis, cannot be removed by scraping. These lesions may be confused with hairy leukoplakia.

Diagnosis of hyperplastic candidiasis is made from the histological appearance of hyperkeratosis and presence of hyphae.

Angular cheilitis: It appears clinically as redness, ulceration, and fissuring either unilaterally or bilaterally at the corners of the mouth. It may appear alone or in conjunction with another form of candidiasis.

Herpes simplex virus: Recurrent intraoral HSP lesions occur more commonly on poorly keratinised tissue like the buccal and labial mucosa, an uncommon site in healthy individuals.

Oral hairy leukoplakia: It appears as an asymptomatic adherent white patch with vertical corrugations, most commonly on the lateral borders of the tongue and may spread to cover the entire dorsal surface. They may also spread downward onto the ventral surface of the tongue, where they form usually flat lesions. Rarely, lesions occur on the soft palate. The surface is irregular and may have prominent folds or projections, some times markedly resembling hair. Hairy leukoplakia lesions vary in size and appearance and may be unilateral or bilateral. Oral hairy leukoplakia has since been shown to be associated with a localised (Epstein-Barr virus) infection and occur in individuals whose CD4 lymphocyte count is less than 200/mm^3.

Histologically, parakeratosis and koilocytes are seen with little or no underlying inflammation.

In one study hairy leukoplakia is seen in 19% of HIV positive patients with oral lesions.

Human papilloma virus (HPV): The most common genotypes found in the mouth of patients with HIV infection are 2, 6, 11, 13, 16, and 32.

Syphilis

Several studies have shown that syphilis may manifest as unusual skin and mucosal lesions in HIV infected patient usually associated with aggressive evolution of the disease. These unusual manifestations of syphilis are also often associated with unusual clinical and laboratory findings.

Waldeyer's ring lymphoid hyperplasia is a symptomatic complication of HIV infection.

Characteristically, the process is accompanied by a scattering of multinucleated giant cells adjacent to the tonsillary crypt of surface epithelium.

Kaposi's sarcoma

Kaposi's sarcoma may occur intraorally, either alone or in association with skin and disseminated lesions. Intraoral lesions have been reported at other sites and may be the first manifestation of late stage HIV disease (AIDS). Kaposi's sarcoma occurs most commonly in men but also has been observed in women.

Clinical features

Site: Most common oral site is the hard palate, but the lesions may occur in any part of oral mucosa, including the gingival, soft palate and buccal mucosa.

Kaposi's sarcoma can appear as a red, blue, or purplish lesion. Occasionally, yellowish mucosa surrounds the Kaposi's lesion. Oral Kaposi's lesions may enlarge, ulcerate, and become infected.

Lymphoma: Diffuse, undifferentiated non-Hodgkin's lymphoma (NHL) is a frequent HIV- associated malignancy. Most are of B cell origin, and Epstein-Barr virus occurs in cells from several cases. Lymphoma can occur anywhere in the oral cavity and there may be soft tissue involvement with or without involvement of underlying bone. The lesion may present as firm, painless swelling that may be ulcerated.

Neutropenic ulcers: Neutropenic ulcerations are very painful ulcerations that can appear on both keratinised tissues and are associated with absolute granulocyte counts of less than 800/ul. These lesions are being found with increasing frequency in the HIV-infected population, although the cause of this increase in frequency remains unknown.

Waldeyer's ring lymphoid hyperplasia is an often-symptomatic complication of HIV infection.

Characteristically, the process is accompanied by a scattering of multinucleated giant cells adjacent to the tonsillary crypt of surface epithelium. These cells, which harbor significant amounts of HIV, exhibit histiocytic markers and probably belong to the accessory immune system.

Laboratory diagnosis of HIV infection

The laboratory tests employed to establish the diagnosis of HIV infection consists of:

I. Specific tests for HIV infection

A. Demonstration of HIV antigen

B. Demonstration of antibodies

C. Isolation of virus.

II. Tests for proviral DNA

III. Tests to establish immunodeficiency

A. Total leukocyte count and lymphocyte count

B. Reversal of T4:T8 lymphocyte ratio

C. B-2 macroglobulin

D. Platelet count: Marked thrombocytopaenia

E. Raised IgG and IgA levels.

Demonstration of viral antigen

1. ELISA can detect P24 antigen in the serum in 30% of patients during window period in 10% of asymptomatic patients and 50 to 60% of AIDS patients. As the antibody response builds up antigen tests become negative. However, late in the infection, P24 antigen may reappear until most of the patients with AIDS give a positive test. Detection of P24 antigen indicates active HIV infection.
2. HIV proviral by PCR is very sensitive but expensive. Using oligonucleotides directed as highly conserved regions of the viral genome uses HIV DNA RCR to detect HIV-1 provirus in mononuclear cells. This test can be performed within 24 hours of infection and has sensitivity and a specificity of 95% and 97%, respectively. Although it is more sensitive than viral culturing, the diagnostic performances of the 2 methods are equivalent.
3. Plasma HIV type I RNA can be detected and quantitated by RT-PCR; this is by far the most sensitive method available in laboratories for diagnosis of HIV infection.
4. RNA transcription.
5. An enzyme labelled probe binds to the immobilised probe.

Demonstration of antibody

Antibodies to HIV are far easier to detect than the virus itself, their presence or absence in the blood stream is the basis for the most widely used test of HIV infection.

A person whose blood contains HIV antibodies is said to be seropositive, meaning that she or he is infected with HIV.

1. ELISA
   a. **Rapid HIV tests**, followed by confirmatory HIV tests, which provide results in minutes, simplify and expand the availability of HIV testing. Their sensitivity is as high as 100%.
   b. **Western blot:** This is a highly specific confirmatory test. Specificity when combines with ELISA > 99.99%. It is based on detecting specific antibody to viral core antigen (P24) and envelops glycoprotein (gp41). This is a more difficult test to perform, very costly and requires trained and experienced laboratory workers to interpret the results.
   c. **Immunofluorescence:** In this test, HIV infected cells are acetone fixed on slides and then reacted with test serum followed by fluorescein conjugated anti-human gamma globulin. A positive reaction appears as apple-green fluorescence of cell membrane under fluorescence microscope.
   d. Radio immunoassay (RIA).
   e. Viral cultures are obtained by co-cultivating potentially infected and uninfected mononuclear cells together promote viral replication. Every few days' culture is assayed for P24 antigen detection assays indicate infection. This technique required a mean 7-14 days to perform, but it may require as long as 28 days.
   f. **HIV viral load tests**.

These tests measure the amount of actively replicating virus. It correlates with disease progression and response to antiretroviral drugs.

Indirect tests

1. Differential T4 (CD4) and T8 (CD8) cell counts: T4 : T8 ratio is reversed. The most widely used marker is the absolute CD lymphocyte count. People with healthy immune system usually have more than 950 CD4 cells /μl of blood. People with AIDS have CD4 cell count below 200 cells/μl.

2. CD4 lymphocyte percent: Percent may be more reliable than CD4 count. Risk of progression to an AIDS opportunistic infection or malignancy is high with percentage < 20%.

3. Beta-2 microglobulin is increased in AIDS patients, with progressive disease, particularly with opportunistic infections. It is a cell surface protein indicative of macrophage-monocyte stimulation. Levels > 3.5mg/dl associated with rapid progression of disease.

4. Complete blood examination: There is anaemia, neutropaenia, and thrombocytopaenia, common with advanced HIV infection.

Treatment

Treatment of AIDS

There is currently no publicly available vaccine for HIV or cure for HIV or AIDS.

Anti-HIV (also called antiretroviral) medications are used to control the reproduction of the virus and to slow or halt the progression of HIV related disease. When used in combinations, these medications are termed Highly Active Antiretroviral Therapy (HAART).

Current treatment for HIV infection consists of highly active antiretroviral therapy or HAART.

Standard goals of HAART include improvement in the patient's quality of life, reduction in complications, and reduction in HIV viremia below the limit of detection.

Anti-retroviral drugs are expensive, and the majority of the world's infected individuals do not have access to medications and treatments for HIV and AIDS.

HAND, FOOT AND MOUTH DISEASE (HFMD)

Human syndrome caused by intestinal viruses of picorna viridae family. Most common strains causing HFMD are Coxsackie A virus and Enterovirus 71(EV 71).

HDMD is highly infectious. It can spread from one person to another through direct contact with discharge from the nose and throat, saliva, infected stools, or fluid from a blister.

Hand, foot and mouth disease is a common viral illness of infants and children. The disease causes fever, and blister like eruptions in the mouth and or a skin rash. They begin as small red spots that blister and then often become ulcers. The sores are usually located on the tongue, gums, and inside of the cheeks. Mouth ulcers will heal in about 7 days.

MEASLES

This paramyxovirus infection is endemic worldwide. Measles is a serious disease in the malnourished, vitamin deficient or immunocompromised.

Clinical features

Measles is the commonest and the most infectious of childhood exanthemata.

Infection is by droplet spread with incubation period of 14 days to onset of rash. The prodromal phase begins with bad cold, running nose, fever, sore throat, cough and upper respiratory infection.

A few days later a bright red blotchy, rash breaks out on the forehead, face and to the body, arms and legs, by which time the rash will begin to fade from face.

Skin rashes show dilated dermal capillaries, edema and lymphocytic infiltrates. Waethin-Finkeldoy giant cells are seen in all tissues.

Generalised lymphadenopathy, hepatitis, encephalitis, keratitis, bronchitis (croup), otitis media, and diarrhoea are common, with bacterial pneumonia in approximately 4% of cases. A rare late complication is 'subacute sclerosing pancephalitis'.

Oral manifestations

Koplick's spots named after Henry Koplick, an American pediatrician, who first described them in 1896.

Koplick spots are pathognomonic for early stage measles.

They are located on the buccal mucosa in the premolar and molar area. Koplick spots consist of bluish-grey specks against an erythematous background. The lesions are plaque like or nodular and oval or round. If they are numerous, the entire buccal and labial mucosa may give a look of mottled erythema.

The tongue is usually furred. Bleeding and hypertrophy of gingivae occur frequently.

Prevention

The way to prevent measles is by administering measles vaccine at 9 months of age. The standard MMR (mumps, measles and rubella) vaccine is given in two dosages. The first dose should be at 12-15 months of age. The second vaccination should be at 4-6 years of age.

Management

The child is isolated and excluded from school for about 10 days. Antibiotics are given only if there is a bacterial infection. To prevent itching of rashes a calamine lotion may be applied. Antihistaminics may also help.

INFECTIOUS MONONUCLEOSIS (GLANDULAR FEVER)

Epstein-Barr virus infectious mononucleosis is also known as Pfeiffer's disease or kissing disease. Emil Pfeiffer described the syndrome as an infectious process in 1889.

Clinical features: Infectious mononucleosis is an acute self-limited disease usually affecting young adults. The infection is characterised mainly by fever, sore throat, generalised lymphadenitis, splenomegaly, hepatitis and haemolysis.

Mode of infection: Spread of infection is by close contact. The virus colonises in pharyngeal epithelium and is present in the throat washings and saliva shortly after infection. The infection spreads via saliva and has an incubation period up to 8 weeks. The virus is thought to be transmitted by kissing.

Oral lesions: Lesions of oral cavity may be the first manifestation of disease. These consist of gingivostomatitis, gingival bleeding and multiple pinpoint petechiae at the junction of the hard and soft palates, tonsillar exudates, uvular edema, diffuse erythema of the oral mucosa and rarely ulcers.

Sore throat, pharyngitis and tonsillitis may also occur in association with oral lesions.

Diagnosis

(i) An increase of lymphocytes in blood, many of which have an atypical morphology.

(ii) The Paul-Bunnel test is positive in high dilutions, agglutinating the sheep's red blood cells due to the presence of heterophile antibody for EBV antigen.

(iii) Antibodies to viral capsid antigen (i.e., VCA-IgG and VCA-IgM) are produced slightly earlier than the heterophile antibody and more specific for infection.

FUNGAL INFECTIONS OF ORAL CAVITY

MONILIASIS

Oral candidiasis is common in infants and occurs in adults with lowered resistance. Well-defined white patches develop on the mucosa of the cheeks, tongue, gum, tonsils, or pharynx.

Causes

Candida does not become a problem until there is a change in the chemistry of the oral cavity that favours candida over the other microorganisms that are present.

1. These changes can occur as a side effect of taking glucocorticoids antibiotics or drug treatment as chemotherapy.
2. These changes can also be caused by certain conditions such as diabetes, drug abuse, anaemia, and malnutrition.
3. As a consequence of immune deficiencies relating to old age or infection, such as AIDS.

TABLE 9.4
CLASSIFICATION OF ORAL CANDIDIASIS

A. Acute
- (i) Acute pseudomembranous (thrush)
- (ii) Acute atrophic erythematous

B. Chronic
1. Chronic hyperplastic
   - (i) Chronic oral candidiasis (oral leukoplakia)
   - (ii) Endocrine candidiasis syndrome
   - (iii) Chronic localised
   - (iv) Chronic diffuse
2. Chronic atrophic oral erythematous
3. Chronic familial mucocutaneous

Four clinical forms of candidiasis

1. **Moniliasis or thrush:** White, creamy or yellow spots with red background that appear in the inner surface of the mouth. If the white membrane is removed, a raw, bleeding surface is exposed.
2. **Erythematous:** Red peeling patches, most commonly on the palate and tongue.
3. **Hyperplastic:** Extra tissue that cannot readily be wiped off and may appear discoloured because of staining caused by foods or tobacco.
4. **Angular cheilitis:** Red cracks at the corners of mouth often covered by a pseudomembrane. Angular cheilitis can occur with other forms of candidiasis or appear separately.

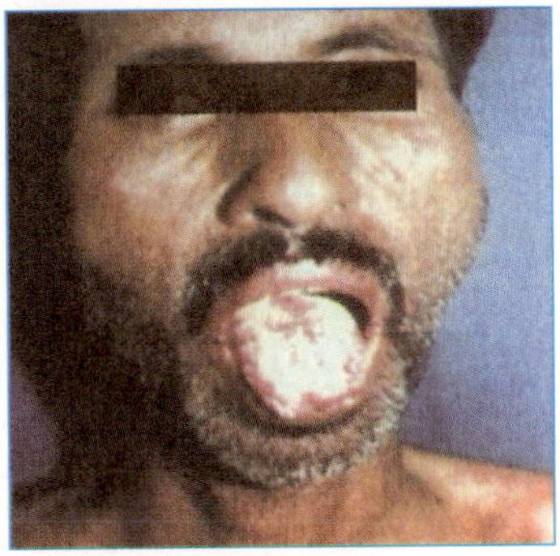

Fig.9.10: Showing thrush in a case of AIDS

Microscopically: The lesion reveals mucosal ulceration and an acute inflammatory exudate and fibrin beneath. There are necrotic cells, keratin and dense network of candida organisms in the form of hyphae and spores. The fungi can be identified within these pseudomembrane as boxcar-like chains of tubular cells producing, pseudohyphae from which bud ovoid yeast forms, typically 2 to 4 μm in greatest diameter.

MUCORMYCOSIS

Paultaufi first described Mucormycosis in humans in 1885.

Mucormycosis (zycormycosis) is a rare yet life-threatening and serious infection of fungi of Mucorales order usually affecting face or oropharyngeal cavity. The most common fungi responsible for mucormycosis in humans are Mucor, Albsida, and Rhizopus.

Opportunistic fungal infections such as mucormycosis usually occur in immunocompromized patients but can infect healthy individuals as well. The predisposing factors are uncontrolled diabetes, malignancies such as lymphomas, and leukaemias, renal failure, organ transplant, long term corticosteroid and immunosuppressive therapy, cirrhosis, burns, protein energy malnutrition and AIDS.

Mucormycosis is one of the most rapidly progressing and lethal forms of fungal infection in humans, which usually begins in the nose and paranasal sinuses. The fungus invades the arteries, forms thrombi within the blood vessels that reduce blood supply and cause necrosis of hard and soft tissues. Once entered into the arteries, the fungus can spread to orbital and intracranial structures.

Usually mucormycosis presents as an acute infection and manifests as rhinocerebral, pulmonary, gastrointestinal, cutaneous, or disseminated form.

Symptoms of rhinocerebral mucormycosis include pain, fever, and orbital cellulitis, with bulging of the affected eye (proptosis). The roof of the mouth (palate), the facial bones, surrounding the eye socket or sinuses, or the septum of the nostrils may be destroyed by the infection. Infection of the brain may cause seizures, palatal paralysis, and coma.

Mucormycosis of lung causes fever, cough, and sometimes difficulty in breathing.

Complications may include loss of neurologic function, blindness, or blood clots in the brain and lung vessels.

Oral manifestations

Palatal ulceration and necrosis are the most characteristic oral lesions. The ulcer is sharply demarcated with a black necrotic Escher while the bone is exposed. Ulcers from mucormycosis have also been reported on gingival, lip, and alveolar ridge. Teeth loosen and spontaneously exfoliate.

Microscopically

Biopsy from tissue shows non-septated, 90-degree broad branching hyphae with neutrophilic infiltrate. Pathogen invades the vessel walls causing vascular occlusion, thrombosis, infarction and tissue necrosis.

Management

If mucormycosis is suspected, prompt amphotericin B therapy should be administered due to rapid spread and mortality rate of the disease. Infected tissue—and especially dead tissue—may be removed by surgery.

RHINOSPORIDIOSIS

Rhinosporidiosis is an infectious disease caused by aquatic protozoan previously considered to be a fungus.

It is caused by Rhinosporidium seeberi.

Geographic distribution: More than 90% of cases have been reported from India, Sri Lanka, and South America. In India, sporadic cases occur all over but endemic foci exist in part of Orissa, Andhra Pradesh, Kerala, Chennai, and Raipur.

Rhinosporidium seeberi has not been cultured and animal inoculation is also not possible. Nothing definite is known about the mode of transmission of infection. However, it has been suggested that the organism is transmitted in dust or water. It is believed that fish may be the natural hosts of Rhinosporidium seeberi.

Infection is more common in:

- Person bathing in muddy stagnant pools of water.
- Those who dive into streams to collect sand from river beds.
- Paddy cultivators.
- In dry areas, after dust storm and eye injury.

Clinical features

It chiefly affects the mucus membrane of the nose, conjunctiva, cheek, vulva, lacrimal sac, ear, larynx, bronchus, penile urethra, rectum, and skin. Disseminated form of disease is reported in literature.

Rhinosporidiosis is a chronic disease characterised by the development of large polyps or wart-like lesions. The lesions are soft, friable and highly vascular.

Oral manifestations

Commonest site is soft palate and cheek.

There is polypoidal mass, soft in consistency, pink in colour and excessive mucus discharge. The polyp is highly vascular and bleeds easily.

Microscopically

Large numbers of cysts typically lie just beneath the hyperplastic epithelium. The lesion is composed of large numbers of fungal spherules embedded in a stroma of connective tissue and capillaries. In tissues the organism forms large sporangioma approaching 300 μ in diameter that contains spores that mature at different rates. Mature sporangiospores are approximately 8-9 μ in size and escape through a pore that develops in the sporangial wall. On rupture of a sporangium, the spores are discharged into submucosa or on the surface of the mucosa. The intervening tissue consists of inflammatory granulation tissue (plasma cells, lymphocytes, histiocytes, neutrophils and foreign body type of giant cells).

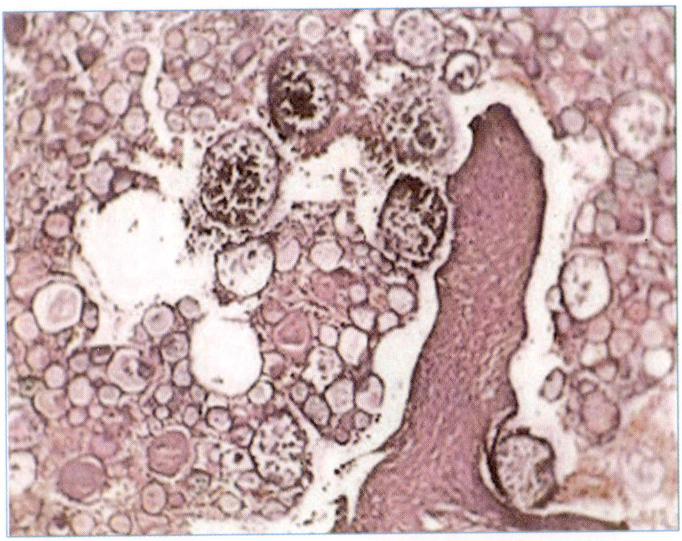

Fig.9.11: Microscopic appearance of rhinosporidiosis showing sporangia with sporangiospores

Diagnosis

Excised macerated tissue or discharge is mounted in 10% KOH for examination. Spherules and large number of free endospores are typically present.

ASPERGILLOSIS

Aspergillosis is caused by inhalation of Aspergillus conidia or mycelial fragments, which are present on vegetation (nuts and grains) decaying matter, soil and air.

Clinical features

Aspergillus is a ubiquitous fungus, which may cause an allergic pulmonary response to otherwise healthy individuals. This is also known as Brewer's lung or belongs to the group of diseases known by the term extrinsic allergic alveolitis.

Aspergillus can produce allergic asthma, allergic pulmonary aspergillosis, extrinsic allergic alveolitis, aspergilloma, and invasive aspergillosis. It can cause endocarditis, hepatocellular carcinoma, and otomycosis.

Disseminated or invasive aspergillosis occurs in immunocompromised individuals. The fungus first establishes in lung tissue and disseminate to involve other organs—particularly brain, kidney, nasopharynx, cornea, gastrointestinal tract, and skin.

Oral manifestations

Orofacial lesions caused by aspergillosis species include invasive aspergillosis of the antrum, indolent chronic sinusitis, allergic sinusitis and oral lesions.

Oral lesions of aspergillosis are seen predominantly in some immunocompromised patients with invasive aspergillosis. Yellow or necrotic ulcers typically appear on the palate or occasionally on the posterior tongue. Palatal ulcer is painful and surrounded by a ring of black necrotic tissue.

HISTOPLASMOSIS

Histoplasma capsulatum causes the commoner form of histoplasmosis and has a global distribution with particularly high prevalence in South USA, Africa, Australia, and scattered reports are available from Asian countries.

The fungus is present in soil enriched with excreta of birds, chicken, and bats.

Dr Samuel Darling first recognized the disease in Canal Zone of Panama.

Clinical features

Acute histoplasmosis

Irregular fever, enlargement of lymph nodes, splenomegaly, hepatomegaly, anaemia, ulcerative lesions of buccal mucosa, nose, intestine, anus and genitalia characterise it.

Chronic pulmonary histoplasmosis

Unilateral or bilateral apical infiltrate are seen in the lungs that progressively enlarge and cavitate.

Oral manifestations

Oral lesions are sometimes isolated—and have also been recorded—in apparently healthy persons. Oral lesions are usually ulcerative or nodular, have been found on the tongue, palate, buccal mucosa, or gingival, and rarely invade the mandible or maxilla. The lesion can closely simulate tuberculosis or squamous cell carcinoma.

Microscopically

Yeast like bodies of 2-5μ diameters are seen in macrophages and there are usually epitheloid-cell granulomas with or without caseation.

Diagnosis

Biopsy: Demonstration of Histoplasma capsulatum in sputum, bone marrow aspirate, peripheral blood, scrapings from dermal or mucosal ulcers, and biopsies of lymph nodes and other organs.

PARACOCCIDIOIDOMYCOSIS

It is also known as South American Blastomycosis.

A dimorphic fungus known as Paracoccidiodes Brasilensis causes it. The fungus has been isolated from soil and is introduced into the mouth due to the habit of cleaning the teeth with twigs, or inhaled.

Oral manifestations

It produces prominent oral manifestations, as chronic, progressive granulomatous inflammatory lesions of the lips, cheeks, floor of mouth, tongue, and pharynx. Yeast phase is present in tissues. It consists of large round or oval cells with multiple budding.

COCCIDIOIDOMYCOSIS

Coccidioidomycosis infection is also known as 'California valley fever', 'Desert fever' or 'Coccidial granuloma', 'San Joaquin Valley fever'.

It is endemic in certain parts of Arizona, California, Nevada, New Mexico, Texas, Utah, and North Western Mexico.

The disease is caused by coccidioides immitis.

The spores produced by the fungus become airborne, which are usually inhaled leading to infecion.

In the lung, arthroconidia form spherules (30-60 μm diameter). These contain numerous endospores, 2-5 μm diameter. The mature spherules have double wall measuring 2 μm in thickness. At maturity, the spherules rupture and their endospores are released which develop to form spherules in adjacent tissue.

Clinical features

Pulmonary coccidioidomycosis has two forms: Primary and progressive:

1. In chronic form of disease, that usually involves lungs, is seen in 5-10% of infected individuals. There are presence of pulmonary nodules or peripheral thin-walled cavities in lungs. Primary pulmonary infection spreads by haematogenous route to mucus membranes of mouth, nose, lymph nodes, and adjacent skin.
2. Progressive disseminated coccidioidomycosis form of the disease is associated with marked systemic upset and features of lobar pneumonia.

Rarely, the endospores may be carried by the blood stream to the bones, adrenals, meninges, joints, skin, thyroid, pericardium, gastro-intestinal tract and central nervous system.

Primary coccidioidomycosis of skin

Oral manifestations

Lytic lesions of bones of jaw may develop.

Diagnosis

1. The fungal infection can be demonstrated by microscopic detection of diagnostic cells in body fluids, exudates, sputum, and biopsy tissues.
2. With specific nucleotide primary C immitis DNA can be amplified by PCR.
3. It can be detected in culture by morphological identification or by using molecular probe that hybridise with immitis RNA.

BLASTOMYCOSIS

Blastomycosis is caused by inhalation of spores of blastomyces dermatitis.

Blastomycosis infection is clustered in States adjacent to the Mississippi and Ohio rivers and the Lakes of regions. In India, cases have been reported from Delhi and Madhya Pradesh.

Clinical features

Men aged 30-50 years are affected most commonly.

Males have been found to be affected more often than females (10 : 1). Constitutional symptoms include fever, chills, night sweats, weight loss, malaise and myalgia. After inhalation of spores they are converted into yeast and invade the lungs to produce granulomatous caseating lesion in the lower lobes. Hilar lymph nodes may become involved. These lesions usually heal or become chronic.

Skin lesions: Skin lesions appear on hands, face, feet, wrists, ankles, and unexposed surfaces.

Oral manifestations

Oral lesions exhibit regular, erythematous or white intact surface. The lesions should be differentiated from squamous cell carcinoma.

Diagnosis

- Microscopic examination and culture of sputum for demonstration of fungus.
- Serological diagnosis of blastomycosis antigen using complement fixation antibodies.
- Immunodiffusion (ID): Precipitin bands are obtained after immunodiffusion.
- Recently developed immunoassay with the A-antigen of blastomyces dermatitis has been shown to be more sensitive than complement fixation and immunodiffusion tests.
- Chemiluminescent DNA probes are available for identification of B dermatitis.

Treatment

Intravenous amphotercin, oral itraconazole are the drugs of choice, respectively for severe and mild forms of disease.

PARASITIC LESIONS OF ORAL CAVITY

ENTAMOEBA GINGIVITIS

Entamoeba gingivalis—morphologically very similar to Entamoeba histolytica—is often found in the mouth where it lives as a commensals. This species show great proliferation when associated with microorganisms. Oral infection may be suspected in the presence of generalised dental mobility, especially in young patients, enlarged tongue, fetid halitosis, vivid red colour, frequent haemorrhages and pruritis of gingiva. Oral lesions caused by entamoeba histolytica although extremely uncommon when present are characterised by a single or few very painful nonspecific serpiginous and destructive ulcers.

Diagnosis: Entamoeba gingivalis may be recovered from dental plaques.

MYIASIS

The furunculoid myiasis is characterised by the presence of one or more papules or nodules housed with larva.

LEISHMANIASIS

Flagellate protozoa of genus Leishmania cause the disease. Transmission is by the bite of sandfly. It is endemic in Tropics, Subtropics and Southern Europe.

The flagellates of the genus Leishmania are named after the British army surgeon Sir William Leishman.

Leishmania organisms, which represent a protozoon, appear in a section as round to oval bodies from 2 to 40 μm in size. They have no capsule. Within the body there is relatively large, deeply basophilic, round nucleus about 1μm in diameter and in addition, a small rod-like paranucleus or kinetoplast. They are also known as Leishman Donovan bodies (LD bodies). They cause three kinds of diseases in man—visceral, cutaneous, and mucocutaneous.

MUCOSAL LEISHMANIASIS

Post-kala-azar Leishmaniasis

It is also called American Leishmaniasis and caused by Leishmania brazilensis and and L. panamensis.

The condition affects the hard palate and the dorsum of the tongue forming granulomatous nodules occasionally with ulcers at both the sites.

Clinically: The surface becomes rough, nodular and may even ulcerate by breaking down the nodules.

Nasal mucosa shows infiltrative, ulcerative, vegetating, and atrophic-crusted lesions. Involvement of upper lip and nasal region gives a taperoid appearance.

Gingival Leishmaniasis is unusual and is mainly observed in immunocompromised patients.

Diagnosis

Biopsy from the gingival lesions present an intense inflammatory infiltrate permeated by polymorphs. Amastigote forms of parasites can be demonstrated inside the macrophages by using Giemsa stain.

TRYPANOSOMIASIS/CHAGAS' DISEASE

It is also known as South American trypanosomiasis.

South American trypanosomiasis is caused by a haemoflagellate, Trypanosoma cruzi, and transmitted by reduviid bugs of family Triatomie.

Routes of transmission are:

1. It can be transmitted by blood transfusion.
2. Transplantation of organs from infected blood cultures have been reported.
3. Infections transmitted through laboratory accidents with infected blood culture have been reported.
4. The congenital form is discovered in 2% of abortions and premature births.
5. Infections also have been transmitted through breastfeeding and contaminated food.

Recently Chagas' disease has been reported in patients with acquired immunodeficiency syndrome.

Clinical features

The symptoms start after 1-2 weeks of incubation and consist of fever and malaise. Acute disease is fatal in about 10% but subsides without treatment.

Main features of Chagas' disease is myocarditis, chronic dilatation of esophagus, and colon, stillbirth, bronchiectasis, dilatation of stomach, duodenum, gallbladder and ureter.

Oral manifestations

Mouth lesions are mainly seen on the lips and are similar to the skin chagoma. They are characterised by an erythematous nodule, swelling or ulcer at the site of inoculation, which, in general, heals spontaneously in about three weeks.

Diagnosis

Detection of trypanosomes in peripheral blood smears.

Amplified parasite DNA in blood or tissue fluid can be detected by PCR.

TOXOPLASMOSIS

Toxoplasmosis is caused by Toxoplasma gondii, a coccidian of the class sporozoa that affects one-third of world population.

Nicolle and Manceaux described the parasite in 1908 in smears made from spleen and liver of a North African rodent gundi.

Toxoplasma gondii exists in three forms—oocyst, tachyzoites, and tissue cyst.

Transmission

A. Ingestion of contaminated food.

Human infection occurs from two sources:

1. Infection can also occur by eating raw or undercooked meat containing tissue cysts, most commonly lamb, pork, or beef.
2. Ingestion of food, vegetables and drink contaminated by infective oocyst from cat faeces.

B. Transplacental: Foetus is infected in utero through transplacental route.

C. Contaminated blood transfusions, organ transplants, and accidental inoculation by handling of infected mice and culture in the laboratory.

Toxoplasmosis occurs as a result of an infection with the protozoan Toxoplasma gondii. Cervical lymphadenitis is the most common form of acquired toxoplasmosis.

Toxoplasmosis is typically classified as:

1. **Congenital toxoplasmosis:** If mother was infected prior to current pregnancy, virtually no risk of fetal transmission exists. If the mother becomes infected during pregnancy, the fetus is at risk regardless if mother is asymptomatic. Fetal infection with T. gondii may result in stillbirth or abortion. Congenital infection is more severe if acquired in the first—or, in some cases, second—trimester. Infection during the second and third trimesters tends to be symptomatic.

   Disease in the newborn may be severe, with jaundice, rash, and hepatomegaly, followed by a characteristic tetrad of abnormalities, chorioretinitis, cerebral calcifications, hydrocephalus or microcephaly and psychomotor retardation.
2. **Acquired toxoplasmosis in the compromised patients:** Toxoplasma myocarditis with or without coexistent poliomyelitis is the third most common complication.
3. **Toxoplasmosis in the immunocompromised host**.
4. **Neurotoxoplasmosis:** It occurs in immunocompromised patients (cell mediated immunity). This is a common complication in 90% of HIV patients. It can be subacute or acute onset of neurological symptoms. Most common symptoms are focal neurological deficient such as headache, hemiparesis, speech abnormalities and altered mental status and seizures. Fever may or may not be present.
5. **Ocular manifestations:** Focal retinitis and secondary granulomatous inflammation of the choroids occur.

Oral manifestations

Oral and perioral manifestations are seldom seen. Tongue, larynx, or pharynx myositis as well as parotid swelling may occur in the acquired forms. Enamel hyperplasia can be observed in congenital infection.

Diagnosis

1. CT scan/MRI shows ring-enhancing lesions.
2. A rising titer of IgM antibody indicates recent infection.
3. Polymerase chain reaction (PCR amplication of T. gondii gene is possible).

TRICHOMONIASIS

Trichmoniasis is a venereal disease transmitted by a flagellate protozoan trichomonas vaginalis. Trichomoniasis also can be present in the urethra, prostate gland, and epididymis with a lower frequency than in the vagina. Trichomonas vaginalis is a leaf-shaped, or globular flagellate that measures about 8 to 30 μm long with a nucleus near the rounded anterior pole, and the axostyle. Its locomotive organs include four anterior flagella and an undulating membrane.

Clinical features

The incidence of trichomoniasis is at its peak in the age group 16 to 35 years.

Female patients may have urethritis, cystitis, cervicitis, or infection of Skene's duct and Bartholin gland. Trichomonas vaginalis, which infects the glands of the urethra and endocervix, causes a mild persistent vaginitis with a green frothy watery discharge. Itching is severe.

Vaginal examination usually reveals strawberry appearance caused by marked congestion, and petechial haemorrhages in the vaginal mucosa and portiovaginalis of cervix.

Oral manifestations

This parasite has been frequently related to lesions of peridontium, the tissue that surrounds the tooth. Its abnormal proliferation is associated to the development of periodontal pockets, chronic inflammatory reaction, and eventually destruction and loss of teeth in severe cases.

CYSTICERCUS CELLULOSAE

Cysticercosis, a helminthic disease commonly seen in India, Latin America, Estern Europe, and Southern Africa, results from extra-intestinal encystations of the larval form of Taenia solium.

Life cycle of Taenia solium

The adult worm lives in the small intestine of man. The eggs or gravid segments are passed out with faeces on the ground. The pig ingests them.

On reaching the alimentary system of intermediate host, the radially striated wall of the eggs rupture and oncospheres are liberated. These penetrate the gut wall with the aid of their hooks and gain entrance into the portal vessels or mesenteric lymphatics, finally reaching the systemic circulation. Usually, they travel via the portal vein and successfully reach the following organs: the liver, the right side of heart, lungs, and systemic circulation. The naked oncospheres are filtered out from the circulating blood into the muscular tissues where they ultimately settle down and undergo further development.

The tissues involved are subcutaneous tissues, brain, muscle, and heart.

The oncospheres lose their hooks on reaching their destinations, the cell wall, the cells in the centre liquefies, and in about 8 days after infection each oncosphere forms an oval vesicle gradually increasing in size, containing at its bottom the larva referred to as cysticercus.

The infection usually occurs through oral route by ingestion of uncooked pork infested larva of parasites.

Cysticercosis in the oral tissue such as the tongue, labial mucosa, buccal mucosa—and floor of the mouth has also been reported.

Oral cysticercosis is uncommon, but when present mainly involves the tongue and cheek.

Cysticercosis of tongue usually takes the form of numerous firm elastic round painless nodules or papules about 2 cm in diameter when fully developed. The cysts are ovoid and white to opalescent. The cysticerci are composed of a single, invaginated protoscolex in a fluid filled cystic cavity. They are 1.5 cm long and 0.8 cm in diameter. The cyst cavity is lined by fibrous tissue with inflammatory cells, and contains fluid and the larval stage of parasite.

Microscopy may demonstrate suckers, refractile hooklets, and a branched tract in protoscolex. Inflammatory response comprises lymphocytes, plasma cells, macrophages, epitheloid cells and giant cells. When cysticercus dies the lesion may become scarred and calcified.

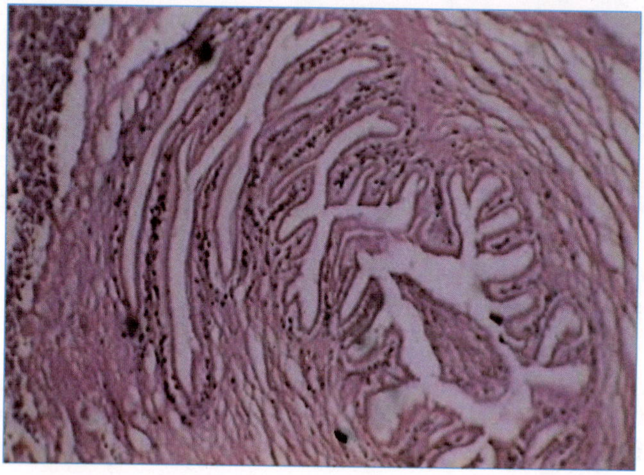

Fig.9.12: Shows cysticercus cellulosae with coelomic cavity

Diagnosis

Demonstration of larval stage of parasite in a biopsy specimen. The most popular serologic test is enzyme linked immunosorbent assay.

HYDATID DISEASE

Hydatid disease is caused due to the larval stage of parasite Echinococcus granulosus a small tapeworm. The canine animals like dogs and wolf are the definite hosts as they harbour the original parasite, the gravid segment of the parasite is passed out in the faeces of the dog and eating of vegetation contaminated with ova results the development of hydatid disease in intermediate hosts like cattle and humans.

TRICHINOSIS

Trichinosis is a worldwide zoonotic disease closely related to cultural and dietary habits.

Trichinella spiralis is a nematode that parasitises rats and pigs and is only transmitted to humans if they eat particularly cooked infected pork usually as sausage or ham.

When infected meat is ingested humans digest the cyst wall, and trichinella larvae attach to the wall of the duodenum or jejunum.

Larvae are released from cysts in ingested muscle and sexually mature into adult worms in the ileum.

The larvae mature and produce additional larvae, which then migrate from the gut into the general circulation. These larvae localise in striated muscles.

Clinical features

The clinical effects depend on the intensity of infections: 90% of infections are light, but symptoms usually develop when there are more than 10 larvae per gram of skeletal muscle: they include the clinical picture of acute myalgia, facial edema, and fever.

Larval migration may cause acute myocarditis, pneumonitis and encephalitis, and are sometimes fatal.

Oral manifestations

As in other parts of the body, encystations are in the striated muscles and in the oral cavity this is predominantly in the tongue and masseter muscle. The usual cycle of events is that they invade the tongue and masseter muscle, where calcification will take place after about 6 months and lead to the death of the larvae.

Microscopically

Biopsy may disclose trichuris spiralis larvae (100 x 6 μm) coiled within a muscle fibres host nurse cell surrounded by capsule.

Inflammatory infiltration includes monocytes, plasma cells, eosinophils and T lymphocytes.

Management

Treatment is with albendazole 20 mg/kg daily for 7 days. Given early in the infection this may kill newly-formed adult worms in the submucosa and thus reduce the number of larvae reaching the muscles. Corticosteroids are necessary to control the serious effects of acute inflammation.

INFECTIOUS DISEASE DUE TO INFECTED PROTEINACEOUS PARTICLE PRION DISEASE

Oral manifestations: The oral manifestations of human form of prions disease are characterized by development of dysphagia, dysesthesia, or paresthesia or disturbed taste.

Bibliography

Anantnarayan R and Panikar Jayaram CK: *Textbook of Microbiology*. 2005. 7th edition. Orient Longman.

Coogan M.M et al: *Oral Lesions in Infection With Human Immunodeficiency Virus*. Bull World Health Organization 2005 Sep; 83 (9): 700-6.

CO Envonwu, Falkter WA Jr, EO Idigbe, BM Afolabi, M Ibrahim, D Onwujekwe, O Savage and VI Meeks: *American Journal of Tropical Medicine and Hyg* 60 (2) 1999, PP 223-232.

Hansen LS, Allard RH: *Encysted Parasitic Larvae In The Mouth*. J American Dental Association 1984; 108 (4): 632-6.

Sharma AB, Laishram DK, Sarma: *Primary Tuberculosis Of Tongue*. Indian Journal of Pathology and Microbiology Volume 51(1) 2008 P 65.

CHAPTER

10

OSTEOMYELITIS

INTRODUCTION

The word **'osteomyelitis'** originates from the ancient Greek words *osteon* (bone) and *muelinos* (marrow) and means infection of medullary portion of the bone.

Definition: Osteomyelitis is defined as inflammation of bone, bone marrow, periosteum, and Haversian canal.

Jaw bones are relatively more frequently affected by osteomyelitis than other skeletal bones. Odontogenic infection is the most common cause of osteomyelitis of the jaws, even though other causes, such as injury, malignancy, malnutrition, diabetes, chronic systemic disease or disease occurring in hypovascularised bone and soon may be associated with osteomyelitis. The incidence of osteomyelitis is more common in mandible than in the maxilla because the distribution of blood vessels is poorer in mandible than in maxilla and the cortical bone mandible is thicker and more compact than the maxilla.

TABLE 10.1
CLASSIFICATION OF OSTEOMYELITIS

- **I. Acute osteomyelitis**
  - i. Acute suppurative osteomyelitis
  - ii. Acute subperiosteal osteomyelitis
  - iii. Acute periosteitis
- **II. Chronic osteomyelitis**
  - i. Non-specific type
    - a. Chronic intramedullary osteomyelitis
    - b. Chronic focal sclerosing osteomyelitis

Contd.

Contd.

c. Chronic diffuse sclerosing osteomyelitis
d. Chronic osteomyelitis with proliferative periosteitis
e. Chronic subperiosteal osteomyelitis
f. Chronic periosteitis

ii. Specific type
a. Tuberculous osteomyelitis
b. Syphilitis osteomyelitis
c. Actinomycotic osteomyelitis

III. Radiation induced osteomyelitis

IV. Idiopathic osteomyelitis

Osteomyelitis is mainly of three types: Acute, subacute, and chronic.

ACUTE OSTEOMYELITIS

Age: Acute haematogenous osteomyelitis is primarily a disease in children. Direct trauma and contagious focus osteomyelitis are common among adults and adolescent than in children.

Site: The maxilla is involved in infancy, and mandible is involved in adolescent.

Organisms: It is due to staphylococci, Escherichia coli, Klebseilla, pseudomonas, group B streptococci, haemophilus, proteus, and brucella. In patients with sickle cell anaemia, osteomyelitis due to salmonella is very common. Osteomyelitis may be caused by Actinomyces israelii.

Predisposing factors: Predisposing conditions that affect host resistance and play a role in development of osteomyelitis jaw include diabetes mellitus, agranulocytosis, leukaemia, sickle cell disease, fibrous dysplasia, and Paget's disease.

Pathology

Organisms reach the bone by one of three routes:

(i) Haematogenous dissemination.
(ii) Direct extension from a focus of acute infection in the adjacent joint or soft tissue.
(iii) Traumatic implantation after compound fracture or orthopedic surgical procedure.

The organisms settle down under the periosteum and pus is produced. If pus accumulates beneath the periosteum, perforation through it usually takes place. Proteolytic enzymes, necrosis by arterial thrombosis, destroy bone. There is decalcification of bone due to hyperaemia and bone is absorbed by activity of osteoclasts.

Medullary abscess can spread to subperiosteal space, joint cavity or medullary cavity.

Clinical features

(i) Pain at the site of involvement.
(ii) Fever and malaise are seen but in early phases.
(iii) Redness, swelling are late signs and suggest the presence of pus.
(iv) There is regional lymphadenitis.
(v) There may be anaesthesia and paraesthesia of the lip when pus extends to the mental foramen due to pressure neuritis.
(vi) The teeth in the affected segment of the jaw may become loose and tender.
(vii) Sinus formation with discharge of pus may occur in later stages.

Macroscopically

Sequestrum is white, dry irregular piece of bone with granular surface. The sequestrum is surrounded by a subperiosteal shell of new bone formed around the focus of inflammation. The new bone shell is called the involucrum.

Microscopically

Section shows dense, diffuse, infiltration of the marrow by neutrophils.

Investigations

1. Magnetic resonance imaging (MRI) can be extremely helpful in unclear situations. Ultrasonography and computed tomography scanning may be helpful in the evaluation of suspected cases of osteomyelitis.
2. **X-ray:** In the early stages no radiographic changes. In the late stages shows metaphyseal abscess. There is periosteal lifting giving an onion peel appearance, moth-eaten erosions of medulla and cortex with sequestrum formation.
3. **Blood:** Polymorphonuclear leukocytosis, raised erythrocyte sedimentation rate, elevated C reactive protein and positive blood culture during the first 5 days in about 50% of cases.
4. Pus culture is positive in aspirate.

Complications

General complications include anaemia, amyloidosis, and septic embolization leading to septicaemia.

Local complications

1. Acute osteomyelitis, if inadequately treated, progresses to chronic osteomyelitis.
2. Pyaemia frequently complicates the picture, as a result of dissemination of septic thrombi, pericarditis, endocarditis, pyaemic abscess of the kidney, and the spleen.
3. Pathological fracture due to corticomedullary erosion. In neglected cases, this can occur where subperiosteal bone has failed to form.
4. Sympathetic effusion of neighbouring joint.
5. Occasionally there is development of squamous cell carcinoma in the epithelial lined wall of a sinus. Rarely, osteogenic sarcoma develops from draining sinus.

Management

- General symptomatic measures should include intravenous fluids and analgesics.
- Aggressive antibiotic therapy should be instituted.
- Flucloxacillin is often the antibiotic of choice.
- Treatment usually require surgery for debridement, drainage of abscesses, and removal of sequestra.

ALVEOLAR OSTEITIS

It is also called dry socket, localised acute alveolar osteomyelitis, alveolitis sicca dolorosa, and alveolagia.

The frequency of occurrence for dry sockets, when considering for all tooth extractions collectively is roughly on the order 1 to 3%. Dry socket occurs in as many as 20% of cases involving the extraction of mandibular (lower) impacted wisdom teeth.

Predisposing factors

- Dental patients who have experienced dry sockets with past tooth extractions are at greater risk for developing a dry socket with future tooth extractions.

- **Age:** The age of the dental patient may be related to the risk for experiencing dry sockets. Younger patients are at less risk for dry sockets than comparative older patients.
- **Location of teeth:** In general, there is a greater incidence of dry sockets with molars as opposed to front teeth. The greatest risk of dry socket formation seems to be associated with lower wisdom teeth, especially impacted lower teeth.
- **Traumatic tooth extraction:** Traumatic tooth extractions are more likely to result in dry socket formation. The general hypothesis is that the traumatised bone in the area of extractions site releases compounds (tissue activators)which diffuse into the blood. These tissues activators cause the blood clot to disintegrate, thus leading to the delayed healing of the socket. It is also thought that some of the compounds released as a result of this blood clot disintegration are kinins—a type of compound known to stimulate pain receptors, hence causing much of the pain associated with dry sockets.
- **Smoking:** Patients who smoke tend to have a greater risk of dry socket formation.
- **Oral contraceptives:** Women who use oral contraceptives tend to have a greater risk of dry sockets
- Bacterial contamination of the socket, premature loss of blood clot and difficult and prolong extraction gives rise to dry socket.
- For the first 24 hours after extraction the dental patient should avoid vigorous ringing, refrain from actions like sucking on a straw or cigarette, alcohol and tobacco use in general, minimise physical stress and exercise, and avoid hot liquids such as coffee or soup.
- Dry socket is more common in diabetes.

Clinical features

Alveolar osteitis is a painful phenomenon that most commonly occurs a few days following the removal of mandibular (lower) wisdom teeth. It occurs when the blood clot within the healing tooth extraction site is disrupted. In rare cases, the removal of the upper wisdom teeth can also result in alveolar osteitis.

A dry socket typically presents as a sharp and sudden pain commencing 2-5 days following extraction of a mandibular molar, most commonly the third molar. The pain, which often radiates up and down the head and neck, can be extremely unpleasant for the patient. It will cause pain in the ear as well. It can also be accompanied by a foul taste or smell.

On examination, there is absence of a clot in the socket of a recently extracted tooth; however, the socket may contain food debris and, when looking down into the socket, exposed bone is visible. The term ***'dry socket'*** is derived from this empty socket appearance. The lymph nodes in the patients jaw or neck may become enlarged.

Management

- Mild pain in case of dry socket is usually treated asymptomatically with mild pain-killers.
- The extraction socket is irrigated with chlorhexidine/betadine or normal saline.
- Any food debris in the extraction socket must be removed.
- Zinc oxide eugenol dressing, along with symptomatic pain-killers, is usually the treatment of choice.
- Non-steroidal anti-inflammatory drugs like aspirin and brufen are usually the most preferred painkillers.
- Acute pain despite using pain-killers may be treated temporarily by a nerve block with local anaesthesia.

CHRONIC OSTEOMYELITIS

It is a sequelae of (i) neglected, acute intramedullary and/or subperiosteal osteomyelitis (ii) infection following open fracture (iii) post-operative infecting iatrogenic osteomyelitis (iv) in Paget's disease and osteopetrosis (v) association of debilitating condition (e.g., malnutrition, diabetes, uremia) (vi) Possibility of syphilis, tuberculosis, and actinomycosis.

Clinical features

The patient with chronic osteomyelitis has a typical history of intermittent acute exacerbation with pain, temperature, redness, and discharging sinuses. The tissues are thickened and puckered, especially at the sinuses or scars, where they are attached to the bone.

Microscopic examination of chronic intramedullary osteomyelitis shows areas of acute and subacute inflammation in the cancellous spaces of the necrotic bone. Active osteoclastic resorption of bone is noted in the more peripheral portion. There is fibre rich granulation tissue, new bone formation of bony trabeculae and thickening of trabeculae.

X-ray findings: Chronic osteomyelitis of mandible often shows an irregular-shaped radiolucent area with poorly defined borders and/or mottled and increased radioopacity is also demonstrated as a mixture of osteolysis and osteosclerosis in equal parts.

CT scan findings: CT scan findings observed are areas of bone-defect pattern, frosted-glass pattern and compact-bone pattern.

Management

Chronic osteomyelitis is more difficult to manage unless all necrotic bone and organisms are removed. Occasionally, resection of larger parts of mandible is necessary to achieve this goal.

CHRONIC FOCAL SCLEROSING OSTEOMYELITIS

The focal type is also known as periapicalosteitis/osteomyelitis or condensing osteomyelitis.

Definition: Chronic focal sclerosing osteomyelitis is a reaction of bone to a mild bacterial infection, often the result of carious tooth, in persons with a high degree of tissue resistance, results in localised radiopacity.

Etiology

It represents a hyperplastic reaction of bone to a mild bacterial infection. The portal of entry is through an inflamed or necrotic pulp that has developed in a tooth secondary to a deep carious lesion, a large restoration or, less frequently, a cracked tooth.

Clinically

Chronic focal sclerosing osteomyelitis is most often seen in young adults although it can occur at any age.

There is no sex predilection. Chronic focal sclerosing osteomyelitis occurs frequently in the mandible, with most cases appearing in the premolar/molar region. The mandibular first molar is most commonly involved.

Chronic focal sclerosing osteomyelitis is asymptomatic and is typically discovered during radiographic examination. This lesion is always associated with pulpal death and necrosis and, consequently, the involved tooth is always non-vital.

Microscopically

Biopsy tissue includes normal bone marrow exchange with fibrous tissue, occasionally accompanied by inflammatory cell infiltration, de novo bone formation, and presence of bone sequestration. It also includes dense trabeculae with limited area of bone marrow, reduced in size thus resembling compact bone. The bone tissue includes osteoblasts, while bone marrow contains lymphocytic infiltrate.

Radiologically

X-ray shows uniform, dense, radioopaque mass of sclerotic bone surrounding the apex of the root. The borders of the lesion are smooth and well-defined, or appear to blend into the surrounding bone with the loss of lamina dura apically. The adjacent tooth exhibits a continuous, thickened periodontal ligament and, sometimes, a concurrent apical inflammatory lesion.

CHRONIC DIFFUSE SCLEROSING OSTEOMYELITIS (CDSO)

Definition: Chronic diffuse sclerosing osteomyelitis of the jaws is a proliferative reaction of bone to a low-grade infection of the jaws.

Etiology

Chronic diffuse sclerosing osteomyelitis is a disease of obscure origin. There have been many hypotheses for the cause of this disease, but the etiology is still unknown. Institute has been able to demonstrate actinomyces and eikenella as the etiologic factors in chronic diffuse osteomyelitis in number of patients.

Clinical features

Although this condition may affect any age, sex or race, it tends to occur more often in middle-aged Afro-American females.

Chronic diffuse sclerosing osteomyelitis is seen predominantly in adult Caucasian men. Chronic diffuse sclerosing osteomyelitis typically is found in the mandibular body, angle and ramus. Generally it is unilateral, but it may be bilateral. The disease shows an insidious onset, lacking an acute stage. Frequently there is history of a past toothache, recent dental extraction, or infection of a flap of tissue over an erupting tooth. The absence of pus, fistula, and sequestration are characteristics of chronic diffuse sclerotic osteomyelitis.

Radiologically

There is an alteration of the normal trabecular pattern. The lesion demonstrates increased density and appears as an opaque segment of the mandible. The borders are defined poorly, blending into the normal trabecular pattern.

Microscopically

Section from lesion characteristically consists of trabeculae of bone that are arranged in a linear parallel orientation (mosaic pattern). The trabeculae exhibit irregular size and shape. The intervening stroma is composed of fibrous connective tissue generally devoid of inflammatory cells or only sparsely infiltrated with lymphocytes and plasma cells. Sequestra show typical features of necrosis. There may be subperiosteal thickening, because of the formation of new bone.

CHRONIC PROLIFERATIVE OSTEOMYELITIS

It is also called Garre's osteomyelitis, periosteitis osssificans.

Chronic osteomyelitis with subperiosteal new bone formation results from periosteal reaction to chronic inflammatory/infectious stimulation. In the maxillofacial region, it is traditionally termed Garre's osteomyelitis and, more recently, periosteitis ossificans.

Garre sclerosing osteomyelitis is a chronic, non-suppurative sclerosing osteomyelitis. It occurs in young patients secondary to dental infection. A localised, hard, non-tender swelling of mandible characterises it. It involves the body of the mandible from the alveolus to the inferior border and may extend into the ramus. It is commonly associated with carious tooth, usually a lower first molar. The infection spreads towards the surface of the bone, resulting in inflammation of the periosteum and deposition of new bone underneath the periosteum. This peripheral formation of reactive bone results in localised periosteal thickening.

Microscopically

It consists of sclerotic bone, necrotic foci, coarse or thin trabeculae and granulation tissue.

Radiologically

Radiographs show a local area of calcified proliferation of bone that is smooth; often has a laminated or onion peel appearance.

TUBERCULAR OSTEOMYELITIS

The involvement of the mandible by tuberculous infection is extremely rare as it contains less cancellous bone. Sixty percent of all cases of tuberculosis of jaw occur in children below the age of 16 years, although cases of affected adults are also described. The mandibular involvement is more frequent than maxilla and the alveolar and angle regions have greater affinity.

The infection may extend to the mandible by:

1. Direct transfer from infected sputum or infected raw milk of cow through
   a. An open pulp of carious tooth
   b. An extraction wound
   c. Gingival margin or perforation of an erupting tooth.
2. Regional extension of soft tissue lesion to involve the underlying bone.
3. Haematogenous route.

Bacilli are possibly transferred from a primary focus in another part of the body and localised in the jaw, after trauma.

Tuberculosis of the jaw causes slow necrosis of the bone and may involve the entire mandible.

X-ray findings: The destruction of the bone in radiographs appears as blurring of trabecular details with irregular areas of radiolucency. There is erosion of the cortex with little tendency to repair. It gives characteristic **'worm eaten'** appearance. Gradually the bone is replaced by soft tubercular granulation tissue. Caseation appears at places followed by softening and liquefaction.

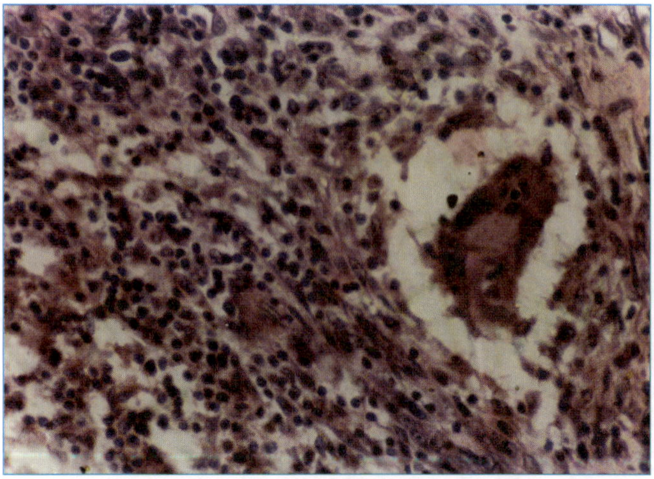

Fig.10.1: Shows caseation, Langhan's giant cell, lymphocytes and fibrosis in a case of tubercular osteomyelitis

A subperiosteal abscess then forms presenting a painless, soft swelling. This cold abscess may burst—either intra or extra orally—forming single or multiple sinuses. Pathological fracture of mandible and sequestration may also occur.

Chronic mandibular osteomyelitis results from odontogenic infection, post extraction complication, trauma, and the subsequent inadequate treatment of a fracture mandible.

Age and Sex: The typical age of presentation is in the fifties to the sixties, with males more likely to be affected. The commonest site is the posterior body of the mandible.

The incidence—outside of those who have received head and neck radiotherapy and the immunocompromised—is increased in patients who have poor oral hygiene and are abusers of alcohol or tobacco.

SYPHILITIC OSTEOMYELITIS

Occasional cases of syphilitic osteomyelitis involving the mandible and, less commonly, the maxilla, have been described. The condition represents a gummatous involvement of bone with extensive necrosis.

Clinically: The condition is characterised by pain, swelling, suppuration and sequestration and—clinically and radiologically—the condition may resemble pyogenic osteomyelitis. X-ray shows radiolucent areas commonly seen in hard palate.

RADIATION OSTEOMYELITIS

Radiation causes severe damage to the blood vessels, leading to death of the bone cells. This results in avascularity of the bone, which is an irradiated bone, and may lead to osteoradionecrosis. It is for this reason that extraction of the teeth in the affected area is advisable prior to radiation therapy.

OSTEORADIONECROSIS

Osteoradionecrosis of the jaw bones is common in chronic radium poisoning.

Osteoradionecrosis is a condition of non-vital bone at the site of radiation injury. It is a complication of high-dose radiation therapy for tumours of the oropharynx, and oral cavity.

Causes

Mandibular osteoradionecrosis develops most commonly after local trauma, such as dental extractions, biopsies, related cancer surgery, and periodontal procedures, but may also occur spontaneously.

Predisposing factors

- **Radiation dose:** It has been shown that increasing the external beam of radiation dose above 50 Gray gives a significantly increased risk for osteoradionecrosis. After dose between 60 and 72 Gy using standard fractionation, an incidence of osteoradionecrosis between 5% and 15% is reported.
- **Time to deliver the radiation dose:** Radiation therapy gives a progressive injury to tissues at a cellular and subsequently humoral level. If the entire dose is given in a short period of time, this will prevent the remaining viable local non-tumour cells from recovery and, therefore, will cause more damage.
- **More of delivery:** More localised delivery; by means of, e.g., brachytherapy limits radiation damage to external beam radiation.
- **Location:** Less vascularised part of mandible such as the posterior part or surgically manipulated parts are more susceptible to osteoradionecrosis.
- **Inadequate oral hygiene:** Intraoral tissues are damaged by irradiation, which causes mucositis and xerostomia. These conditions—in combination with poor dental care or a poorly fitting-

tissue borne prosthesis—give rise to odontogenic infections. This again, can leads to osteoradionecrosis.

- **Post-radiation surgery:** Any surgical procedure to the jaws that is performed after irradiation will increase the risk for developing osteoradionecrosis.
- **Pre-radiation surgery:** Since vascularisation of these tissues is impaired, preradiation surgery may cause osteonecrosis. This is due to loss of periosteal blood supply due to a marginal mandibular resection, unstable fixation of mandibular split osteotomy leading to malunion or non-union and inadequate tissue covering of the bone after resection of tumour.
- **Infections:** In an irradicated field, minor insult such as periodontal disease, pulpal infections and procedures such as dental extractions can result in delayed healing and, in some cases, develop osteoradionecrosis.

Pathogenesis

Irradicated mandible, periosteum, and overlying soft tissue undergo hyperaemia, inflammation and endarteritis. These conditions ultimately lead to thrombosis, cellular death, progressive hypovascularity and fibrosis.

Clinical features

Mandible is more frequently involved than maxilla. Clinical symptoms include pain, swelling, trismus, and oral cutaneous fistula formation, difficulty in deglutition, mastication and speech. Teeth become loose.

Microscopically

In general, there are six changes that occur temporarily in relation to radiation exposure. This includes hyperaemia, inflammation, thrombosis, cellular loss, hypovascularity, and progressive fibrosis.

There is intense fibrosis of inferior alveolar artery and periosteal arteries. Normal marrow is replaced by dense fibrous tissue with loss of osteocytes. There is absence of osteoblasts and lack of new bone formation.

CT scan shows cortical disruption, with disorganisation, and loss of trabeculation of the spongiosa of the mandible.

Bibliography

Kasper Braunwald Fauci, Hauser Longo Jameson: *Harrison's Principles of Internal Medicine*, Vol II 16th edition. New York: McGraw-Hill. 2005.

Roddie MN, Macsween Keith Whaley: *Muir's Textbook of Pathology*. 13th edition 1992.

CHAPTER

11

DISEASES OF BLOOD AND BLOOD FORMING ORGANS

DISEASES AFFECTING ERYTHROCYTES

ANAEMIA

Definition: Anaemia is a pathological condition characterised by a reduction in the concentration of haemoglobin in the peripheral blood below for the age and sex of the patient.

Classification of anaemia

Anaemia is broadly classified into two:

I. Morphological classification

II. Etiological classification

TABLE 11.1
MORPHOLOGICAL CLASSIFICATION OF ANAEMIA

- Normochromic normocytic anaemia
  Anaemia of acute blood loss
  Aplastic anaemia
- Hypochromic, microcytic anaemia
  Iron deficiency anaemia
  Thalassaemia
- Normochromic, macrocytic anaemia.
  Pernicious anaemia
  Anaemia due to folate and vitamin B_{12} deficiency
- Normochromic, microcytic anaemia
  Anaemia due to chronic infection

TABLE 11.2
ETIOLOGICAL CLASSIFICATION OF ANAEMIA

I. **Blood loss anaemia**
   A. **Acute blood loss:** Accidents, surgery, antepartum haemorrhage, post-partum haemorrhage, haematemesis, haemoptysis
   B. **Chronic blood loss:** Hookworm infestation, gastrointestinal bleeding, maliganancy, peptic ulcer, bleeding piles, haematuria, and abnormal menstrual bleeding

II. **Impaired red cell production**
   Iron deficiency anaemia
   Vitamin B_{12} deficiency
   Folic acid deficiency
   Protein calorie malnutrition

III. **Depression of erythropoietic activity**
   Anaemia associated with chronic disease
   Infection
   Connective tissue disorders
   Inflammatory disorders
   Disseminated malignancies
   Anaemia associated with renal failure

IV. **Aplastic anaemia**
   Anaemia due to replacement of bone marrow by:
   Leukaemia, lymphoma, myeloproliferative disorders, myelodysplastic syndrome, myeloma

V. **Anaemia due to inherited disorders** e.g., Thalassaemia

VI. **Anaemia due to excessive destruction**
   Anaemia due to intrinsic defect in RBCs
   Anaemia due to extrinsic defect on RBCs

A. IRON DEFICIENCY ANAEMIA

Causes

Causes of iron deficiency anaemia are deficiency of iron in the diet, pregnancy, infancy, poor absorption, and blood loss.

Oral manifestations

1. **Atrophic mucositis:** There is atrophy and loss of keratinisation of buccal mucosa and gingival. In some patients atrophic mucositis of aerodigestive tract or oropharynx may predispose to the occurrence of squamous cell carcinoma.
2. **Atrophic glossitis:** Papillae of tongue especially filiform papillae in the anterior two-third undergo atrophy. In severe cases, fungiform papillae are also affected leaving the tongue smooth and glazed.

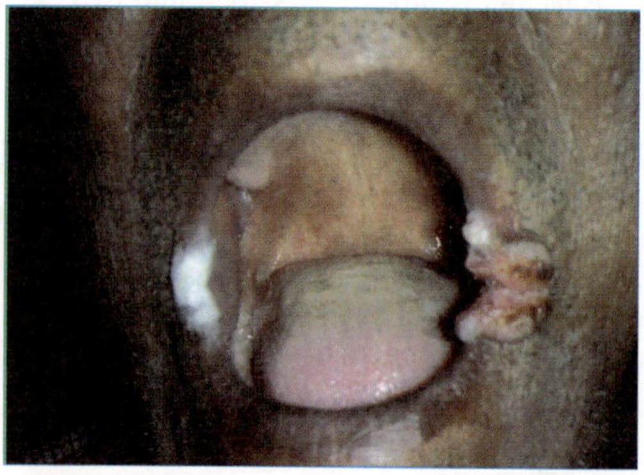

Fig.11.1: A showing features of angular cheilitis

3. **Angular cheilitis:** Atrophic glossitis is associated with fissures and ulcers at angle of mouth. There is reddening and some level of discomfort. It is caused by Candida albicans. There may be pain on opening or stretching, and rarely bleeding from ulcerated area.
4. **Pallor:** Buccal mucosa and gingiva is pale.

5. **Dysphagia:** Mucosa at the junction between esophagus and hypopharynx may form web-like projections into the lumen and leads to dysphagia for solid food (Plummer-Vinson syndrome). The projections are due to subepithelial infiltration with chronic inflammatory cells. Hyper-plastic epithelial activity may appear in some patients and postcricoid carcinoma may develop.

Changes in other tissues

Patient complains of headache, giddiness, tinnitus, dyspnoea on exertion, tingling and numbness of hands and intermittent claudication.

Finger nails become thinned, flattened and finally spoon-shaped (koilonychias). Nails become brittle or ridged.

Atrophic gastritis of variable severity with decrease in gastric juice secretion and hypochlorhydria or achlorhydria occurs in fair number of cases.

Gastrointestinal symptoms: Liver and spleen may be palpable due to fatty changes in organs.

Haematological findings

Haemoglobin, packed cell volume, total RBC counts are low.

Microcytic hypochromic type of anaemia. MCV and MCH are low.

Peripheral smear shows microcytes, hypochromia and pear-shaped RBCs.

Reticulocyte count is increased.

Bone marrow findings: Bone marrow shows erythroid hyperplasia, which is micronormoblastic type. Iron staining of bone marrow shows absence of unstainable iron in reticulin cells and less than 10% normoblasts stain as siderocytes.

Biochemical findings

Serum iron is low (Normal value is 50-180μg/dl). In severe iron deficiency serum iron is less than 50μg/dl.

Total iron binding capacity: Normal level is 250 to 450 μg/dl. In severe iron deficiency it is increased. It may be 500 μg/dl.

Serum ferritin: Normal levels are 20 to 150 ng/ml. It is low. In severe cases it may be < 10 ng/ml.

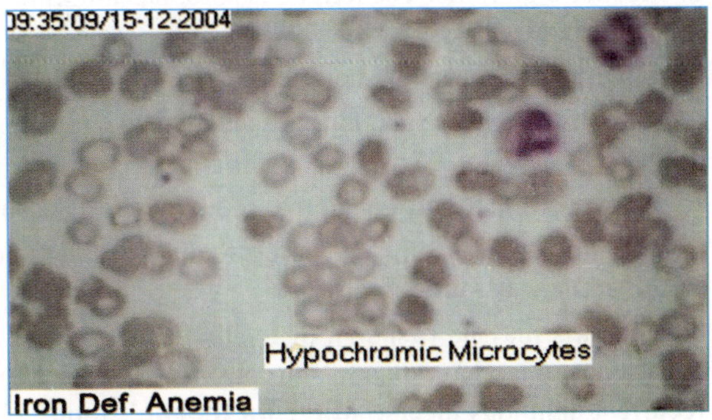

Fig.11.1A: Peripheral smear from a case of microcytic hypochromic anaemia

Other investigations

Examination of faeces

a. **Examination of faeces** for detection of melena. Bright red may be seen in lower gut bleeding.
b. **Occult blood test** present in faeces when gastrointestinal bleeding is intermittent.
c. **Microscopical examination** for ova, parasites and protozoa. Hookworm infection is a potent cause of severe anaemia.
d. **Examination of urine:** Urine examination detects haematuria and kidney disease.
e. **Gastric juice analysis:** Absolute achlorhydria and hypochlorhydria are frequently detected in iron deficiency anaemia.

Management

Anaemic women should take ferrous sulphate tablets. For a child below 12 months a mixture of ferrous ammonium citrate sweetened with glycerine and for children a ferrous ammonium citrate mixture should be given in curing.

In severe anaemia blood transfusion is given, if required followed by and/or parenteral administration and treatment of conditions causing iron deficiency anaemia.

B. VITAMIN B_{12} DEFICIENCY ANAEMIA

PERNICIOUS ANAEMIA

It is also known as Addisonian pernicious anaemia, tend to occur in whites.

Causes

Pernicious anaemia is due to inadequate gastric production or defective function of intrinsic factor.

Hereditary lack of intrinsic factor may occur as autosomal recessive homozygous.

Autoimmune mechanism: Antibodies are present in the serum and gastric juice of most patients of pernicious anaemia.

Blocking antibodies block the binding of vitamin B_{12} to intrinsic factor and binding antibodies react with IF B_{12} complex and prevent it from binding to ileal receptors.

Total gastrectomy, oesophagojejunostomy, and subtotal gastrectomy may lead to pernicious anaemia in course of several years. Corrosive gastritis, gastric carcinoma are rare causes of megaloblastic change.

Clinical features

Oral manifestations

The entire symptom complex of the tongue in pernicious anaemia is referred to as Hunter's glossitis or Moeller's glossitis. The tongue is sore, has a burning sensation, and shows atrophy of the papillae (beef streak).

Fissures and ulcers are common.

Atrophy of mucosa and muscles and disappearance of filiform papillae has been described as 'bald tongue'.

Nonspecific stomatitis: Pernicious anaemia is associated with nonspecific stomatitis.

Megaloblastic anaemias manifest themselves in the oral cavity as a part of megaloblastic changes in the entire gastrointestinal tract.

Glossitis may be first sign of folate or vitamin B_{12} deficiency. Clinically, patients with megaloblastic anaemias have painful atrophy of the entire oral mucus membrane and tongue as well as recurrent aphthous ulcers. **'Magenta tongue'** rather characteristic, may herald a B_{12} deficiency.

Tongue may show lobulations, which may be secondary to decrease in saliva production.

Oral mucosa shows greenish yellow discolouration at the junction of hard and soft palate due to increased serum bilirubin (jaundice).

Microscopically: Oral epithelial cells in pernicious anaemia reveal giant hyperchromatic nuclei with prominent nucleoli, pleomorphism, and serrated nuclear membrane. There is atrophy of epithelium with intra and or subepithelial chronic inflammatory cell infiltration.

Laboratory findings

Haematological findings

Haemoglobin and total RBC count is reduced. RBC count is less than 3 million/cubic millimetre.

MCV is more than 100 femto litres, low MCH and MCHC.

There is pancytopaenia, red blood cells, granulocytes and platelets are all reduced in number.

Peripheral smear: Anaemia is macrocytic hypochromic type with polychromasia, punctate basophilia, Howell-Jolly bodies and presence of nucleated RBCs. Megaloblasts may be present in peripheral blood. Polymorphs show hypersegmented nuclei (more than 5 lobes).

BONE MARROW

Macroscopic findings: Increased red marrow in all long bones, which appears red and gelatinous (red currant jelly). Red marrow extends into shaft of long bones and replaces yellow marrow.

Microscopically

Megaloblastic reaction is pathogenomic of pernicious anaemia. Bone marrow is hypercellular with megaloblastic erythropoiesis. Megaloblast is a large cell with large nucleus. Chromatin has an open pattern being arranged in a fine reticular fashion giving the nucleus-stippled appearance. Nuclear chromatin lags behind cytoplasm haemoglobinisation, with the result that megaloblasts with eosinophilic cytoplasm may still show nuclei with fine reticular chromatin. One or two Howell-Jolly bodies may be present.

Laboratory findings

Serum level of Vitamin B_{12}: It may be markedly decreased. Normal level is 16-64 µg/percent.

Intrinsic factor in gastric juice: In pernicious anaemia it is usually zero and never exceeds 10 units/ml.

Histamine fast achlorhydria and presence of IF antibodies in serum are detected.

Management

Most of the patients should be given vitamin B_{12} parenterally. The standard dosage is 100 mg intramuscularly every 30 days. Some of the cases are treated with massive oral dose of vitamin B_{12}.

C. HAEMOLYTIC ANAEMIA

Definition: The haemolytic anaemia comprises a group of disorders characterised by an increased rate of red cell destruction with a shortening of mean red cell life span.

TABLE 11.3
CLASSIFICATION OF HAEMOLYTIC ANAEMIA

A. Hereditary causes
1. Abnormal shape of RBCs
   a. Hereditary spherocytosis
   b. Hereditary elliptocytosis
2. Red cell enzyme defect
   a. G6PD deficiency
   b. Pyruvate kinase deficiency
3. Haemoglobinopathies
   a. Synthesis of abnormal haemoglobin chain Hb S, D, I, J, K.
   b. Defective globin chain synthesis thalassaemia syndrome

B. Acquired causes
1. Autoimmune haemolytic anaemia
   a. Warm antibody type
   b. Cold antibody type
2. Isoimmune haemolytic anaemia
   a. Haemolytic transfusion reaction
   b. Haemolytic disease of newborn
3. Drug induced immune haemolytic anaemia
   Penicillin, phenacetin, sulphonamide, quinidine

Contd.

Contd.

4. Haemolysis due to toxins and chemicals
   a. Bacterial toxins: Cl. welchii, Streptococci
   b. Chemicals: Lead, arsenic, copper
   c. Vegetable compounds: Fava bean
   d. Insects: Spider venom, snake venom
5. Red cell fragmentation syndrome
   a. March haemoglobinuria
   b. Microangiopathic haemolytic anaemia
6. Hypersplenism
7. Paroxysmal nocturnal haemoglobinuria
8. Parasitic invasion of red cell: Malarial parasite

SICKLE CELL ANAEMIA

This is a hereditary disease due to presence of haemoglobin S in patient's red blood cells. This is the abnormal haemoglobin of sickle cell disease and is much more insoluble in the reduced form than as oxycompounds. It is characterised by sickle-shaped erythrocytes due to presence of an abnormal type of haemoglobin (haemoglobin S).

Geographical distribution

In India, Lehmann and Kutbush first discovered this disease in tribes of South India.

This condition occurs in Nigeria, Uganda, America, West Indian Negroes, South Italy, Greece, Turkey and India. In India it is common in tribal and backward communities. This condition is described in Gond, Mahar, Kundbi, Teli, Munda, Bhil, Konda, Koya, and Kurmi community.

According to Indian Council of Medical Research this occurs in workers of tea garden in Assam, people living at the bank of Godawari river, workers of bidi karkhana in Maharashtra, tribals of Bihar, Orissa, Rajasthan, and Chattisgarh. In Madhya Pradesh— it is seen in Jhabua, Mandala, and Betul district.

Cause

In normal individuals, haemoglobin A is present in RBCs but in sickle cell disease red blood cells contain haemoglobin S. Haemoglobin S differs from haemoglobin A, glutamic acid which is normally present in 6th position at beta chain is replaced by valine, therefore the RBCs which are normally biconcave become sickle shaped and are destroyed by reticuloendothelial system. The haemoglobin S moves slower on electrophoresis gel and polymerises into an insoluble linear crystalloid that induces fatal changes in the red cells that have been exposed to low oxygen.

Classification

Sickle cell anaemia is classified into different types:

1. Homozygous sickle cell anaemia
2. Heterozygous trait
3. Sickle cell thalassaemia
4. Haemoglobin S/E disease
5. Haemoglobin S/C disease

Homozygous sickle cell anaemia: It is a hereditary disorder. In child, genes through parents transmit HbS. If mother and father both have haemoglobin S then the child suffers from homozygous sickle cell anaemia.

Heterozygous sickle cell trait: If mother or father has haemoglobin S then, in 50% of individuals, HbS replaces HbA.

Homozygous sickle cell anaemia

Clinical features

It is common in females. Symptom appears at the age of 6 months. The high level of haemoglobin F in the newborn protects the child for first 4 to 6 months.

Patients have stunted growth, loss of weight, kyphosis, less height, prominent frontal bones, and mongoloid facies.

Sometimes there is severe pain in abdomen with rigidity. In such cases, if surgery is performed due to wrong diagnosis of acute abdomen, leads to death.

There is increased susceptibility to infection due to decreased resistance (depressed immunity).

Renal medullary necrosis and ischaemic medulla gives rise to haematuria.

Haemolytic crisis

Dehydration, exercise, anoxia, excessive cold, mental tension and ingestion of sulpha drugs causes sickling of RBCs inside body, this causes excessive haemolysis of RBCs—leading to anaemia and jaundice.

Sickling in arteries lumen causes obstruction of blood flow and causes infarction of bones, brain, spleen and kidney.

In sickle cell anaemia large indolent and deep ulcers are formed most commonly around the ankle of the older child. Stasis of RBCs has a major role. Sickle cell dactylitis presents as a hand-foot syndrome early in life. Painful swelling of both hands and feet due to avascular necrosis of phalangeal bones is characteristic of this condition.

Obstruction of cerebral blood vessels causes infarction, and haemorrhages gives rise to headache, convulsion, hemiplegia, and mental abnormality. Most of the patients expire before reaching puberty.

There is enlargement of heart, tachycardia, and systolic and diastolic murmur. Severe abdominal pain, muscle and joint pain, high temperature results in circulatory collapse.

Oral manifestations

(i) In sickle cell disease, oral mucosa may be pale or yellowish due to haemolytic jaundice.

(ii) There is anesthesia of the mandibular nerve, pulpitic pain and pulpal necrosis, which can be ascribed to the microvascular occlusions that tend to affect organs with terminal circulation.

(iii) The patients with sickling disorders are more likely to have pain which is indistinguishable from toothache, presumably due to pulpal infarcts.

(iv) In areas of osteoporosis and erosion followed by osteosclerosis in mandible there is Salmonella osteomyelitis.

(v) Dental mal-occlusion may be present secondary to expansion of the bone marrow space.

(vi) There is greater incidence of caries in young patients, but no increase in periodontal disease.

(vii) Craniofacial features such as maxillary protrusion and more forward growth of the mandible with significantly retruded maxillary and mandibular incisors have been documented in children with sickle cell disease.

(viii) X-ray skull shows widening of medullary spaces, thinning of cortical bone, and sparseness of trabeculae, which produces a hair-on-end appearance. Intraoral periapical radiographs reveal 'step ladder' like trabeculae between contagious posterior teeth. There is osteoporosis and appearance of large irregular areas of radiolucency.

(ix) Mongoloid facies with high cheek bones and bimaxillary proganthism, flat face, swelling over eyelid and depressed nose is present.

Diagnosis

Laboratory features of haemolysis are unconjugated bilirubinaemia, urobilinogenuria, haematuria, increased alkaline phosphatase and isoenzymes—both bone and liver.

Peripheral smear shows normocytic normochromic anaemia, sickle cells in peripheral smear, normoblasts, target cells, Howell-Jolly bodies, spherocytes, polychromasia, basophilic stippling and pappenheimer bodies after splenectomy. Reticulocyte count is markedly increased.

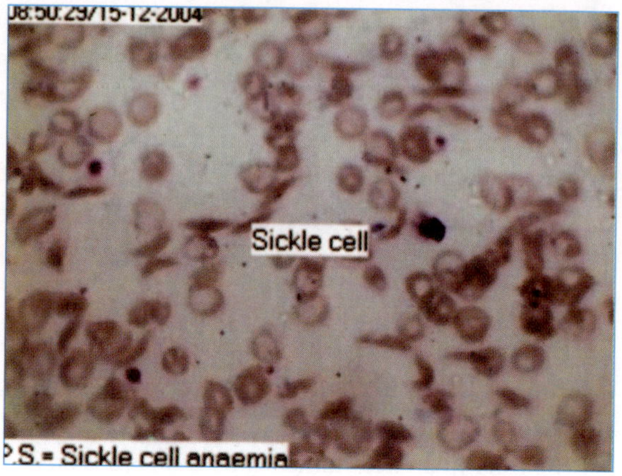

Fig.11.2: Peripheral smear from a case of sickle cell anaemia showing presence of sickle cells

Sickling test: When patient's blood is mixed with 2 percent sodium metabisulphite the red blood cells become sickle shaped.

Haemoglobin electrophoresis stabilises the diagnosis.

Management

A. **Prevention:** Patients with haemoglobin S should avoid dehydration, anoxia, excessive exercise, and prevention from cold, mental tension, air journey, high altitude, and ingestion of sulpha drugs.

B. **Treatment**
   1. Repeated blood transfusion
   2. Splenectomy causes improvement in many cases
   3. Administration of folic acid for regenerating bone marrow
   4. Ingestion of Na bicarbonate and sodium citrate
   5. Antibiotics and vaccination for prevention from infections
   6. Bone marrow transplantation
   7. Gene therapy for the treatment is under trial.

THALASSAEMIA

Nomenclature: Thalassaemias are also known as Cooley's anaemias or Mediterranean anaemia. These hereditary globinopathies are common around the Mediterranean Sea, hence the name Thalassaemia. It is derived from Greek word which ***'Thalassos'*** means the sea.

Definition: Thalassaemias are a diverse group of hereditary disorders in which there is reduced rate of synthesis of one of more of the globin polypeptide chains.

Geographical distribution: Thalassaemias are worldwide and occur in nearly all-ethnic groups. But they are particularly prevalent in Mediterranean region, the Indian subcontinent and South East Asia. Thalassaemias were originally described in Italians, Greeks, Spanish, and Sind area of Gujarat.

Classification

Depending upon whether the genetic defect or deletion lies in transmission of alpha or beta globin genes the thalassaemias are classified into two:

Alpha thalassaemia: The patients with alpha thalassaemia have structurally normal alpha chains but their production is impaired.

Beta thalassaemia: In patients with beta thalassaemia, β globin chain is structurally normal but their production is decreased.

Alpha thalassaemias

Alpha thalassaemias are due to deletion of one or more genes located on short arms of chromosome 16.

Alpha thalassaemias are mainly of two types:

Heterozygous alpha thalassaemia

Homozygous alpha thalasaemia

Haemoglobin H disease: Haemoglobin H is beta chain tetramers. Haemoglobin β4 is functionally absent. In newborn, 1 to 2% is haemoglobin Bart. After one year it is absent. Patient with HbH disease presents with haemolytic anaemia, splenomegaly and cholelithiasis.

Oral changes: There is severe alveolar bone loss, pronounced spacing of maxillary anterior teeth and mongoloid facies.

Diagnosis

Vital staining with brilliant cresyl blue induces blue inclusion bodies HbH which precipitates in many red blood cells. Haemoglobin electrophoresis shows presence of haemoglobin H.

Haemoglobin Bart: Haemoglobin Bart is gamma globin chain tetramers γ4, which has low oxygen affinity leading to severe tissue hypoxia. Haemoglobin Bart hydrops foetalis is incompatible with life due to severe tissue hypoxia. This condition is either fatal in utero or the newborn dies shortly after birth. If born alive, severe haemolytic anaemia is present.

Beta thalassaemia

A single gene on chromosome 11 codes for beta chains. Mutation in this gene results in a failure to synthesise beta chain or reduced synthesis of beta chains. Failure to synthesise beta chain leads to an excess of alpha chains within the red cells, which gets precipitated and damage the erythrocyte.

Depending upon the extent of beta chain synthesis there are three types of beta thalassaemias:

Thalassaemia major or homozygous.

Thalassaemia intermedius homozygous

Thalassaemia minor or heterozygous.

Clinical features

It is a disease of childhood. Thalassaemia major causes death before adolescence is reached. Pallor starts appearing within 4-6 months. Patients first presents with pallor of the skin, jaundice, fever, chills, malaise and generalised weakness.

There may be marked hepatosplenomegaly and cholelithiasis.

Death is generally due to intercurrent infection, cardiac arrhythmias, haemosiderosis of cardiac muscle, heart block and congestive cardiac failure.

Oral manifestations

The child is ill nourished and the head is enlarged, with a typical mongoloid facies (chipmunk) i.e., sunken bridge of the nose, puffy eyelids, with an epicanthic fold. Mongoloid facies is due to expansion of marrow in the molar bones. There is protrusion of the upper molar teeth.

Rodent facies: There is marked over-development of maxilla associated with hyperplasia of alveolar process, which results in anterior open bite and prominent cheek bone producing characteristic **'rodent facies'**.

X-ray findings: As a result of marrow hyperplasia there is thinning of the cancellous bone of entire skeletal system. There is rarefaction and absorption of cortex demonstrable by X-ray and may precede skull changes. The calvarium shows a typical **'hair on end'** or so-called sunray appearance. This is probably due to separation of diploe by hyperplastic marrow associated with new bone formation on the outer table of skull showing multiple perpendicular striations.

Jaw bones show coarsening of some bony trabeculae and blurring or disappearance of others, it often produces a typical radiographic appearance called **'salt and pepper'** effect.

There is delayed pneumatization of the paranasal sinuses, especially the maxillary sinuses.

Diagnosis

MCHC is low but MCHC may be normal.

There is microcytic hypochromic anaemia.

Peripheral smear shows anisocytosis, poikilocytosis, target cells, and normoblasts.

There is presence of foetal haemoglobin (10-20%). It may be up to 90%.

Haemoglobin electrophoresis shows presence of increased amounts of haemoglobin F and A2 and almost complete absence of HbA.

Antenatal diagnosis is possible by the techniques of polymerase chain reaction for thalassaemia gene on cells obtained by amniocentesis, chorionic villus biopsy or direct fetal blood sampling.

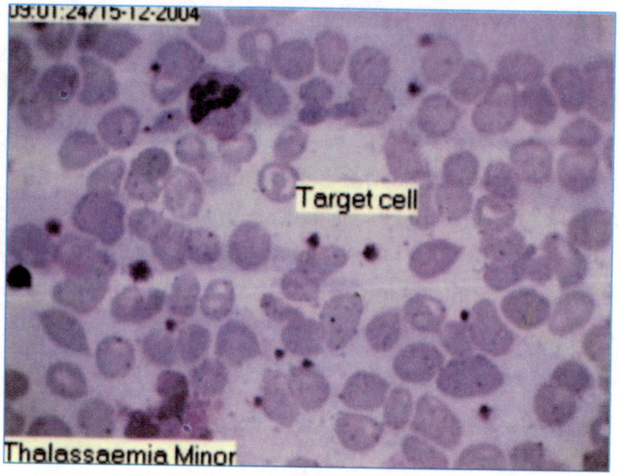

Fig.11.3: Peripheral smear shows presence of target cells in a case of thalassaemia

Treatment

1. Patient requires repeated blood transfusion, folic acid supplement to maintain increased demand of hyperplastic marrow.
2. Splenectomy in selected cases may show a temporary improvement of the blood picture.
3. Prevention and treatments of iron overload is being done in some centres with fair success rate by chelating agents.
4. Bone marrow transplantation is being done in some centres with fair success rate.

CONGENITAL ERYTHROPOIETIC PORPHYRIA

The porphyrias are largely genetic (and heritable); rarely they may be acquired disorders of haem synthesis due to deficiencies of specific enzymes in the haem-synthetic pathway.

Congenital erythropoietic porphyria (CEP) is due to deficiency of enzyme uroporphyrinogen III cosynthase. The bone marrow is usually affected.

Clinical features includes haemolytic anaemia, splenomegaly, photosensitivity leading to bullae, crusting, scars, sclerodermatoid change, hyper- and hypopigmentation.

Dental changes

There is erythrodontia (red teeth). The colour of the teeth varies from yellow to brown-red with occasional shades of pink and purple. The teeth contain uroporphyrin I and show red fluorescence.

HAEMOLYTIC DISEASE OF NEWBORN

Erythroblastosis fetalis

In first pregnancy fetal red blood cells commonly enter the maternal circulation shortly before or during labour, in the course of obstetric manipulations and during abortion. Anti Rh antibodies produced in maternal blood are incomplete, IgG type and capable of crossing placental barrier in subsequent pregnancies. The maternal anti Rh antibodies reaches the fetus via placenta; it reacts with the fetal agglutinogens—as a result there will be continuous haemolysis of RBCs.

Clinical features

There is still-birth. Infant is born with severe anaemia, jaundice, edema, and ascitis. There is severe anoxia in utero with cardiac failure and hepatosplenomegaly due to extramedullary erythropoiesis.

Kernicterus: When unconjugated bilirubin is more than 15mg/dl brain damage occurs due to deposition, staining and necrosis of the basal nuclei.

Changes in teeth

The deciduous teeth usually present black, yellow-brown or blue discolouration. In some cases typical ring-like defect appears which is known as Rh hump. It usually involves the incisal edges of the anterior teeth and middle portion of the deciduous cuspid and first molar crown.

Laboratory diagnosis

RBCs count varies from normal to less than 1,000,000 cells per cubic millimetre.

Peripheral smear shows large number of normoblasts, polychromasia, and spherocytes.

Serum bilirubin is very high.

Hereditary Elliptocytosis

It is inherited as an autosomal trait. It is due to abnormality in the spectrin molecule. There is haemolysis of RBCs leads to haemolytic anaemia.

Peripheral smear shows prominent elliptocytosis (more than 40%). There is normocytic normochromic anaemia.

Glucose 6 phosphate dehydrogenase deficiency

It is one of the most common of all genetic defects with a high frequency (4 to 40%) among persons of Mediterranean, Asian and African regions. Incidence is low in Europeans and Japanese. Deficiency is more common in areas where malaria is endemic.

Inheritance of defect is sex-linked, affecting male and carried by females.

Normally intracellular glutathione GSH inactivates oxidants. The erythrocytes and its membrane are vulnerable to injury by endogenous or exogenous oxidants. Principal effects of a deficiency is a decrease in reduced glutathione; in consequence oxidants are free to damage cellular constituents, and haemoglobin is readily oxidised to methaemoglobin intracellular precipitate of which is seen as Heinz bodies.

Clinical features

Persons with G6PD deficiency normally enjoy good health but are liable to haemolysis in response to oxidants stress. Haemolysis is precipitated by acute bacterial infection, infection of compounds, e.g., fava bean. Certain drugs, e.g., antimalarials, sulphonamide, antitubercular drugs, phenacetin, and antihelmintics cause severe haemolysis.

Severe intravascular haemolysis accompanied by pain in abdomen and kernicterus.

Diagnosis

Estimation of G6PD gives confirmative diagnosis.

There is considerable reticulocytosis.

Blood film shows fragmented and contracted red blood cells with Heinz bodies.

D. APLASTIC ANAEMIA

Definition: Aplastic anaemia is a disorder or a group of disorders characterised by decrease in production of erythrocytes, leukocytes, and platelets leading to pancytopaenia; anaemia, leukopaenia and thrombocytopaenia. Anaemia is due to suppression of bone marrow.

Clinical features

Aplastic anaemia affects persons of all ages and sexes and onset is insidious. Primary aplastic anaemia may be very acute, ending in a fatal issue within a few weeks or may last for some months. Patients may feel weakness after slight physical exertion, dyspnea and exhibits pallor of the skin. Haemorrhages due to thrombocytopaenia at various sites such as skin (ecchymosis and petechiae) nose, gums, vagina, bowel and occasionally central nervous system. Granulocytopaenia and agranulocytosis causes fever with chills and prostration.

Chronic infections, recurrent chest infection, pneumonia, and septicemia are common complications.

Splenomegaly is characteristically absent in aplastic anaemia but lymphadenopathy may be seen in some cases.

TABLE 11.4
CLASSIFICATION OF CAUSES OF APLASTIC ANAEMIA

A. Hereditary or idiopathic (primary)
- Fanconi anaemia
- Diamond Blackfan syndrome
- Schwachman syndrome,
- Dyskeratosis congenital.

B. Acquired (secondary)

1. Chemical and dose related
- Alkylating agents
- Benzene
- Hair dye
- Chloramphenicol
- Cytotoxic drugs

Idiosyncratic reactions
- Chloramphenicol
- Antidiabetic drugs

Contd.

Contd.

- Antibiotics-Sulphonamides, Streptomycin, Isoniazid
- Organic chemicals
- Thiouracil
- Dinitrophenol
- Trinitrotolulene

2. Physical agents
   - External: Irradiation, X-ray, Gamma rays
   - Internal: 33p, $51_{cr,}$ 131_{I}
3. Infection
   - Viral: HIV, Hepatitis A, B, C, cytomegalovirus Epstein-Barr virus, parvovirus, B_{19}
4. Long continued wasting diseases: Nephritis
5. Metabolites: Pancreatitis, cachexia, and pregnancy
6. Immunity: Host versus graft reaction
7. Paroxysmal nocturnal haemoglobinuria
8. Tumours: Thyroid tumours, metastatic carcinoma, aleukaemic leukaemia, Multiple myeloma, Ewing's sarcoma.

Oral manifestations

1. Oral manifestations in aplastic anaemia include intraoral petechiae (gingival, soft palate), ecchymoses, haematomas and spontaneous bleeding of gingival.
2. Intraoral erythematous candidiasis is common.
3. Viral infections seen in aplastic anaemia are herpes simplex, herpangina, and varicella zoster.
4. Tongue and oral mucosa is pale due to anaemia.
5. There is ulceration and necrosis of oral mucosa. Large ragged ulcers covered by grey or black necrotic membrane may be present, which are as a result of generalised lack of resistance to infection and trauma.
6. Some workers reported hyperplasia of gingival tissue.

POLYCYTHAEMIA

Definition: Polycythaemia denotes an increase in number of red blood cells per cubic millimetre. It is also defined as increase in a haemoglobin level above normal for age and sex of the patients.

The term polycythaemia rubra vera is used for primary or idiopathic polycythaemia.

Secondary polycythaemia is due to high altitude, congenital heart diseases and malignant neoplasm.

TABLE 11.5
CLASSIFICATION OF POLYCYTHAEMIA

A. Relative polycythaemia
- a. Diminished plasma volume: Dehydration shock
- b. Spurious polycythaemia (stress polycythaemia, Gaisbock syndrome)

B. Absolute polycythaemia

I. Secondary polycythaemia (increased erythropoietin)
- a. Appropriate erythropoietin production

Contd.

Contd.

1. Arterial oxygen unsaturation; high altitude, pulmonary disease, cyanotic heart disease, smoker's polycythaemia, methaemoglobinaemia HbM
2. High oxygen affinity haemoglobinopathy
b. Inappropriate erythropoietin production
1. Neoplasm: Renal cell carcinoma, cerebellar haemangioma, hepatoma, uterine fibroids, adrenal cortical neoplasm
2. Renal pathology: Cysts, hydronephrosis, transplantation
c. Familial polycythaemia
II. Polycythaemia vera

In polycythaemia total RBCs count is 6,500,000 to 8,000,000/ cu mm.

In both primary and secondary forms the oral mucous membrane may be raspberry or purple in colour, and spontaneous gingival bleeding may occur.

II. DISEASES AFFECTING LEUKOCYTES

A reduction in the number of granulocytes in blood is known as neutropenia or sometimes, when severe, as agranulocytosis.

TABLE 11.6
CAUSES OF NEUTROPAENIA

A. Decreased production

a. **Drug-induced:** Alkylating agents, antimetabolites, many noncytoxic agents like routinely used antibiotics, antihistamines, anticonvulsants, anti-psychotics, anti-platelet agents.

b. **Haematological diseases:** Idiopathic, cyclic neutropaenia, Chediac-Higashi syndrome, aplastic anaemia, infantile genetic disorders like Kostmann's syndrome.

c. **Tumour infiltration and myelofibrosis.**

d. **Infections:** Tuberculosis, typhoid fever, brucellosis, tularemia, measles, infectious mononucleosis.

e. **Nutritional deficiencies:** Folate deficiency, vitamin B_{12} deficiency.

B. Peripheral destruction

a. **Isoimmune:** ANCA-opsonised engulfment by splenic and alveolar macrophages

b. **Autoimmune:** Rheumatoid arthritis, Felty's syndrome, SLE, etc.

c. Drugs acting as haptens-aminopyrine, phenylbutazolidine.

d. Vasculitis, as in Wegner granulomatosis.

C. Peripheral pooling (transient)

a. Overhelming Gram-negative bacteraemia.

b. Cardiopulmonary bypass.

c. Haemodialysis.

d. Leukopheresis.

AGRANULOCYTOSIS

Clinical features

The initial symptoms are often fever, sore throat, painful mouth ulcers, malaise, and chills, followed by marked weakness, fatigability and reduced immune response.

Agranulocytosis is the term given to the clinical effects of severe neutropaenia, namely fever, prostration and ulceration, particularly of the gingivae and pharynx.

Oral manifestations

Oral ulcers are oval and variable in size. In addition, gingivitis or periodontitis is a frequent finding with ulcerations located on the attached gingivae. Pain is a feature of these lesions.

Infections constitute the major problem; they commonly present as ulcerating, necrotising lesions of gingival, floor of the mouth, buccal mucosa, pharynx, or other sites in oral cavity. In agranulocytosis there are many oral ulcers with numerous microorganisms and few inflammatory cells.

Microscopically: The epithelium is lacking and there is an eosinophilic fibrin surface, Underlying the pseudomembrane and imperceptibly merging with it is a zone of amorphous necrotic tissue, which is strikingly devoid of neutrophils.

Complications of agranulocytosis include pneumonia, septicemia, bacterial and fungal infection.

Bone marrow: There is marked decrease in maturing granulocyte precursors in the marrow.

CYCLIC NEUTROPAENIA

Discovery have been reported showing autosomal dominant forms of cyclic neutropaenia, and some sporadic cases of cyclic neutropaenia have mutations of ELA_2.

Cyclic neutropaenia is present in children but acquired form of cyclic neutropaenia in adulthood exists.

Patients manifest fever, sore throat, stomatitis, and regional lymphadenopathy, as well as arthritis, cutaneous infection and conjunctivitis.

Otitis media, joint pain and headache are often present during the neutropaenic phase.

Oral manifestations

1. Oral ulcers that are multifocal are located primarily on movable mucosa, appear every 20 to 25 days, persist for 5-8 days and reappear on a periodic basis—probably represent oral manifestations of cyclic neutropenia.
   The ulcers are shallow, may show erythematous halo, and vary in size.
2. Coexistant periodontal lesions are common.
3. The gingival papillae are erythematous and edematous, and may be ulcerated.
4. Vertical alveolar bone loss with pocket formation is encountered in many regions throughout both dental arches.
5. Gingival recession leading to tooth mobility.

LEUKAEMIAS

Rudolf Virchow, the renowned German pathologist, coined the term leukaemia in 1886.

Definition: Leukaemia is a malignant state of haemopoietic tissue characterized by widespread proliferation of leukopoietic cells in the bone marrow with or without appearance of abnormal premature leukocytes in the peripheral blood.

Classification

Based on rate of progress

A. **Acute leukaemia:** It is of sudden onset and life expectancy without treatment is short (3-4 months). It tends to affect younger people. The symptoms develop rapidly, and it can quite quickly become life threatening if not treated.

B. **Chronic leukaemia:** It is of gradual onset and patients have usually been unwell for years and survive a much longer time. It tends to affect older people.

On the basis of cell type leukaemias may be

Acute myeloblastic leukaemia

Acute lymphoblastic leukaemia

Chronic myeloid leukaemia

Chronic lymphatic leukaemia

Hairy cell leukaemia.

Etiology of leukaemia

Oral manifestations in patients with leukaemia have been described in all subtypes of acute myeloid leukaemia, chronic myeloid leukaemia, acute lymphoblastic leukaemia, and chronic lymphocytic leukaemia.

Etiology

Genetic factors: Several congenital conditions may increase the risk of leukaemia. Most common are Down's syndrome, Bloom's syndrome, Klinefelter syndrome, and Wiskott-Aldrich's syndrome, Fanconi's anaemia and ataxia telangiectasia.

Environmental factors: A number of risk factors for developing leukaemia have been identified.

1. **Preleukaemic blood disorders** such as myeloproliferative syndromes or myelodysplastic syndromes can evolve into leukaemia, exact risk depends on the type of MDS/MPS.
2. **Drugs:** Exposure to anti-cancerous chemotherapy, in particular alkalyting agents, can increase the risk of subsequent development of AML. The risk is highest about 3-5 years after chemotherapy. Other chemotherapeutic agents—specifically epipodophyllotoxins and anthracyclines—have been associated with treatment related leukaemia.
3. **Ionising radiation** exposure can increase the risk of leukaemia. Survivors of the atomic bombings of Hiroshima and Nagasaki had an increased rate of leukaemia, as did radiologists exposed to high levels of X-rays to the absorption of modern radiation safety practices.
4. **Occupational chemical exposure** to benzene and other aromatic organic solvents is controversial as a cause of leukaemia.
5. **Infections:** Viruses have also been linked to some forms of leukaemias, e.g., certain cases of ALL are associated with viral infections by either human immunodeficiency virus (HIV or T lymphocytic virus HTLV-1and 2) causing adult T-cell leukaemia, lymphoma.
6. **Genetic and chromosomal factors:** Philadelphia chromosome is found in about 15% of cases of chronic myeloid leukaemia. Scientific research has shown that malignancies are due to subtle or less subtle changes in DNA that lead to unimpaired cell division and breakdown of inhibitory processes.

ACUTE LEUKAEMIA

ACUTE MYELOID LEUKAEMIA

TABLE 11.7
MORPHOLOGICAL SUBTYPES OF ACUTE MYELOID LEUKAEMIA

Subtypes	Common name	Morphology
M0	Undifferentiated	Primitive cells
M1	AML without maturation	Myeloblasts predominate, distinct nucleoli, few granules
M2	AML with maturation	Myeloblasts and promyelocytes predominate, Auer rods +/-
M3	Acute promyelocytic leukaemia	Promyelocytes predominate, hypergranular, often with multiple auer rods per cell
M4	Acute myelomonocytic leukaemia	Monocytoid appearing cells in peripheral blood: M4 with eosinophilia is subtype
M5	Acute monocytic leukaemia	Two subtypes identified: (a) differentiated with 80% Promonocytes and monocytes
M6	Acute erythroleukaemia	Predominance of erythroblasts and markedly dysplastic erythroid precursors
M7	Acute megakaryocytic leukaemia	Pleomorphic, undifferentiated blasts react with antiplatelet antibodies and contain platelet peroxidase

ACUTE LYMPHOBLASTIC LEUKAEMIA

TABLE 11.8
MORPHOLOGICAL SUBTYPES OF ACUTE LYMPHOBLASTIC LEUKAEMIA

Subtype	Common name	Morphology
L1	Acute lymphoblastic leukaemia (ALL)	Small round blasts with scanty cytoplasm
L2	ALL	Pleomorphic larger blasts with more cytoplasm and prominent nucleoli
L3	ALL	Large blasts cells with basophilic vacuolated cytoplasm and vesicular nuclei; undifferentiated cell type

Clinical features in acute leukaemias

It is more common in children and young adults between the age of 15 and 39 years. Males are affected more commonly than females with a ratio of 3 : 2.

A. Symptoms due to bone marrow failure

1. Symptoms due to anaemia: Pallor, fatigue, weakness and dyspnea.
2. Infections are due to reduction in normal lymphocytes. Infections are quiet common and include those of mouth, throat, skin, respiratory, perianal and other sites.

3. Bleeding from gum due to thrombocytopaenia, haemorrhages in the skin, retina, pleura, pericardium, peritoneum, pelvis of the kidney and bleeding from other sites are due to thrombocytopaenia.

B. Due to organ involvement

1. Lymphadenopathy and enlargement of lymph nodes are common in ALL.
2. **Splenomegaly:** Moderately enlarged, sinuses are filled with leukaemic infiltration. Splenic infarction, subcapsular haemorrhages, and rarely splenic rupture may occur.
3. **Hepatomegaly:** There is enlargement of liver due to leukaemic cell infiltration with variable portal fibrosis.
4. Pain and tenderness of bones result from marrow expansion with infiltration of the periosteum.
5. **Nervous system:** There is leukaemic cell infiltration of brain nerve roots, and meninges. Meningeal infiltrates more common in children in lymphoblastic variety. Haemorrhages are seen in extra- and intra cerebral areas which give rise to paralysis.
6. **Respiratory system:** Infiltration of various parts with leukaemic cells, which may be migratory. Miliary lesions are common.

Oral manifestations

Gingival infiltration of leukaemic cells is commonly seen in acute monocytic leukaemia (M5) and myelomonocytic leukaemia (M4).

Common oral findings in acute leukaemia include

(i) **Swelling:** Gingival swelling as a result of low-grade infection at the gingival margins but lack of effective white cells.

(ii) Spontaneous gingival haemorrhaging and small petechial haemorrhages or bruising of the oral soft tissue is secondary to thrombocytopaenia. There may be ecchymoses with necrosis of the oral mucosa.

(iii) Leukaemic patients are more prone to oral candidiasis, herpetic infections, and neutropaenic ulcerations. These ulcers are typically deep, punched out lesions with a grey-white necrotic base. They occur commonly after chemotherapy, related to mucosal trauma and/or opportunistic infections.

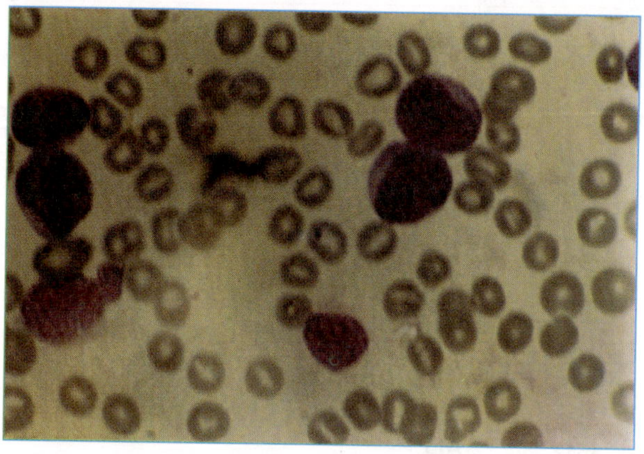

Fig.11.4: Peripheral smear from a case of acute myeloid leukaemia

(iv) Anaemia, mucosal pallor may be noticeable, and is an important sign in children among whom anaemia is otherwise common.

(v) Profuse bleeding follows tooth extraction.

The gingivae become packed and swollen with leukaemic cells—particularly in acute myelogenous leukaemia in adults.

Microscopically: Sections prepared from oral lesions in chronic lymphocytic leukaemia show a dense infiltration by lymphocytes or with slightly larger round hyperchromatic nuclei.

Haematological findings

Leukocyte count is usually raised, often 100,000/cumm.

Peripheral smear shows large number of primitive blast (lymphoblast or myeloblast).

There is thrombocytopaenia.

Bone marrow is hypercellular, and is tightly packed with immature cells. There is an associated anaemia, thrombocytopaenia, and decreased functioning of neutrophils.

CHRONIC LEUKAEMIA

CHRONIC MYELOID LEUKAEMIA (CML)

Clinical features

CML is generally seen in young or middle aged adults, with a peak incidence at 55 years. This disease can occur at any age. Chronic leukaemia begins insidiously and exhibits few clinical sign and symptoms.

Symptoms: Half of patients have no symptoms at all when they are diagnosed. CML presents mostly in the chronic phase. Main features of chronic phase are tiredness, weight loss, headache, and visual disturbances, night sweat, and bone pain. Patients may present with abdominal discomfort and rarely persistent painful erection (priapism).

Signs: There is usually massive enlargement of spleen, which may exceed 3 kg, and often causes great discomfort. There is hepatomegaly and lymphadenopathy.

Patients with chronic leukaemia may exhibit a pale oral mucosa and prolonged bleeding time.

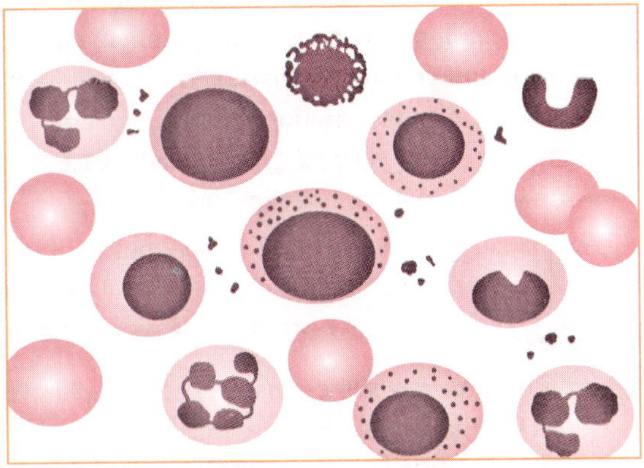

Fig.11.5: Peripheral smear from a case of chronic myeloid leukaemia leukaemia

Haematological findings

RBCs: Anaemia is moderate, normocytic and normochromic type. Smear shows presence of small number of normoblasts.

WBCs: Total leukocyte count is very high and may reach up to 500,000/cumm or even more. Most of the cells are mature neutrophils. Myeloblasts, myelocytes, metamyelocytes, promyelocytes, and band cells are present in the smear. Neutrophilic alkaline phosphatase activity is markedly decreased.

Chronic myeloid leukaemia is associated with the presence of chromosomal abnormality, e.g., Philadelphia chromosome.

CHRONIC LYMPHATIC LEUKAEMIA

Clinical features

Chronic lymphatic leukaemia usually presents in an indolent fashion in older patients. The disease occurs during the age of 45 to 70 years. It is never seen in children. CLL is common in males than in females.

Symptoms: Clinically symptoms usually develop gradually. Patients of CLL complain of tiredness, loss of weight, fever, loss of appetite, lethargy, night sweats, and breathlessness. They have bleeding and bruising including frequent or severe nose bleeding, bleeding from gums, and petechiae. Patients may experience frequent infections of skin, lungs, and kidney.

Signs

Generalised enlargement of lymph nodes is a prominent feature. Cervical, axillary, inguinal, abdominal, mediastinal, post-auricular, submaxillary and pectoral group of lymph nodes are enlarged, firm, discrete, and painless. Splenomegaly and hepatomegaly is frequent. Tongue, tonsil, nasopharynx is hypertrophied and form large masses. There is hepatosplenomegaly.

Skin shows two different types of lesions:

(i) **Erythroderma:** Reddening, edema, and thickening.

(ii) **Leukaemia cutis:** Localized or generalised yellow brown or purple nodules, which may ulcerate, are present in CLL.

Oral findings: There is bruising, bleeding from gums and presence of petechiae in oral mucosa.

Haematological findings

Blood picture

RBCs show moderate anaemia. Normoblasts are rarely seen. Anaemia is haemolytic type of autoimmune nature.

WBCs: Leukocyte count is usually near 100,000/cumm.

Peripheral smear: 80 to 90% cells are small lymphocytes. Naked nuclei without cytoplasm are quiet common. The neoplastic lymphocytes are fragile and frequently disrupted mechanically during smear preparation, producing characteristically smudge cells. Occasionally CLL transforms into polymphocytic leukaemia.

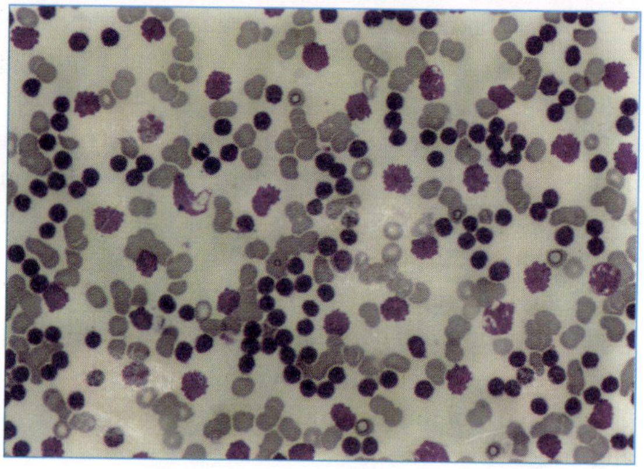

Fig.11.6: Peripheral smear from a case of chronic lymphatic leukaemia shows small lymphocytes with naked nuclei

The small lymphocytes differ from normal lymphocytes by possessing looser chromatin network. There is often a narrow rim of pale blue cytoplasm.

Bone marrow

1. Bone marrow shows an excess of lymphocytes and gradually replaces the normal haemopoietic cells. Eventually the fatty marrow is also replaced by lymphocytes and shaft of the long bones become filled with pale leukaemic cells.
2. Reduced myeloid precursor.
3. Replacement of erythroid element by infiltrating lymphocytes.
4. Megakaryocytes usually decreased.

MULTIPLE MYELOMA

Synonyms: Multiple plasmacytoma, Plasma cell myeloma, and Kahler's disease.

Multiple myeloma is a malignant tumour of bone marrow. It is defined as a chronic, progressive, and neoplastic proliferation of plasma cells.

Etiology

This is unknown. Risk factors include exposure to pesticides and herbicides (in farm workers), ionising radiation, prolonged use of hair colouring agents and chronic antigenic stimulation.

Clinical features

More than 80 percent of cases occur in patients past 45 years of age. Some patients have pathological fractures:

1. **Pain:** Bone pain is an important clinical feature of myeloma. It is due to lytic lesions which weaken bone, causing compression with or without collapse, may compress nerve roots in spine. Release of osteoclast activating factor (OAF) contributes to lysis.
2. **Infections** due to decreased ability to produce specific antibody, hypogammaglobulinaemia, and neutrophilic dysfunction (especially bacteria causing pneumonia, and pyelonephritis).
3. **Hyperviscosity syndrome** due to high levels of immunoglobulin, producing microcirculatory impairment; typically seen in plasmacytoid lymphoma producing IGM (macroglobinemia) but may occur with myeloma producing IgG or IgM.
4. **Bleeding tendency:** These can occur—such as purpura or mucosal bleeding. They are due to thrombocytopaenia, platelet dysfunction and antibodies against clotting factors.
5. **Anaemia:** Fatigue, weakness, and pallor result from anaemia. Anaemia can result from replacement of bone marrow by myeloma cells, suppression of normal lymphocytes by myeloma cells and neutropaenia secondary to marrow infiltration are responsible.
6. **Neurological symptoms** include lethargy, weakness, depression, and confusion.
7. **Renal failure:** This occurs in 50% of patients. Its causes are—formation of light chain casts in renal tubules, hypercalcaemia, amyloid deposits, and pyelonephritis.

Oral manifestations

Tongue: The most common manifestation of amyloidosis (in multiple myeloma) is macroglossia, which occurs in 20% of patients.

Burning mouth syndrome is the initial sign of multiple myeloma.

When multiple myeloma involves the oral cavity, it is usually a late manifestation of lesions within the jaws, most often the mandible. The mandible is involved far more frequently than the maxilla, especially the most active haemopoietic areas—the ramus, angle and molar region of the mandible. These lesions cause swelling of the jaws, pain, numbness, mobility of teeth and pathologic fractures. The incidence of joint involvement in multiple myeloma averages about 15%.

Since multiple myeloma results in immunosuppression, a variety of infections may be present, including oral hairy leukoplakia and candidiasis.

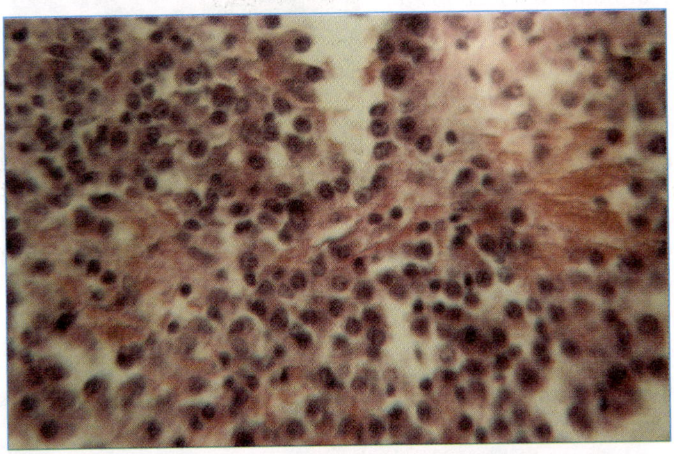

Fig.11.7: Shows microscopic appearance of myeloma (myeloma cells)

Pathogenesis

Many myeloma cells express membrane phenotype of plasma cells, e.g., cytoplasmic immunoglobulin, PC-1, PCA-1 and CD 38. Multiple myeloma arises from malignant transformation of a B-lymphoid stem cell committed to produce plasma cells. Interleukin-6 (IL-6) is an essential growth factor for plasma cells.

Haematological findings

WBC count is normal, rises, or moderately reduced, but moderate leukopaenia is the most common finding.

Anaemia is usually normocytic, normochromic, occasionally macrocytic or leukoerythroblastic.

Bone marrow: Normal bone marrow is replaced by soft grey gelatinous tumour, often likened to red gelatinous jelly with haemorrhage and there is erosion and destruction of cortical bone.

Cellularity is markedly increased.

Malignant plasma cells are present in parts of the bone marrow involved. They may form clumps or sheets, which replace the marrow, or may be scattered among the normal haematopoeitic cells.

Myeloma cell varies in size, from 15-25μm, the cytoplasm has a deep blue colour, is non-granular and usually shows a pale perinuclear clear area or **'hof'** representing Golgi zone. The nucleus is generally eccentric but may be situated centrally within the cytoplasm but lacks the cartwheel appearance. The nuclear chromatin appears to be in the form of a loose mesh; several nucleoli may be discernable and are usually more obvious in the myeloma cells. Russell bodies consisting of hyaline globules of immunoglobulin are present in the cytoplasm. Binucleated or multinucleated plasma cells are present. Intracellular accumulations of immunoglobulins may produce distinctive morphological features such as Mott cells or Morula cells (numerous **'grape-like'** pale bluish-cytoplasmic inclusions).

Urine examination: The light chains pass through glomerular filtrate appearing in urine as Bence Jones proteins (precipitates during heating, redissolves between 90°-100°C). During passage through the tubules the protein precipitates as casts and also damages the epithelial cells (myeloma kidney).

The presence of monoclonal spike (M protein) is seen in the serum or urine. The presence of single type of immunoglobulin is reflected in the electrophoresis pattern.

X-ray skull shows small-circumscribed areas of rarefaction of the bone (cannon ball). Bone changes consist of either diffuse decalcification or localised areas of bone destruction or a combination of the two. Classically, the lesions are seen as punched out defects in the bone.

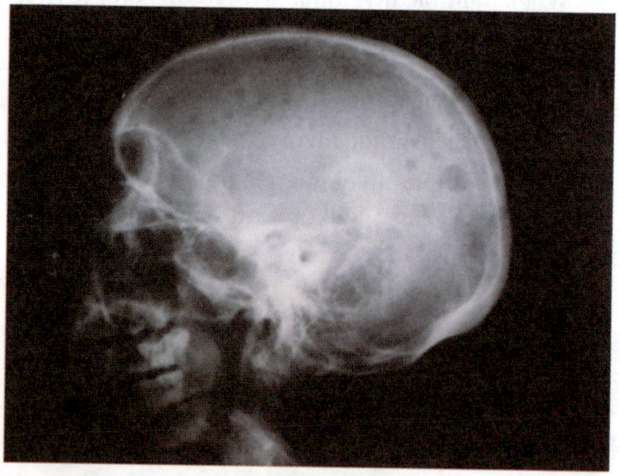

Fig.11.8: X-ray skull from a case of multiple myeloma. Multiple punched out lesions are seen

LANGERHANS' CELL HISTIOCYTOSIS

Langerhans' cell histiocytosis (LCH), previously known as histiocytosis X, is a rare proliferative disorder in which accumulation of pathologic Langerhan's cells leads to local tissue infiltration and destruction. The three syndromes are:

- Eosinophilic granulomas—unifocal and multifocal.

- Letterer-Siwe disease.
- Hand-Schuller-Christian disease.

I. EOSINOPHILIC GRANULOMA

The sex incidence is predominantly male. The bony lesion is usually solitary. It is seen in older children and young adults. Mandible is usually involved. Pain, swelling and fractures are the presenting symptoms. The bones frequently involved are ribs, pelvis, and flat bones of skull, mandible and long bones.

X-ray shows well-defined radiolucent defects within the bone.

Microscopically: The lesion is granulomatous and shows reticulum cells, a large number of eosinophils, plasma cells, neutrophils and cholesterol. The eosinophilic component ranges from scattered mature cells to sheet-like masses of cells. Occasionally, areas of bone necrosis may interrupt the cellular infiltrate. The foamy cells may also be amassed in clumps.

II. ACUTE DISSEMINATED LANGERHAN'S CELL HISTIOCYTOSIS (Letterer-Siwe disease)

It usually occurs before 2 years of age but occasionally may involve adults.

There are osteolytic bony lesions. Extensive infiltration of the marrow often leads to anaemia, thrombocytopaenia, and predisposition to recurrent infections.

Patient complains of sore mouth, halitosis, bad taste, gingivitis, aphthae, bleeding from gums, loss of teeth, oral candidiasis, swelling of jaws, and osteolytic lesions in gingival. Diffuse destruction of bone of maxilla and mandible—which may result in loosening and premature loss of teeth.

The lesions arc disseminated in nature with involvement of skin, mucus membrane, lymph nodes, liver, spleen, eyes, bones and pulmonary parenchyma.

Microscopically: The section from the lesion shows lymphocytes, plasma cells, reticuloendothelial cells and giant cells. Fibrosis may also be present.

III. HAND SCHULLER CHRISTIAN DISEASE

A more localised variant, primarily referred to as Hand Schuller Christian disease, or multifocal eosinophilic granuloma, is a childhood disease that consists of the triad of diabetes insipidus, lytic bone lesions, and proptosis. It is the result of error of metabolism of cholesterol and its esters.

The age group involved is more than 3 years of age. It is more common in boys than girls 2 : 1.

Oral manifestations include

(i) Irregular ulceration of the hard palate, which may be the manifestation of the disease.

(ii) Gingival infiltration and ulcerated nodules, difficulty in chewing and foul-smelling breath also occurs.

(iii) Loose and sore teeth with precocious exfoliation and failure of healing of tooth socket following extraction.

Microscopically: The lesion shows large number of foam cells, lymphocytes, plasma cells, eosinophils, neutrophils and an occasional giant cell. Langerhan's cells contain rod-shaped cytoplasmic structure called Birback granules.

HAEMORRHAGIC DISORDERS

THROMBOCYTOPAENIA

A platelet count of less than 100,000 per cumm in peripheral blood is usually considered as thrombocytopaenia (normal count is 150000/cumm to 400,000 per cumm).

Primary thrombocytopaenia is defined as primary process of unknown etiology and referred as idiopathic thrombocytopaenic purpura.

Secondary thrombocytopaenic purpura is secondary to variety of clinical conditions. It is caused due to drugs, diseases of bone marrow, abnormal destruction of platelets, excessive consumption of platelets, loss of platelets from circulation and congenital thrombocytopaenia.

TABLE 11.9
CLASSIFICATION OF THROMBOCYTOPAENIA

I. Primary thrombocytopaenia

Idiopathic thrombocytopaenic purpura

II. Secondary thrombocytopaenia

A. Platelets defects

1. Drug induced: Antidiabetics, antihistaminics, sedatives, antimicrobial, and phenylbutazone
2. Diseases of bone marrow: Leukaemia, multiple myeloma, metastatic carcinoma
3. Anaemias
   a. Megaloblastic anaemia
   b. Paroxysmal nocturnal haemoglobinuria
   c. Aplastic anaemia
   d. Viral infections: Measles, rubella, influenza
4. Bacterial infection

B. Abnormal destruction of platelets

A. Incompatible platelet transfusion
B. Immunological reactions
   i. Immunohaemolytic anaemia
   ii. Leukaemia
   iii. Lymphoma
   iv. Rheumatoid arthritis
   v. Hyperthyroidism

C. Excessive consumption

i. Thrombotic thrombocytopaenic purpura
ii. Episodic thrombocytopaenia
iii. Haemolytic uraemic syndrome
iv. Cavernous haemangioma

D. Defective regulation of thrombopoiesis

Episodic thrombocytopaenia

E. Congenital thrombocytopaenia

i. Congenital megakaryocytic hypoplasia
ii. Hereditary thrombocytopaenia

F. Loss of platelet from circulation

i. Hyperthyroidism
ii. Hypothermia
iii. Haemorrhage
iv. Massive exchange transfusion
v. Post-surgery.

Idiopathic thrombocytopaenic purpura

Etiology

Idiopathic thrombocytopaenic purpura (Werlhof's disease, purpura haemorrhagica and autoimmune thrombocytopaenic purpura) is a disease of obscure etiology:

1. Autoimmune thrombocytopaenia may also occur in association with other autoimmune disorders, e.g., systemic lupus erythematosus, or myasthenia gravis, and autoimmune haemolytic anaemia. It may complicate lymphoma and chronic lymphatic leukaemia.
2. It is also common in persons infected with AIDS.
3. Idiopathic thrombocytopaenic purpura is a quantitative disorder of platelets caused by antibodies directed against platelet or megakaryocytic antigens. The presence of antibodies, often directed against platelet membrane glycoprotein IIb-IIIa, causes the premature removal of platelet by the monocyte macrophage system. Occasionally, antigen antibody immune complexes adhere to platelets as their Fc receptor—resulting in their premature removal from the circulation.

The coated platelet are segregated and destroyed in the spleen and, to a degree, in the liver. Oestrogen increases the destruction of the platelets in the spleen explaining why chronic idiopathic purpura is more common in women.

A transient thrombocytopaenic purpura may occur in newborn infants born to mother with idiopathic thrombocytopaenic purpura suggesting the transplacental passage of an anti-platelet factor—mother to fetus.

There are two forms of ITP, acute and chronic:

Acute ITP: It is a self-limiting disease, occurs most commonly in children between 2-6 years of age and accounts for most cases in children. It is characterised by acute onset with haemorrhages into skin and mucus membranes with an average platelet count of 20,000/cmm blood. In about 80% of cases there is a previous history of viral respiratory tract infection 1-3 weeks prior to onset of petechiae.

Chronic ITP: Chronic ITP is a disease of young to middle-aged females. Onset is less abrupt and undergoes remissions and replaces alternating over long periods.

Pathological changes are described under three headings:

I. Skin and mucus membrane changes

The skin is the most common site of haemorrhage. When platelet count falls sufficiently in idiopathic thrombocytopaenic purpura, purpura is evident in the skin. Petechiae appears first in the skin and mucus membrane. Purple or red dots less than 0.5 cm across caused by bleeding most common in the skin over bony prominences. They characteristically occur in groups or crops. Sometimes bleeding into the skin is more extensive with ecchymoses or haematoma. Minor trauma causes bruising. Haemorrhagic vesicles sometimes develop in the children with the acute form of the disease.

Epistaxes, menorrhagia, haematuria, haematemesis or malena are common manifestations.

Oral lesions: The lesions are most prominent in the oral cavity and consist of gingival bleeding, petichae, and ecchymoses.

Mucosa is pale due to anaemia.

Haemorrhagic bullae may be present.

II. Other organs

Central nervous system: Sometimes there is severe intracranial haemorrhage.

Spleen is enlarged two to three times than normal, weigh 300 to 400 grams.

Microscopically, There is hyperactivity and enlargement of splenic follicles characterised by increased mitotic and phagocytic activity.

Pulp is infiltrated with scattered neutrophilic and eosinophilic leukocytes and megakaryocytes may be present in the sinuses and sinusoidal walls. If thrombocytopaenia is unusually severe, macrophages filled with cholesterol or ceroid derived from phagocytosed platelets appear in red pulp.

III. Haematological findings

Platelet count: Reduced—may be as low as 10,000/cumm.

Erythrocytes: Anaemia develops due to haemorrhage. In the early stages it is normocytic normochromic type, later on becomes microcytic hypochromic type with prolonged bleeding.

Blood film shows only occasional platelets, which are often large (giant platelet), small and atypical form.

Bone marrow

Megakaryocytes

1. Many young megakaryocytes—single nucleus, scanty or moderate cytoplasm, and few granules.
2. Exceptionally large megakaryocytes—non-lobulated nucleus, vacuolated cytoplasm, a few granules.
3. Megakaryocytes appear to be rounded-up with more or less hyaline border and cytoplasm with decreased granularity.
4. Platelets are few around the megakaryocyte.

Bleeding time prolonged.

Clot retraction—poor, may not form at all.

Coombs' test is positive in many cases.

Anti-platelet IgG antibodies are present.

About 30% of cases have positive **anticardiolipin antibody**.

Platelet life span is reduced.

THROMBOTIC THROMBOCYTOPAENIC PURPURA

Thrombotic thrombocytopaenic purpura is a rare blood condition characterised by thrombus in the circulation, which results in consumption of platelets and, thus, a thrombocytopaenia. The TTP syndrome is characterised by microangiopathic haemolysis, platelet aggregation/hyaline thrombi whose formation is unrelated to coagulation system activity. Platelet microthrombi predominate, they form in the microcirculation (i.e., capillaries throughout the body, causing partial occlusion of vessels). The thrombi partially occlude vascular lumina with overlapping proliferative endothelial cells.

Organ involvement: Endothelia of the kidney, brain, heart, pancreas, spleen, and adrenal are particularly vulnerable to TTP. The lungs, liver, gastrointestinal tract, gallbladder, skeletal muscles, retina, pituitary gland, ovaries, uterus, and testes are also affected to a lesser extent. No inflammatory changes occur.

Pathogenesis

1. In TTP, vWF is synthesised normally initially as UlvWF, but its subsequent break down (cleavage) is defective. This is due to a lack of enzyme activity, called vWF-cleaving protease that breaks down von Willebrand factor in the blood. The deficiency may be inherited (genetic), in which case it will be revealed in childhood, or it can be acquired in life.
2. Most adult onset TTP appears to be secondary to the development of an antibody that inhibits this enzymatic activity. Both mechanisms result in the presence of ultra-large von Willebrand factor within the circulation.

Laboratory findings

1. Thrombocytopaenia and anaemia.
2. Microangiopathic haemolytic anaemia with negative Coombs' test.
3. Peripheral smear shows fragmented RBCs, normoblasts, and polychromasia.
4. **LDH level:** Extremely elevated, mostly as a consequence of LDH from ischaemic or necrotic tissue cells rather than haemolysis.
5. **Biopsy:** Bone marrow or gingival biopsy samples yield diagnostic lesions (hyaline thrombi in arterioles, capillaries and venules) in 30 to 35% cases. The intravascular thrombi are composed of loose aggregates or platelets that becomes organised into amorphous plugs, which are often replaced by fibrin. These fibrin deposits more readily seen in PAS stain.

DISORDERS OF PLATELET FUNCTION

GLANZMANN THROMBASTHENIA

It is initially described by Glanzmann in 1918, is an autosomal recessive disorder with no sex difference affecting one of two genes, either platelet membrane glycoprotein IIb or glycoprotein IIIa. GPIIb and GPIIIa exist together as a dimer and joined together, referred to as GPIIb/IIIa. GPIIb/IIIa once activated will bind to one end of fibrinogen. This allows the formation of a large collection or aggregates of platelets, commonly called clot. In GpIIb/GpIIIa, the platelet can no longer bind one another, and clot fails to form.

Glanzmann thrombasthenia is a rare haematological disorder with oral manifestations affecting platelets and clotting. Spontaneous bleeding from mucosal tissues and excessive bleeding from skin damage characterise it.

HAEMOPHILIA

1. CLASSICAL HAEMOPHILIA OR HAEMOPHILIA A

Haemophilia A is the commonest of all congenital disorders, resulting in deficiency and reduced activity of functional plasma coagulation factor VIII-C.

Haemophilia figured prominently in the history of European Royalty and is thus known as ***'the Royal disease'***.

Queen Victoria passed the mutation to her son Leopold and through several of her daughters to several Royal families. It has an incidence of 1 in 10,000 of the population and occurs in all ethnic groups.

Pathogenesis

Haemophilia A is caused by quantitative reduction of factor VIII in 90% of cases, while 10% cases have reduced activity of factor VIII-C. Some patients lack plasma factor VIII-C whereas other have a non-functional factor VIII-C molecule present in normal concentration. Majority of haemophiliacs have family history with an X-linked inheritance pattern. In 25% of cases, the mutation of the factor VIII gene may be new. A haemophiliacs patient's daughters will be carriers and all sons will be normal. Since factor VIII-C (AHF) is determined by a defect on X-chromosome, hemizygous males are primarily affected.

HAEMOPHILIA B

Haemophilia B or Christmas disease is a clotting disorder caused by mutation of the factor IX gene. The factor IX gene is located on X-chromosome Xq 27.1—q27.2. It is inherited as X-linked recessive.

Mostly males are affected. It is second most common form of haemophilia. It is called Christmas disease after Stephen Christmas, the first patient described with this disease.

The factor IX deficiency leads to an increased prepotency for haemorrhage. This is in response to mild trauma, or even spontaneously, such as in joints or muscles. Children with severe haemophilia B often begin to show increased prepotency for haemorrhage. This is in response to mild trauma, or even spontaneously, such as in joints or muscles. Children with severe haemophilia B often begin to show increased bruising around the age of one year. It may present earlier if the child undergoes surgery, or after trauma, including immunisation.

Haemophilia C: Haemophilia C is the result in the synthesis of PTA factor X (plasma thromboplastin antecedent).

Clinical features

Although the defect is present at birth, bleeding manifestations are uncommon during the neonatal period and usually appear only when the child begins to crawl. Individuals with haemophilia experience recurrent haemarthroses in large joints. These usually begin spontaneously without apparent trauma and most commonly affect knees, elbows, ankles, and hips. The joint is hot, swollen and painful.

Muscle haematomas are also characteristic of haemophilia. They occur most commonly in the calf and psoas muscles. Other haemorrhagic sites include central nervous system, gastrointestinal system, genitourinary system, pulmonary system, and cardiovascular system.

Patients who acquire HIV, hepatitis, or other viruses suffer from maladies associated with those infections.

Oral manifestations

There is persistent bleeding from frenum of lip and tongue. Bleeding may occur from alveolar sockets after tooth extractions and lacerations of tongue. Physiological processes of tooth eruption and exfoliation may be associated with severe and prolonged haemorrhage. Haematoma of the floor of the mouth occur which extends to the larynx and produces haematoma—with consequent respiratory distress.

von WILLEBRAND'S DISEASE

von Willebrand's disease is an autosomal disorder characterised by deficiency of von Willebrand factor leading to decreased platelet adhesion to vessel wall. von Willebrand's disease has been classified as congenital or acquired.

Clinical features

Superficial bruising, epistaxis, and menorrhagia, gastrointestinal bleeding episodes, and postoperative bleeding are common. Some patients may present with large ecchymoses and haematoma.

Oral manifestations

Mucosal, gum and post-extraction bleeding are the most common oral manifestations.

Haematological findings

1. Normal platelet count.
2. Bleeding time is prolonged.
3. Reduced von Willebrand factor level.
4. von Willebrand (vWF) antigen can be measured by quantitative immunoelectrophoretic assay, which measures the amount of vWF protein in the plasma, while enzyme linked immunosorbent assay reflects the number of binding sites.

Bibliography

Ambill R, Nandkumar K: *Glanzmann Thrombasthenia. A Hematological Disorder With Oral Manifestations. A Case Report*: J Contem Dental Pract 2008 July, (9) 5 107-113.

Malin MA, Bagan JV, Jimenezy et al: "Langerhans cell restricted to oral mucosa". *Oral Surgery, Oral Medicine, Oral Patho, Oral Radiol*, Endod. Jan 2001 91 (1) 76-9.

CHAPTER

12

SKIN DISEASES MANIFESTED IN ORAL MUCOSA

ERYTHEMA MULTIFORME

Erythema multiforme is a rapidly progressive vesiculobullous eruption of unknown etiology that most commonly affects young adults.

Etiology

Erythema multiforme may be induced by:

1. **Infections:** It is commonly associated with a preceding Mycoplasma pneumoniae, herpes simplex virus infection, histoplasmosis, typhoid, leprosy and acute respiratory tract infection.
2. Drugs like sulphonamides, trimethoprim, nitrofurantoin, phenylbutazone, digitalis, birth control pills, and penicillin.
3. It is also seen in several internal malignancies (carcinoma and sarcoma) as well as autoimmune diseases like systemic lupus erythematosus, polyarteritis nodosa and dermatomyositis.
4. **Immunological:** It is caused by cytotoxic T-cells that may be targeting cross-reactive antigens in or near the basal cell layer of the skin and mucosae.

Clinical features

The disease occurs more commonly in males in the age group of 20 to 30 years of life. Often the disease is accompanied with prodromal symptoms, e.g., fever, malaise, headache, cough, sore throat occurring one week before onset.

Patient presents with a polymorphic eruption of erythematous macules, blisters, urticarial plaques, vesicles, bullae, erosions and target lesions (concentric, circular erythematous rings resembling a target or bulls eye). Target lesions are dusky round; maculopapules appear suddenly in a symmetric pattern on the backs of hands and feet and the extensor aspect of forearms and legs.

Microscopically: There is intercellular edema and dyskeratosis. Epidermis shows mild to moderate necrosis. Occasionally subepidermal bullae may be seen. Around the blood vessels there is infiltration of lymphocytes, eosinophils and neutrophils. The infiltration is seen at dermoepidermal junction also. The endothelial cells of the blood vessels will be swollen. There will be perivascular fibrin exudates and focal areas of fibrinoid necrosis.

Oral lesions

There is haemorrhagic crushing of the lips, tongue and buccal mucosa, floor of mouth and palate. There are erythematous patches with erosions and painful ulcerations difficult to examine.

Microscopically: Section shows vesicles, epithelial necrosis, basal cell liquefactive degeneration, perivascular mixed inflammation including eosinophils. The infiltrate is seen at dermoepidermal junction. There is intercellular edema, dyskeratosis and mild to moderate epidermal necrosis.

Types of erythema multiforme:

1. Erythema multiforme major
2. Erythema multiforme minor
3. Stevens-Jonhson's syndrome
4. Toxic epidermal necrolysis
5. Oral erythema multiforme.

STEVENS-JOHNSON'S SYNDROME

Stevens-Johnson syndrome is a life-threatening condition affecting the skin in which cell death causes the epidermis to separate from the dermis. Stevens-Johnson syndrome is a rare condition, with a reported incidence of around 2.6 per million people.

Stevens-Johnson syndrome, also called erythema multiforme major, is a symmetric, severe vesicobullous eruption on at least two mucus membranes (oral, anorectal, and ocular membranes, lips) with frequent atypical target lesions affecting in some cases up to 15% of the body surface area.

Disease occurs at any age, but more common above 40 years.

Pathogenesis

Drug-specific activation of T-cells has been shown in vitro on peripheral blood mononuclear cells of patients with drug eruptions. The nature of antigens that drive the cytotoxic cellular immune reaction is not well-understood.

Skin findings

Skin lesions are variable. Erythematous papules, small vesicles on dusky purpuric macules, or erythema multiforme target lesions can appear.

Microscopically

Early stage: Vacuolisation of basal keratocytes and individual cell necrosis throughout the epidermis.

Late stage: Full thickness epidermal necrosis and detachment with formation of subepidermal split above basement membrane. There is little or no inflammatory infiltrate in dermis.

Oral manifestations

Mucus membranes are strongly affected, most commonly mouth and lips. Lips may be edematous, bloody, or crusted. Bullae and shallow ulcers resembling aphthous ulcers are common. Bullae rupture, mucosal lesions become deeply erythematous erosions, often covered by grey pseudomembranous exudates.

On the oral mucosa, bullae erode and result in grey-yellow fibrinous exudates with thick haemorrhagic crust. Mouth lesions are painful, and tender.

Ocular form: In the ocular form there is conjunctivitis with or without purulence. Bullae, corneal ulceration, and uveitis may occur.

About one-third of patients have pulmonary involvement with cough and patchy infiltrates on chest X-ray. In fatal cases, pneumonia and renal failure may occur.

TOXIC EPIDERMAL NECROLYSIS

Toxic epidermal necrolysis is a potentially life-threatening skin disorder that is most commonly drug-induced. However, the disorder has other potential etiologies, including infections, malignancy, and vaccinations.

Toxic epidermal necrolysis may occur in all age groups. The mean age of the patients with toxic epidermal necrolysis is reported to be between 46 and 63 years. The lesion is very extensive, e.g., epidermal detachment is more with severe mucosal involvement scarring as sequelae.

Treatment

Therapy for oral erythema multiforme is mainly palliative consisting of oral analgesics and lidocaine rinses.

In moderate to severe cases 30 mg/day prednisolone or methyl prednisolone for several days and tapered after symptoms subside.

PSORIASIS

Psoriasis is a common and chronic skin disorder.

Clinical features

The disease usually presents in second and third decades of life; however, it may be present in young children and, occasionally, elderly. It is more severe in winter and less severe in the summer as a result of increased exposure to ultraviolet light.

Patches of circular to oval shaped red plaques that itch or burn are typical of plaque psoriasis. The patches are usually found on the arms, legs, trunk or scalp but may be found on any part of the skin. The most typical areas are the knees and elbows. It is characterised by pink to red papules and plaques. Plaque is covered by loosely adherent scales that are characteristically silver-white in colour.

Clinical types

- **Stable plaque psoriasis:** Most common form of the disease usually forming scales. The lesions are red with dry silvery-white scaling, which may be obvious only after scraping the surface.
- **Guttate psoriasis:** Appears as small red spots on the skin.
- **Erythrodermic psoriasis:** Intense redness over large areas.
- **Pustular psoriasis:** White blisters surrounded by red skin. It is a severe form of psoriasis with eruption of minute pustule with shedding of nails is common.
- **Inverse psoriasis:** Shiny red patches occur in the area of friction, e.g., in groin, arm-pits and skin folds or under breast.
- **Psoriatic arthritis:** Causes, pain, stiffness and swelling in and around the joints. Psoriatic arthritis characteristically involves the terminal interphalangeal joints but frequently large joints may be affected.

Oral manifestations

Oral lesions are reported on lip, buccal mucosa, palate, gingival, and floor of the mouth. Oral manifestations of psoriasis are rare, but whenever these occur, they have been reported to manifest varied clinical pictures ranging from whitish areas or plaques, red areas or even ulcerations.

Usually, four types of oral manifestations occur in patient with psoriasis:

- The first type consists of minute well-defined grey to yellowish-white lesion that is round or oval.
- The second type is characterised by white, elevated, lacy, circular, lesion on the oral mucosa including the tongue.
- The third type consists of a fiery red erythema of the oral mucosa, including the tongue.
- The fourth type of oral lesion described in psoriasis is a geographic tongue that occurs most frequently among the patients with psoriasis.

Nail changes occur in 30% of cases of psoriasis and consist of yellow-brown colouration. Along with skin lesions there may be arthritis, myopathy, enteropathy, spondylitic heart disease, diabetes, vitiligo, and acquired immunodeficiency syndrome.

Microscopically

Histological findings demonstrates:

1. Confluent parakeratosis.
2. Acanthosis with regular elongation of the rete ridges with thickening in their lower portion.
3. Thinning of the suprapapillary epidermis with the occasional presence of small spongiform pustules.
4. Munro microabscess of neutrophils superficially.
5. Pallor of the upper layer of epidermis.
6. Diminished to absent granular layer.
7. Elongation and edema of dermal papillae.
8. Chronic inflammation of sub-epidermal layer with polymorphonuclear leukocytes, lymphocytes, and histocytes.
9. Dilated and tortuous blood vessels high in the submucosa.

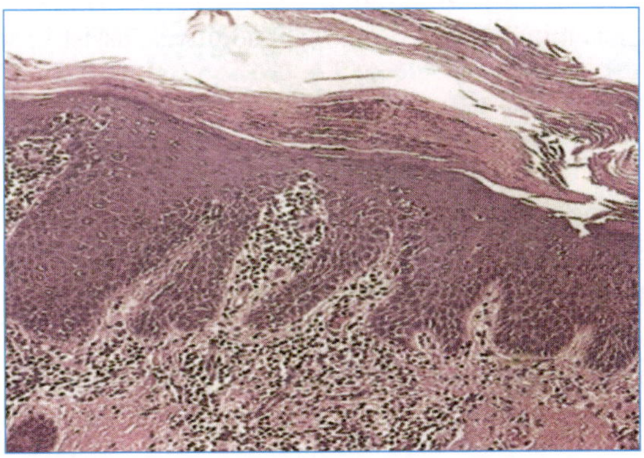

Fig.12.1: Section of psoriasis showing engorgement of papillae and Munro abscesses

Pathogenesis

Pathogenesis of psoriasis has seen all types of theories and postulates.

They are:

Genetic predisposition is well-known. Familial clustering, concordance in twins, and association with HLA-CW6 and HLA-DR7, B13, B17 is associated with psoriasis. Recent evidence states that there is a psoriatic gene on chromosome 1q21 that is responsible for epidermal proliferation.

Immunological: Research indicates that the disease may result from a disorder in the immune system. In psoriasis, the T-cells abnormally trigger inflammation in the skin. These T-cells, abnormally, also cause skin cells to grow faster than normal to pile up in raised patches on the outer surface of skin.

The cytokines released by lymphocytes leading to stimulation of keratocytes, lymphocytes trafficking, vascular change, and neutrophil chemotaxis. This alteration brings hyperproliferation of keratocytes.

Certain factors may trigger psoriasis:

a. Injury to the buccal mucosa due to infection, inflammation, and excessive scratching can trigger psoriasis.
b. Sunlight aggravates the symptoms.
c. Streptococcal infection may cause a type of plaque psoriasis.
d. HIV psoriasis typically worsens after an individual has been infected with HIV.
e. **Drugs:** Lithium, beta-blockers, anti-malarials and non-steroidal anti-inflammatory drugs aggravate psoriasis.
f. Emotional stress, alcohol, and menopause worsen the condition.

Treatment

Topical therapy

- Emollients (moisturisers) help soften scales and reduce discomfort.
- Steroid cream and ointments help to reduce inflammation. They range in strength from very potent to mild.
- Tazatotene (Tazorac) is a topical retinoid for treating mild to moderate plaque psoriasis.
- Anthralin or other coal tar preparations help to slow skin cell production.
- Vitamin D_3 calcipotriene (Dovonex) reduces the thickness of plaque.
- Retinoid diminishes the induration, scaling and redness of plaque.
- Bath solutions, such as mineral salts or oatmeal additives, assist in soothing skin and encouraging healing.

Phototherapy

- Ultraviolet light B (UVB), either outdoors or from a light box in a physician's office, helps to heal lesions.
- Psoralen and ultraviolet light A (UVB) involves the combined use of photosensitising medication, called psoralen and a long-wave ultraviolet light (UVA).
- Eximer lasers may be used to treat a small, localised area of psoriasis. They are a way to deliver UVB light directly to the psoriasis without exposing normal skin.
- **Internal medicines:** Methotrexate, cyclosporin A and Retinoid therapy helps to reduce inflammation.

PEMPHIGUS

It is an autoimmune disease involving the skin and mucosa and characterised by intraepithelial vesicles or bullae formation.

Different types of pemphigus are:

1. Pemphigus vulgaris
2. Pemphigus foliaceous
3. Pemphigus vegetans

4. Pemphigus erythematosus
5. Endemic pemphigus foliaceous
6. Paraneoplastic pemphigus.

PEMPHIGUS VULGARIS

Pemphigus vulgaris is a rare autoimmune mucocutaneous disorder characterized by blistering of skin and mucus membrane.

Clinical features

Pemphigus vulgaris occurs most commonly in fourth and sixth decades of life but has been even reported to occur in a 3-year old. Male to female ratio is 1 : 1, with whites more commonly affected.

In the skin, scalp, face, axilla, groin, trunk and points of pressure are involved. The lesions are superficial vesicles and bullae. They rupture easily and leave shallow erosions, covered with dried serum and crust. Intact blisters are persistent. Suprabasal acantholytic blister is a characteristic feature of vulgaris.

Oral lesions

The typical lesion is a small or large, clear fluid blister which breaks rapidly in the mouth to leave a flat white, somewhat tender ulcer with a thin red line around it.

In 50–70 percent of patients pemphigus vulgaris blisters occur on the mucus membranes. Most patients with oral involvement develop ill-defined, irregular erosions appearing on the gums, buccal cavity or upper palate. There is little or no erythematous inflammatory halo and fresh lesion may retain epithelial tags at its periphery. The base of a pemphigus ulcer is not concave saucerised and there is considerably less associated pain. Gingival involvement may manifest as desquamative gingivitis.

Microscopically shows intraepithelial bullae, acantholysis, and a mild to moderate infiltrate of eosinophils. The basal keratocytes, although separated from one another through the loss of attachment, remain firmly attached to the dermis like a ***'row of tomb stones'***.

Etiology

- **Genetic:** The aetiology of pemphigus vulgaris is uncertain. In some cases it may have a strong genetic basis as it has been more frequently in certain racial groups, for example the Ashkenazi Jews and those of Mediterranean descent. Strong association with certain HLA class alleles (DRBI 0402 and DQBI 0503) has been demonstrated in pemphigus vulgaris.
- **Immunological:** Pemphigus is characterised by blistering due to antibodies against desmosomes results in forming of blisters.

  Immunologic attack on desmosomes results in forming of blisters. Pemphigus vulgaris patients have serum IgG antibodies to desmogleins 1 and 3 (Dsg1 and Dsg3), which can be demonstrated by direct immunofluorescence on normal squamous epithelium.
- **Drugs:** Pemphigus-like oral eruption may occur in patients after drug therapy or with lymphoreticular malignancies (paraneoplastic pemphigus).
- **Physical agents** like burns, ultraviolet light and ionising rays, surgical and cosmetic procedures, contact allergens, dietary factors (tannins) causes pemphigus vulgaris.
- The emotional stress is the endogenous factor that plays a role as a predisposing factor.

PEMPHIGUS FOLIACEOUS

Pemphigus foliaceus is an autoimmune dermal blistering disease characterised by crusted lesions.

Clinical features

It occurs in a seborrheic distribution on the face or first appears on the scalp, chest, or upper back. Intact blisters are not usually seen. The vesicle roof is so thin that it ruptures.

Microscopically shows an intraepidermal bulla, acantholysis in the dermis and a mild to moderate eosinophilia. Histologic features of pemphigus foliaceous may have three patterns—(i) Acantholytic keratocytes (ii) A subnormal blister with dyskeratocytes (iii) Granular layer.

Immunoglobulin (IgG) and often complement C3 are found in the intercellular substance areas of the epidermis.

In direct immunofluorescence, serum immunoglobulin G (IgG) antibodies are present in approximately 75% of patients with active disease.

Brazilian pemphigus: It is also known as Fogo Selvagen. It is speculated that the disease is somehow related to arthropod, borne infectious agent. More than 1,000 new cases per year are estimated to occur in the endemic regions. This form of pemphigus resembles clinically to pemphigus foliaceous and is endemic to Brazil. It is seen in children and frequently in family groups.

PEMPHIGUS VEGETANS

Clinical features

Pemphigus vegetans is a rare form occurring in only 1 to 3% of individuals. The clinical lesions are not usually blisters. They are large, moist, verrucous, vegetating plaques studded with pustules. These fungoid lesions become covered by purulent exudates and exhibit inflamed borders. These lesions are found in nose, mouth, groin, axilla, and flexural surfaces.

It has two variants:

(i) Neumann type

(ii) Hallopeau type.

Neumann type: Lesions of Neumann type occur as flaccid bullae that rupture, leaving denuded areas or may develop pustules.

Microscopically, shows verrucous, vegetative epidermal hyperplasia with broad papillae are apparent. Intradermal abscesses are composed of almost entirely of eosinophils, zones of acantholysis may be small and difficult to observe.

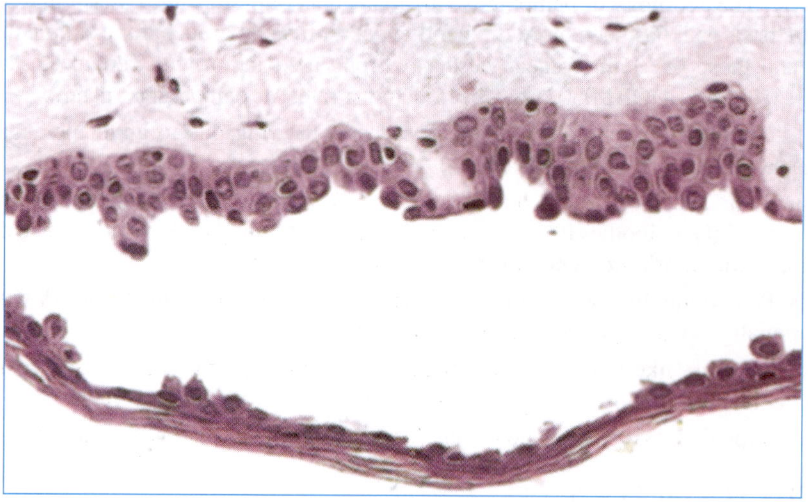

Fig.12.2: Section shows epidermal bullae (pemphigus)

Hallopeau type: Hallopeau type that clinically manifests as pustules initially rather than vesicles and bullae, also develop into verrucous vegetations.

Acrodermitis contina of Hallopeau is a rare, chronic, recurrent disorder classified as a form of pustular psoriasis, the most cases affect one or two digits. It tends to be resistant to both topical and systemic treatments for psoriasis.

PEMPHIGUS ERYTHEMATOSUS

It is also called Senear-Usher syndrome. In pemphigus erythematosus, the lesions are more superficial than those in the foliaceous variant.

Patients present with vesiculobullae or superficial eroded lesions, which may ooze and crust, particularly in sun-exposed areas, such as the face, the upper part of chest, and the back. Pemphigus may be photosensitive.

On the face, pemphigus erythematosus presents on the bridge of the nose and on malar areas as in the butterfly distribution seen in lupus erythematosus.

PARANEOPLASTIC PEMPHIGUS (PNP)

Mucus membrane is primarily and most severely involved. Most prominent clinical findings consist of several oral and conjunctival erosions in a patient with underlying neoplasm—usually lymphoma, sarcoma, and lung cancer. Other associated malignancies and conditions include CLL, Castleman disease, Waldenstrom macroglobulinaemia.

Anhalt has proposed the following new, minimal criteria for the diagnosis of paraneoplastic pemphigus:

- Painful progressive stomatitis.
- Histopathologic changes of acantholysis or lichenoid/interface dermatitis.
- Demonstration of antiplakin antibodies.
- Demonstration of an underlying lymphoproliferative neoplasm.

Oral manifestations

The earliest and most constant clinical finding in paraneoplastic pemphigus is painful oral erosions. Of those patients who present with a skin eruption, all go on to develop mucositis at some point during the course of the disease. Some patients only experience oral lesions. The erosions can occur anywhere in the mouth, including the buccal, labial, gingival, and lingual mucosae. All surfaces of the oropharynx can be affected.

Management

Corticosteroids, immunosuppressive drugs, plasmapheresis can manage the disease, and administration of 8-methoxypsoralen followed by exposure of peripheral blood to ultraviolet light.

BULLOUS PEMPHIGOID

It is self-limiting and rarely lasts over 5 years. It occurs commonly in the elderly age group with equal sex predilection. Site of occurrence include the inner surfaces of the forearms, axillae, groin, and lower abdomen. Oral involvement is present in up to one-third of patients.

Bullous pemphigoid is an uncommon subepidermal blistering disease typically presenting on the flexor surface of elderly patients. Begins with a localised area of erythema or with pruritic urticarial plaques. Plaques turn dark red in 1 to 3 weeks as vesicles and bullae rapidly appear on their surfaces.

Bullous pemphigoid may present with several distinct clinical presentations as:

- **Generalized bullous form:** It is the most common presentation. Tense bullae arise on any of skin surface, with a predilection on the flexural areas of the skin. The bullae can occur normal-appearing, as well as erythematous skin surfaces.

- **Vesicular form:** The vesicular form is less common. It manifests as groups of small, tense blisters, often on an urticarial or erythematous base.
- **Vegetative form:** The vegetative form is very uncommon, with vegetating plaques in intertriginous areas of the skin, such as axillae, the neck, the groin, and infra-mammary areas.
- **Generalised erythroderma form:** This rare presentation can resemble psoriasis, generalized atopic dermatitis, or other skin conditions characterised by an exfoliative erythroderma.
- **Urticarial form:** Some patients with bullous pemphigoid initially present with persistent multiracial lesions that subsequently convert to bullous eruptions.
- **Nodular form:** This rare form is termed pemphigoid nodularis, has clinical features that resemble pruarigo nodularis, with blisters arising on normal appearing or nodular lesional skin.
- **Acral form:** In childhood-onset bullous pemphigoid associated with vaccination, the bullous lesions predominantly affect the palms, the soles, and the face.
- **Infant form:** The blisters tend to occur frequently on the palms, soles, and face—affecting genital areas rarely.

Oral manifestations

Oral lesions are present in 10 to 40 percent of cases.

Oral mucosal involvement is uncommon and begins as bullae, they tend to rupture and results in large ulcerations.

Gingival lesions consist of generalised edema, inflammation, desquamation and localised areas of discrete vesicle formation.

Microscopically: Subepidermal bullae in dermis and bullae cavity show lymphocytes or eosinophilic infiltration. These cells are chiefly perivascular and are predominantly eosinophils. In severe inflammation, the basal keratocytes of mesenchymal demonstrates spongiosis. There is basal layer vacuolation. The vacuolated basal layer eventually gives rise to a fluid-filled blister.

Pathogenesis

There is linear deposition of immounoglobulin IgG autoantibodies and complement in the basement membrane zone.

IgG autoantibodies bind to the skin basement membrane of patients with bullous pemphigoid.

The antigen concerned in these lesions is named as ***'Bullous pemphigoid antigen'*** **(*BP230 BpAg1*)** and ***BP180*** **(*BPAg2*)**. It is present at dermoepidermal junction.

Direct immunofluorescence shows immunoglobulin G (IgG), complement C3, or both, in a linear band at the basement membrane zone.

Management

Systemic steroids in lower doses, for short period, combined with immunosuppressive drugs and dapsone.

CICATRICAL PEMPHIGOID

Cicatrical pemphigoid (CP) refers to a group of rare chronic autoimmune blistering diseases that predominantly affect the mucus membranes, including the conjunctiva and occasionally the skin.

It is also called benign mucus membrane pemphigus. It is an autoimmune disease. Autoantibodies in patients with cicatrical pemphigoid include bullous pemphigoid antigen BPAG 2, type VII collagen, integrin subunit B4 M168 and laminin.

Clinical findings

Cicatrical pemphigoid is a rare disease, largely of the elderly, that leads to blisters that rupture easily and also to primary erosions resulting from epithelial fragility in the mouth, orpharynx, and, more rarely, the nasopharyngeal, oesophageal, genital and rectal mucosae.

Ocular involvement may initially manifest as unilateral or bilateral conjunctivitis with burning, dryness and foreign body sensation as the first symptom. There is sensation of grittiness or pain. Conjunctivitis may lead to impaired vision or blindness. Lesion forms, erode and heal to leave scar tissue.

Skin lesions: Blisters on the skin develop in 25-30% of patients manifesting as tense vesicles or bullae that may heal with scarring or milia. Scalp involvement may lead to alopecia. Pruritis at the site of blisters or generalised pruritis develops.

Oral manifestations

Mouth involvement presents as recurrent, painful erosions. The gingivae are most commonly involved, followed by the palate, and the buccal mucosa, however, any mucosal site in the mouth may show blisters. Involvement of the oropharynx may present with hoarseness or dysphagia. Progressive scarring disease may lead to esophageal stenosis requiring dilatation procedure. Supraglottic involvement may lead to airway obstruction compromise requiring tracheostomy.

Treatment

The primary aim of treatment is to stop blister formation, promote healing and prevent scarring. Cicatrical pemphigoid is a particularly difficult disease to treat as it can affect so many different parts of body.

Topical steroid creams/ointments are used.

In few cases, intralesional steroid injections and, in severe cases, short burst of oral corticosteroids are used.

EPIDERMOLYSIS BULLOSA

Epidermolysis bullosa is rare disorder caused by a mutation of the keratin gene. The disorder is characterised by the presence of extremely fragile skin and recurrent blister formation, resulting from minor friction or trauma.

Epidermolysis bullosa can be classified on the basis of level of blister formation as:

a. Epidermolytic (EB simplex)
   (i) Generalised form
   (ii) Localised form (Weber-Cockayne syndrome)
b. Dermatolytic (dystrophic) epidermolysis bullosa
   (i) Recessive
   (ii) Dominant
c. Junctional epidermolysis bullosa
d. Epidermolysis bullosa acquista.

Epidermolysis bullosa simplex

The estimated prevalence of epidermolysis bullosa simplex is 1: 30,000 to 50,000 people.

Mutations in the KRT14 and KRT5 genes cause epidermolysis bullosa simplex.

Clinical features

Epidermolysis bullosa simplex is one of the major forms of epidermolysis bulllosa. Blistering may primarily affect the hands and feet in milder cases, and the blisters usually heal without leaving scars.

Severe cases of this condition involve widespread blistering that can lead to infection, dehydration, and other medical problems. Severe cases may be life-threatening in infancy.

Clinical types of epidermolysis bullosa simplex are:

Weber-Cockayne type: The mildest form of epidermolysis bullosa simplex known as Weber-Cockyane type is characterised by skin blistering that begins anytime between childhood and adulthood and is usually confined to hands and feet. Later in life, skin of the palms and soles of the feet may thicken and harden (hyperkeratosis).

Koebner type: In Koebner type, blisters appear at birth in early and are more widespread.

Epidermolysis bullosa simplex with mottled pigmentation is characterised by patches of darker skin on the trunk, arms, and legs that fade in adulthood. This form of the disorder also involves skin blistering from early infancy, hyperkeratosis of palms and soles, and abnormal nail growth.

Dowling-Meara type is the most severe form of epidermolysis bullosa simplex, extensive severe blistering can occur anywhere on the body, including inside of mouth, and blisters may appear in clusters.

Oral manifestations

Bullae of the oral cavity are reported in occasional cases of generalised epidermolysis bullosa simplex, but teeth are not affected.

Microscopically: There is degeneration of basal keratocytes cells with intrabasal separation as a result of blister formation at a lower level in epidermis. Vesicles and bullae are developed as a result of destruction of basal and suprabasal cells so that some nuclei may persist on the floor of the blister.

Epidermolysis bullosa dystrophic dominants

Clinical features

Generalised blistering present at birth. Blistering becomes localised to hands, feet, elbow or knees as child grows older and in response to friction. Small white spots called milia are often present at healed but scanned sites.

The autosomal dominant forms of dystrophic epidermolysis bullosa have 2 subtypes—albopapuloid type occurs as atrophic scars that are hypopigmented, and exhibit lichenoid-like papules. In hypertrophic form, the scarring tends to be hypertrophic.

Oral manifestations

Teeth are unaffected. Bullae can be seen. Sometimes, oral milia can be present.

Microscopically: There is a cleavage beneath lamina densa thus separating the skin at this level. The lamina densa, lamina lucida and basal cell plasma membrane along with hemidesmosome are intact on blister roof.

Epidermolysis bullosa dystrophic recessive

Clinical features

It may present severe blistering. Generalised severe blistering is more common and involves large areas of skin and mucus membranes. Blisters heal but with scarring and deformity causing limited movement as fingers and toes may be fused together (mitten hands). Complications such as infection, malnutrition and dehydration may cause death in infancy and those who survive are at great risk of developing squamous cell carcinoma.

Oral manifestations

Autosomal recessive dystrophic type bullae, which are markedly fragile and haemorrhagic are found in all patients at the junction between the hard and soft palates. Oral ulceration as well as blistering can be observed at birth or shortly thereafter.

The major dental complication in epidermolysis bullosa dystrophic recessive type is an increased risk of caries. Hypoplastic and pitted enamel affecting principally the molars is also seen. Enamel formation is abnormal, leading to extensive caries.

Patients present with a distinct oral involvement consisting of microstomia, ankyloglossia and vestibule obliteration.

Oral involvement may lead to fusion of the tongue to the floor of the mouth and progressive diminution of the size of the oral cavity.

Esophageal erosions can lead to webs and strictures that can cause severe dysphagia.

Microscopically: Section shows normal keratocytes beneath a thickened stratum corneum. The lower margin of the mitten was formed just below the lamina densa of the basement membrane at a level similar to that of the usual blister formation in this condition. A substantial portion of the mitten, however, consisted of necrotic keratocytes without an intact basement membrane.

Junctional epidermolysis bullosa

Clinical features

Subtypes of junctional epidermolysis bullosa are:

1. Herlitz type: Generalised and most severe form of junctional epidermolysis bullosa where blisters appear all over the body and often involve mucus membranes and internal organs. May only present at birth with small single blisters but becoming widespread soon after. Most cases are lethal within the first 12-24 months of life.

Complications such as infection, malnutrition and dehydration usually lead to early death in infancy.

2. Non-Herlitz type: Generalised blistering and mucosal involvement present at birth or soon after scalp, nails, and tooth more involved.

Complications such as infection, malnutrition and dehydration may cause death in infancy but those who survive clinically improve with increasing age.

3. Generalised atrophic benign epidermolysis bullosa.

Mild generalised blistering present at birth, usually with scalp, nail and teeth involvement. Blisters heal with a distinctive atrophic appearance. Blisters worsen in warmer climates.

4. Epidermolysis bullosa with pyloric stenosis: Severe generalized blistering in conjugation with pyloric atresia at birth. Prognosis is poor and usually results in death during infancy.

It has onset at birth, absence of scarring, milia, pigmentation and death within 3 months of age.

There is mutation in the gene encoding the protein, e.g., defects in α_3 subunit of laminin 5 involve LAMA 3 gene.

Oral manifestations

Oral bullae are frequently very extensive and, because of their extreme fragility, produce serious feeding problems. Severe disturbances in enamel and dentin formation of deciduous teeth also occur.

Oral mucosa is involved and teeth exhibit a highly dysplastic enamel defect that gives teeth ***'pitted or cobble-stone'*** appearance.

Other oral manifestations may include anodontia, neonatal teeth and dental caries.

Microscopically: It is similar and identical to those occurring in the dystrophic recessive disease.

Epidermolysis bullosa acquista

Clinical features

Epidermolysis bullosa acquista is a heterogenous disorder characterised by non-inflammatory bullae. The etiology is unknown, but trauma and sun exposure have been implicated. Autoimmune/systemic diseases show some association.

Microscopically: Histological sections of skin show separation of the epidermis from the dermis in a subepidermal plane. There are subepidermal bullae—early vacuolation in dermal papillary tips. There is absence of a significant inflammatory response. The adjacent epidermis is normal.

Management

Oral antibiotics are given if there is secondary infection. Treatment of this condition comprises of wound care and prevention of wound infection. After pricking the large blisters the fluid is released and they are dressed properly to minimise reaction.

SCLERODERMA

Scleroderma is an autoimmune disease of the connective tissue. The word scleroderma comes from Greek words ***'Sclero'*** meaning hard ***'derma'*** meaning skin.

Systemic sclerosis is characterised by progressive fibrosis of skin and multiple organs.

Etiology: Vascular and environmental factors are found to play a major role in the isolated cases of this disease.

Scleroderma is a rare, chronic autoimmune disease of connective tissue, which afflicts an estimated 150,000 to 500,000 Americans, primarily females who are 30 to 50 years old at onset.

Types of scleroderma: There are two main types of scleroderma: Localised and systemic.

Systemic forms can affect any part of the body (skin, blood vessels, and internal organs).

Localised scleroderma

A. **Morphea is scleroderma skin** that is localised to a patchy area of the skin and becomes hardened and slightly pigmented.

B. **Linear scleroderma** is located usually to a lower extremity, frequently presenting as a strip of hardening skin down the leg of a child. Linear sclerodermas in children can staw bone growth of the affected limb. Sometimes linear scleroderma is associated with ***'satellite'*** area of a patch of localised scleroderma skin, such as on the abdomen.

C. **Juvenile scleroderma:** When any form of scleroderma—either localised or systemic—occurs in children, it is also called childhood scleroderma or juvenile scleroderma.

D. **CREST variant:** This form of scleroderma is milder disease than generalised scleroderma; it is characterised by:

C—Calcinosis

R—Raynaud's phenomenon

E—Esophageal dysfunction

S—Sclerodactyly

T—Telangiectasia

Organs affected

Skin: The skin is always involved, usually first in the hands. Thin epidermis overlies compact bundles of collagen that lie parallel to epidermis. Finger-like projections of collagen extend from the dermis into subcutaneous tissue and bind the skin to the underlying tissue. Dermal appendages are atrophied and rete pegs are lost. Activated fibroblasts themselves produce cytokines, and growth factors, such as IL-1, prostaglandin E (PGE), TGF-B, and PDGF, which may, in turn serve to activate other fibroblasts.

Joints: A characteristic finding is a thick layer of fibrin overlying and within the synovium. Later in the disease the synovium may become fibrotic. Fibrinous deposits appear on the surfaces of tendon sheaths and in the overlying fascia and may lead to audible cracking over moving tendon.

Muscles: Some patients develop myositis like that of polymyositis. Contractures of fingers and toes are quite common with long-standing disease.

Kidney: Scleroderma affects the kidneys causing glomerular disruption and intimal proliferation, medial thinning, and increased collagen deposition in the adventitial layer of small interlobular renal arteries. Secondary changes (e.g., fibrin thrombi, fibrinoid necrosis, immune reactions, increased vasomotor tone) contribute to renal dysfunction symptoms and signs. Proteinuria develops in 50% of patients with scleroderma, but is usually mild. Malignant hypertension occurs in 20% of patients with systemic sclerosis.

Lungs: Some patients can develop pulmonary hypertension or elevation in the pressures of the pulmonary artery. This can be progressive and lead to right-sided heart failure. Other pulmonary complications in more advanced disease includes pleuritis, aspiration pneumonia, pulmonary haemorrhage, pleural effusion and pneumothorax.

Heart: Inflammatory and fibrotic disease of heart in systemic sclerosis includes pericarditis, myocardial fibrosis, and contraction band necrosis of coronary vessels. The myocardial lesions result from focal myocardial necrosis, which may reflect focal ischaemia secondary to a Raynaud's-like activity of the coronary microcirculation.

Maxillofacial and oral manifestations

1. **Reduced mouth opening:** Loss of skin folds around mouth giving rise to mask like appearance of the face atrophied nasal alae giving rise to *mouse facies.*

   Crenations are seen along the buccal mucosa with severe buccal mucosal fibrosis.

   There may be rigidity of tongue and lips. Reduced mobility of the tongue may affect chewing, swallowing and, sometimes, speech.

   The lip of a patient with scleroderma may appear to be pursed due to constriction of the mouth aperture—thus making it difficult to open the mouth.

   There is loss of attached gingival and multiple areas of gingival recession.

2. **Dental caries:** It is due to destruction of the tooth substance by acids produced by dental plaque.

3. **Dry mouth (xerostomia):** Some patients with scleroderma can develop dry mouth as a consequence of some destruction of the salivary glands. Dry mouth can cause difficulties in speech, and swallowing, increase the liability of caries, gingivitis, fungal infection of the mouth, and bacterial infection of salivary glands.

   The lining of the mouth can become sore or burning. A lack of saliva can give rise to an unpleasant taste, and food may become bland in taste. Finally, a lack of saliva can lessen the retention of upper dentures.

4. **Mouth ulcers:** When mouth ulcers occur, they can be very painful and may be associated with thrush, or can develop due to normal movements of the tongue against the sharp dry edges of the teeth, fillings or dentures, cheek biting due to lack of saliva can also cause ulcers.

5. **White patches:** White patches on the lining of the mouth (oral mucosa) can arise as a result of some drugs. The white patches are usually painless.

6. **Salivary gland enlargement:** Patients with long standing dry mouth can have recurrent enlargement of one or more salivary glands. When painless, this usually is a consequence of inflammation of the glands.

7. **Gingivitis:** Gingivitis may be more common in scleroderma as a result of any accompanying dry mouth, and difficulty in tooth-cleaning due to limited mouth opening. The frequency and severity of periodontitis is not notably increased in scleroderma.

8. **Mandibular resorption:** Taveras first reported mandibular resorption in scleroderma in 1959. Mandibular resorption in progressive systemic sclerosis is relatively uncommon and reported in 10% of cases. Scleroderma can loosen teeth by causing the ligament around the teeth to expand due to collagen deposition. When the ligament expands, the teeth are less supported by bone structure.
9. **Temporomandibular joint involvement:** Scleroderma can cause temporomandibular joint involvement. Reduced opening of mouth and fixation of jaw are results of involvement of peri-temporal mandibular joint tissue.
10. **Tongue cancer:** Sixty-fold increase in the incidence of squamous cell carcinoma of the tongue in patients with systemic sclerosis. Potential causative agents may be chemical substances ingested through the oral route, possibly triggering both cancer and systemic sclerosis. Oral viral infections are due to immunocompromised state of systemic sclerosis.
11. **Sjogren's syndrome:** About twenty percent of patients with systemic scleroderma also have secondary Sjogren's syndrome. Symptoms of Sjogren's syndrome include dry eyes, and dry mouth.

Roentgenographic feature: Extreme widening of periodontal ligament, i.e., two or four times the normal thickness is a characteristic features of scleroderma. It occurs in 10-37% of cases.

Management

Systemic glucocorticoids may be of benefit for limited periods early in the disease. Other systemic treatments (EDTA, aminocaproic acid, D-penicillamine, para-aminobenzoate, colchicines, immuno-suppressive drugs) have not been shown to be lasting benefit. Currently interferon-gamma is being tested clinically, as is photopheresis.

DERMATITIS HERPETIFORMIS

Dermatitis herpetiformis is a rare, chronic, intensely pruritic vascular dermatosis associated with a gluten sensitive enteropathy.

The prevalence is 11 to 39 per 100,000. It is rare in Africans and Asians.

It is also called ***Duhring- Brocq*** disease.

Clinical features

Gastrointestinal changes: This chronic condition usually appears after the age of 30. The male and female ratio is 2 : 1.

Gastrointestinal involvement is usually asymptomatic.

Malabsorption of fat, D-xylose or iron occurs in less than 20% of patients. There is increased risk of small bowel lymphoma and non-intestinal lymphoma.

Skin changes: Dermatitis herpetiformis is characterised by intensely itchy, chronic papulovesicular eruptions usually distributed symmetrically on extensor surfaces (buttocks, back of neck, scalp, elbows, knees, back). The condition is extremely itchy and the desire to scratch can be overwhelming. This sometimes leading to excoriation of blisters before a doctor examines them. The blisters vary in size from very small up to 1 cm across.

Microscopically: The epidermal bulla is filled with serous exudates and contains leukocytes, the majority of which are neutrophil polymorphs, and eosinophils. There is also perivascular infiltrate of lymphocytes. The tips of dermal papillae are separated from the overlying epidermis to form a cleft. There is vacuolation of basal cells overlying the microabscesses.

Hypothyroidism or thyroid disorders may be associated with skin lesions.

Oral manifestations

The characteristic findings are presence of vesicles and bullae at any intraoral site. The bullae rupture rapidly to leave areas of superficial ulceration.

Pathogenesis

It is speculated that an individual with genetic background may develop IgA antibodies in the gut to components of dietary gluten. The disease shares a strong association with class locus antigen HLA DRw3, HLA-B and HLA-DQw2, alleles DQA 10501 and B 10201 of chromosome 6.

Diagnosis

IgA anti-endomysial antibodies (IGA-EmA) are found in 70% of patients not on a gluten free diet. Serum IgA-EmA titers correlate with the severity of jejunal villus biopsy.

By direct immunofluorescence, dermatitis herpetiformis shows granular deposits of IgA and C3 selectively localised in the tips of the dermal papillae, where they are deposited on anchoring fibrils.

Management

A gluten-free diet can control the disease alone.

Medication: Dapsone, 100 to 150 mg/day orally, typically relieves itching and burning within 48-72 hours.

DERMATOMYOSITIS

It is one of the autoimmune disorders being a subset of polymyositis.

Frequency: The estimated incidence of dermatomyositis/polymyositis is 5.5 cases per million population.

Age: Dermatomyositis can occur in persons of any age, but the most common age of onset is in the fifth and sixth decades of life.

Sex: Women are affected twice as often as men.

Race: Whites are more frequently affected. However, the rise in the incidence of African- Americans is greater than that of whites.

Two variants are recognised:

1. Childhood variant
2. Adult variant.

Childhood variant: It is a self-limiting disease, may be complicated by contractures of muscles as also by calcinosis cutis.

Adult variant: Prolonged progressive course unless treated adequately. One-third of these patients may have underlying malignancies.

Clinical features

Dermatomyositis is a collagen disease, equally affecting both the sexes, mostly in the fifth decade of life.

This involves both skin and muscles.

The most characteristic lesion is a reddish-purple erythema of the upper eyelids with occasional scaling is called ***'heliotrope erythema'***. Women with dermatomyositis have a slightly increased risk of developing visceral cancers.

Gottron sign: Scaly erythematous plaques on the knuckles, knees, elbows, interphalangeal or metacarpophalangeal joints and other areas.

Gottron papule: Erythematous, and atrophic papules are found over the knuckles and pressure points.

Microscopically: There is widespread patchy necrosis and inflammation, often affecting the peripheral fibres of muscle fascicles. The inflammatory infiltrate, which is often perimysial, is composed of lymphocytes, macrophages and eosinophils. Both regenerating and degenerating muscle fibres are seen. Muscle fibres show edema, swelling, loss of striations, hyaline and vascular changes.

Nail fold changes consist of periungual telangiectases and/or a characteristic cuticular change with hypertrophic area.

Oral manifestations

The oral mucosa may show dark red or bluish erythema. In the early stages, tongue is markedly swollen and, later, becomes harder. In the late phase, tongue is atrophic.

ACANTHOSIS NIGRICANS

These lesions (velvety, hyperpigmentation and thickening of the skin) usually restricted to flexural areas like axillae, inguinal regions, and neck, are of many types:

I. Benign

1. As an autosomal dominant trait with variable penetrance
2. Acral acanthosis nigricans
3. Unilateral acanthosis nigricans
4. Syndromic acanthosis nigricans
5. Drug-induced acanthosis nigricans
6. Mixed type.

II. Malignancy associated acanthosis nigricans

III. Psudoacanthosis nigricans: In association with obesity or endocrine abnormalities and diabetes.

Oral manifestations

Oral manifestations of malignancy-associated nigricans involve the lips, tongue, and palate. Gingival hyperplasia may also occur. Non-pigmented hypertrophy of the papillae along the dorsal surface and lateral edge of the tongue yield a characteristic fissured and shaggy texture. The lips are also subject to these papillomatous growths and swelling. The buccal mucosa shows some papillae, but more commonly velvety, white plaques are present along with the uneven appearance. Intradental gingival may become so hyperplastic that it interferes with eating as it covers the teeth.

Microscopic features: Biopsy from lesion shows hyperkeratosis, papillomatosis and mild acanthosis with minimal or no melanin pigmentation. There is thinning of adjacent epidermis and presence of horn cyst.

HEREDITARY HAEMORRHAGIC TELANGIECTASIA

It is also known as ***'Osler's Weber-Rendu'*** disease. The disease is inherited as an autosomal dominant trait and manifested by multiple capillary microaneurysms in the skin and mucus membrane. Other sites which may be involved are conjunctiva, bronchi, gastrointestinal tract, renal tract and vagina.

Rarely, these lesions rupture, causing serious nose-bleeds, bleeding into the gut, or haematuria.

Clinical features

Skin: As Rendu described in his hallmark work, typical lesions appear as ***'small purple stains'***, of the size of a pinhead, the largest reaching the size of a lentil. The typical telangiectasia is smaller than 5 mm and found beneath the skin or mucosal surfaces.

Colour changes from bright red to violaceous to purple. Macular, papular, or punctate lesions are typical, linear or spider-patterned are rarely present.

Oral manifestations

Within the oral tissues the lesions occur more on the lips, tongue, cheeks, and palate.

Telangiectasias are prominent on the tongue, palate, nasal mucosa, palms, soles, and nail beds. The spots from 1-3 mm are non-pulsatile, and blanch on pressure. Oral bleeding is observed as a frequent complaint after tooth-brushing.

A thin layer of endothelial cells lines telangiectases; because of their thinness they bleed easily.

Management

Electrocautery and pulse dye laser is used to destroy cutaneous and accessible mucosal lesions. Estrogens have been used to treat recalcitrant bleeding.

PITYRIASIS ROSEA

Pityriasis rosea (*pityrias* = fine scales, *rosea* = pink or rose)

In the United States overall prevalence of pityriasis rosea has been calculated to be 0.13% in males and 0.14% in females. It has also been seen in United Kingdom, Nigeria, Sudan, Brazil, Lagos, Singapore, Turkey, Kuwait, and Hong Kong.

Cause

Pityriasis rosea is a rash of unknown cause, which lasts about six weeks.

Herpes virus 6 and 7 (HHV-6 and HHV-7) has sometimes been associated with pityriasis rosea.

Drugs such as bismuth, barbiturates, captopril, gold, organic mercurials, metronidazole, ketotifen have been implicated as causing drug induced pityriasis rosea.

It may occur at anytime of year, but pityriasis rosea is more common in the spring and fall.

Clinical features

Pityriasis rosea most often affects teenagers or young adults.

In most cases there are no other symptoms but, in some cases, rash follows a few days after an upper respiratory viral infection.

Pityriasis rosea usually starts with pink or tan oval area (sometimes called a *herald or mother patch*) on the chest or back. The main patch is followed by smaller pink or tan patches elsewhere on the body—usually the back, neck, arms and legs. The rash lasts approximately 2-6 weeks.

The herald patch measures few mm to 1-2 cm in diameter. The patch is characterised as oval or round with a central, wrinkled, salmon-coloured area and a dark peripheral area. The patches are oval and may form a pattern over the back that resembles the outline of ***'Christmas tree'***. Borders are raised.

Rash may be accompanied by low-grade fever, nausea, headache, and fatigue.

Microscopically: There is absence or decrease of the granular cell layer, extravasation of red blood cells in papillary dermis and partly into the epidermis, dyskeratosis, liquefaction of basal cells, homogenisation of papillary collagen, intraepidermal vesicles in apparently dry skin. There is edema, hyperaemia, and perivascular infiltration by lymphocytes, plasma cells, and histiocytes.

Oral lesions

Pityriasis rosea usually avoids the face, although sometimes a few spots spread to the cheek.

Oral lesions of various types have been reported with pityriasis rosea, including erythematous plaques, haemorrhagic puncta, papulo-vesicles bullae, and ulcers. Most studies reported the incidence between 10-16%.

Treatment

If the rash itches, treatment with steroid cream or ointment usually brings prompt relief. Extensive or persistent cases can be treated by phototherapy.

EHLER'S-DANLOS SYNDROME

Ehler's-Danlos syndrome (EDS), also known as ***'cutis hyperplastica'*** is a group of inherited connective tissue disorders, caused by a defect in the synthesis of collagen.

The syndrome is named after two doctors—Edward Ehlers of Denmark and Henri-Alexandre Danlos of France.

This is a rare autosomal dominant disorder; characterised by increased capillary fragility, increased elasticity of skin and hyper-extensibility of joints.

It affects approximately 2 to 5 in 100,000 people.

Clinical features

Skin: The skin is usually white and soft, and underlying vessels are sometimes visible. The skin is easily hyperextensible. It is easy to pull and, once released, returns to its original state.

Molluscoid pseudotumours consist of fat surrounded by a fibrous capsule. Fragility of dermal skin is common with frequent bruises and lacerations.

Extensive scarring or unusually wide scars, particularly at the knee, elbow, forehead, and chin.

The basic defect in connective tissue may lead to serious internal complications, including rupture of colon and large arteries, ocular fragility, with rupture of cornea and retinal detachment and diaphragmatic hernias.

Oral manifestations

Gums: The fragility of gingival can be detected by following treatments such as prophylaxis, periodontal surgery, or extraction. Early onset of periodontitis is one of the most significant oral manifestations of the syndrome. This can lead to the premature loss of deciduous and permanent teeth.

Teeth: Some studies have reported enamel hypoplasia, stunting of root growth, and pulp stones. Premolar and molar teeth can present with deep fissures and long cusps. Teeth seem to be fragile and microdontia is sometimes present. Hypodontia of permanent teeth, delayed eruption and dentin dysplasia is reported in cases of Ehler's-Danlos syndrome.

Joint: Hypermotility of temporomandibular joint resulting in repeated dislocations of the jaw have been reported.

Tongue: Tongue is supple.

Palate is commonly vaulted.

WHITE SPONGE NEVUS

Cannon described it in 1935.

It is also known as Cannon's disease or hereditary leukokeratosis of mucosa; appears to follow hereditary pattern as an autosomal dominant trait.

Cause

It is caused by mutation of keratin 4 and keratin 13 genes.

Clinical features

White sponge nevus almost always presents during childhood and there is no gender predilection.

It presents in the mouth, most frequently as a thick bilateral white plaque with a spongy texture, usually on the buccal mucosa, but sometimes on the labial mucosa, alveolar ridge, or floor of the mouth. The gingival margin and dorsum of the tongue are almost never affected.

Individual lesions are seen as a relatively thick, white, often corrugated plaque, which may cover most of the oral mucosa. Usually asymptomatic, rare examples of mild discomfort have been reported from secondary infection.

Microscopically: There is marked intercellular edema of the superficial epithelial cells, predominantly within the spinous layer. The nuclei are typically pyknotic and the cells may mimic the koilocytes of viral infection. Edematous cells may be organised into inverted triangles with broad bases along the surface, and there may be a thickened parakeratin layer.

Management

There is no specific treatment for this disease.

ECTODERMAL DYSPLASIA

It is also known as ***'hereditary hypohydrotic ectodermal dysplasia'***.

Cause

It is a X-linked, recessive Mendelian character. It results from aberrant development of ectodermal deviation in embryonic life.

Clinical features

Hair: Hair manifest as fine, sparse, and with reduced density in eyebrows and eyelashes.

Skin: The skin may be lightly pigmented. Skin sustaining injury may grow back permanently hypo-pigmented. In some cases, red or brown pigmentation may be present.

Nails: Fingernails and toenails may be thick, abnormally shaped, ridged, slow growing, or brittle. The cuticles may be prone to infections.

Sweat glands: The sweat glands aplasia leads to intolerance to heat and deregulation of body temperature.

Oral manifestations

Dental features: It may include hypodontia or anodontia, malformed, rudimentary or pegged teeth, and/or enamel defects and frequent dental caries.

There is midfacial hypoplasia that results in protuberant lips.

The palatal arch is frequently high and cleft palate may be present.

INCONTINENTA PIGMENTI

A genetic skin pigmentation disorder characterised by eye, teeth, bone, nail, and hair malformations as well as central nervous system abnormalities and mental deficiency.

Cause

Incontinenta pigmenti is caused by mutations in the NEMO/IKK-gamma gene, which is located on chromosome Xq28.

Clinical features

Skin lesions: Characteristic skin lesions compatible and by with the early, vesicular and/or vesicular stages of incontinenta pigmenti are present at birth few years of life in approximately 90% of patients. The cutaneous manifestations of the hyperpigmented stage develop during infancy.

Skin features occurs in four stages:

Stage 1 (vascular): It is characterised by the development of red papules and vesicles on an erythematous base that follows Blaschko lines.

Stage 2 (verrucous): Thickened warty-appearing linear and whorled plaques on an erythematous base that follow Blaschko lines characterise it.

Stage 3 (hyperpigmented) is characterised by streaks and whorls of brown or slaty-grey colour pigmentations.

Stage 4 (atrophy) is characterised by hypopigmented, atrophic, and reticulate and linear patches observed on the lower extremities, usually involving calves.

Hair changes include, scarring, alopecia and are seen in 28-38% of patients.

Nail feature include nail dystrophy, which ranges from mild pitting or ridging of the nail plate to hyperkeratosis and oncholysis.

Ophthalmologic findings: Loss of visual acuity and blindness are significant complications. Retinal manifestations include retinal detachment, proliferative retinopathy, vitreous haemorrhage and atrophy.

Neurological: Mental retardation, seizures, microcephaly, and cerebral atrophy.

Oral manifestations

Dental abnormalities and jaw changes are seen in 80% of patients and involve both deciduous and permanent teeth. Dental abnormalities are permanent and thus serve as a very useful diagnostic finding in older patients.

It includes delayed tooth growth, tooth decay, missing teeth, hypodontia, microdontia, malformed teeth, round, conical and pegged teeth, cleft lip, cleft palate, delayed tooth eruption micrognathia, pronathia and gothic palate.

Poor enamel quality leading to an increased incidence of dental caries has been reported. Nasty metallic taste, loss of appetite is common symptom. Areas of hypermineralisation and decreased enamel mineralisation can also occur.

Treatment

There is no specific treatment. Genetic counselling for carrier females is advisable. Associated systemic defects are to be addressed.

POROKERATOSIS MIEBELLI

Porokeratosis is a clonal disorder of keratinisation characterised by one or more atrophic patches surrounded by a clinically and histologically distinctive ridge like border called coronoid lamella.

Porokeratosis occurs in fair-skinned individuals. It is rare in darker-skinned populations.

Etiology

It is autosomal dominant disease. Several risk factors for the development of porokeratosis have been identified; these factors include genetic inheritance, ultraviolet radiation and immunosuppression.

Clinical features

Porokeratosis Miebelli usually appears in childhood, but lesion may be present at birth or may first occur at puberty or later.

The face, genitalia, oral mucosa and cornea may also be affected. Porokeratosis Mibelli most often affects the limbs, particularly the hands and feet, the neck and shoulders, the face, genitals, and the cornea, although any part of the body may be affected including the mucus membrane.

Lesions start as small, light brown scaly papules that may join into one or more plaque is separated from the surrounding skin by a warty rim with well-defined thin furrows running in its centre.

Skin cancer can develop within porokeratosis Meibelli. This may be either basal cell or squamous cell carcinoma. Lesions appear most often on the limbs and show a tendency to centrifugal spread.

Oral manifestations

There is delayed tooth eruption, peg and cone shaped crowns, congenitally missing teeth, malformed teeth and additional cusps.

Microscopically: Section from lesion shows typical coronoid lamella, band-like infiltration beneath the epidermis, liquefaction degeneration of the basal layer, and subsequent coagulative necrosis of the keratocytes.

KERATOSIS FOLLICULARIS

Keratosis follicularis, also known as Darier's disease or Darier's white disease. French dermatologist Ferdihard-Jean-Darier type and White first reported the disease in 1889.

Darier's disease, or keratosis follicularis, is a pruritic autosomal dominant inherited disease with multiple discrete scaling, crusted, and pruritic papules; it is malodorous and disfiguring and also involves the nails and mucus membrane. It is characterised by premature and abnormal keratinisation and loss of epidermal adhesion with acantholysis. It usually persists throughout the lifetime of patients.

Clinical features

The age at onset varies from children through adulthood, though it typically appears between 8 and 15 years of age.

The lesions start as pinhead to pea-sized flesh coloured papules. The disease is characterised by greasy crusted papules on the scalp, face, neck, seborrheic areas of the trunk and flexures of extremities. Patients with keratosis follicularis experience pruritis and sometimes pain in the affected skin areas.

Nails changes provide important diagnostic clues. White and red longitudinal nail ridges, longitudinal splitting, and subungual hyperkeratosis are frequently found.

Oral manifestations

Mucosal lesions are detected in 15% of cases. White, centrally depressed papules present on mucosa of cheeks, hand and soft palate and gums (*'cobblestone' lesions*). These lesions resemble leukoplakia. At times, oral lesions may affect the salivary glands and cause obstruction. Overgrowth of gums is also reported.

Management

There is no specific treatment for Darier's disease. Patients are instructed to avoid sun exposure, heat, and humidity.

HEREDITARY BENIGN INTRAEPITHELIAL DYSKERATOSIS

It is also known as Witkop-von Sallman syndrome.

Hereditary benign intraepithelial dyskeratosis (HBID) is a rare autosomal dominant disorder characterised by elevated epibulbar and oral plaques and hyperemic conjunctival blood vessels. The condition is predominantly seen in Native Americans belonging to the Haliwa-Saponi tribe located in Northern North Carolina.

Clinical features

It is most commonly seen in children with no sex predilection.

Eye manifestations: About the limbus—both nasally and temporally—there are foamy gelatinous plaques, more superficial than pterygia, on a hyperemic bulbar conjunctiva. The dyskeratosis may involve the cornea, producing blindness from shedding and resultant vascularisation of cornea. Photophobia and itching of the eyes, especially in children, are common.

Oral manifestations

Orally the lesions are localised at the commissures, buccal mucosa, tongue, palate, gingival and lips.

The buccal mucosa is affected symmetrically. The lesion acquires a thick, whitish, spongy, macerated aspect with or without folds, resembling the white sponge nevus.

Microscopically: There is hyperplastic-stratified squamous epithelium with an overlying multilayered parakeratotic mantle containing rounded cells with dense cytoplasm and pyknotic nuclei. A mild to moderate lymphoplasmatic infiltrate within the subepithelial stroma beneath the affected epithelium. Scattered throughout the hyperplastic epithelium from the basal layer to the surface are rounded isolated cells with pyknotic or crenated nuclei surrounded by dense eosinophilic cytoplasm, leading appearance defined as intraepithelial dyskeratosis. The adjacent conjunctival epithelium may vary from normal to a thickened stratified squamous type.

Management

Electrocautery and pulse dye laser is used to destroy cutaneous and accessible mucosal lesions. Estrogens have been used to treat recalcitrant bleeding.

LINEAR IGA DERMATOSIS

Linear immunoglobulin A (IgA) dermatosis is an autoimmune vesiculobullous disease that may be idiopathic or drug induced.

The incidence of adult linear IgA dermatosis in Southern England has been estimated to be 1 case in 250,000 populations per year. Children and adults are affected.

Skin lesions are annular, grouped, papules, vesicles, and bullae. Skin lesions may also include erythematous plaques, blanching macules, and papules or targetoid erythema-multiform like lesions. Bullae may be discrete arranged in a herpetiform pattern, often described as the cluster of jewels.

Oral manifestations

Oral lesions are seen in 5 to 70 percent and present on palate, tonsillar pillars, tongue and buccal mucosa. Oral lesions include vesicles, ulcerations, erythematous patches, erosions, desquamative gingivitis, and erosive cheilitis and they may precede skin lesions. Oral desquamative gingivitis may secondarily damage teeth. The oral lesions heal by scarring. Oral lesions show erosions and scarring.

Microscopically: Section shows subepidermal blisters with neutrophils.

Immunochemistry: Linear IgA is seen at basement membrane zone. Low titres of IgA antibodies are present against basement membrane zone.

Treatment

Most patients with linear IgA disease improve or clear with Dapsone 50 to 100 mg daily. Other medications that have been reported to help individual patients include corticosteroids, tetracycline, erythromycin, sulfapyridine, colchicines and mycophenolate mofeti.

Bibliography

Edwin T Park, Henry Lancaster: *Oral manifestations of systemic diseases*. Dermatology Clinic 2003:21:171-82.

James, William, Berger, Timothy, Elston, Dirk: (2005), *Andrew's Diseases of the Skin: Clinical Dermatology*. (10th edition). Saunders.

Klaus Wolff, Richard Allen Johnson, Dick Summoned: *Fitzpatrick's Colour Atlas and Synopsis of Clinical Dermatology*: 5th edition McGraw-Hill. 2005.

Lever's Histopathology of Skin: 8th edition LippinCott Raven.

Makee PH 1999: *Essential Skin Pathology*. 2nd edition. Mosby.

Palle Holmstrup, Anne HP, Lone A, et al: Oral Infections and Systemic Diseases. Dental Clinic N. America 2003; 47:575-98.

Silverman S, Gorky M, Lozada-Hur F: *A prospective follow up study of 570 Patients With Oral lichen Planus: Persistence Remission, and Malignant Association. Oral Surg, Oral Med, Oral Pathol* 1985: 60: 30-4

Thomas P Habif: *Skin Diseases Diagnosis and Treatment*. Mosby 2001.

Weinberg, Neil S Prose, Leonard Kristal: *Colour Atlas of Pediatric Dermatology*. 4th edition. 2008.

CHAPTER 13

ORAL ASPECTS OF METABOLIC DISEASES

DIABETES

Diabetes mellitus is a chronic disorder of carbohydrate, fat, and protein metabolism. A relative or absolute deficiency in insulin secretory response, which translates into impaired carbohydrate (glucose use), is a characteristic feature of diabetes mellitus, as is the resulting hyperglycemia.

TABLE 13.1
ETIOLOGICAL CLASSIFICATION OF DIABETES MELLITUS

I. **Primary diabetes**
   - A. Type I diabetes (insulin-dependent diabetes mellitus)
     1. Immune mediated
     2. Idiopathic
   - B. Type II diabetes (non-insulin diabetes mellitus)
   - C. Maturity-onset diabetes of the young (MODY)
   - D. Obese
   - E. Non-obese

II. **Secondary diabetes**
   - A. Genetic defects of beta cell function characterised by mutation in:
     1. Hepatocyte nuclear transcription factor (TNF) 4a
     2. Glucokinase
     3. Hepatocyte nuclear transcription factor la
     4. Insulin promoter factor

Contd.

Contd.

B. Genetic defects in insulin action

C. Diseases of exocrine pancreas

Pancreatitis, pancreactomy, neoplasia, cystic fibrosis, haemochromatosis

D. Endocrinopathy

Pheochromocytoma, Cushing's syndrome, Acromegaly, hyperthyroidism, glucagonoma, somatostatin

E. Drugs and chemicals

Corticosteroids, Thiazide, diuretics, phenytoin, thyroxine

F. Infections

Congenital rubella, cytomegalovirus

Coxsackie virus

G. Uncommon forms of insulin mediated diabetes 'stiff man syndrome'. anti-insulin receptor antibodies.

H. Other genetic syndromes associated with diabetes

Down's syndrome, Klinefelter's syndrome, Turner's syndrome

Huntingson's syndrome

I. Impaired glucose tolerance

J. Gestational diabetes.

TABLE 13.2
DIFFERENCES BETWEEN TYPE I AND TYPE II DIABETES

No.	Features	Type I diabetes	Type II diabetes
1.	Age	Below the age of 25 years	Above the age of 25 years
2.	Type of onset	Sudden and severe	Gradual and insidious
3.	Frequency	10-20%	80-90%
4.	Weight	Wasted	80% are above over-weight
5.	HLA	HLA genes DQB1 0302, DQA1 0301, DQA1 0501 and DQB1 0201	No HLA association
6.	Family history	< 20%	About 60%
7.	Genetic locus	Unknown	Chromosome 6
8.	Diabetes in identical twins	40% in concordance twins	100% in concordance twins
9.	Pathogenesis	Autoimmune disease, deficient β cells of Langerhans	Normal
10.	Islet cell antibodies	Autoantibodies present in 85% of cases	No islet cell antibodies
11.	Blood insulin level	Severe insulin deficiency	Insulin level normal or increased or relative deficiency

Contd.

Contd.

12.	Islet cell changes	Insulitis, marked atrophy, fibrosis, lymphocytic infiltration	
13.	Amylin	No amylin deposition	Amylin deposition surrounding β cells
14.	Complications	Develop ketoacidosis	Hyperosmolar non-ketotic
15.	Treatment	Insulin + diet	Diet + exercise + anti-diabetic drugs + insulin

Clinical features

Patients complain of polydipsia (excessive intake of fluid), polyuria (excessive passing of urine), and polyphagia (excessive appetite).

There is increased susceptibility to bacterial and fungal infections, sometimes complicated by pyelonephritis.

Atherosclerosis develops early and causes myocardial infarction, cardiovascular disease and peripheral vascular disease.

Somatic neuropathy, automatic neuropathy, atherosclerosis and pressure on abnormal locations give rise to ischaemic foot.

Proliferative retinopathy causes visual impairment or total blindness.

Diabetic neuropathy can cause distal sensory/motor polyneuropathy.

Diabetic ketoacidosis occurs in type I diabetes mellitus with absolute deficiency of insulin.

Oral manifestations

No specific oral lesions associated with diabetes. However, there are number of problems by presence of hyperglycaemia.

Generally, the symptoms are more severe, and the rate of their progression appears to be more rapid in those patients who have poorly controlled with insulin, or in those with non-insulin-dependent diabetes (NIDDM).

Periodontal disease

It is due to:

- Microangiopathy altering antigenic challenge
- Altered cell mediated immune response
- Increased Ca^+ and glucose lead to plaque formation
- Increased collagen breakdown.

Salivary glands

Xerostomia: About one-third of diabetic patients complain of xerostomia, which may be due to an overall diminished flow of saliva and an increased salivary glucose level.

Sialadenitis: Concomitant diffuse non-tender, bilateral enlargement of the parotid glands— called diabetic sialadenitis—may be seen in patients.

Tenderness, pain and burning sensation of tongue.

Dental caries: It has been well-documented that there is a higher incidence of dental caries in patients with poorly controlled diabetes.

- It is due to xerostomia and increased saliva glucose.
- Hyperglycaemia state shown a positive association with dental caries.

Increase risk of infection

- Reasons unknown but macrophage metabolism altered with inhibition of phagocytosis.
- Peripheral neuropathy and poor peripheral circulation.

Immunological deficiency

- It is due to high sugar medium.
- Decrease production of antibodies.

Candidiasis and mucormycosis

Candidial infections are more common adding effects with xerostomia.

Erythematous candidiasis presents as central papillary atrophy of the dorsal tongue papillae, and has been reported in up to 90% of cases.

Mucormycosis and benign migratory glossitis have also been shown to have a higher incidence in IDDM than in general populations.

Delayed healing of wounds

- Due to microangiopathy and utilisation of protein for energy, may retard the repair of tissue.
- It is due to increased prevalence of dry socket.

Miscellaneous conditions

- **Pulpitis:** It is due to degeneration of blood vessels
- **Neuropathies:** May affect cranial nerves (facial, trigeminal)
- **Drug side effects:** Lichenoid reaction may be associated with sulphonyl urea (chlorpropamide)
- **Ulcers:** Oral mucosal lesions such as traumatic ulcers and irritation fibromas are seen in diabetes
- Glossodynia may also be present in diabetes, resulting in painful mastication and swallowing.

Diagnosis

Incisional and gingival biopsy is the most reliable technique for definite diagnosis. For evaluation of mucosal changes in patients with diabetes, some studies have used gingival biopsies showing an increase in thickness and hyalinisation of small capillaries.

ADDISON'S DISEASE

Addison first described it in 1885. It is called chronic adrenal insufficiency of the adrenal cortex.

Causes

Addison's disease is a condition of hypoadrenalism associated with bilateral destruction of the suprarenal cortex often due to tuberculosis, amyloidosis, metastatic carcinoma, haemochromatosis, adrenal infarction, fatty change, congenital adrenal hypoplasia, and cytotoxic contraction of adrenal.

Clinical course

1. The outstanding features of Addison's disease are weakness, lethargy, loss of appetite and weight, and dizziness.
2. The blood pressure that falls further when standing—causing dizziness or fainting.
3. Gastrointestinal disturbances are common and include anorexia, nausea, vomiting, weight loss, and diarrhoea.
4. Skin changes in Addison's disease, with areas of hyperpigmentation, or dark tanning, covering exposed and non-exposed parts of the body, this darkening of the skin is most visible on scars, skin folds, pressure points such as elbows, knees, knuckles, and toes, lips and mucus membranes. There is increase in amount of melanin in deeper layers of rete Malphighi and mel-

anophages of the dermis are lodged with coarse granules of melanin. The diminished adrenal activity stimulates an increased production of melanin stimulating hormone (MSH).

5. Addison's disease can cause irritability and depression.
6. Because of salt loss, craving of salty foods also is common.
7. Hypoglycaemia or low blood glucose is more severe in children than in adults.
8. In women, the menstrual periods may become irregular or stop.

Oral manifestations

Sites: Patches of pigmentation is found on the mucous membrane of the lips, buccal mucosa, gingiva and tongue.

Microscopically: Section reveals an excessive amount of melanin in the basal layers of the epithelium.

Diagnosis

A diagnosis of Addison's disease is made by laboratory tests.

ACTH stimulation test: This is most specific test for diagnosing Addison's disease. In this test, blood cortisol, and urine cortisol, or both, are measured before and after a synthetic form of ACTH is given by injection. In the so-called short or rapid ACTH test, measurement of cortisol in blood is repeated 30 to 60 minutes after an intravenous ACTH injection. The normal response after an injection of ACTH is a rise in blood and urine cortisol levels. Patients with either form of adrenal insufficiency respond poorly or do not respond at all.

Corticotrophin releasing hormone (CRH) stimulation test: When the response to the short ACTH test is abnormal, a **'long'** CRH stimulation test is required to determine the cause of adrenal insufficiency. In this test, synthetic CRH is injected intravenously and blood cortisol is measured before and 30, 60, 90 and 120 minutes after the injection. Patients with primary adrenal insufficiency have high ACTH but do not produce cortisol.

ADRENAL INSUFFICIENCY

TABLE 13.3
CAUSES OF ADRENAL INSUFFICIENCY

Acute
Waterhouse-Friderichsen syndrome
Sudden withdrawal of long-term corticosteroid therapy
Stress in patients with underlying chronic adrenal insufficiency
Chronic
Major Contributors
Autoimmune adrenalitis
Tuberculosis
Acquired immunodeficiency syndrome
Metastatic disease
Minor Contributors
Systemic amyloidosis
Fungal infections
Haemochromatosis
Sarcoidosis

Predisposing factors

1. Following stress such as physiological or psychological stress.
2. Massive adrenal haemorrhage may destroy the adrenal cortex sufficiently to cause acute adreno-cortical insufficiency.
3. Surgical removal of bilateral adrenals in treatment of selected breast cancers, cortical hyper-function or hypertension.
4. Sudden withdrawal of long-term corticosteroid therapy.

Waterhouse-Friderichsen syndrome

Waterhouse-Friderichsen syndrome is named after Rupert Waterhouse, an English physician and Carl-Friderichsen, a Danish pediatrician, who independently described it in early 1900s.

Cause

This occurs in septic shock due to many virulent organisms—Neisseria meningitides, Pseudomonas, Pneumococci, Haemophilus, Staphylococci, Cytomegalovirus, and hypovolemic shock.

Clinical features

The disease occurs in children but also in adults. The onset of illness is non-specific with fever, rigors, vomiting, and headache, diarrhoea, extensive purpura, cyanosis and circulatory collapse, usually accompanied by meningitis and haemorrhage into the adrenal glands.

Treatment

Ceftriaxone is an antibiotic commonly employed today. Hydrocortisone can sometimes reverse the hypoadrenal shock. Sometimes reverse plastic surgery and grafting is needed to deal with tissue necrosis.

HYPERCORTICOLISM (CUSHING'S SYNDROME)

Cushing's syndrome, or hypercorticolism, results from a sustained increase in blood glucocorticoids levels.

The syndrome is produced by an excess of circulating the glucocorticosteroid due to the over action of cells of zona fasciculata. It was discovered by American physician, surgeon, and endocrinologist Harvey Cushing (1869-1939) and reported by him in 1932.

Clinical features

1. Painful obesity confined over face (*full moon face*) central and truncal obesity, thin arm and legs, prominence of fat over shoulders (*buffalo hump*).
2. Loss of libido, impotency, and oligospermia in males and sterility, menstrual disorder amen-orrhoea in females.
3. Increased protein breakdown resulting in wasting and thinning of skeletal muscle.
4. Thinning of the skin (which causes easy bruising) and other mucus membrane, purple or red striae on the trunk, buttocks, arm, legs or breast. Increased frequency to bacterial infection is common.
5. Kyphosis, generalised osteoporosis and wasting of skeletal muscles.
6. High fasting blood sugar and glycosuria in 20% of patients.
7. Hypertension in 80% of cases because of associated retention of sodium and water.
8. Increased protein breakdown resulting in wasting and thinning of skeletal muscles.
9. Arrest of growth in affected children with mental confusion and psychoses. Depression and anxiety including panic attacks are common.

10. Women with Cushing's syndrome usually show some features of virilism, e.g., masculine distribution of hair, acne, oligomenorrhoea enlargement of clitoris and deepening of voice.
11. Increase tendency to bacterial infections and poor healing of wounds.

Oral manifestations

Pathological fractures of mandible, maxilla, and alveolar bone may occur upon low impact of trauma due to osteoporosis. In children, growth and development including skeletal and dental age may be retarded.

Healing of fractures as well as healing of alveolar bone and soft tissues after dental extraction is delayed.

Etiopathogenesis

There are four major types of Cushing's syndrome:

1. **Adrenal Cushing's syndrome:** It is associated with cortical adenoma, carcinoma, and cortical hyperplasia. The average age of onset is about 3rd and 4th decades.
2. **Pituitary Cushing's syndrome:** Is seen in 60 to 70% cases, occurs due to pituitary basophilic adenoma, multiple micro-adenomas, bilateral adrenal hyperplasia and elevated plasma ACTH. This form of syndrome, known as Cushing's disease, affects women five times more frequently than males.
3. **Ectopic Cushing's syndrome:** Some benign or malignant tumours that arise outside the pituitary can produce ACTH. This condition is known as ectopic ACTH syndrome. Lung tumours cause over 50% of these cases. Men are affected 3 times more frequently than women. The most common forms of ACTH producing tumours are oat cell or small cell lung cancers, which accounts for about 25 percent of all lung cancer and carcinoid tumours. Other less common types of tumours that can produce ACTH are thymomas, pancreatic islet cell tumours and medullary carcinoma.
4. **Iatro Cushing's syndrome:** Occurs when the body's tissue are exposed to excessive levels of cortisol for long period of time. Many people suffer the symptoms of Cushing's syndrome because they take glucocorticoid hormones such as prednisolone for asthma, rheumatoid arthritis, lupus or other inflammatory diseases.

Management

Treatment depends on the specific reason for excess of cortisol and may include surgery, radiation, chemotherapy, or use of cortisol reducing agents.

Certain drugs—such as metyrapone or ketoconazole—can lower cortisol levels and can be used while awaiting more definitive treatment such as surgery.

Metyrapone in dose of 2-6 g per day in divided doses by mouth.

HYPERPARATHYROIDISM

Hyperparathyroidism is defined as elevated serum parathyroid hormone (PTH) due to increased secretion. It is one of the most common causes of hypercalcaemia in the hospital setting. However, in India and other countries where there is vitamin D deficiency, the classical manifestations of primary hyperparathyroidism are seen more commonly.

Primary hyperparathyroidism (PHPT): It is characterised by inappropriately increased secretion of PTH. It is usually due to adenoma (85%), hyperplasia, and, rarely, carcinoma.

Secondary hyperparathyroidism: It is associated with chronic hypocalcaemia most commonly associated with chronic renal failure and malabsorption syndrome.

Tertiary hyperparathyroidism: In a patient with reactive hyperplasia, the glands may become autonomous. Usually it is detected when a patient in chronic renal failure on dialysis gets a transplant and has persistently elevated PTH levels causing hypercalcaemia.

Clinical features

Hyperparathyroidism can become evident at any age. About 70% patients are women. Most are over 40 years old:

1. **Urinary calculi:** Urine calcium is increased owing to increased filtration of calcium, despite the fact that calcium reabsorption in distal tubule is also increased. The patients are more prone to develop renal stone and nephrocalcinosis. The stones consist of calcium oxalate, calcium phosphate, or some mixture of the two.
2. **Skeletal changes:** The skeletal manifestations of primary hyperparathyroidism may range from the relatively mild to crippling bone disease. There may be osteitis fibrosa cystica, brown tumours, single or multiple bone cysts, pseudotumour and pathological fractures.

   Microscopically: The bones usually show thinning of their trabeculae, with an increase in osteoclastic activity.
3. **Metastatic calcification:** It is common in soft tissues, lungs, heart, stomach, and blood vessels. There may be foci of calcification in the conjunctiva. Calcification in cornea can cause hazy bands of opacity concentric with the limbus—an appearance called band keratopathy.
4. **Gastrointestinal:** Nausea, vomiting, anorexia, and weight loss may be seen in hyperparathyroidism. Peptic ulceration may be seen. Peptic ulcer is attributed to increased secretion of gastrin, secondary to elevated serum levels of calcium or PTH. Pancreatitis is also seen, which may be due to calcium stones in pancreatic ducts.
5. **Nervous system:** Lethargy, listlessness, personality change, irrational behaviour and memory loss may be seen. If the hypercalcaemia becomes high then confusion, stupor, or coma is common.

Oral manifestations

Oral manifestations are:

1. Enamel hyperplasia
2. Failure of tooth eruption caused by hyperparathyroidism early in life
3. Candidiasis syndrome
4. **Skeletal changes:** The skeletal manifestations of primary hyperparathyroidism may range from the relatively mild to crippling bone disease. There may be osteitis fibrosa cystica, brown tumours, single or multiple bone cysts, pseudotumours, and pathological fractures.

Brown tumour

Brown tumour is a non-neoplastic lesion resulting from abnormal bone metabolism in hyperparathyroidism.

It represents the terminal stage of the bone remodeling process during secondary hyperparathyroidism. Brown tumours in hyperparathyroidism commonly affect jaw bones.

The term brown tumour comes from the colour of lesion, which results from vascularity, haemorrhage, and deposits of haemosiderin.

Histopathology shows network of ovoid- to spindle-shaped mesenchymal cells with focal aggregates of multinucleated giant cells diffusely present throughout the lesion.

Oral radiographic manifestations of hyperparathyroidism include a generalised loss of the teeth, loss of lamina dura surrounding the roots of the teeth, loss of cortication around the inferior alveolar canal and maxillary sinus, and of the trabecular patterns of jaw.

Laboratory findings

Serum calcium level is raised and serum phosphorus level is decreased. In occasional cases, radioimmunoassay of PTH may be necessary. Serum alkaline phosphatase level is elevated.

Treatment

Treatment with large calcium supplements, vitamin D, and restriction of phosphate is necessary. Surgical excision of adenoma if required.

HYPOTHYROIDISM

Deficiency of thyroid hormone is called hypothyroidism.

Primary hypothyroidism: When primary hypothyroidism cause, due to pathology of thyroid gland.

Secondary hypothyroidism: When the pituitary or the hypothalamus is the cause.

Decreased secretion of thyroid hormone results in cretinism if deficiency is present since birth and myxoedema, if it develops in adults.

Cretinism

Causes of cretinism

1. Failure of development of the thyroid (thyroid agenesis).
2. Failure of hormone synthesis due to severe iodine deficiency in the diet of both mother during pregnancy and the baby after birth.
3. Failure of hormone synthesis due to presence of dietary substances (goitrogens) that block hormone synthesis.
4. Failure of hormone synthesis due to autosomal recessive enzyme deficiency.

Clinical features

The symptoms may be present at birth, but appears during the first month or two of life.

Clinical features of cretinism include impaired development of the skeletal system and central nervous system, with severe mental retardation, short stature and coarse facial features.

The infant has dry rough skin, widely set eyes with periorbital puffiness, broad nose, deficient hair and teeth, pot-belly with umbilical hernia and protruberant tongue.

Long-standing hypothyroidism in early life results in retardation of both growth and maturation of the skeleton with severe dwarfing.

Myxedema

Clinical features

Many organ systems in the body are affected but all are hypo-functional. It is more common in women than men and occurs between 40-50 years of age. Basal metabolic rate is decreased.

Skin shows loss of hair all over the body, but typically in the scalp and eyebrows. Hydrophilic mucoprotein ground substance accumulates in the dermal connective tissue causing coarsening of the features. There is firm non-pitting edema of the supraclavicular fossae and dorsum of the hands.

Nervous system: Commonly the patient becomes dull, listless, or drowsy. It is due to direct effect of lack of thyroid hormone on the brain. There is delayed tendon reflexes and carpel tunnel syndrome. This is as a result of stiffness due to the direct effect of lack of thyroid hormone.

Heart is flabby and microscopically shows interstitial edema and swelling of the myocytes. The pulse is slow. There is mild diastolic hypertension and breathlessness. It is due to low cardiac output and decreased ventilatory function. The incidence of atherosclerotic cardiovascular disease is increased in hypothyroidism. Cold intolerance is due to diminished blood supply and vasoconstriction.

Radiograph finding includes cardiomegaly.

Gastrointestinal tract: Bowel motility is decreased, resulting in constipation.

Upper aero-digestive tract: Airway obstruction due to goitre, enlarged tongue, pharyngeal muscle dysfunction, and myxoid polyps of larynx.

Reproductive system: Women with hypothyroidism can suffer ovulatory failure, progesterone deficiency, and irregular and excessive bleeding. It is due to suppressed gonadal function.

Myxedema coma: A long-standing hypothyroidism can present with life-threatening situation, and this is called myxoedema coma.

Oral manifestations

Common oral findings in hypothyroidism include:

1. Macroglossia, dysgeusia.
2. Poor periodontal health, and delayed wound healing.
3. Salivary gland enlargement.
4. Enlargement of the lips and tongue is due to the accumulation of glycosaminoglycans. Due to enlargement, tongue may protruded continuously and such protrusion may lead to malocclusion of teeth.
5. There is failure of eruption of teeth though the formation is normal.
6. Maxilla is overdeveloped and mandible is underdeveloped. Retarded condylar growth leads to characteristic micrognathia and open bite relationship.

Laboratory findings

1. The level TSH is increased in primary hypothyroidism. Low T_4 (FT_4) and T_3 (FT_3) is diagnostic.
2. The thyroid autoantibodies (anti-TPO, anti microsomal and anti-thyroid globulin) are usually positive in autoimmune disease.
3. There is hyperlipidaemia.
4. Hypochlorhydria or achlorhydria.
5. Blood cholesterol and lipid levels are increased.

Management

Supplements are either natural hormones extracted from the thyroid glands of animals or synthetic hormones (such as levothyroxine).

Although treatment provides the necessary hormone control, hypothyroidism often continues throughout life, and the patient may require life-long follow-up and medication to control the condition.

HYPERTHYROIDISM

Hyperthyroidism is also called thyrotoxicosis; it is a syndrome in which there is excessive production of thyroxin in thyroid glands.

Cause

Hyperthyroidism occurs in Grave's disease, toxic adenoma, and toxic nodular goitre. Rarely, hyperthyroidism may be caused by hypersecretion of pituitary TSH because of a pituitary tumour or due to hypersecretion of thyrotrophin releasing hormone. Excessive thyroxin causes generalised increase in metabolic rate of all body tissues.

Graves' disease is an autoimmune disorder in which a variety of autoantibodies may be present in the serum. The occurrence of this disorder is strongly associated with the inheritance of human leukocyte antigen (HLA)-DR3.

Clinical features

Women are affected up to seven times more often than men. It is common in between 20 to 40 years of age.

Cardiovascular system: Heart is a target organ for hyperthyroidism. Patient presents with palpitation and dyspnea. Auricular fibrillation is due to direct action of thyroid hormone on the heart and is more common in the older patients with thyrotoxicosis. Patients may show tachycardia and heart failure. Mitral valve prolapse is a common abnormality found in patients with Graves' disease.

Central nervous system: Symptoms include restlessness, tremors, insomnia, anxiety disorders, depression mania and difficulty in getting up from sitting position.

Thyrotoxic storm: Severe acute systemic states with delirium, coma, and convulsion may occur with thyrotoxicosis. Cardinal manifestations include fever, tachycardia, gastrointestinal dysfunction and central nervous system related symptoms.

Gastrointestinal system: Stimulation of gut results in hypermotility, malabsorption, vomiting and diarrhoea. There may be jaundice in these cases.

Reproductive system: There is amenorrhoea and short menstrual cycle.

Eye: Eye manifestations are wide, staring gaze and lid lag are present owing to sympathetic overstimulation of the levator palpebrae muscle.

Skin: Skin is soft, warm and flushed. Heat tolerance and excessive sweating is common.

Oral manifestations

Oral findings in hyperthyroidism include increased susceptibility to caries, periodontal disease, enlargement of extraglandular thyroid tissue, (mainly in the lateral posterior tongue), maxillary or mandibular osteoporosis, accelerated dental eruption and burning mouth syndrome. Early jaw development and alveolar bone atrophy.

There is hyperplasia of all lymphoid tissue bearing areas in the oropharynx and tonsillar regions.

There is hypomotility of tongue.

Investigations

1. There is an increase in T_3 and T_4 and TSH levels are increased.
2. The radioactive iodine uptake is usually very high showing that the thyroid is producing excessive hormone.
3. Thyroid stimulating immunoglobulin (TPI) is also positive.

Management

Currently, there are three principal ways to treat hyperthyroidism: Drug therapy, radioactive iodine therapy, and surgery.

Drug therapy: Topazole or propyroid thiouracil pills are antithyroid agents. Betablockers such as propranolol (Inderal) may be prescribed to block the action of the circulating thyroid hormone.

Radioactive iodine therapy: The patient is given a capsule or a drink of water containing radioactive iodine.

HYPERPITUITARISM

Gigantism

If a growth hormone-secreting adenoma occurs before epiphyses close, as in the case of prepubertal children, excessive levels of growth hormone result in gigantism.

By far most people with gigantism have growth hormone secreting pituitary adenomas or hyperplasia. Although gigantism is typically an isolated disorder, rare cases occur as a feature of other conditions, such as multiple endocrine neoplasia (MEN) type I, MacCune-Albright syndrome (MAS), neurofibromatosis and tuberous sclerosis.

Clinical features

Clinical features include tall stature, mild to moderate obesity, soft tissue hypertrophy, frontal bossing, hyperhidrosis, osteoarthritis and peripheral neuropathy. Complications of gigantism are diabetes mellitus, hypogonadism, hypothyroidism, and adrenal insufficiency.

Oral manifestations

Oral manifestations are microcephaly, coarse facial features, prognathism and macroglossia.

Acromegaly

If elevated levels of growth hormone persist, or present after closure of the epiphyses, patients develop acromegaly, in which growth is most conspicuous in soft tissues, skin and viscera and bones of the face, hands, and feet.

Clinical features

Clinical features of growth hormone excess include increased hand and foot size, heel-pad thickness, increased size requirement of shoe, glove, rings and collars, large fleshy nose, hyperhydrosis, oily skin, carpel tunnel syndrome, arthritides, and acanthosis nigricans.

Other features include generalised visceropathy—heart, thyroid and liver. There is cardiomyopathy, arrhythmias, left ventricular hypertrophy, hypertension, sleep apnoea, secondary diabetes, and respiratory failure.

Kyphosis is usually present due to irregular vertebral atrophy, and hypertrophy commonly results.

Oral manifestations

Protracted chin with massive body of mandible, thick and extruded lower lip, broad lower jaw, wider lower face, more or less quadrangular shape of the lower jaw (lantern jaw) indicated acromegalic jaw (hyperpituitarism). Mandibular condylar growth is very prominent. The palatal vault is usually flattened and the tongue increases in size and may cause crenation on its lateral border.

Laboratory findings

Plasma level of growth hormone are usually raised, sometimes only slightly, e.g., 5-10 μg/litre.

HYPOPITUITARISM

Hypopituitarism, which commences after puberty, is called Simmond's disease.

The term hypopituitarism means the combined deficiency of any of the anterior pituitary hormones. This most commonly results from the destructive effect of pituitary macroadenoma.

Clinical features

The presentation is highly variable and depends on the underlying lesion and pattern of resulting hormone deficiency:

1. The growth hormone deficiency produces lethargy, muscle weakness, and increased fat mass.
2. Gonadotrophin secretion becomes impaired within male, loss of libido and in female oligomenorrhoea, and amenorrhoea. In male there may be gynaecomastia and decreased frequency of shaving.
3. Loss of ACTH resulting in symptoms of cortisol deficiency. There may be postural hypotension and dilutional hyponitraemia.

4. Decrease in thyrotrophic hormone leads to myxedema and of growth hormone to dwarfism and infantilism.

Oral manifestations

Dental arch is smaller than normal and, thus, cannot accommodate all the teeth—resulting in crowding and subsequent malocclusion.

PROGERIA

It is also known as Hutchinson-Gliford progeria syndrome. The term progeria is derived from the Greek word *geras* meaning old age. Very few cases are reported from India (Bihar, Mumbai, Pondicherry, Karnataka) and 97% of patients have been Caucasians.

Cause

Huchinson-Gliford-progeria syndrome is a childhood disorder caused by a point mutation in position 1824 and the LMNA gene, replacing cytosine with thiamine, creating an unstable form of the protein lamin A.

Clinical features

Progeria affects between 1 in 8 million children, with a total reported incidences of just over 100 in the last century, since it's been identified and most affected children have a life span of around 20 years.

Clinical features include dwarfism, wrinkled and pinched nose. Mental growth is equivalent to other children of the same age. The disease is characterised by thin, atrophic, shiny skin with sclerodermoid changes, sparse to absent scalp hair, eyebrows and eyelashes, craniofacial disproportion, a sculpted beaked nose, short stature, pyriform thorax, thin limbs, musculoskeletal and cardiovascular manifestations.

Oral manifestations

Micrognathia, and delayed eruption of the permanent teeth are common features. The mandibular angle may be increased. The plane angle is steep and the anterior fontanel is open. There are no frontal sinuses and mastoid development is poor. Teeth have been irregular in form, small, discoloured, and deficient in number in most of the cases. Microscopic evidence of senile changes in dental pulp has been reported.

Bibliography

Lindsay RS and Toft AD: 1997. *Hypothyroidism.* Lancet 349:413.

Bruce M Wenig, Clara S Heffness, Carot F Adare: 1997: *Atlas of Endocrine Pathology*: 1st edition. Saunders.

Seymour I Schwartz, Shires G Tom, Granck C Spencer, et al: *Principles of Surgery* (6th edition). McGraw Hill, 1994.

Wilson JD et al: 1998 William *Textbook of Endocrinology*, 9th edition. Philadelphia: Saunders.

CHAPTER

14

DISEASES OF BONES AND JOINTS WITH ORAL MANIFESTATIONS

OSTEOPOROSIS

It is a generic term referring to a state of decreased mass per unit volume of a normally mineralised bone due to loss of bone protein.

Localised osteoporosis

Disuse atrophy is found in immobilised or paralysed limbs, e.g., following poliomyelitis or in the old courses of treatment for bone tuberculosis.

Primary generalised osteoporosis

Primary generalized osteoporosis is associated with aging.

Factors responsible for etiology of primary osteoporosis are:

Hormonal factors (Postmenopausal): Hormonal factors play a significant role in the development of osteoporosis, especially in postmenopausal women. The bone loss associated with estrogen deficiency may be caused by a combination of increased bone resorption and decreased bone formation.

Senile: Senile osteoporosis occurs in adults of both sexes and increases in severity with age. Testosterone deficiency is present in about one-third of men with senile osteoporosis.

Genetic: Certain variations of the vitamin D receptor gene are associated with a lower maximum bone density, presumably because they impair the bone-forming effects of vitamin D.

Secondary generalised osteoporosis could be secondary to other known states or diseases.

Causes of secondary osteoporosis

a. **Endocrine:** Hyperparathyroidism, hyperprolactinaemia, hyper- or hypothyroidism, ovarian or adrenal failure, pituitary tumours, insulin dependent diabetes mellitus and Cushing's syndrome.
b. **Neoplasia:** Multiple myeloma, carcinomatosis, osteolytic metastases.

c. **Gastro-intestinal diseases:** Malnutrition, malabsorption, vitamin C and D deficiencies, and chronic liver diseases.

d. **Drug-induced osteoporosis:** Corticosteroids, oral contraceptives, anticoagulants, chemotherapy, alcohol.

e. **Mechanical factors:** Reduced physical activity is associated with accelerated bone loss.

f. **Others:** Rheumatoid arthritis, psoriatic arthritis.

Clinical features

Vertebral changes may be particularly striking with bulging of the intervertebral disc through the weakened end plate (Schmorl's nodes), increased concavity of the vertebrae, collapse with wedging, or less commonly—uniform flattening.

Bony trabeculae are thinner and more widely separated than usual, resulting in an increased susceptibility to fractures. The bone trabeculae are thin so that marrow spaces are wider.

The thin trabeculae do not show much osteoblastic activity though foci of osteoclastic resorption may be met with.

Osteomyelitis may occur due to relatively avascularity and there may be severe bony pain.

Oral manifestations

Osteoporosis may lead to tooth loss, because the density of the bone supporting the teeth may be decreased. There may be fracture of jaws during tooth extraction. Osteoporosis has been reported to be risk factors for periodontal disease. Teeth are poorly calcified and are more prone to caries. In osteoporosis there is delayed eruption and early loss of teeth, missing teeth and malformed teeth. Patients are more prone to osteomyelitis.

Investigations

Serum calcium: Normal

Serum phosphorus: Normal

Alkaline phosphatase: Normal

Urinary calcium: High or normal.

Radiographic measurements of bone density by techniques such as dual-energy X-ray absorptionmetry (DEXA).

OSTEOGENESIS IMPERFECTA

It is also called fragilitas ossium or brittle bone disease and Lobstein disease. It is a group of hereditary conditions characterised by abnormal development of type I collagen. Most cases are due to mutations in type I collagen genes (CoLIA1, CoLIA2) causing either reduced collagen production or formation of abnormal collagen molecules that are rapidly degraded. It represents as a hereditary autosomal dominant trait.

Clinical features

The subject is often stillborn.

Osteogenesis imperfecta type I: It is characterised by multiple fractures after birth, blue sclerae, and hearing abnormalities. The initial fractures usually occur after the infant begins to sit or walk. Other features seen in all the types of osteogenesis imperfecta with variable degrees of severity are joint laxity, aortic incompetence, mitral valve prolapse, arterial ruptures etc.

The severity varies from neonatal lethal (type II) through very severe with multiple fractures in infancy and childhood (type III and IV to mild type I), which is classically accompanied by blue sclerae, and in which bone deformity is less marked.

Oral manifestations

The maxilla and the mandible are affected.

In patients with dental abnormalities, deciduous and permanent teeth are opalescent, and amber or blue-grey on eruption. There is increased constriction at the coronal-radicular junctions and pulps become obliterated with secondary dentin. However, pulps may be wider than normal during early development. Roots are thinner and shorter than normal. Some researchers described ***'thistle-tube'*** or ***'flame shaped'*** pulps in several patients with osteogenesis imperfecta.

Some patients have normal coloured teeth. In some cases, abnormalities of the teeth are conspicuous. Permanent teeth may be bell-shaped and fragile. Because of hypoplasia of the dentin and pulp, the teeth are misshapen and bluish yellow.

Histological features

Sections of bone reveal thinner cortical plates than normal. Trabeculae of the spongy bone also exhibit fractures. The calcification of the bone is normal.

In osteogenesis imperfecta the foetal collagen is not converted into mature bone.

Radiologically: The bones are extremely thin, delicate, and abnormally curved. When a fracture occurs the fracture callus may be so extensive as to resemble a tumour.

Diagnosis

Diagnosis of these cases, molecular diagnosis by mutation screening of the CoLIA1 and CoLIA2 genes can be performed, but this is not widely available.

Management

Treatment of osteogenesis imperfecta is mid-disciplinary in nature. Orthopedic surgery is required for the treatment of fracture and correction of limb deformities while physiotherapists and occupational therapists play an important role in rehabilitation of patients and in managing the consequences of bone deformity.

CLEIDOCRANIAL DYSPLASIA

Cleidocranial dysplasia (*cleido* = collar bone + *cranial* = head + *dysplasia* = abnormal forming), also known as cleidocranial dystosis and Marie-Sainton disease, is a condition characterised by defective development of the cranial bones and by the complete or partial absence of the collar bones.

Characteristics include

- Delayed closure (ossification) of the space between the bones of the skull.
- Premature closing of the coronal sutures.
- Protruding jaw (mandible) and protruding brow bone (frontal bossing).
- Wide nasal bridge due to increased space between the eyes (hypertelorism).
- High arched palate or possible cleft palate.
- Short stature.
- Scoliosis of the spine.
- Dental abnormalities failure—to lose the baby teeth at the expected time; slow eruption of secondary teeth; extra teeth; delayed or absent formation of teeth.

CRANIOFACIAL DYSOSTOSIS (CROUZON'S SYNDROME)

The syndrome is named after Octave Crouzon, a French physician, who first described this disorder.

It is inherited as autosomal dominant. Incidence is 1 : 25,000.

Clinical features are

- Craniosynostosis
- Maxillary hypoplasia
- Ocular proptosis due to shallow orbits resulting in conjunctivitis and keratitis
- The eyes show hypertelorism, and divergent strabismus
- Conductive hearing deficiency
- Spina bifida occulta is reported in some cases.

Oral and facial features

- The palate is high arched and cleft palate in some cases
- Mandibular prognathism (chin appears to protrude despite normal growth of mandible) and gives the effect of the patients having a concave face
- Unilateral and bilateral cross-bite
- Anterior open bite
- Supernumerary teeth
- Maxillary crowding
- Ectopic eruption or maxillary first permanent molars (47%)
- Shoved shaped maxillary incisors.

MARFAN'S SYNDROME

The prevalence of Marfan's syndrome is estimated to be 2 to 3 per 10,000.

Marfan's syndrome is characterised by skeletal disproportion (arm span greater than height), arachnodactyly (long, thin spider fingers), sternal depression, generalised hypermotility of joints, lens dislocation, spina bifida and a high arched palate. It results from mutations of fibrillar gene, (FBN1) a component of extracellular matrix.

Ectopia lentis may lead to severe myopia and retinal detachment.

The serious complications are in the cardiovascular system, with mitral valve prolapse, aortic incompetence and aortic dissection.

In addition to these features, Marfan's syndrome patients have defects in the skin, skeletal muscles and lungs. ***'Stretch marks'*** occur in areas of flexural stress; muscle appears myopathic with loss of and hypotonia; damage to the connective tissue in lungs may manifest as spontaneous pneumothorax.

DOWN'S SYNDROME

It is also called ***'Mongolism'*** and ***'Trisomy 21 syndrome'***.

It is a genetic disorder caused by the presence of all or part of an extra 21st chromosome. It is named after John, L. H. Down, the British doctor who described it in 1886. Down's syndrome is associated with some impairment of cognitive ability and physical growth as well as facial appearance. Down's syndrome is usually identified at birth but they are obvious in children older than 1 year.

Down's syndrome is the most common autosomal abnormality and occurs in approximately 1 case per 700 live births.

Types

1. In 90% of Down's syndrome children have trisomy 21 47, XX+21.
2. Rest of the patients have translocations; several translocations are possible: t(14q 21q), t(15q,21q), and t(21q, 21q).
3. Mosaic type 46, XX/47, XX+21.

Clinical features

The children affected are mentally retarded. Many of the common physical features of Down's syndrome also appear in people with standard sets of chromosomes. They include a single transverse crease, shorter limbs, and poor muscle tone.

Characteristic head appearance—Small head, (brachycephaly), flat facies, with increased interocular distance (hypertelorism), depressed nasal bridge, flat occipit, and broad short neck.

Health concerns of individuals with Down's syndrome include a higher risk for gastroesophageal reflux disease, recurrent ear infections, and obstructive sleep apnoea and thyroid dysfunction. Almond shaped eyes caused by an epicanthic fold of the eyelid. There are white spots on the iris known as Brushfield spots. The fingerprints have characteristic pattern.

Skeletal anomalies—Short stature, broad, short hands, feet, and digits, short curved fifth finger, clinodactyly of the fifth finger, dysplasia of the pelvis and joint laxity.

Patient with Down's syndrome presents with intestinal stenosis, umbilical hernia, and premature aging with Alzheimer-like senile degeneration.

It is interesting to note that Down's syndrome is often associated with acute megakaryocytic leukaemia. About 30% of the patients have a congenital malformation of the heart, most often inter-auricular and inter-ventricular septal defect and tetralogy of Fallot's.

Oral manifestations

Small mouth with protruding tongue and enlarged tongue near the tonsils. There is difficulty in eating and speaking, scrotal tongue, hypoplasia of maxilla, delayed tooth eruption, hypodontia, juvenile periodontitis, and cleft lip or palate. Teeth are malformed, enamel hypoplasia and microdontia. Fissuring and thickening of lips, and angular cheilitis are frequent.

OSTEOPETROSIS

Nomenclature: Osteopetrosis, literally ***'Stone Bone'***, is also known as marble bone disease and Albers-Schonberg disease.

Osteopetrosis is a clinical syndrome characterised by the failure of osteoclasts to reabsorb bone, leading to impairment of bone modeling and remodeling. This result in skeletal fragility despite increased bone mass, and it also causes bone marrow failure, disturbed tooth eruption, nerve entrapment syndromes, and growth impairment.

Etiology

Osteopetrosis is an uncommon hereditary disorder caused by deficient osteoclastic activity. In some of these patients the osteoclast lacks carbonic anhydrase II—an enzyme needed to acidify the milieu within the Howship's lacunae for proper lytic function. They have been shown to express the creb gene, somehow making them dysfunctional. An ability to produce super-oxide anion has also been documented.

Clinical features

It is usually found in adults between 20 to 40 years old.

Osteopetrosis is commonly seen at the base of the skull.

Two main forms exists:

1. Recessively inherited severe osteomyelitis.
2. Dominantly inherited mild form.

Presentation

Severe osteopetrosis

(i) Infant is short with a large head and frontal bossing, knock-knees.

(ii) Nerve compression causes blindness and deafness.

(iii) Reduction in bone marrow space causes anaemia, thrombocytopaenia, and an increased susceptibility to infection.

(iv) There may also be hydrocephalous, delayed eruption of teeth, and fractures.

Mild osteopetrosis

Ranges from asymptomatic and discovered incidentally on X-ray.

Investigations

1. **X-ray** shows a homogeneous, intensely dense, marble appearance, instead of normal structure of the bone.
2. The principle features are:
    (i) The entire skull is thickened and dense, especially at the base.
    (ii) Narrowing of the cranial foramina, which may cause optic atrophy or other cranial nerve involvement.
    (iii) Hydrocephalus.
    (iv) Interference with dentition.
    (v) Bones may be club-like or appear like a bone within a bone.
    (vi) There may be evidence of osteomyelitis or fractures.
    (vii) Sinuses are small.
3. In severe cases of osteopetrosis, the plasma calcium is reduced, and acid phosphatase and calcitriol are raised.

Treatment

The treatment of osteopetrosis is difficult. Interferon gamma treatment can improve blood counts and reduce frequency of infections, but, in severe cases, bone marrow transplantation may be required to provide a source of normal osteoclasts that resorb bone normally.

OSTEITIS DEFORMANS (PAGET'S DISEASE)

Paget's disease is named after the British surgeon, Sir James Paget, who first identified the disease in 1877.

Paget's disease of bone is a common disease of unknown etiology affecting bones in the elderly. About 90% of patients with Paget's disease are over 50 years of age.

Males are affected slightly more often than females.

Cause

Current opinion is that this disease is a result of a slow-virus infection by a virus belonging to the paramyxoviruses, atypical measles, or defective respiratory syncytial virus. These infected osteoclasts seem to be more responsive to IL-6 and show exaggerated osteolysis.

Paget's disease of bone tends to appear in families. It is also common in people of Anglo-Saxon descent and those who live in England, the United States, Australia, New Zealand, and Western Europe. Familial Paget's disease is linked to long arm of chromosome 18.

Oral manifestations

In Paget's disease, one or both the jaws may be affected. There is progressive enlargement of the jaws, and widening of alveolar process (alveolar ridge in edentulous).

The mucosa is always intact over the lesion.

Mobility, migration, and interdental spacing are frequently seen in dentulous areas.

If the patient is a denture wearer he complains of the denture getting tight very soon after they are remade.

PATHOLOGY

Macroscopically: The bone is soft, porous, light, has the feel of dry bread and can easily be sliced by knife. Paget's disease may present as a solitary lesion (monostatic) or may be multifocal (polyostatic).

Microscopically: In the vascularised connective tissue, woven bone is laid first which is later converted in lamellar bone but there is delay in the mineralisation of the newly laid down osteoid. The disorganisation in the structure of the lamellar bone leads to the formation of cement lines.

Malignant tumour, usually osteosarcoma, may develop in areas of long-standing active Paget's disease.

Investigations

1. Serum alkaline phosphatase level is increased.
2. High levels of serum calcium.
3. X-rays commonly show abnormalities of bone turnover, including areas of increased and areas of decreased bone deposition.
4. Urinary hydroxyproline a measure of collagen breakdown is increased.

FIBROUS DYSPLASIA

Fibrous dysplasia is a bone disorder in which scar-like fibrous tissue develops in place of normal bone.

Fibrous dysplasia is a chronic disorder in which bone expands due to abnormal development of fibrous tissue, often resulting in uneven growth of bones, pain, brittle bones and bone deformity.

The lesion is usually a swelling of a part of the body that arises during periods of bone growth in older children and adolescents; and is slowly growing.

Cause

Exact cause of fibrous dysplasia is not known, but it is believed to be due to a chemical irregularity in a specific bone protein. It appears to be a developmental defect in bone formation. Over-expression of the FOS photooncogene and somatic mutations in the gene coding for a stimulatory G protein (Gsa) located on chromosome 20 have been described in polyostotic form.

Types

It occurs in three forms:

(i) Monostotic

(ii) Polyostotic

(iii) Albright's syndrome.

MONOSTOTIC FIBROUS DYSPLASIA

Monostotic form is the most common, and is usually diagnosed in early adulthood. Approximately 70-80% of fibrous dysplasias are monostotic.

There are no signs and symptoms.

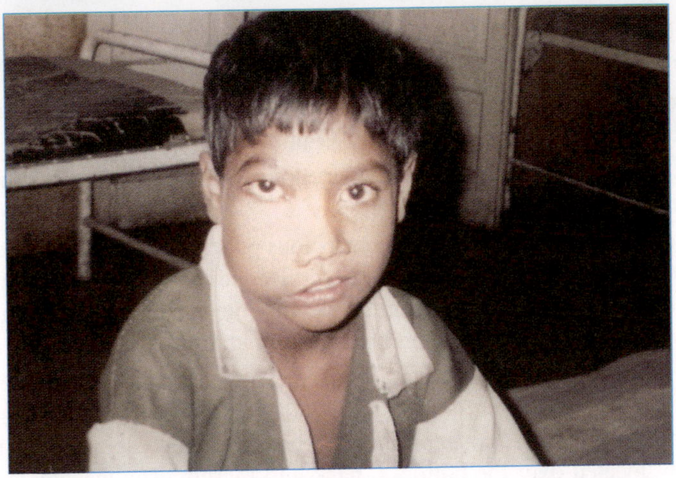

Fig.14.1: Showing fibrous dysplasia in maxilla in a 10-year male

The lesions are commonly found in a rib, the jaw, femur or tibia, though any bone may be involved. Deformity and exophthalmos may occur when the maxilla or facial bones are affected.

Oral manifestations

The jaws are involved very frequently in monostotic fibrous dysplasia.

Children are most commonly affected with maxillary lesion. In monostotic fibrous dysplasia there is displacement of teeth due to the expansion of the alveolar process. Teeth mobility may ensue at later stages. Dental anomalies such as supernumerary teeth have been reported in connection with the monostotic fibrous dysplasia.

POLYOSTOTIC FIBROUS DYSPLASIA

Two-third of patients are symptomatic before 10 years.

Polyostotic dysplasia may be unilateral or bilateral and it may involve several bones of a single limb with or without skeleton involvement. Polyostotic fibrous dysplasia may occur as multiple lesions in the adjacent bones. Fibrous dysplasia can occur in any bone. The sites of involvement are femur, tibia, pelvis, ribs, skull, and facial bones (50%), upper extremities, lumbar spine, clavicle and cervical spine.

More severe fibrous dysplasia may cause: Bone pain, difficulty in walking, bone deformities, fractures and scoliosis.

Sarcomatous changes (osteosarcomas or fibrosarcoma, chondrosarcoma and malignant fibrous histiocytoma) have been observed in about 0.5% of cases of polyostotic fibrous dysplasia. The polyostotic form is occasionally associated with myxomas of skeletal muscle (Mazabraud form).

Oral manifestations

Craniofacial involvement is common and, when present, may cause significant facial deformity. The commonest lesions are in the mandible and periorbital bones. Expansion and deformity of jaw, disturbed eruption pattern of teeth and because of loss of normal support of developing teeth and endocrinal disturbances affecting the timing of eruption of the teeth.

Management

Several studies have shown that bisphosphonates are useful in alleviating chronic pain in patients with fibrous dysplasia.

McCUNE-ALBRIGHT'S SYNDROME

In 50% of cases of fibrous dysplasia, the skeletal lesions are associated with skin pigmentation and endocrine dysfunction in which case the McCune-Albright syndrome is applied. It is caused by mutations in the GNAS1 gene, which erodes the stimulatory G-protein Gsα.

This condition is characterised by endocrine dysfunction including acromegaly, Cushing's syndrome, hyperthyroidism, and vitamin D resistant rickets.

The most common endocrine abnormality is precocious puberty in girls (boys rarely have McCune-Albright syndrome). Vaginal bleeding has been noted. Secondary sexual characteristic such as pubic and axillary hair and development of breasts are evident by the age of 5 years. As a result, premature closure of the growth plates may lead to abnormally short stature.

The most frequent extra-skeletal manifestations of McCune-Albright's syndrome are characteristic skin lesions. These are pigmented ***'café-au-lait'*** (literally coffee made with milk—the light brown colour of this) spots with irregular (*'coast of Marine'*) borders, which do not cross the midline of the body and are usually located over the buttocks, back and sacrum. The macules have a tendency to overlie the skeletal changes.

Fibrous dysplasia has some associated endocrine (hormonal) problems including precocious puberty and areas of increased skin pigment called café-au-lait marks.

Microscopically: The normal bone is sharply demarcated from the whitish, gritty, fibrous tissue (sandy to touch), often containing cysts and small nodules of cartilage, which expands the bone.

Histological features: The lesion mostly constitutes of fibres and proliferating fibroblasts. The stroma constitutes of interlacing collagen fibers. Chinese character pattern or ***'lobster claw'*** or ***'fish hook'*** of arrangement of the bony trabeculae of non-lamellar, woven bone with irregularly scattered osteoclasts and cartilage may be present. Trabeculae can also be C shaped.

Diagnosis

Imaging shows focal osteolytic lesions on X-ray and focal increases on bone scan.

Management

Removal of affected bone followed by bone grafting. Treatment is symptomatic with orthopedic treatment of fracture and deformity. Intravenous pamidronate has been reported to help bone pain and healing of lytic lesions.

CHERUBISM

Cherubism is a rare genetic disorder that causes prominence in the lower portion in the face. The name is derived from the temporary chubby- cheeked little angel resemblance, often confused with cherubs, in Renaissance paintings.

The condition is inherited in an autosomal dominant pattern.

Mutations in the SH3BP2 gene have been identified in about 80% of people with cherubism. In most of the remaining cases, the genetic cause of the condition is unknown.

X-ray: Radiologic characteristic of cherubism shows bilateral relatively symmetric jaw involvement that is limited to maxilla and mandible.

Imaging typically shows expansive remodeling of the involved bones, thinning of the cortexes and multilocular radiolucencies with a coarse trabecular pattern.

ACHONDROPLASIA

It is the most common genetic form of dwarfism—1 : 15,000 live births, and is inherited as an autosomal dominant.

Cause

Insufficient or disorderly formation of bone in the region of the epiphyseal cartilage interfering with the growth of long bones results in a condition called achondroplasia.

Achondroplasia is an inherited disòrder characterised by impaired maturation of cartilage in the developing growth plate.

A vast majority of cases of achondroplasia are caused by dominant mutations involving the gene coding for fibroblast growth factor receptor 3 ($FGFR_3$) located on the short arm of chromosome 4.

Clinical features

Head of affected patients appear usually large, compared with the bones formed from cartilage of the face. The forehead is bulging and the roof of nose is indrawn. The indrawing of nose results from a shortening of the base of the skull due to imperfect ossification, sometimes accompanied by premature union of the basisphenoidal and sphenoidal sutures.

Microscopically: The zones of proliferation and hypertrophy are narrowed and disorganised and contain clusters of large chondrocytes instead of well-formed columns. At the base of growth plate, there is premature deposition of horizontal shrufs of bone which seals the plate and prevents further growth. Chondrocyte development is defective; the orderly longitudinal growth of bone is disrupted, resulting in stunting of bones.

PIERRE-ROBIN SEQUENCE

Pierre-Robin sequence is a congenital condition of facial abnormalities in humans.

The heterogeneous birth defect has a prevalence of approximately 1 per 8,500 livc births. The male female ratio is 1 : 1.

Causes

It is not known just how this abnormality occurs in infants, but one theory is that, at sometime during the stage of the formation of the bones of the fetus, the tip of the jaw (mandible) becomes stuck in the point where each of the collar bones (clavicle) meet the sternum, effectively preventing the jaw bones from growing. It is thought that, at about 12 to 24 weeks' gestation, when the fetus begins to move, the movement of the head causes the jaw to 'popout' of the collar bones. From this time on, the jaw of the fetus grows as it would normally, with the result that, when born, the jaw of the baby is much smaller than it would have been with normal development, although it does continue to grow at a normal rate until the child reaches maturity.

Clinical features

Pierre-Robin sequence is characterised by an unusually small mandible (micrognathia), posterior displacement or retraction of the tongue (glossoptosis) and upper airway obstruction. Incomplete closure of the roof of the mouth (cleft palate), is present in the majority of patients, and is commonly U-shaped. Macroglossia and ankyloglossia are relatively rare findings.

Natal teeth (teeth appearing when the baby is born), recurrent ear infections, and small opening of roof of the mouth, cause choking.

Treatment

Infants with this condition should not be put on back, so that the tongue does not fall back into the airway.

A tracheostomy is sometimes required.

CAFFEY- SILVERMAN SYNDROME

It is also known as Caffey's disease, Caffey's syndrome, and familial subperiosteal bone formation. It was first described in detail in 1945.

Clinical features

Infantile cortical hyperostosis is believed to exist in two forms—familial and sporadic.

Familial form seems to have an earlier onset; 24% of these cases occur at birth. Incidence of mandibular involvement is less than that observed in the sporadic form.

Sporadic form is becoming less common. It has a higher incidence of mandibular involvement than does the familial form.

Infantile cortical hyperostosis is a proliferative bone disease of infants under 6 months of age. The average age at time of diagnosis is 9 weeks.

Peculiar to this disease is bilateral subperiosteal new bone formation, most commonly involving mandible. Less commonly, the clavicle, tibia, ulna, femur, ribs, humerus and fibula were involved with periodic proliferation in the first 3 months of life. The disease follows fever, usually appearing before 6 months of age and disappearing during childhood.

Oral manifestations

Puffy jaws and cheeks give the face a characteristic appearance. Enamel hypoplasia may be present.

Radiological findings: Typical radiologic feature is a marked periosteal new bone formation surrounding the diaphysis of long bones. The new bone becomes lamellated as the activity of the condition subsides and the bone becomes normal.

Histological findings

1. Overlying periosteum shows inflammatory infiltrate.
2. The superosteal bone shows immature lamellar bone formation.

GENERALISED CORTICAL HYPEROSTOSIS

Generalised cortical hyperostosis is an inherited skeletal dysplasia characterised by enlargement of lower jaw and thickening of the long bones and the top of the skull.

Generalised cortical hyperostosis or Van Buchem's disease is inherited as an autosomal recessive trait.

The disease is characterised by generalised thickness of the cortical table throughout the skeleton, primarily the tubular bones, the calvaria, and the mandible.

The hyperostotic changes become evident during the second decade of life. The jaw is squared and enlarged. Thickening of cranial base may eventually lead to foramina narrowing with attending neurologic deficits including facial paralysis, optic atrophy and hearing loss.

MASSIVE OSTEOLYSIS

It is also called Vanishing bone disease, Phantom bone disease, Gorham's disease and Graham-Stout disease.

Garham-Stout disease is a rare condition of unknown etiology that is thought to result from a localised endothelial proliferation of lymphatic vessels resulting in destruction and absorption of bone.

Graham's disease is an extremely rare bone disorder; fewer than 200 cases are reported in the medical literature. It is characterised by bone loss (osteolysis) often associated with swelling or abnormal blood vessel growths (angiomatous proliferation).

Clinical features

Condition affects both sexes equally. It is most commonly seen in children and young adults.

Head and neck area is affected in 30 percent of cases. The most commonly affected bones are the clavicle, scapula, humerus, ribs, ischium and sacrum. Bone loss can occur in just one bone or spread to soft tissue and adjacent bone.

Oral manifestations

The reabsorption of interior border of mandible and floating teeth within the bone have been reported. Maxilla is less commonly affected.

Microscopically: The mandibular body, ramus and coronoid processes are completely replaced by fibrous tissue, but inferior alveolar nerve and artery are intact.

Management

1. Surgical intervention has been suggested as the method of choice.
2. Radiotherapy acts by accelerating sclerosis of the proliferating blood channels and prevents regrowth of these vessels.

SKELETAL FLUOROSIS

Skeletal fluorosis manifestations are seen in the young as well in adults. The usual complaints of the patient, viz. pain in the neck, back, joints, and rigidity, begin in the regions where cancellous bones predominate as it is recorded that cancellous bone accumulates more fluoride compared to cortical bone.

X-ray reveals increased girth, thickening and density of bone. In certain patients, due to calcium deficiency, osteomalacia type changes occur, revealing weak bone with trabecular pattern instead of dense bone; calcified membrane/ligaments may be observed.

Acute toxicity: There is nausea, vomiting, pain in the stomach, bloated feeling/gas formation in the stomach, constipation followed by diarrhoea, may be due to fluoride toxicity, polyuria and polydypsia, if detected, may be due to fluoride toxicity manifestations. Muscle weakness, fatigue, anaemia, with very low haemoglobin level may be due to fluoride toxicity.

Chronic toxicity: In severe cases of fluorosis, there is complete rigidity of joints resulting in stiff spine, described as ***'bamboo spine'***, and immobile knee, pelvic and shoulder joints.

Crippling deformity is associated with rigidity of joints and includes kyphosis, scoliosis, and flexion deformity of knee joints, paraplegia, and quadriplegia. Fluorosis begins with vague pain in the back and extremities.

Bibliography

Emanuel Rubin, John L Farber: *Pathology*. 3rd edition. Lippincott-Raven. 1998.

John Ebnezar: *Textbook of Orthopaedics*, 3rd edition. Jaypee. 2006.

Kasper Braunwald Fauci, Hauser Longo Jameson: *Harrison's Principles of Internal Medicine*, Vol II. 16th edition. New York: McGraw-Hill. 2005.

Roddie MN, Macsween Keith Whaley: *Muir's Textbook of Pathology*. 13th edition. 1992.

Vinay Kumar, Ramzi S Cotran, Stanley L Robbins: *Basic Pathology*. 7th edition. Saunders. 2003.

CHAPTER

15

ORAL MANIFESTATIONS OF IMMUNOLOGICAL DISORDERS

INTRODUCTION

Primary immunodeficiencies have many oral manifestations. The clinical presentation of these diseases demonstrates the roles of different immune cells for the maintenance of oral health.

TABLE 15.1
INFECTION SUSCEPTIBILITIES & ORAL MANIFESTATIONS IN T- AND B-CELL DEFICIENCIES

T- AND B- DEFICIENCIES CELL DEFECTS		
Immune system defects	**Examples**	**Oral manifestations**
Decreased numbers of both T- and B-cells	Severe combined Immunodeficiency	Candidiasis, herpes infections, oral ulcerations and severe necrotising gingival stomatitis
T-CELL DEFECTS		
Immune system defects	**Examples**	**Oral manifestations**
CD8+T cell defects	Major histocompatibility complex or MCH, Class I deficiency	Not described
CD4+T cell defects	MCH class II deficiency	Candidiasis and herpetic infections
CD4+T cell defects	Hyper IgM syndrome	Candidiasis, herpes infections, cleft palate, hypertelorism, and enamel hypoplasia

Contd.

Decreased number of T cells	DiGeorge velocardiofacial syndrome	Candidiasis, herpes infections, cleft palate, hypertelorism and enamel hypoplasia
B – CELL DEFECTS		
Immune system defects	**Examples**	**Oral manifestations**
No immunoglobulin production	X-linked agammaglobulinemia	Possible septicemia from odontogenic infection
Severely decreased or no immunoglobulin G antibody production	Common variable immunodeficiencies	Possible septicemia from odontogenic infection, some patients, however, are asymptomatic
Severely decreased or no IgA antibody deficiency	Severe IgA deficiency	Candidiasis, oral ulcerations, Others report no oral changes

Infectious complications of DiGeorge syndrome include oral candidiasis, herpetic infections, pneumonia, chronic rhinitis and susceptibility to all viral and opportunistic infections such as pneumocystis carinii.

SJOGREN'S SYNDROME

It is a triad syndrome with keratoconjunctivitis sicca, xerostomia, and arthritis.

Age and sex: Approximately 90 per cent of Sjogren's syndrome cases occur in women between the ages of 35 and 45 years.

Sjogren's syndrome mainly involves the salivary glands. There is symmetrical bilateral enlargement of parotid glands, submandibular glands, and lacrimal glands.

Microscopically

There is destruction of the intraglandular ducts, often, with hyperplasia of the duct, epithelium form masses containing pale staining hyaline material and dense infiltration with lymphocytes (primarily activated CD4+T cells) and plasma cells. The glandular tissue shows various degrees of atrophy, perhaps due to obstruction.

Etiology and pathogenesis

Several lines of evidence suggest that Sjogren's syndrome is an autoimmune disease in which the ductal epithelial cells of the exocrine glands are the primary targets.

Investigations

(i) There is usually hypergammaglobulinaemia and associated rheumatoid arthritis and rheumatoid factor is positive in serum in 52 per cent of cases.

(ii) Anti-SS-A and anti-SS-B are present in a majority of primary type of Sjogren's syndrome cases.

(iii) Anti-salivary duct antibodies are present in a majority of cases of the secondary type.

AMYLOIDOSIS

Synonyms: Lardaceous disease (1842), Amyloid disease (Virchow 1963), B-fibrillosis (Glenner 1974).

Definition: Amyloidosis is defined as a diverse group of disease process characterised by extracellular tissue deposits, in one or many organs, of protein materials, which are genetically termed amyloid.

TABLE 15.2
BIOLOGICAL BASED CLINICO-PATHOLOGICAL CLASSIFICATION OF AMYLOIDOSIS

A. Systemic generalized amyloidosis
1. Primary generalised amyloidosis (AL)
2. Secondary reactive/inflammatory amyloidosis (amyloid AA)
3. Haemodialysis-associated (AB2 M)
4. Heredofamilial (ATTR).
B. Localised amyloidosis
1. Senile cardiac
2. Senile cerebral
3. Endocrine
4. Tumour forming (AL).

Organs most commonly involved are kidneys, spleen, liver, heart, gastrointestinal tract, and adrenals. Tumour forming amyloidosis is seen in skin, eye, lung, urogenital tract, larynx, trachea, tongue, and nasal septum.

Amyloid may also be seen in pheochromocytoma, islet cell tumours, medullary carcinoma of thyroid, and type II diabetes.

Amyloidosis of oral cavity

Amyloid deposits occur in the buccal mucosa, tongue, palate, gingival and floor of the mouth.

Primary systemic generalised amyloidosis: The most common oral manifestation of amyloidosis is macroglossia, which occurs in between 15 to 20 per cent of patients with light chain diseases. The tongue can grow in massive proportions and can be smooth or possess a variety of polypoid appendages, which form as the tongue grows against gaps in the teeth. The tongue becomes adynamic, firm and friable—and may cause problems with deglutition, speech, and breathing.

Secondary systemic generalised amyloidosis: It occurs as a result of some long continued tissue-destroying process such as tuberculosis, lung abscess, osteoarthritis, chronic skin abscesses, leprosy, bronchiectasis, rheumatoid arthritis, and malignant tumours such as Hodgkin's lymphoma and renal cell carcinoma. It is characterised by extracellular tissue deposition of fibrils that are composed of serum amyloid A (SAA) protein, a major acute reactant protein, produced predominantly by hepatocytes.

Amyloid deposits occur in the gingival; and a gingival biopsy may be used as an aid in diagnosis. The gingival may be infiltrated and may be bluish, spongy and hypertrophied.

Tumour forming localised amyloidosis

Clinical features are

1. The enlarged tongue demonstrates lateral ridging due to teeth indentation.
2. Although pain is not usually present, enlargement, firmness, and loss of mobility are common.
3. Interference with taste has been reported in some patients.

Macroscopically: Tongue may be firm and appear relatively normal or it has yellow nodules on the lateral surface.

Microscopically: Biopsy material stained by Haematoxylin and Eosin shows extracellular homogeneous, structureless and eosinophilic hyaline material.

Stains used to demonstrate amyloid in tissues

Hematoxylin and Eosin stain

Special stains

van Gieson stain: Amyloid takes a khaki colour while the background is yellow.

Congo red stain: Amyloid appears red under the light microscope and gives a green fluorescence under polarising microscope.

Fluorescent stain: Thioflavin T gives a yellow fluorescence under ultraviolet light.

Electron microscopy: Regular fibrillar structure as observed by electron microscopy.

CONTACT STOMATITIS AND DERMATITIS (STAMATITIS VENENATA)

TABLE 15.3
CLASSIFICATION OF CAUSES OF CONTACT STOMATITIS AND DERMATITIS

A. Food and food adhesives	
• Candies	• Cinnamon
• Chewing gum	• Cough drops
B. Cosmetic preparations	
• Lipsticks	• Sunscreen
• Lip balm	
C. Dental preparations	
• Dentifrices	• Mouth washes
• Denture powder	
D. Denture materials	
• Colophony	• Acrylic monomers in denture
• Gold, mercury, copper, nickel	• Bisphenol
E. Dental therapeutic agents	
• Menthol	• Eugenol
• Benzocaine	• Silver nitrate
• Iodides	• Volatile oils
• Alcohol	• Antibiotics

Stomatitis is defined as inflammation of the mucous membranes of any structure in the mouth, which involve the cheeks, gums, tongue, lips and roof or floor of the mouth.

Contact stomatitis is an inflammation of the oral mucosa as a result of contact allergy.

Contact dermatitis is a common cause of eczematous cheilitis. Usually presents in third and fourth decades of life. More females are affected than males. This is probably due to frequent use of cosmetics and lip preparations among office-workers.

Clinical features

Possible manifestations include erythema, angioneurotic oedema, burning sensations, and loss of taste, numbness, erosion, ulcerations and vesicles. Small areas of ulceration erosion are formed as a result of rupture of vesicles. The irritant reaction is usually due to heat and chemical injury. Allergic stomatitis may be accompanied by cheilitis. Oral lichen planus, while often idiopathic, may be caused by allergy to dental materials.

Colophony is an ubiquitous contact steriliser, which may be present in dental materials such as periodontal dressings, impression materials, cements fix adhesives and varnishes. Exposure to a steriliser in a hypersensitive person may initiate allergic contact dermatitis/stomatitis.

Management

- Removal of causative agent is essential in contact stomatitis.
- Systemic steroids are rarely required for contact stomatitis.
- Intraoral topical steroids are prescribed in severe cases of contact stomatitis.
- Sucking on ice cubes provides temporary relief from contact stomatitis.

RECURRENT APHTHOUS STOMATITIS

Aphthous stomatitis is also known as canker sore—an illness that causes small ulcers to appear in the mouth, usually inside the lips, on the cheeks, or on the buccal mucosa or on the tongue.

Recurrent aphthous ulcer occurs worldwide and is reported on every populated continent. Recurrent aphthous ulcers affect 31-66% of the international population.

Etiology

- **Bacterial infection:** The fact that chemical compounds typically associated with bacterial and viral infections have been isolated from canker sores suggested that bacteria or virus could be a causative agent in the formation of these mouth ulcers. Several infectious agents have been identified in association with aphthous ulcer lesions, including human herpes virus (HHV-6 and HHV-8), varicella zoster virus, human papilloma virus (HPV), cytomegalovirus (CMV), Epstein-Barr herpes virus (EBV), herpes simplex virus(HSV-1, HSV-2), helicobacter species, and L-forms of streptococci. However, authorities generally agree that aphthous ulcers and recurrent aphthous ulceration do not represent acute infections and are not contagious.

  Immunological abnormalities: Cytotoxic action of lymphocytes and monocytes on the oral epithelium seems to cause ulceration, but the trigger remains unclear. Approximately 66% of patients who are HIV positive have herpetiform and major recurrent aphthous ulcers.
- **Haematinic deficiency:** Deficiency of iron, folic acid (folate), or vitamin B_{12} in up to 20% of cases.
- **Hereditary:** A family history of recurrent aphthous ulcers is evident in some patients. Recurrent aphthous ulcers is highly correlated in identical twins. Association between specific HLA haplotypes and recurrent aphthous ulcer has been investigated.

Predisposing factors

- Trauma to the mouth is the most common trigger of aphthous ulcers. Physical trauma, such as that caused by toothbrush abrasions, laceration with sharp or abrasive foods such as (toast), or objects, accidental biting after losing teeth or dental braces can cause aphthous ulcers by breaking the mucous membrane.
- **Endocrine conditions:** Endocrine factors in some women whose recurrent aphthous stomatitis is clearly related to the fall in progesterone level in the luteal phase of their menstrual cycles.
- **Psychic factors or stress:** Stress underlies RAS in many cases. RAS are typically worse at examination times.
- Cessation of smoking may aggravates or precipitate RAS.
- **Immunological deficiency:** Ulcers similar to RAS may be seen in HIV and other immune defects.
- Gastrointestinal disorders—particularly celiac disease (gluten-sensitive enteropathy) and Crohn's disease in about 3% of cases.
- Sodium lauryl sulphate is a detergent in some healthcare products may produce oral ulceration.

Types of aphthous ulcers

Aphthous ulcers are classified according to the diameter of the lesions:

Minor aphthous ulcers, which comprise more than 80% of recurrent aphthous cases, are less than 1 cm in diameter and heal without scarring within 7-10 days. At any time, one or more ulcers can be seen.

They occur mainly in the 10-40 years old age group.

They are found mainly on the non-keratinised mobile mucosa of the lips, cheeks, floor of the mouth, sulci or ventrum of the tongue. They are only uncommonly seen on the keratinised mucosa of palate or dorsum of the tongue.

The lesion is usually surrounded by an erythematous hollow and is covered by a yellowish fibrinous membrane.

Major aphthous ulcers are also known as Sutton's ulcer periadenitis mucosa necrotica. They are found on any area of the oral mucosa, including the keratinised dorsum of the tongue or palate. They are over 1cm in diameter, take longer to heal, and often scar on healing. They are well-circumscribed and round, with indurated margins. They may coalesce upon healing, which may take as long as 6 weeks. Scars may result in decreased mobility of the uvula and tongue and destruction of portions of the oral mucosa.

Herpetiform ulcerations are considered a distinct clinical entity that manifests as recurrent crops of dozens of small ulcers throughout the oral mucosa. This least common form (5-10% of cases) has the smallest aphthae, commonly no larger than 1cm in diameter. They are found in a slightly older age group than the other forms of recurrent aphthous stomatitis and are found mainly in females.

Microscopic findings: CD4 + lymphocytes are found in submucosa and perivascular regions in the preulcerative stage. These cells predominate early but soon are outnumbered by CD8 + lymphocytes (95%) when the ulcerative stage develops. Macrophages and mast cells are common inhabitants of the ulcer bed.

REITER'S SYNDROME

Reiter described it in 1916 as triads of symptoms consist of non-specific urethritis, conjunctivitis, and arthritis. It commonly occurs as a postenteric condition in Scandinavia and France.

Oral manifestations: Oral lesions occur in 20-40% of the cases. They appear as papules and ulceration on the buccal mucosa, gingival and lips. In the oral cavity painless aphthous-like ulcers are found. Lesions on the tongue resembles 'geographic tongue'.

Reactive arthritis is associated with human leukocyte antigen HLA-B27. The infectious trigger is usually one of shigella, salmonella, chlamydia, yersinia, campylobacter etc. Recurrence and chronicity are common features.

SARCOIDOSIS (BESNIER -BOECK-SCHAUMANN'S DISEASE)

Sir Jonathan Hutchinson (1865-75) first described the disease sarcoidosis. Sarcoidosis is a multisystem granulomatous disorder. The condition is more commonly seen in colder parts of Northern Europe where the incidence is approximately 40/10,000 (1 in 250). In North America it tends to be more common, and more aggressive in Afro-Caribbean populations.

Etiology and pathogenesis

Sarcoidosis most commonly affects adults between 20 and 40 years of age and is rare below 10 years of age.

Immunological

1. Studies underscore that lymphocytes interact with macrophages. Some postulate that CD4 + T helper cells, in concert with macropages produce a cascade of cytokines and chemotactic

factors which result in tissue changes and granulomatous lesions that affect many tissues and allow for multisystem.

2. The macrophages release interleukin 1(IL-1), interleukin 6 (IL-6), tumour necrosis factor (TNF), 1: 25-dihydroxyvitamin D and angiotensin covering enzyme.
3. There is also an increased production of T_{H1} cytokines, such as interferon.

Genetic: A recent theory has advanced that African Americans are associated with certain HLA genotypes (e.g. class I, HLA 1), HLA-DR 11, 12, 14, 15, 17, and HLA-B8

Sarcoidosis is a chronic granulomatous inflammation of unknown etiology, characterised by the formation of multiple discrete granulomas in many tissues. It usually starts in lungs and lymph nodes. Sarcoidosis involves skin, eyes, liver, CNS, bone marrow, kidneys, skeletal muscles, heart, and endocrine organs.

Lungs: Sarcoid granulomas can involve any part of the lung. They can be found in airways of any size, in the walls of the blood vessels, and in the pleura. Fibrosis is seen in 20% of cases of pulmonary sarcoidosis. Chronic disease progresses to end state of honey-comb lung.

Clinical features: Patients are mostly asymptomatic and the disease is recovered on routine chest X-ray.

Pulmonary symptoms are in the form of breathlessness, cough (dry) and vague chest pain. Non-pulmonary manifestations are erythema nodosum, arthralgia, fever, skin nodule, superficial lymphadenopathy, uveitis, cardiac arrhythmia, cranial nerve palsy, lassitude, fatigue, hypercalcemia, and even diabetes insipidus.

Eye lesions

Patients diagnosed with systemic sarcoidosis have 20% incidence of ocular involvement. The most prevalent ocular sign is unilateral anterior, granulomatous uveitis. Less common presentations include unilateral non-granulomatous uveitis, bilateral intermediate uveitis and bilateral chronically smoldering low-grade granulomatous inflammation (Lofgren's syndrome).

The common clinical ocular findings associated with sarcoid uveitis include decreased or hazy vision, pain, photophobia, lacrimation, conjunctival infection, cells and flare in the anterior chamber, granulomatous iritis with large **'mutton fat'** keratic precipitation scattered over the back surface of the corneal endothelium, iritis, spill over leading to anterior vitritis, true vitritis with white exudative debris in the region of the ora serrata (snowball or snowbank retinopathy) with retinal vasculitis and phlebitis.

Lymph nodes

Lymph nodes that are commonly enlarged in sarcoidosis are the intrathoracic lymph nodes at the hilum of the lung. The enlargement of these nodes is invariably bilateral and almost symmetrical, and can be associated with diffuse pulmonary infiltration.

Macroscopically: Capsule of the node is thick and fibrous. The affected lymph nodes may be greatly enlarged, greyish or pinkish in colour.

Microscopically: Granulomas resemble those occurring in tuberculosis except for the absence of caseous necrosis in sarcoid granulomas. There is no necrosis within the follicles, but some contain laminated black calcified Schaumann bodies.

Oral manifestations

Oral manifestations include multiple, nodular painless ulcerations of the gingival, buccal mucosa, labial mucosa and palate. Rarely sarcoidosis may involve the tongue including swelling, enlargement and ulceration. Non-tender well-circumscribed brownish-red or violaceous nodules with superficial ulceration have been reported on the lip in patients with sarcoidosis.

Other oral manifestations include asymptomatic swelling of the involved mucosa, gingivitis and ulcers.

Parotid glands involvement is usually bilateral, non-tender, and occurs approximately in 6% of the cases.

Microscopically

Sarcoid granuloma is characterized by tight clusters of epitheloid cells with a variable number of Langhans giant cells and foreign body type of giant cells. Caseation is absent.

The cytoplasm of sarcoid giant cells may contain inclusion bodies of three types:

1. Small laminated couch shaped calcified concretions called Schaumann bodies or conchoidal bodies.
2. Asteroid bodies are star-shaped inclusions of unknown composition.
3. Residual bodies, which may be transformed Schaumann bodies.

Diagnosis

1. **Radiologically:** The four following radiological abnormality can be distinguished:
   a. Hilar node enlargement with normal lung fields.
   b. Hilar node enlargement with pulmonary infiltration.
   c. Pulmonary infiltrations without hilar node enlargement.
   d. Pulmonary fibrosis with honeycomb lung.
2. **Kvein test:** 0.1 ml intradermal injection of suspension of human sarcoid spleen in the skin produces small papule at the site 4-6 weeks.
   The biopsy of the papule shows typical sarcoid granuloma on histology.
3. Serum hypercalcaemia and increased secretion of calcium in urine.
4. The cells in the granuloma release angiotensin-converting enzyme into the serum; the detection of elevated levels of the enzyme in serum is a useful test for sarcoidosis.

MIDLINE LETHAL GRANULOMA

Definition: It is a rare condition involving progressive destruction of the midface region, which includes the nose, sinuses, palate and even the eyes.

Midline granuloma is also known as midfacial lymphoma, Stewart's granuloma, malignant granuloma, granuloma gangraenescens, polymorphous reticulosis, angiocentric T-cell lymphoma.

Under the term lethal **'midline granuloma'** three varieties may be included: the essentially inflammatory, or idiopathic midline granuloma; the obviously neoplastic, or polymorphic reticulosis which is a lymphoproliferative disorder; and a lymphoma with low-grade malignancy.

Clinical features

Chronically, ill-patients present with fever, flu-like syndromes and malaise. Patients complain stuffy nose, persistent rhinitis, cough, loss of sense of smell, nasal discharge, blood in nasal discharge, and epistaxis.

There is destruction of nasal septum, hard palate, lateral nasal walls, paranasal sinuses, skin of the face, orbit and nasopharynx. Maxillary sinus shows an enhancing soft tissue mass destroying nasal septum and medial wall of sinus, and polypoidal enhancing lesions. There is involvement of the right superior alveolar ridge and adjacent palate with total erosion of anterior hard palate. There is saddle nose deformity, nasal ulceration and cutaneous sore.

Unless treated it ends fatally within 12 to 18 months.

Microscopically

Biopsy from the lesion shows mixtures of small, medium and large size lymphoid cells, along with tissue necrosis.

Immunochemical study shows that these abnormal lymphoid cells are CD^+, CD3, CD4, CD5, CD15, CD56, and CD79.

WEGENER'S GRANULOMATOSIS

Wegener's granulomatosis is named after the German physician who described it in 1936. The triad of lesions in Wegner's includes:

1. Acute necrotising granulomas of the upper and lower respiratory tract such as nose, nasal sinuses, nasopharynx, tongue, trachea, bronchi and lungs.
2. Focal necrotising granulomatous vasculitis involving small arteries, veins, capillaries, arterioles.
3. **Renal disease:** Focal necrotising cresentric glomerulonephritis often associated with interstitial necrotising vasculitis and granulomas in extraglomerular space.

Clinical features

Men are affected more often than women. Average age is about 40 years.

The disease begins in two third of patients with upper respiratory symptoms. Cutaneous lesions are present in the early stage of disease in about one-fourth of patients, and oral lesions occur in nearly all patients. Other features include skin rashes, muscle pains, articular involvement, mononeuritis or polyneuritis. Proteinuria and haematuria develop in 85% of cases.

Oral manifestations

The gingival shows ulceration, enlargement and friable granular lesions.

Microscopically

Two types of lesions are present:

1. Variously sized, often confluent areas of fibrinoid necrosis surrounded by polymorphous infiltrate containing neutrophils, lymphoid cells and plasma cells characterise necrotising granulomas. There are variable numbers of giant cells.
2. Vessels show intimal thickening and necrotising vasculitis.

Diagnosis

Anti-neutrophilic cytoplasmic antibody is found in over 90% of patients and is of a high titre.

The titre comes down with immunosuppressive therapy. Probably Wegener's granulomatosis is caused immunologically, though the mechanisms involved are uncertain. The prevalence of HLA-BS and HLA DR2 is increased in patients with the syndrome.

POLYARTERITIS NODOSA

In 1886 Kussumaul and Maier first described polyarteritis nodosa (PAN), a disease of small sized and medium sized arteries. Only 1 : 1,000,00 persons contracts PAN and they are usually men. Although any organ can be affected PAN most commonly involves the skin, joints, peripheral nerves, gastrointestinal tract and kidney.

Causes

PAN is also observed as a complication of hepatitis B (HB) and hepatitis C (HC) infection.

Antineutrophil cytoplasmic antibodies (ANCA) appear to play a significant role in causing endothelial damage. ANCA can active neutrophils to adhere more to endothelial cells and to stimulate neutrophils that have been primed with tumour necrosis factor (TNF-α) to lyse-Cultured endothelial cells. Two types of ANCA exist. Perinuclear (P-ANCA-antimyeloperoxidase) are often in patients with microscopic polyarteritis or MPA).

Pathology

Blood vessels: Lesions are segmental and tend to involve bifurcation of branches of arteries. Involvement of venules is not seen with classic PAN. Characteristic of PAN is a necrotising vasculitis characterised by transmural inflammation of medium sized to small arteries. Predominant cellular infiltration is by neutrophils, eosinophils and lymphocytes.

Ocular manifestations: Retinal vasculitis, retinal detachment, and cotton wool spots (cytoid bodies) are signs of PAN.

Skin: The most common skin lesions are palpable purpura, ulceration, infarction and livedo reticulosis.

Renal lesions: In 85% kidney is most frequently involved. There are multiple small intrarenal aneurysms. Aneurysms may disappear (thrombosis) or appear in new locations. Arterial narrowing and thrombosis causes multiple small cortical infarcts. PAN is associated with hypertension and renal failure.

Oral manifestations

1. Ulceration of vasculitis nature can be found in the buccal mucosa and soft palate.
2. The patient presents with a diffusely inflamed, orange red tongue that has burning sensation.
3. Orally erythema of lips, buccal mucosa and tongue.

Clinical features: Classic PAN often presents with systemic symptoms like myalgia, malaise, fever, weight loss, melena, predominantly motor peripheral neuropathy, and renal intestinal disease and hypertension.

Diagnosis

1. Antineutrophilic cytoplasmic autoantibodies are present in the serum in a minority of cases.
2. Histologic confirmation by biopsy of acutely affected tissue such as muscle or kidney.

CROHN'S DISEASE

Crohn's named after an American physician who described it in 1932.

Crohn's disease is uncommon in India and other poorer countries. The disease is more common in North America and Northern Europe. It is seen in patients in the third decade of life; another peak in the sixth decade.

Etiology

The etiology is unknown. Several possibilities have been suggested, including infectious, immunologic, environmental, and genetic.

Cause

1. **Infection:** Infections like mycobacterium paratuberculosis and M. avium, atypical mycobacteria, measles, and Yersinia enterocolitic have been implicated.
2. **Immunological:** Abnormalities in the immune system have often been involved as being causes of Crohn's disease.

   Crohn's disease is thought to be an autoimmune disease with inflammation stimulated by an over-active T1 cytokine response. However, more recent evidence has shown that T_h17 is of greater importance in the disease.

3. **Genetic:** Research has indicated that Crohn's disease has a strong genetic link. Mutations in the CARD 15 gene (also known as the NOD2 gene) are associated with Crohn's disease.

   Although the disease can affect any part of gastrointestinal tract from the mouth to the anus, the great majority of lesions are seen in the distal small bowel or colon.

PATHOLOGY

Macroscopically

The disease characteristically shows skip-lesions, affecting a segment of the small bowel with areas of normal mucosa in between. The affected mucosa usually shows linear or laciform ulceration with intervening mucosal swelling producing a 'cobblestone' appearance. The lumen is narrowed. Often fat from the mesentery beneath the serosa surround the involved segment of bowel the lesion feels like a hosepipe or a dead eel.

Microscopically

1. The inflammatory process typically involves all layers of the gut wall (i.e. it is transmural) and may extend into the mesentery.
2. The mucosa shows diffuse hyperemia, acute inflammation, abnormal villus pattern and shallow aphthous ulceration.
3. Ill-defined clumps of lymphocytes and plasma cells are scattered in the submucosa and subserosa. Germinal centre is present in the exudate.
4. Discrete, non-caseating granulomas, mostly in the submucosa, is also often present. In many cases ulceration is associated with metaplasia of gastric type.
5. The regional lymph nodes show non-caseating granulomas or reactive hyperplasia with prominent lymphoid follicles.

Complications of Crohn's disease are:

1. Structure formation leading to intestinal obstruction.
2. Fibrous adhesions leading to intestinal adhesion. Fistulae to bowel, bladder, and vagina may be seen.
3. Perforation of the bowel by the deep-fissured ulcers causing intra abdominal abscesses.
4. Increased incidence of carcinoma of the bowel after many years.
5. Rarely there can be significant bleeding from areas of ulceration.
6. Malabsorption, especially of bitamin B_{12}.
7. Gynaecological disease is in the form of dyspareunia and rectovaginal fistula.
8. Cholelithiasis is common in patients with ileal Crohn's disease especially those with intestinal resection for the disease. The proposed mechanism is due to the interruption of the enterohepatic circulation of bile salt.

Extraintestinal complications include arthritis, and arthralgia, uveitis and iritis, hepatitis and pericholangitis, and erythema nodosum and pyoderma.

Oral manifestations

Oral involvement occurs in 8-9% of Crohn's disease. Oral manifestations of Crohn's disease include:

1. Diffuse labial, or mucosal swelling
2. Diffuse swelling of one or both lips with associated angular cheilitis
3. 'Cobble-stoning' of the buccal mucosa with hyperplastic rigid mucosa
4. Aphthous ulcers

5. Deep linear ulcers, pseudopolyps and/or labial swelling and induration
6. Mucosal tags
7. Granulomatous cheilitis
8. Gingival and alveolar lesions are granular and erythematous abscess or vegetation and areas of intense erythema. These many small projections are red or pink in colour, but careful examination may show tiny pustules beneath the epithelium, which liberate purulent material when ruptured.

Investigations

Imaging: Small bowel disease is best detected by barium meal and follows:

1. Mucosal irregularities and ulceration.
2. Strictures—Especially the string sign of contour.
3. Skip lesions with apparently normal bowel in between them.
4. Intestinal fistulae.

B. Biopsy may also be obtained from the mucosa of right side of the colon and terminal ileum at colonoscopy.

C. **Serological markers:** Anti-saccharomyces cerevisiae antibodies (ASCA) positive in over 80% of patients. Antibodies may develop, that cross-react with red cell antigens and cause haemolysis.

RHEUMATOID ARTHRITIS

Rheumatoid arthritis is one of the collagen diseases. Rheumatoid arthritis term is derived from Greek for a flowing stream or river. It is an autoimmune disease.

Age incidence: The disease usually begins between 25 and 55 years but may affect both older and younger people.

Sex incidence: Rheumatoid arthritis affects about 3% of female and 1% of the male population in temperate people.

Sites of occurrence: Rheumatoid arthritis typically presents as symmetric arthritis affecting the small joints of the hands, and feet, ankles, knees, wrists, elbows and shoulders. Proximal interphalangeal joints, metacarpophalangeal joints are particularly involved.

Rheumatoid arthritis is a chronic systemic disease of unknown etiology involves tissues other than joints and tendons.

Pathological changes

Synovium: Histology: The synovial lining of affected joint is inflamed and hyperplastic and proliferates to form swollen, congested, thick villus processes which project into the joint space. Hypertrophy of synovial membrane occurs, with the formation of lymphoid follicles resembling immunologically active lymph nodes. There are foci of fibrinoid necrosis and fibrin deposition.

Articular cartilage: Prominent pannus may form over the articular cartilage, which may undergo organization, leading to fibrous ankylosis and sometimes-bony ankylosis. In some patients with rheumatoid arthritis, chronic inflammation leads to the destruction of cartilage, bone and ligaments causing deformity of joints.

Synovial fluid analysis: It is less viscous than normal. Joint fluid analysis usually reveals a WBC count of 2000-50,000/cumm. The concentration of protein in fluid is increased.

EXTRA-ARTICULAR LESIONS

Rheumatoid nodules: In rheumatoid arthritis nodules 1-2 cm diameter often develop in the subcutaneous tissues, often in the skin at the elbows. The rheumatic nodules, which are usually found in areas of pressure, are movable, firm rubbery and occasionally tender. A large nodule may ulcerate. They are granulomas, consisting of a central sheet of deeply eosinophilic fibrous tissue, which has undergone fibrinoid necrosis, surrounded by palisaded histiocytes, plasma cells, lymphocytes and macrophages.

Cardiovascular lesions: Asymptomatic pericarditis occurs in approximately 30% of patients with seropositive RA with pericardial effusions and constrictive pericarditis being complications. Rarely aortic regurgitation or a conduction defect occurs.

Rheumatoid vasculitis may occur when severe it gives rise to skin ulceration and gangrene.

Lung: In the lungs, rheumatoid arthritis often causes pleurisy, less frequently interstitial pneumonitis, fibrosis, Caplan's nodules or vasculitis.

Lymph nodes are often hyperplastic, showing many lymphoid follicles with large germinal centers and numerous plasma cells in the sinuses and medullary cords.

Amyloidosis: About 20% of cases of chronic rheumatoid arthritis have some evidence of amyloid disease affecting the spleen, liver and kidney.

Muscles of the part undergo atrophy; especially the extensor of the fingers and the swollen fingers show characteristic flexion. The atrophy is the result of inflammatory nodular polymyositis involving widely separated muscles.

Eye involvement is presented in the form of kerotoconjunctivitis and uveitis.

Less than 1% develops scleritis or episcleritis.

Oral manifestations

1. Oral manifestations include jaw pain on chewing, clicking, hypermobility, and condylar resorptions with recession of chin.
2. Ulceration of vasculitis nature can be found in buccal mucosa and soft palate.
3. Erythema of lips, buccal mucosa and tongue.
4. Occasionally arthritis of the temporomandibular joint may interfere with mouth opening.

Clinical features

The onset of the disease may be acute, slowly progressing, or insidious. Diseased joints are frequently warmed, swollen, and painful. There may also be constitutional symptoms such as weakness, malaise, low-grade fever, weight loss and myalgia.

The most common presentation is with a gradual onset of symmetrical arthralgia and synovitis of small joints of the hands, feet and wrists. In young patients there is morning stiffness, polyarthritis, and pitting edema.

Vasculitic involvement of the extremities may give rise to Raynaud's phenomenon and chronic leg ulcers.

Cervical cord compression can result from subluxation of the cervical spine at the atlantoxial joint or at a subaxial level.

Neurological: Peripheral neuropathy and mononeuritis multiplex may occur. The most common problem is Carpal tunnel syndrome due to compression of the median nerve by swelling around the wrist.

Osteoporosis classically occurs in RA around inflamed joints. It is postulated to be partially caused by inflammatory cytokines.

Lymphoma: The incidence of lymphoma is increased in RA as it is in most autoimmune conditions.

ETIOPATHOGENESIS

1. Rheumatoid arthritis is one of the autoimmune disorders characterised by presence of an IgM type circulating autoantibody called rheumatoid factor produced against the portion of autolous IgG. A negative rheumatoid factor does not rule out RA rather, the arthritis is called seronegative. Various other antibodies are found in some patients with RA, notably antinuclear antibodies, usually in lower titre and antibodies to various cytoplasmic constituents and to collagen.
2. Because of low specificity of Rheumatoid factor a new serological test has been developed in recent years, which test for the presence of anticitrullinated protein antibodies (ACPA). It is positive in 80% of patients.
3. Cigarette smoking is a risk factor for Rheumatoid arthritis and the positivity for rheumatoid factor in RA subjects.
4. Immunological reactions play a major role in the pathogenesis of rheumatoid arthritis. An autoimmune response is triggered by an infectious event. Once triggered the response causes inflammation of the synovium, leading to edema, vasodilatation and infiltration by activated CD4 cells in nodular aggregates and CD8 cells in diffuse infiltrate. Early and intermediate molecular mediators of inflammation include tumour necrosis factor Alpha (TNF-alpha) interferon (IF Y) and interleukin IL1, IL8 and IL15, fibroblast growth factor, platelet-derived growth, transforming growth factor beta.
5. Infectious agents such as EBV, cytomegalovirus or rubella virus, Borrelia species, Erysipelothrix, mycoplasma, parvovirus and mycobacteria may cause rheumatoid arthritis.

There are many variants of RA characterised by non-suppurative inflammatory synovitis and arthritis.

1. **Juvenile Rheumatoid arthritis** (Still's disease): It is characterised by Rheumatoid arthritis in young adolescent with generalised lymphadenopoathy and hepatosplenomegaly. Some cases are associated with HLA-B27.

2. **Felty's syndrome** is named after the American physician who described it in 1924. Patient develops splenomegaly, neutropaenia, anaemia, and thrombocytopaenia.

3. **Ankylosing spodylitis** (Marie Strumpell disease): In rheumatoid involvement of the spine, particularly sacroiliac joints in young male patients.

Laboratory studies

1. The anaemia is normocytic normochromic type. Thrombocytosis may be present.
2. ESR is elevated.
3. Plasma protein shows decreased albumin and a rise in globulin and fibrinogen and a moderate increase of C reactive protein.
4. Serum rheumatoid factor (RF) is positive in approximately 70% of patients.
5. **Latex agglutination test:** It is as reliable as the sheep's cell agglutination test. In this, a suspension of latex particles mixed with borate buffer and gamma globulin is used. It is mixed with a drop of serum and positive test is indicated by agglutination of latex particles visible to the naked eye.
6. **Coon's fluorescent antibody technique:** It has been utilised by Mellor et al to determine the site of origin of rheumatoid factor.
7. Radiologically, there are 'melon seed' bodies due to inflammatous villus projections, which hang into the joint cavity from thickened synovial membrane covering the cartilage.

ANGIONEUROTIC EDEMA

It is also known as angioedema, Quinck's edema, and giant urticaria.

Henrich Quince first described the clinical picture of angioedema in 1882.

Angioneurotic edema: Angioneurotic edema is most commonly the result of mast cell granulation, which may be spontaneous or triggered by the allergic IgE mediated response. However, other important causes include drug reactions, e.g., to ACE (angiotensin-converting enzyme) inhibitors and CI inhibitor deficiency. The fluid leaks into deeper tissues under the skin, which causes the tissues to swell. The swelling of angioneurotic edema can occur anywhere in the body but most commonly affects eyelids, lips, and genitals. Involvement of larynx and tongue may cause ill-threatening respiratory tract obstruction, and edema of the intestine may cause abdominal pain and distention.

Etiology

Allergic edema: Angioedema most frequently occurs as part of an IgE mediated, allergic response and a specific trigger such as food, animal dander and insect venom should be sought. Physical stimuli such as heat, cold or vigorous exercise may also cause spontaneous mast cell granulation and angioedema, which is associated with dermatographism. Angioedema is characterised by painless, non-pruritic, non-pitting and well-circumscribed areas of edema due to increased vascular permeability.

Drug-induced angioedema is common. It is most frequently associated with ACE inhibitors, aspirin, and non-steroidal anti-inflammatory agents, radiocontrast media, opiates and antibiotics.

Hereditary angioneurotic edema is characterised by recurrent self-limited attacks involving the skin, subcutaneous tissue, upper respiratory tract or gastrointestinal tract. Attacks may be precipitated by dental procedures and last for several hours to 2-3 days.

Oral manifestations

In angioneurotic edema there is edematous swelling of the upper lip, face, tongue, floor of the mouth, palate and periorbital area. Skin of the face, normally around the mucosa of the mouth and/or throat as well as tongue, swell up over a period of minutes to several hours. Swelling can also occur elsewhere, typically in hands and feet. There may also be slightly decreased sensations in the affected areas due to compression of nerves. Urticaria may develop simultaneously. In advanced cases, angioedema progresses to complete airway obstruction and death caused by laryngeal edema.

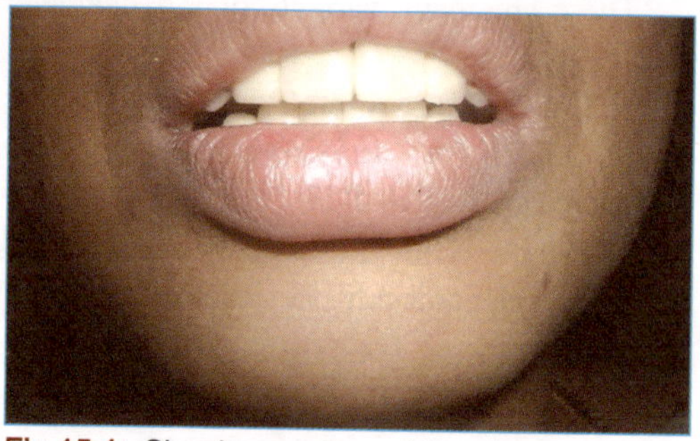

Fig.15.1: Showing swelling of lips due to angioneurotic edema

CONTACT STOMATITIS AND DERMATOSIS

Patients may present with dry, flaky, skin, on their lips or lip swelling. This is most likely due to contact allergy.

BEHCET'S SYNDROME

Behcet's disease is named after Hulusi Behcet (1889-1848), the Turkish dermatologist and scientist who first recognised the syndrome in one of his patients in 1924.

It is also called ***'oculo-oro-genital'*** syndrome, Marbus Behcet and Silk Road disease. A triad of aphthous, genital ulceration and uveitis characterises it. There may also be lesions of the skin, joints, and central nervous system. Disease is prevalent in Japan (1 : 10,000), South East Asia, the Middle East, and Southern Europe. It is rare in Northern Europe and the United States.

Pathogenesis

Several studies have investigated the involvement of immunological mediators such as tumour necrosis factor, interleukin IL-1, IL8, IL-12, and some growth factors, in patients, with Behcet's disease. The lesions are the result of leukocytoclastic (acute) and lymphocytic (late) vasculitis. The disease appears to be linked to HLA-B 51 alloantigens especially seen in Eastern Mediterranean and individuals of Japan. Symptoms appear to be milder when HLA-27 is present.

Clinical features

The disease begins between 10 and 45 years of age, with a mean age of occurrence of 30 years.

Oral manifestations

Oral ulcers are present in all cases. Painful ulcers erupt in a cyclic fashion in the oral cavity and/ or genital mucus membrane. Oropharyngia and oral ulcers may persist/recur weeks to months before other symptoms appear.

The edge of the ulcer is characteristically punched out. They may range from several millimetres to 3 centimetre in diameter. Punched out ulcers with rolled or overhanging borders and necrotic base; red rim; occur in crops (2 to 10) on oral mucus membrane.

Microscopically: Microscopy of lesional tissue shows vasculitis and thrombosis. T-lymphocytes are predominant neutrophil infiltrates in which cells appearing within the vessel walls have been described.

Neurological

Onset delayed, occurring in one-quarter of patients. Meningoencephalitis, benign intracranial hypertension, cranial nerve palsies, brain stem lesions, pyramidal/extrapyramidal lesions, and psychosis.

Cutaneous lesions

Cutaneous lesions are common and may include acneiform lesions, nodules, erythema nodosum, superficial thrombophlebitis, pyoderma gangrenosum-type lesion and palpable purpura.

Gastrointestinal

Abdominal discomfort, abdominal pain and diarrhoea with intestinal ulcers, occurring primarily in the ileum and colon closely resembling Crohn's disease may occur.

Other lesions include erythema nodosum, arthritis, vasculitis, and intestinal ulceration.

Treatment

Thalidomide gives a quick relief from mucocutaneous lesions.

Bibliography

Pepys M B. Amyloidosis Annual Rev med 2006, 57: 223-41

Pickens MM: **The changing concept of amyloid**. Arch pathol lab medicine125: 38-43, 2001.

CHAPTER

16

NUTRITION AND ORAL CAVITY

PROTEIN DEFICIENCY

Severe protein energy malnutrition is a serious, often lethal, disease. The most common victims of PEM worldwide are children. A child whose weight falls to less than 80% of normal life is considered malnourished. When the level falls to 60% of normal weight for sex, height, and age, the child is considered to have marasmus.

MARASMUS

Marasmus is due to continued restrictions of dietary energy and protein as well as other nutrients.

Marasmus is a serious worldwide problem and involves more than 50 million children younger than 5 years.

Causes

The major factors that cause a deficit of calorie and protein intake include:

1. Marasmus can also be due to improper feeding habits, metabolic abnormalities, or congenital malformations that will not permit ingestion, digestion, or absorption of sufficient food.
2. Transition from breast-feeding to nutrition—poor foods in infancy.
3. Acute infections of gastrointestinal tracts.
4. Chronic infections such as HIV and tuberculosis.

Clinical features

Marasmus occurrence increases prior to age 1. The afflicted are often fretful, irritable, and voraciously hungry.

A child with marasmus looks emaciated. Body weight may be reduced to less than 80% of the normal weight or height.

In marasmus there is generalised wasting of muscle mass, loss of adipose tissue, stunting of growth but no edema.

There is depletion of subcutaneous fat in the arms, chest wall, shoulders, or metacarpal regions.

The skin and mucus membranes may be dry and atrophic.

Diarrhoea is frequent, many infants are hungry but some are anorexic.

Brain, skeleton and kidney are preserved, whereas liver, heart, pancreas, and digestive tract are first affected.

Investigations

A moderate normochromic or slightly hypochromic anaemia is usually present.

Serum albumin levels are either normal or only slightly reduced.

KWASHIORKOR

Kwashiorkor is due to a quantitative and qualitative deficiency of protein, but in which energy intake may be adequate.

Geographical distribution

It is seen in Southern and Central Africa, West Indies, tropical America, and India.

Causes

The disease is frequently precipitated by outbreaks of febrile illness, such as malaria, measles, or gastroenteritis.

Clinical features

1. It is characterised by retarded growth of the child with mental apathy, edema of feet and general symptoms of anorexia, vomiting and loose bulky stool.
2. Hair is light, dry, and brittle, with marked depigmentation or discolouration in Africa but in India there is diffuse alopacia.
3. Children with kwashiorkor have characteristic skin lesions with alternating zones of hyperpigmentation, areas of desquamation, and hypopigmentation, giving a *'flaky paint'* appearance. Skin shows hyperkeratosis, atrophy of epidermis, parakeratosis. The lower limbs, buttocks, and perineum are usually most affected but ulcers can occur over pressure points and deep cracks in skin folds.
4. Muscles are always wasted and, as a result, many children may not be able to crawl.
5. The liver shows extensive fatty change with little inflammatory exudates.
6. There is atrophy of pancreas.

Oral manifestations

Papillary atrophy: The tongue is smooth, glazed or waxy due to atrophy of papillae.

There is bilateral angular stomatitis and fissuring of lips.

Bright reddening of tongue.

Biochemical changes

Plasma concentration of essential amino acids and tyrosine are low.

Plasma albumin level is low owing to failure of synthesis in the liver. Plasma transferrin is lowered.

DISTURBANCES OF LIPID METABOLISM

GAUCHER'S DISEASE

This uncommon condition was described by Gaucher in 1882.

This disease is the most common lysosomal storage disorder.

Gaucher's disease is heredofamilial and shows autosomal recessive inheritance.

Pathogenesis

It is due to deficiency of glucocerebrosidase. As a result, glucocerebroside accumulates principally in the reticuloendothelial cells, but sometimes also in the central nervous system neurons. In the cerebroside molecule, the kerasin is characterised by glucose replacing galactose.

Clinical features

Three main types of Gaucher's disease are recognised affecting adult, infants, and juveniles, respectively:

Type I is non-neuropathic and adult form.

There is lymphadenopathy, splenomegaly, and hepatomegaly, and bony lesion consisting of decalcification, osteosclerosis, moth-eaten appearance.

The skin may show hyperpigmentation. In later stages, Gaucher's cells may form aggregate in skin and also in the conjunctiva where they may be seen as wedge-shaped yellow-brown patches, termed pingueculae.

There is pancytopaenia, or thrombocytopaenia secondary to hypersplenism.

The femur, vertebrae and sternum are mainly affected.

In the femur it produces a bottle-shaped, conical swelling of lower part of shaft, eroding the cortex.

Type II: The disease starts within the first 2 to 3 months. The conspicuous features are muscular rigidity, strabismus, trismus, dysphagia, and laryngeal spasm.

Glucocerebrosides accumulate not only in macrophages but also in neurons and death occurs in infancy from the effects of central nervous system.

Type III is also known as the juvenile form. The features are intermediate between in infants and adult types and death results in a few years.

Microscopically

Gaucher's cell is a large cell (20 to 80μm) round, oval, or polygonal and contains one or more nuclei. The cytoplasm is filled with a fine or coarse fibrillar material, which gives the appearance of crumpled tissue paper. The Gaucher's cells are found in liver, spleen, bone marrow, lymph nodes, tonsils, thymus, and Peyer's patches.

When the bone is involved bone marrow shows numerous large, foamy, slightly granular cells with small round pyknotic nuclei.

Gaucher's cells are fat-negative. Periodic acid Schiff staining is usually intensely positive.

Diagnosis

The diagnosis in homozygous can be made by measurements of glucocerebrosidase activity in peripheral blood leukocytes or extracts of cultured skin fibroblasts.

Treatment

Replacement therapy with recombinant enzymes is effective but extremely expensive.

Bone marrow transplantation has been attempted.

NIEMANN-PICK DISEASE (SPHINGOMYELINOSIS)

Niemann-Pick's disease primarily affects Ashkanazi Jews.

This systemic lipidosis is characterised by the accumulation of sphingomyelin predominantly and gangliosides in small amounts in reticuloendothelial cells in visceral organs.

On the basis of organ involvement and nature of enzyme deficiency Niemann Pick's disease is divided into five tentative groups—A, B, C, D, and E.

Group A variant: This is the severe infantile form with extensive neurologic involvement, marked visceral accumulations of sphingomyelin, and progressive wasting—early death within the first 3 years of life.

Group B: Visceral, non-neuropathic form.

Group C: Subacute or juvenile form. Type C occurs when the body cannot properly break down cholesterol and other lipids (fats). This leads to too much cholesterol in the liver and spleen and excessive amounts of other lipids in brain.

Group D: It is the Nova Scotian form, with late onset, but with eventual severe CNS defects. It involves a defect that interferes with the movement of cholesterol between brain cells. This type of Niemann Pick disease has also been found in the French Canadian population of Yamouth County, Nova Scotia.

Group E occurs in adults.

Niemann-Pick disease types A and B are autosomal recessive disorders equally affecting males and females.

Type C and type D occur due to mutation of NPC-1 gene involved with cholesterol processing.

Clinical features

The clinical findings are:

1. Enlarged liver and spleen may cause reduced appetite, abdominal distension and pain.
2. Mental retardation is fatal in early lifc.
3. Anaemia, leukocytosis, and thrombocytopaenia.
4. The nervous system is affected. Sphingomyelin accumulation in the central nervous system results in ataxia, slurring of speech and discordinated swallowing (dysphagia).
5. Cholesterol deposits in the tissue.
6. A cherry red spot may be seen over the retina.

Diagnosis

Type A and B are diagnosed by measuring the amount of ASM in white blood cells.

A skin biopsy is usually used to diagnose type C and type D Niemann Pick disease.

Other tests might include:

1. Slit lamp eye examination
2. Liver biopsy and bone marrow examination for presence of Niemann-Pick cells.
3. Sphingomyelin assays.

TAY-SACHS DISEASE (GANGLIOSIDOSIS, HEXOSEAMINIDASE SUBUNIT A SUBUNIT DEFICIENCY)

Tay-Sachs disease is named after Warren Tay (1843-1927) and Bernard Sachs (1858-1944).

Tach-Sachs disease, like other lipidoses, is most common among Ashkenazi Jews, in whom the frequency of heterozygous carriers is estimated to be 1 in 30. Infants who are born suffer from mental retardation, dysfunctions that lead to certain death within 2 or 3 years.

Cause

Tay-Sachs disease is an autosomal recessive disease caused by mutations of both the alleles of a gene (HEXA) on chromosome 15. HEXA codes for the alpha subunit of the enzyme β-hexosaminidase.

Clinical features

This disease is characterised by the increased accumulation of gangliosidosis (Gm_2) in brain and spleen.

The characteristic clinical features are:

1. Mental retardation, blindness, muscular weakness, seizure, hearing loss, intellectual disability and paralysis.
2. A cherry red spot appears in the muscular region of the eye within first year of life.
3. At about two years of age, the circumference of the head becomes 50% greater than normal.

Diagnosis

Tay-Sachs defects can be diagnosed before birth by amniocentesis and chorionic villus biopsy.

DISTURBANCES IN CARBOHYRATE METABOLISM

HURLER'S SYNDROME (MPS I)

It is also called Pfaundier-Hurler's disease, gargolism, dyostosis multiplex and lipochondrodystrophy.

Pathogenesis

Hurler's syndrome is a genetic disorder that results in the buildup of mucopolysaccharides due to a deficiency of alpha-L-diuronidase, an enzyme responsible for the degradation of mucopolysaccharides in lysosomes.

Clinical features

The features of Hurler's syndrome include dwarfism, skeletal deformities, a characteristic facies, mental deficiency, corneal opacities and hepatomegaly. Affected children have a life expectancy of 6 to 10 years. Death is due to cardiac complications resulting from the formation of raised endothelial and endocardial lesions by the deposition of mucopolysaccharides in the coronary arteries and heart valves.

Oral manifestations

The facies is ugly and grotesque like a gargoyle (projecting spout, conveying the water from roof-gutters of buildings). Without this enzyme, a buildup of heparan sulphate and dermatan sulphate occurs in the body.

Distinct facial features (including flat face, depressed nasal bridge, and bulging forehead) become more evidence in the second year.

Dental complications can be severe and include unerupted dentition, dentigerous cyst-like follicles, mal-occlusion condylar defects and gingival hyperplasia.

A large head, short neck, corneal opacity, open mouth associated with enlarged tongue, enlargement of skull and a long antero-posterior dimension are the main characteristic features.

Laboratory findings

1. The deposited glycosaminoglycans are extracted in the urine and can be recognised by chemical analysis.
2. Prenatal diagnosis using amniocentesis and chorionic villus sampling.

Treatment

Gene therapy: There is currently a great deal of interest in treating MPS1 with gene therapy.

HUNTER'S SYNDROME

Hunter's syndrome or mucopolysaccharidosis type II is a lysosomal storage disease caused by a deficient (or absent enzyme iduronate-2 sulphatase).

Hunter's syndrome is X-linked inherited disorder that primarily affects males. The 12S gene is located on X-chromosome.

Clinical features

The symptoms appear after 1 year of life.

Early symptoms in Hunter's syndrome are:

1. Abdominal hernia
2. Ear infections
3. Running noses and colds
4. Hepatosplenomegaly

Skin lesions: Ivory coloured skin lesions are present in the upper back, and sides of the upper arms and thighs.

Cardiac lesions: There is thickening of the heart valves along with the walls of the heart can result in progressive decline in cardiac function.

Lungs: There is obstructive airway disease.

Bony changes in Hunter's disease include:

1. Joint stiffness and limited motion in wrist, elbows, shoulders, hips and knees.
2. Patient is unable to pick small objects.
3. Difficulty in walking.
4. Carpal tunnel syndrome.
5. As a result of bone deformities there is short stature.

Brain: There is mental retardation.

Oral manifestations include prominent forehead, a nose with flattened bridge, and enlarged tongue.

Diagnosis

The most commonly used laboratory screening test for an MPS disorders is a urine test for GAG (glycosaminoglycans).

Prenatal diagnosis is routinely available by measuring 12S enzymatic activity in amniotic fluid or in chorionic villus tissue.

DISTURBANCES IN MINERAL METABOLISM

ACRODERMATITIS ENTEROPATHICA

It is also known as Brabdt syndrome, Dan-Cross syndrome, and congenital zinc deficiency.

Incidence: 1 in 500,000 people in Denmark are affected.

Acrodermatitis enteropathica is an autosomal recessive metabolic disorder affecting the uptake of zinc, characterised by periorificial and acral (in the limbs) dermatitis, alopecia, and diarrhoea.

A mutation of the SLC 39A4 gene on chromosome 8 q24.3 is responsible for this disorder.

Clinical features

Features of acrodermatitis enteropathica start appearing in the first few months of life, as the infant discontinues breast milk.

Paronychia as well as loss of scalp hair, eyebrows, and eyelashes may occur.

The lesions may become secondarily infected with Staphylococcus aureus and Candida albicans.

Skin lesions: There are eczematous patches and plaques of dry scaly skin.

Infants may also experience withdrawal, photophobia, and loss of appetite.

Oral manifestations

Erythematous, confluent, sharply demarcated, symmetric, erosive, scaly and crusted plaques are seen on face.

Candidiasis is common in large number of children.

The lesions, predominantly located on the perioral region extended over cheeks and submental area. Atrophic glossitis, stomatitis, and stomatitis producing thrush-like picture and superficial aphthous-like erosions are also found occasionally.

The typical location of lesion is perioral area, where angular cheilitis may appear, but rarely areas of erythema with white macules of edematous lesions with erosions may develop in the oral mucosa. There may be papillomatous lesions on the tongue with severe halitosis.

Without treatment, the disease is fatal and affected individuals may die within a few years.

Laboratory tests

1. Laboratory test confirming the diagnosis is the measurement of zinc concentration.
2. Serum alkaline phosphatase is low in patients with acrodermatitis enteropathica.
3. Urinary zinc excretion may be reduced.
4. Blood count may reveal anaemia.

Treatment

There is no cure for the condition. Treatment includes lifelong dietary zinc supplementation in the range of greater than 1-2 mg/kg of body weight per day.

DISORDERS OF VITAMINS

VITAMINS

Vitamins are organic substances with key roles in certain metabolic pathway; they are required in small amounts in food because they are not synthesised in the body. Certain vitamins can be synthesised endogenously—vitamin D from precursor steroids, vitamin K and biotin by the intestinal microflora, and niacin from tryptophan, an essential amino acid.

Some vitamins have antioxidant activities and may be associated with diseases like atherosclerosis and cancer. Vitamins are essential for the normal growth and maintenance of life.

Classification

Fat-soluble Vitamins: Vitamin A, D, E, and K.

Water-soluble Vitamins: Vitamin C, and B-complex (B_1, B_2, B_3 B_6, B_9 B_{12}), niacin, pantothenic acid, biotin, lipoic acid, and inositol.

FAT-SOLUBLE VITAMINS

VITAMIN A

Vitamin A deficiency is considered a public health problem in India. The prevalence rate of 6.01 percent in children fewer than 6 years of age was recorded. Vitamin A is fat-soluble vitamin. Retinol is the most important form of vitamin A. It is the transport form, and the storage form being retinal ester. In the human being the diet, vitamin A is derived from the preformed vitamin (retinal) and the provitamin carotenoids; β carotene has the highest vitamin A activity.

More than 90% of the body's vitamin A reserves are stored in the liver. Vitamin A is found in foods such as milk, liver, eggs, green vegetables (spinach and amaranth), and an orange fruits.

Functions

(i) Its steady supply is needed for dim light vision.

(ii) It is necessary for maintaining the integrity of normal functioning of glandular and epithelial tissues which line intestinal, respiratory and urinary tracts as well as the skin and eyes.

(iii) It helps in the preservation of the structural integrity and normal permeability of cell membranes as well as the mitochondria, lysosome, etc.

(iv) Other functions include bolstering of immune mechanism. Concomitant keratinisation of epithelial cells and loss of immune power together makes the subject susceptible to various infections (e.g., respiratory tract infections and gastrointestinal infections).

(v) It accelerates the normal function of bones and teeth.

(vi) Vitamin A is required for growth, reproduction and life.

Deficiency of vitamin A

Causes of vitamin A deficiency are malabsorption, inadequate diet, malnutrition, and certain lipid lowering medications.

Eyes

1. **Night blindness** or nyctalopia is the commonest sign of vitamin A deficiency. Normally vitamin A is necessary for synthesis of visual purple in cells of retina and cone vision.
2. **Xerophthalmia:** The eyes becomes dry, the condition is called xerophthalmia from Greek *xeros* (dry) and *ophthalamos* (eye). Xerophthalmia leads to keratomalacia and then blindness. Each year, about 500,000 persons in the whole world become blind due to vitamin A deficiency.
3. **Bitot's spots** (opaque white patches) of keratinised epithelium on conjunctiva at the canthus.
4. **Keratomalacia:** The cornea becomes dry followed by keratomalacia and corneal ulcer. In keratomalacia the cornea (part or whole) may become soft and may burst open. Vitamin A deficiency causes squamous metaplasia and keratinisation of the eyes and other organs.
5. **Epithelial changes:** Squamous metaplasia occurs extensively in the respiratory and paranasal sinuses. Squamous metaplasia in the urinary bladder and renal pelvis, with calculus disease, is also seen in many patients. Squamous metaplasia in the ducts of the lacrimal glands obstructs the flow of blood.

A kraurosis vulva is a precancerous condition, which appears at menopause due to deficiency of vitamin A with keratinisation and atrophy of vulva.

Skin: The skin becomes dry and rough and shows pigmented papules at the root of the hair follicles. Hyperplasia and hyperkeratinisation of the epidermis with plugging of the adenexal glands may produce follicular or papular dermatosis (toad skin).

Bone: Imbalance between osteoclasts and osteoblasts causing aberrations in the shape of the bone.

Oral manifestations

Vitamin A deficiency causes hyperkeratosis and hyperplasia of gingival and periodontal pocket formation in the presence of local factors. Defective formation of enamel in teeth occurs in vitamin A deficiency. There is increased caries susceptibility. Histodifferentiation and morpho-differentiation of odontogenic epithelium is not normal; therefore it results in increased rate of cell proliferation.

Other features include impaired healing and tissue regeneration, desquamation of oral mucosa, keratosis, increased risk of candidiasis, gingival hypertrophy, and inflammation, leukoplakia, decreased taste sensitivity and xerostoma.

HYPERVITAMINOSIS A

Acute toxicity: Acute symptoms are developed on the ingestion of very large amounts of vitamin A. These include abdominal pain, drowsiness, sluggishness, severe headache, vomiting and peeling of skin around the mouth and elsewhere. In infants and young children there may be a sudden rise of intracranial pressure and papilloedema.

Chronic toxicity: It may occur following ingestion of 12,000 mcg or more daily for prolonged periods. Continued intake of excessive amounts, especially in children, produces roughness of the skin, irritability, coarsening and falling of hair, anorexia, and loss of weight, headache, hyperesthesia, occasionally anaemia and leukopaenia. There is liver damage and hyperostosis.

Hypervitaminosis vitamin A may particularly seen in well-nutritional affluent pregnant women indulging in self-medication—excessive vitamin A intake. In such cases, teratogenecity (malformation of fetus) can occur.

VITAMIN D

Vitamin D is a steroid hormone. It is represented by a group of steroids that occur mainly in animals but also in plants and yeasts. They give rise to a hormone known as calciferol by various metabolic changes. Vitamin D exists in several forms, each with different level of activity. Calciferol is the active form of Vitamin D. Fortified vegan products contains D2 (ergocalciferol). Food with naturally occurring vitamin D is, however, usually animal derived containing the vitamin D_3 (cholecalciferol). The liver and kidney help to convert vitamin D to its active hormone form. Once vitamin D is produced in the skin or consumed in food, it requires chemical conversion in kidney to form 1, 25 dihydroxyvitamin D, the physiologically active form of vitamin.

Sources

It is also derived from exposure to UV rays of the sunlight on 7- dihydrocholesterol. Which converts the cholesterol in the skin to vitamin D. Dietary sources are deep-sea fish, egg, yolks, milk, butter, plants and grains.

Functions

1. It maintains normal blood level of calcium and phosphorus.
2. It promotes the absorption of calcium and phosphorus from bowels.
3. It enhances mineralisation of bones, collaboration with parathyroid stimulating hormone.
4. Vitamin D stimulates the transcription of mRNA, for calcium-binding protein.
5. Stimulates the PTH-dependent reabsorption of calcium in the distal renal tubules.
6. Research also suggests that vitamin D may help to maintain a healthy immune system and help to regulate cell growth and differentiation.

Deficiency

Nutritional deficiencies are usually the result of dietary deficiency, impaired absorption and utilisation, increased requirement, or increased secretion.

RICKETS

There are four types of rickets:

1. **Type I Vitamin D resistant rickets (VDRR):** There is reduced vitamin D1 alpha-hydroxylase activity and, as a result, no conversion of 25 (OH) D_3 to 1, 25(OH) 2 D_3 takes place. Calcium and phosphates metabolism is deranged, and causes rickets.
2. **Type II Vitamin D dependent rickets (VDDR):** Autosomal recessive disorder where is a single amino acid change in one of the zinc fingers of the DNA binding sites for receptors. Familial occurrence being inherited a X-linked dominant trait.

3. **Renal rickets** due to chronic renal disease. It is caused by defective transport of phosphate by the renal tubules.
4. Chronic liver disease.

Causes

1. Dietary vitamin D deficiency: When an infant is fed exclusively on milk from a vitamin D deficient mother for more than three months, the risk of infantile rickets arises.
2. Malabsorption syndrome like steatorrhoea, celiac disease, and sprue causes rickets due to impaired absorption of calcium.
3. Chronic renal failure.
4. Hypophosphatasia (congenital).
5. Familial hypophosphataemia (Vitamin D resistant rickets).
6. Fanconi's syndrome.
7. Renal tubular acidosis.

Clinical features

1. **Skeletal deformities:**

a. The earlier bony lesions are often cranio tabes—small rounded unossified area in the membranous bones of skull.

b. Bony pain and tenderness over arms, legs, spine, and pelvis.

c. There are presence of bony bumps on the ribs called *rachitic rosary* (bead-like prominences) at the junction of ribs with their cartilages.

d. Later features are bossing of the frontal and parietal bones and delayed closure of the anterior fontanelle.

e. **Extremities:** Knock-knees, bow legs, and coxa vera. The bones are soft due to non-deposition of calcium salts and, hence, they are easily bent by the weight of the body.

f. Forward projection of breast-bone *(pigeon chest)*.

g. **Spine deformities:** Spine curve abnormalities including scoliosis and kyphosis.

The child is restless, fretful and pale with flabby and toneless muscles, which allow the limbs to assume unnatural postures (acrobatic rickets). The abdomen is distended as a result of the weak abdominal muscles, the atony of the intestinal musculature and intestinal fermentation that may arise from excessive carbohydrate in the diet.

Harrison's grooves: The inward pull at the margins of diaphragm creates Harrison's grooves, girdling the thoracic cavity at the lower margin of the rib cage.

Nerves: Nerves are very irritable in low blood calcium. Tetany results, as the blood calcium falls below 7.5mg% characterised by spasm of muscles of hands and feet (carpo-tunnel spasm).

Spasmophilia: It is a triad of tetany, convulsions and laryngismus stridulus.

Respiratory system: Patients are more prone to bronchitis and bronchopneumonia.

Investigations

1. Plasma calcium level is decreased. Normal serum calcium is 9-11mg%.
2. Increased alkaline phosphatase.
3. Low levels of phosphorus.
4. Generalised aminoaciduria except in VDDR.

OSTEOMALACIA

It is prevalent in India, Pakistan, China, and Middle East countries.

Osteomalacia occurs in adults due to vitamin D deficiency. Demineralisation of bone occurs making the bone soft (*osteum* = bones; *malacias* = softening).

Causes

1. Osteomalacia is sometimes found in patients with cirrhosis of liver due to failure to form 25(OH) D.
2. Osteomalacia and bone disorders arise in patients with chronic renal failure. Impaired formation of 1,25 $(OH)_2$ D in the kidney may be responsible.

Clinical features

1. Common features are pain and muscular weakness. The affected sites are the sacrum, ribs, lower lumbar vertebrae, pelvis, and legs.
2. Carpopedal spasm and facial twitching may be manifestation of tetany.
3. The pelvis may become abnormal leading to obstetrical hazards during birth of the child.
4. Pathological fractures may occur.

Oral manifestations

In some cases of osteomalacia, there is increase in incidence of severe periodontitis.

Biochemical changes

1. Plasma calcium level is often not lowered.
2. Elevation of serum alkaline phosphatase to three or more times its normal levels.

VITAMIN E

Vitamin E chemically is tocopherol. Most important lipid-soluble antioxidant nutrients— found in vegetable oils, whole grain cereals, and nuts.

Healing: It prevents the formation of excessive scar tissue and in some instance even melts away unwanted scar tissue.

Causes

Cystic fibrosis, chronic cholecystatic liver disease, abetalipoproteinaemia, short-bowel syndrome, isolated vitamin E deficiency syndrome, and other malabsorption syndromes all may cause varying degrees of neurologic deficits due to related vitamin deficiencies.

Deficiency manifestations

1. Increased susceptibility of erythrocytes to haemolysis by hydrogen peroxide and decrease in the lifespan in human adult males.
2. Anaemia, edema, and skin changes are observed in infants when fed unsaturated oils.
3. Smaller testis and permanent sterility.
4. It causes degenerative changes in muscles. There is necrosis and fibrosis of heart muscles. There is muscle fibre atrophy, which is replaced by connective tissue.

VITAMIN K

Dam named it vitamin K since it is a coagulation-vitamin.

Vitamin K occurs in at least two forms: Vitamin K_1 and K_2. Vitamin K_1 (VK_1) is an essential lipid-soluble vitamin that plays a vital role in the production of coagulation proteins, is found in green leafy vegetables and oils such as soya bean, cotton seed, canola and olive oil. Vitamin K_2 is synthesised by colonic mucosa. Cow's milk is a richer source (60 mgm/L) of vitamin K than human milk. The only biological role of the vitamin K is that of required co-enzyme for a vitamin K dependent carboxylase that catalyses the carboxylation of the amino acid, glutamic acid, resulting its conversion to gamma carboxyglutamic acid (Gia). Gia residues are part of the protein molecules of four of the coagulation factors (II, VII, IX, and X).

Causes of vitamin K deficiency

1. In the newborn, primary deficiency can occur because placental transfer of vitamin K is inefficient, the neonatal bowel has not acquired bacteria and breast milk contains little of the vitamin. It causes haemorrhagic disease of newborn, especially with intracranial and retroperitoneal haemorrhages.
2. Parenchymal liver diseases such as cirrhosis, secondary to viral hepatitis, alcohol intake, hepatic malignancy, amyloidosis, and Gaucher's disease causes vitamin K deficiency.
3. Dietary deficiency occurs in people with malnutrition.
4. Biliary causes, such as common duct obstruction due to stones and strictures, primary biliary cirrhosis, cholangiocarcinoma, and chronic cholestasis, causes maldigestion of fat, the decrease in fat absorption leads to a deficiency of vitamin K.
5. Drugs: Warfarin, antibiotics, coumadin, salicylates, anticonvulsants are some of the common causes of vitamin K deficiency.

Management

It is given in doses of 10-20 mg daily.

WATER SOLUBLE VITAMINS

THIAMINE (B_1)

Thiamine is a water-soluble vitamin. Once absorbed, thiamine mostly concentrates in the muscle tissues. It is not stored in the body. The kidney excretes it.

Functions

1. Thiamine becomes phosphorylated to form thiamine pyrophosphate, involved in many alpha ketoacid decarboxylation and transketolation reactions such as in synthesis of ATP.
2. It may also have role in neuronal conduction.

Sources

It is widely available except in refined foods, e.g., polished rice and white flour. Thiamine is present in adequate amounts in whole grain, spinach, liver, beef, nuts, soyabeans, yeast, and bananas.

Thiamine deficiency

1. Persons may become deficient in thiamine either by not ingesting enough vitamin B through the diet or by excess use—which may occur in hyperthyroidism, pregnancy, lactation, or fever.
2. Prolonged diarrhoea may impair the body's ability to absorb vitamin B_1 and severe liver disease impairs its use.
3. In the deficiency of vitamin B_1, there is impaired conversion of pyruvate to acetyle-CoA. In case of high carbohydrate diet, there is increased plasma concentration of pyruvate and lactate, which may cause life-threatening lactic acidosis.
4. Raw fermented fish, which contains thiaminase and fermented tea leaves, both reduce the availability of thiamine in the diet.
5. Vitamin B deficiency syndrome is common in persons with diets largely of polished rice.
6. It is seen in chronic alcoholics with renal dialysis.

BERI BERI

The name *'Beri'* is from Singhalese word meaning weakness. Deficiency results in any of three polar forms:

1. Cardiovascular (wet beri beri).
2. Neuropathic (dry beri beri).
3. The infantile form.

Dry beri beri

Nervous system involvement is termed dry beri beri. The neurological findings can be peripheral neuropathy characterised by symmetric impairment of sensory, motor, and reflex functions of extremities, especially in the lower limbs.

Microscopically: The lesion comprises of degeneration of myelin in the muscular sheaths without inflammation.

Wernick's encephalopathy

Alcoholics with thiamine deficiency sometimes develop Wernick's disease, named after the German neurologist who described it in 1881. In Wernick's encephalopathy, focal degeneration and haemorrhages have been described in the nuclei surrounding the ventricles, mamillary bodies of the hypothalamus, and dorsal medial areas of thalamus. The earliest change is capillary endothelial proliferation associated with abnormal vascular permeability. There is progressive dementia, ataxia, and ophthalmoplegia. If untreated, the syndrome may progress to coma and death.

Korsakoff's syndrome: Neuronal loss in the cerebral cortex, brain stem, and cerebellum leads to a clinically characteristic psychotic state known as Korsakoff's syndrome—characterised by memory failure and confabulation.

Alcoholic cerebellar degeneration: Thiamine deficiency has also been implicated in the development of atrophy of the superior vermis often seen in alcoholics.

Wet beri beri

Wet beri beri is the term used for the cardiovascular involvement of thiamine deficiency.

The chronic form of wet beri beri consists of three stages:

Ist stage: Peripheral vasodilatation occurs, leading to a high cardiac output state. This leads to salt and water retention mediated through the renin angiotensin-aldosterone system in the kidneys. The resulting fluid overload leads to edema of the dependent extremities.

IInd stage: By the time significant edema occurs, the heart has been exposed to a severely high work load to pump the required cardiac output needed to satisfy end organ requirement.

IIIrd stage: A more rapid form of beri beri is termed acute fulminant cardiovascular beri beri, or Shoshin beri beri. The heart is globular and soft, with dilatation of all chambers. There is interstitial edema, and lymphocytic infiltration. The myocardium reveals parenchymatous, hydropic and fatty degeneration.

Infantile beri beri

It occurs in breast-fed infants, usually between the second and fifth months.

It exists in acute and chronic forms:

Acute form: Cardiac failure may develop abruptly. The infant is restless, cries a lot, oliguria, and shows signs of puffiness. The infant then suddenly becomes cyanosed with dyspnea, tachycardia and die within 24-48 hours.

Chronic form: There is constipation and vomiting. The muscles are soft and toneless. There is often intense pallor of the skin with cyanosis around the mouth. Cardiac failure and sudden death are common.

Laboratory findings

Thiamine blood level: A total blood thiamine level of less than 3.0 μg (normal 3.0 to 9.0 μg per ml).

Vitamin B_2 (Riboflavin)

Riboflavin is nucleoside. In our body riboflavin occurs in two forms: (i) Riboflavin phosphate, also called flavin mononucleotide, (FMA) and (ii) flavin adenine dinucleotide (FAD). Its daily requirement is 2.0 mg.

Sources

It is widely available in meat, dairy products, and vegetables.

Functions

1. Riboflavin is involved in the regulatory function of some hormone connected with carbohydrate metabolism.
2. The free riboflavin present in retina is converted by light to a compound involved in stimulation of the optic nerve.
3. It functions as a coenzyme for a number of flavoprotein enzymes, including cytochrome oxidase.

Causes of deficiency

1. Dietic deficiency of riboflavin occurs in poor persons subsisting on a limited diet with a high cereal content.
2. Rare in secondary deficiency in alcoholic patients and in debilitated (e.g., cancer) patients.
3. Deficiency occurs frequently in conjunction with lack of other B vitamins.

Deficiency manifestations

Seborrheic dermatitis: Scaly, greasy desquamation—chiefly about the ears, nose, and nasolabial folds.

Eye changes: Deficiency may lead to corneal vascularisation and inflammation with interstitial keratitis. There may be itching, watering, burning of eye, photophobia and cataract.

Oral manifestations

Oral mucosa is pale due to anaemia.

Lips: Redness, and shiny appearance of lips is due to desquamation of epithelium.

Cheilosis: Lesions at the mucocutaneous junction at the angle of the mouth leading to painful fissures.

Tongue: Painful glossitis, tongue assuming a red purple (magenta) colour. There is complete atrophy of papillae which gives rise to smooth and glazed tongue.

VITAMIN B_3 (Niacin)

Generic term is nicotinic acid and nicotinamide. Nicotinic acid (P-P factor, niacin) forms a part of coenzymes I (NAD) and II (NADP) as the prosthetic group and is concerned in the transfer of hydrogen in the tissue respiration.

Source

Widely available in grains, beans, and seed oils. It can be endogenously synthesized from tryptophan.

Function

It is widely involved as electron acceptors and hydrogenases.

Pellagra

Pellagra is an Italian word meaning rough skin. It is seen in economically deprived persons.

Causes of deficiency

1. Deficiency can occur from lack of B_3 or lack of tryptophan. It occurs frequently in conjunction with lack of other B vitamins.
2. Deficiency seen usually in chronic alcoholic, in chronic diarrhoea, and debilitating diseases.
3. It is common in persons with diets largely of corn (maize), in which niacin is tightly bound.
4. Carcinoid syndrome, in which there is diversion of tryptophan to make 5-hydroxytryptamine (5-HT); it shows the clinical features of niacin deficiency.
5. In Hartup's disease, many amino acids including tryptophan are not absorbed from the intestine; this condition also leads to pellagra.
6. It is seen in patients with prolonged use of antitubercular drug isoniazid.

Clinical features

Pellagra, the deficiency state, is called the disease of 3 ds—diarrhoea, dementia and dermatitis.

Skin

1. Exposure to trauma or mechanical irritation of the skin, especially over bony prominences, may also determine the site of the lesion.
2. The skin in affected areas is at first red and slightly swollen; it itches and burns.
3. The skin shows erythema with exfoliation and pigmentation.

Digestive system

Oral manifestations

The mouth is sore and often shows angular stomatitis and cheilosis.

The tongue characteristically has a 'raw beef' appearance—red, swollen and painful, though usually without loss of papillae. Secondary infection of the mouth with Vincent's organisms is common. In advanced cases, the tongue loses all the papillae and the reddening becomes intense. Oral ulcers are covered with a grey membrane.

Nervous system

The lesions of the nervous system appear late in the course of the disease. In chronic cases there may be decreased sensation in the feet to touch and loss of vibration and position sense. The loss of position sense may give rise to ataxia.

Pathology

Microscopically: Skin shows edema of the papillae and dilatation of the papillary blood vessels with degeneration of the connective tissue and lymphocytic infiltration of the superficial part of the corium.

Digestive system

The colon is thickened, reddish and may show patchy pseudomembranous change in the mucosa, thickening of the wall with infiltration of the chronic inflammatory cells.

Nervous system: It is characterised by patchy degeneration, mostly of myelin sheath, most commonly involving posterior and lateral columns.

VITAMIN B_6

It is a water-soluble vitamin. Daily requirements are 1 to 2 mg.

Three substances—pyridoxine, pyridoxal and pyridoxamine—together with phosphates are all called pyridoxine. After absorption, pyridoxine, pyridoxal and pyridoxamine are transported into hepatic cells by facilitated diffusion. Pyridoxal kinase phosphorylates pyridoxine and pyridoxamine, after which they are converted to pyridoxal 5-phosphate (PLP) by a flavin-dependent enzyme.

Free pyridoxal is degraded by alkaline phosphatase, hepatic and renal aldehyde oxidase and pyridoxal dehydrogenase. Pyridoxal phosphate acts as a cofactor for many enzymes involved in amino acid metabolism, including transaminases and hydroxylases.

Functions

Pyridoxine is essential for growth of infants.

Muscle phosphorylase contains 70-80% of total body vitamin B_6.

Sources

Pyridoxine, or vitamin B_6 is abundant in yeast, rice polishing, milk, meat, fish, liver, cereals, potatoes, banana and green leafy vegetables.

Deficiency

Causes

1. Deficiency is rare in primary form because B_6 is present in all natural foods, but destroyed in processing.
2. Isoniazid, the antitubercular drug, can produce vitamin B_6 deficiency by forming a hydrazone with pyridoxol.
3. Several congenital defects, e.g., cystathioneuria familial, xanthurenic aciduria and some pyridoxal-responsive anaemias impair the utilisation of pyridoxyl phosphate.

Deficiency manifestations

1. Deficiency gives rise to irritability, convulsions, mental retardation, mental confusion and depression. In some subjects there is lymphopaenia and peripheral neuropathy.
2. Deficiency causes seborrheic dermatitis in the nasolabial folds, less often convulsions, and anaemia.
3. Deficiency causes pellagra like symptoms, microcytic hypochromic anaemia, with sideroblasts in bone marrow, haemosiderosis, resistance to iron therapy, impaired antibodies production, and low immunity.
4. It has been suggested that pyridoxine deficiency may produce arteriosclerosis in man.
5. **Others:** Kidney stones, inflammation of the colon, damage to the pancreas, loss of muscular control, migraine headache, and premature sterility.

Oral manifestations

1. **Angular stomatitis:** Fissures and ulcers develop at the angle of the mouth.
2. **Glossitis:** Tongue is red and swollen due to inflammation of tongue.
3. Tooth decay and halitosis is common.

FOLIC ACID (VITAMIN B_9)

Folic acid is the common name of pteroylmonoglutamic acid consists of pterdine and para-amino benzoic acid coupled to glutamic acid.

Sources

The main dietary sources are green vegetables (spinach), fruits as well as liver, milk, and yeast. Maximum daily requirement is normally 50 μg, which is increased several fold during enhanced metabolic demands, e.g., pregnancy, infancy and lactation.

Normal adults have 5-20 μg folic acid in various body stores, half in liver.

Functions

Folate is necessary for sterility in both men and women. In men, it contributes to spermatogenesis. In women, on the other hand, it contributes to oocyte, maturation, implantation, and placentation.

Causes of deficiency

1. **Dietary deficiency:** It is usually seen in elderly people and infants.
2. **Poor absorption:** Acidic foods and conjugate inhibitors present in beans and other legumes hamper absorption by internal conjugates. Malabsorption disorders (celiac disease, tropical sprue) affect one-third of small intestine and impair absorption of folates.
3. **Increased demand:** Pregnancy, leukaemia, haemolytic anaemia and myeloproliferative disorders.
4. **Drugs:** Drug-induced folate deficiency is commonly seen in methotrexate, phenytoin, therapy and administration of folic acid antagonist.

Clinical features

Deficiency gives rise to megaloblastic anaemia.

Other deficiency manifestations include retardation of growth, weakness, infertility, and inadequate lactation in females.

Symptoms such as weakness, fatigue, irritability, headache, palpitation, and mental retardation occur in folic acid deficiency.

Skin: There is loss of hair, greyish-brown skin pigmentation can also occur.

Reproductive disorders such as spontaneous abortions and difficult labour, and a high infant death rate can also be caused by folic acid deficiency.

Oral manifestations

There is mucositis, oral pain, and ulcerative gingivitis.

Disappearance of filiform papillae and atrophy of mucosa, and muscles in the tongue gives rise to smooth tongue. Tongue appears red and flabby. Atrophy of fungiform papillae occurs in severe cases.

Fissures and ulcers develop at the angle of mouth (angular stomatitis).

Diagnosis

1. Bone marrow shows macrocytosis, and megaloblastic bone marrow.

   Serum level of folate: There are two methods used for measuring serum levels of folates:

   A. Microbiologically—by using lactobacilli casei.

   B. Radioimmunoassay

   Normal level is 6 to 21 μg/l casei method.

3. Red cell folate

   Normal: 160 to 640 μg/l casei method of red cell volume. Serum folate level less than 4 μg/l in folic acid deficiency.

VITAMIN C

It is water-soluble dry crystalline powder. Vitamin C is the most active reducing agent in the aqueous phase of living tissues and is involved in intracellular electron transport.

Sources

Vitamin C, or ascorbic acid, is abundant in citrus fruits, meat, fish, dry pulses, green vegetables, tomatoes, potatoes and other fruits and vegetables.

Function

1. Ascorbic acid also promotes iron absorption, transport and storage, by probably regulating the valency of the iron and maintaining the ratio of ferritin to haemosiderin.
2. Tryptophan, norepinephrine and tyrosine metabolism require vitamin C.
3. It is concerned in the hydroxylation of proline and hydroxyproline, which is an important constituent of collagen.
4. It is essential for the normal regulation of the colloidal condition of intercellular substances including the fibrils and collagen of connective tissue, osteoid tissue, dentin, the intercellular 'cement substance' of the capillaries.
5. It is useful for maintenance of folate pool and mobility and phagocytic activity of neutrophils. It is also necessary for maintenance of bones and proper functioning of the adrenal and thyroid glands.

Causes of vitamin C deficiency

1. Dietary deficiency is due to lack of dietary fruits and vegetables and infant fed exclusively on boiled milk.
2. Increased requirement for vitamin C occurs after trauma, surgery, burns; aspirin, indomethacin, tetracycline ingestion causes deficiency of vitamin C.

Clinical features

1. **Oral manifestations**

   Gums: There is spongy swelling, ulceration and bleeding from gums. The gums are livid in colour, and bleed on slightest touch. There is always some infection by bacteria.

   Teeth: The teeth become loose and easily knocked out.

   There is fetid breath of the patient with fusospirochetal stomatitis.
2. In adults, scurvy begins with hyperkeratosis in the hair follicles, usually first on the limbs.
3. Haemorrhages may occur in the skin, mucus membrane or any other organ and varies from tiny petechiae to haematoma due to increased fragility of capillaries.
4. Defective formation of collagen impairs healing of wounds, and causes capillary haemorrhage and reduced platelet adhesiveness and, clinically, patients have gastrointestinal bleeding and anaemia.
5. Osteoporosis may occur in scurvy, since ascorbic acid is necessary for the synthesis of collagen in all parts of body, including bone.
6. Haematuria, blood in stool, and intracranial haemorrhages occurs in severe cases.
7. Edema of the limbs and face is a frequent finding in severe ascorbic acid deficiency.
8. Deficiency of ascorbic acid distorts the metabolism of tyrosine and phenylalanine and abnormal metabolic products appear in urine.
9. Patient may die of a massive intracranial bleed.

X-ray findings

- Increased density at ends of epiphysis
- Signet ring appearances of epiphysis

- Separation of periosteum from shaft due to subperiosteal haemorrhages
- Ground glass appearance of shaft of diaphysis.

Diagnosis

Blood ascorbic acid determination: Normal concentration in blood plasma is 0.4-1.5 mg/100 ml.

Management

A dose of 250 mg orally daily may saturate the tissues quickly.

CHAPTER

17

DISEASES AFFECTING NERVES AND MUSCLES

NEUROMUSCULAR DISORDERS

DISEASES OF THE NERVES

TRIGEMINAL NEURALGIA (Tic Douloureux)

It is also called prosopalgia, Fothergill's disease, and trifacial neuralgia.

Idiopathic trigeminal neuralgia typically occurs in patients in the sixth decade of life, but it may occur at any age.

Characteristic of trigeminal neuralgia

- Distribution along 1 or more divisions of trigeminal nerve
- Sudden, intense, sharp, superficial stabbing or burning in quality
- Severe pain intensity
- Precipitation from trigger areas or by certain daily activities (e.g., eating, talking, washing the face, cleaning the teeth)
- No symptoms between paroxysms
- Other causes of facial pain excludes by history.

Clinical features

It usually occurs in middle and old age, the disease seldom occurs before 30 years of age. Females are most commonly affected.

This condition causes lancinating pains in the second and third divisions of the trigeminal nerve territory, usually in patients over age of 50 years. Touching trigger zones within the trigeminal territory or by eating may precipitate the pain.

Dysfunction of masticatory apparatus related to spasm of muscles of mastication precipitated by occlusal disharmony or alteration in vertical dimension of the jaws and exacerbated by emotional stress.

It rarely occurs bilaterally.

Clinical features during the attack

Associated symptoms

(i) During the attacks, the face is often thrown into a strong involuntary tonic spasm on the affected side.
(ii) Flushing of face.
(iii) Excessive lacrimation.
(iv) Sometimes secretion of nasal mucus and saliva may occur on the side of the pain.
(v) Popping noise in temporomandibular joint.
(vi) Limitation of jaw motion.

Clinical features in-between the attacks

Trigger zones

Dull continuous pain: Follows paroxysmal pains if severe, usually of a boring character. Skin over the affected region is sore and tender after paroxysms.

Pain in pre-auricular region and muscle tenderness.

Sensory changes: None except for hyperaesthesia.

Skin and hair: After repeated attacks skin becomes shiny and hair in the area may become grey or rubbed away.

Pathogenesis

- The current etiological hypothesis suggests that the neuralgia is most commonly caused by compression of the trigeminal nerve rootlets at their entry to the brain stem by aberrant loops of cerebellar arteries.
- Exciting causes: Spontaneous, or following exposure to cold wind, blow on face, or chewing, or eating, or drinking hot or cold fluid or talking, or washing of face.
- Trigeminal nerve neuralgia appears in advanced stages of multiple sclerosis due to demyelinisation of the nerve.
- It may be caused by damage to the myelin sheath by compression from a tumour.
- There is some evidence that the disorder runs in families, perhaps because of an inherited pattern of blood vessels.

Management

Minimal invasive microvascular decompression surgery can relieve the pain.

Anti-convulsants such as carbamazepine, oxcarbamazepine, topiramate, phenytoin, or garbapentin are generally most effective medications.

GLOSSOPHARYNGEAL NEURALGIA

Causes

Irritation of ninth cranial nerve causes glossopharyngeal neuralgia. In some cases, the source of irritation is never found. Some possible causes for this type of nerve pain are:

- Blood vessels pressing down on the glossopharyngeal nerve
- Growth lesions at the base of the skull
- Tumours or infections of the throat and mouth.

Clinical features

Symptoms usually begin in people over age 40.

Pain is localised to the throat, posterior part of tongue, tonsillar region, nasopharynx, larynx and ear. Glossopharyngeal neuralgia has a tendency towards remissions and exacerbations. Attacks may be triggered by a particular action, such as chewing, swallowing, talking, coughing, or sneezing. The pain may last several seconds to a few minutes and usually affects only one side of throat or tongue.

Management

Treatment is surgical resection of intracranial or extracranial portion of glossopharyngeal nerve.

GENICULATE NEURALGIA (GN)

It is also known as ***'Hunt's neuralgia'***, ***'neuralis facialis vera'***, ***'nervosa intermedius neuralgia'***.

Geniculate neuralgia, also called nervous intermedius neuralgia, is a rare disorder that involves severe pain deep in the ear that may spread to the ear canal, outer ear, mastoid, or eye region. The pain of GN is sharp, shooting, or burning, and can last for hours. Cold, noise, swallowing or touch may trigger painful attacks, but triggers are usually unique to the sufferer.

Females are affected more commonly than males.

BELL'S PALSY

Etiology

1. **Idiopathic:** It is defined as idiopathic, peripheral facial paralysis or paralysis of acute onset.
2. The lesion is within the facial canal and may be due to reactivation of latent herpes simplex virus 1 infection, herpes zoster and Epstein-Barr virus.
3. **Vascular:** It may be primary or secondary. Primary ischaemia is induced by cold or emotional stress. Secondary ischaemia, is the result of primary ischemia which causes increased capillary permeability leading to exudation of fluid, edema, and compression of microcirculation.
4. Risk of Bell's palsy is more in diabetics and pregnant women.
5. **Hereditary:** The fallopian canal is narrow because of hereditary predisposition and this makes the nerve susceptible to early compression with the slightest edema. Ten percent of the cases of Bell's palsy have a positive family history.
6. **Autoimmune disorder:** T lymphocyte changes have been observed.
7. Other important causes of acute facial palsy include suppurative otitis media, head injury, Gullain-Barre syndrome, sarcoidosis and multiple sclerosis.

Clinical features

Paralysis begins suddenly. In many cases, the paralysis occurs at night during sleep. Eye on affected side cannot be closed. On attempting to close the eye, eyeball turns up and out (Bell's phenomenon). Angle of mouth deviated towards the normal side, with dribbling of saliva from the angle of the mouth. Tears flow from the eye (epiphora).

There may be pain behind the ear before and after paralysis. Some complain of noise intolerance (stapedial paralysis) or loss of taste (involvement of chorda tympani).

Management

1. Patients with Bell's palsy should be treated within three days of the onset of symptoms with a seven-day course of oral acyclovir (zovirax) or volacyclovir, plus a tapering course of oral prednisolone.
2. Patients should be monitored for eye irritation and be prescribed eye lubrication. Patients with corneal abrasions should be referred to an ophthalmologist.

3. **Surgery:** Surgical transmastoid decompression of the facial nerve in severe case is being investigated but cannot currently be recommended. Where nerve fails to regenerate, cosmetic surgery to elevate mouth or anastomosis of hypoglossal nerve to the facial nerve may help.

FREY'S SYNDROME

It is also called ***'auriculotemporal syndrome'***, ***'gustatory sweating Baillarger's syndrome, "Duputy's syndrome'***.

The first description of unilateral gustatory hyperhydrosis was done as early as 1757 by the French surgeon M Duphenix and again in 1847 by Baillarger. Frey correlated the unusual physiologic phenomenon (1923) and applied the term ' temporomandibular syndrome'.

Pathogenesis

Frey's syndrome arises as a complication of parotid surgery, usually manifesting several months after the operation. Other causes include injuries to parotid gland, mandibular fracture, obstetric trauma, and parotid abscess. Frey's syndrome has also been reported in cases of diabetic neuropathy.

It is the result of aberrant innervations of sweat glands by parasympathetic secretomotor fibres, which were destined for the parotid. The severed fibres then undergo abnormal regeneration of the cut post-ganglionic cholinergic sympathetics to the sweat glands of the overlying skin. Because of these aberrant neural connections, when salivation is stimulated, local sweat glands are inadvertently activated and patient's cheek becomes flushed and wet.

Clinical features

It is a food related syndrome which can be congenital, or not, and can persist for life.

The symptoms of the Frey's syndrome are redness and sweating on the cheek area adjacent to ear. They can appear when the affected person eats, sees, think, or talks about certain kinds of food which produce strong salivation.

It is characterised by sweating and flushing of the pre-auricular skin during mastication causing nuisance to the person or social embarrassment.

Diagnosis

Observing sweating in the region after eating a lemon wedge may be diagnostic.

Management

Treatment includes:

- Injection of botulism toxin type A
- Surgical transaction of the nerve fibres
- Anticholinergic drug such as scopolamine.

MOTOR NEURON DISEASE

Motor neuron disease is a rare condition causing progressive loss of motor nerve cells.

Three variants are recognised and are categorised by the anatomic location of the neural disturbances.

1. **Progressive muscular atrophy:** Attacks the anterior horn cells.
2. **Amylotrophic lateral sclerosis:** Destroys the motor neurons of the cortico-spinal tracts of cranial nerves motor nuclei.

PROGRESSIVE MUSCULAR ATROPHY (PMA)

Progressive muscular atrophy is a rare subtype of amylotrophic lateral sclerosis (ALS) or motor neuron disease, which affects only the lower motor neuron. PMA occurs in 4% of all motor neuron cases. As a result of motor neuron degeneration, PMA is characterised by muscle atrophy, fasciculations, cramps, muscle twitching and loss of reflexes.

Causes

The cause is not known; though quite a variety of causes have been mentioned by various workers, the most important being hereditary, excessive muscular effort, exposure to cold traumatic injuries to peripheral parts of the body, infectious fever, influenza, diphtheria, measles, and rheumatism.

Clinical features

It occurs in adults between the age of thirty and fifty. It affects males more than females.

PMA starts most frequently with weakness in one hand, although it can be in foot or tongue. The weakness spreads to other muscles as the disease progresses; the affected muscles atrophy and fail to work. Cramps have usually preceded first weakness and muscle twitching occurs at an early stage. Patients do not have spasticity in their muscles nor the very brisk reflexes. Muscles controlling swallowing, chewing, coughing, breathing, and speech may be affected.

AMYOTROPHIC LATERAL SCLEROSIS (ALS)

Amyotrophic lateral sclerosis is a form of motor neuron disease. ALS is sometimes called ***'Maladie de Charcot'*** or ***'Lou Gehring's disease'***. It is a progressive, fatal, neurodegenerative disease caused by the degeneration of motor neurons—the nerve cells in the central nervous system that control voluntary muscle movement.

Approximately 5,600 people in the United States are diagnosed with ALS each year.

Causes

Scientist have not found a definitive cause for ALS. The onset of this disease has been linked to several factors, including a virus, exposure to neurotoxins or heavy metals, DNA defects, immune system abnormalities, occupational factors—such as military service and elite sports and enzyme abnormalities. About 5-10% of cases are inherited. Premature aging of the immune system appears to play a role in the development of amyotrophic sclerosis.

Clinical features

The disease usually strikes between age 40 and 60. More men than women are affected by it.

The earliest symptoms may include twitching, cramping, or stiffness of muscles, muscle weakness affecting an arm or a leg; slurred and nasal speech, and hoarseness of voice.

Some people lose control of one or both legs first. They may have trouble walking and fall.

When muscles in the diaphragm and chest wall fail, patients lose the ability to breathe without ventilatory support. Most people with ALS die from respiratory failure.

Oral manifestations

Cranial involvement produces fasciculation, muscle wasting, and, eventually, paralysis of the tongue, along with the physical complaints of difficulty in chewing, swallowing and speaking. The tongue shrinks and fissures along the dorsal surface become apparent. The initial complaint may be an inability to eat properly or the expelling-off food into the nose during swallowing.

Management

There is no effective treatment for ALS. The drug riluzole (e.g., Rilutek) may add about 3 months to life expectancy. Physical, occupational and speech therapy are helpful. Baclofen and Diazepam may relax the spastic muscles.

PROGRESSIVE BULBAR PALSY (PBP)

The disease was first recognised by French neurologist, G Duchenne, in 1860 and termed **'labio-glossolaryngeal paralysis'** in 1859; Waschsmuth changed the name to progressive bulbar palsy.

Progressive bulbar palsy belongs to a group of disorders known as motor neuron diseases. This specially involves the glossopharyngeal nerve (IX), vagus nerve (X), and hypoglossal (XII) nerve.

Clinical features

Progressive bulbar palsy symptoms can include progressive difficulty with chewing, talking, and swallowing (dysphagia). Patients can also exhibit reduced gag reflexes, weak palatal movements, fasciculation, weak movements of the facial muscles and tongue. In advanced cases of PBP, the patient may be unable to protrude their tongue or manipulate food in their mouth.

TEMPORAL ARTERITIS

It is also known as giant cells arteritis, cranial arteritis, granulomatous arteritis and Harton's disease.

Giant cell arteritis is a vasculitis predominantly involving the large elastic arteries (primarily the extra cranial branches of the carotid artery, commonest being temporal artery). Rarely, aortic arch and its branches are also affected.

Pathogenesis

Autoimmune: The immune system, both cellular and humoral, has been implicated in the pathogenesis of giant cell arteritis. The histopathology of giant cell arteritis has suggested the presence of an antigen driven disease with local T cell and macrophages activation or near elastic tissue in the arterial walls with an important role of the proinflammatory cytokines.

Genetic: Several reports of familial aggregation, association with HLA-DR4 haplotype, and an apparent increased frequency of these conditions in Northern Europe and in persons in the United States with similar ethnic backgrounds suggest a genetic or hereditary predisposition.

Infectious: Some epidemiological observations, reports and studies using DNA detection techniques implicate chlamydia pneumoniae, Mycoplasma pneumoniae and parvovirus B19 as the impetus for the destructive inflammation.

Clinical features

Temporal arteritis is most common in older individuals (55 to 80 years) and rare before the age of 50. Females are affected twice as often as men. In the milder form of giant cell arteritis, patient may complain only of generalised muscle aches, low-grade fever, weakness, weight loss, jaw pains, headache and unusual fatigue. Polymyalgia rheumatica, which is characterised by pain in the shoulders, and hips is closely linked to giant cell arteritis, occurring in about 40-50% of patients. Intermittent claudication occurs in about 50% of cases.

Visual disturbances: The optic nerve head is supplied by the posterior ciliary artery, vasculitis of which leads to occlusion and acute anterior ischaemic optic neuropathy. Damage to the optic nerve results in loss of visual acuity and field, reduced colour perception and papillary defects. Sudden visual symptoms in one eye, leading rapidly to blindness, constitute the most common pattern.

During chewing of firm foods such as meat, fatigue or discomfort of the jaw muscles is noted. In a small percentage of patients, claudication of tongue and throat develops with eating and repeated swallowing.

Most serious complications are blindness, brain stem infarcts, hemiparesis and stroke.

Microscopically

There is marked fibrosis and thickening of intima. External elastic lamina shows fragmentation. Granulomatous inflammation with lymphocytes, macrophages, multinucleated giant cells are frequently observed in later stages of disease.

Laboratory tests

- Erythrocyte sedimentation rate, an inflammatory marker, > 60 mm at the end of 1 hour is seen in most of the cases.
- C-reactive protein, another inflammatory marker is also commonly elevated.
- Platelets may also be elevated.
- Biopsy.

Management

Prompt treatment with corticosteroid medications usually relieves symptoms of giant cell arteritis and may prevent loss of vision.

BURNING MOUTH SYNDROME

Other names are glossodynia, oral galvanism, glossopyrosis, and stomatopyrosis.

Burning mouth syndrome affects upto 4 percent of United State adults.

Burning sensation may be felt either as a continuous or intermittent discomfort which most frequently affect tongue, gums, throat and sometimes the lips or palate.

Causes

The main cause of burning mouth syndrome is yeast infection. Apart from mouth infection, it can be caused due to hormonal imbalance, nerve damage, endocrine disorder, deficiency of vitamin B_{12} and many more reasons.

Clinical features

Women are affected seven times as often as men. It generally occurs in middle-aged or older adults. But it may occur in younger as well.

People with burning mouth syndrome often feel like they burned their mouth with a hot liquid. They may also have a dry or sore mouth; or a bitter or metallic taste in their mouth.

MENIERE'S DISEASE

It is named after the French physician Prosper Meniere, who first reported that vertigo was caused by inner ear disorder in an article published in 1861.

Causes

1. Recently attention has also been focused on the immunologic function of the endolymphatic sac—immune disease may contribute to a substantial percentage with Meniere's disease. Patients with Meniere's disease have a very high prevalence of autoimmune thyroid disease. On the other hand, Ruckenstein and others recently obtained a large number of autoimmune blood test in a group of 40 patients with unilateral Meniere's disease including anti-nuclear antibody, Anti-Jogren, rheumatoid factor, complement, anti-phospholipid antibody.
2. The symptoms of Meniere's disease are associated with a change of fluid volume within a portion of the inner ear known as labyrinth. The labyrinth has two parts: the bony labyrinth and the membranous labyrinth, which are encased by bones, is necessary for hearing and balance and is filled with a fluid called endolymph. An increase in endolymph, however, can cause the membranous labyrinth to balloon or dilate, a condition known as endolymphatic hydrops.
3. The vertigo in Meniere's disease is thought to result from accumulation of excessive fluid pressure in the inner ear. The fluid pressure stretches the membranes. When the membranes are severely stretched, the fluids of the ear may rupture them. This results in mixing of the fluids, one rich in sodium, the other rich in potassium. The mixture of these fluids is thought to bring on the vertigo.

Clinical features

Meniere's disease affects people of all ages, especially those of middle age or older. It is however, uncommon in children.

Meniere's disease is a disorder of the inner ear that can affect hearing and balance. It is characterised by episodes of dizziness and tinnitus and progressive hearing loss, usually in one ear.

Classic Meinere's is considered to comprise the following four symptoms:

- Periodic episodes of rotary vertigo or dizziness
- Fluctuating progressive, unilateral or bilateral hearing loss
- Unilateral or bilateral tinnitus
- A sensation of fullness or pressure in one or both ears.

Symptoms of Meniere's disease come in cycles. The patient suffers multiple episodes lasting several months at a time; it generally subsides. In some individuals, the symptoms seem to be more severe in spring, fall or when under extra emotional stresses. Some people with Meniere's disease find that certain trigger's can set off attacks including overwork, fatigue, emotional distress, additional illnesses, pressure changes, certain foods and too much salt in the diet.

Hearing loss typically fluctuates with hearing being worse some days than others. The hearing loss in Meniere's may lead to severe permanent hearing loss and deafness in the affected ear.

Management

- Symptoms are relieved with antiemetics, antihistamines, or benzodiazepines
- Diuretics and low-salt diet
- Another recently introduced, conservative treatment approach employs a device to deliver a series of low-pressure air pulses designed to displace inner ear fluids. The use of this device is approved for general use by the United States. Food and Drug Administration (FDA) is currently undergoing clinical trials in the United States.

MIGRAINE

Etiology and pathogenesis

The etiology of magraine is largely unknown. There is often a family history, suggesting a genetic predisposition. The great female preponderance and the tendency for some women to have migraine attacks at certain points in their menstrual cycle hint at abnormal hormonal influences.

Causes

Potential migraine triggers include allergy, bright light, loud noises, and certain odour or perfumes, emotional stress, irregular sleep, alcohol, and certain foods.

Clinical features

Migraine may occur at any age, but usually begin between the ages of 10 and 40 and diminish after age of 50. Some people experience a migraine a month, while others have only a few migraines throughout lifetime. Approximately 75% of migraine sufferers are women.

Classical migraine: Patients having paroxysmal headache, nausea and/or vomiting, and an aura of focal neurological events (usually visual) are said to have classical migraine. Approximately one-third of people who suffer migraine headache perceive an aura—unusual visual, factory or other sensory experiences that are a sign that the migraine soon occurs. Typically, a classical migraine attack starts with a non-specific prodrome of malaise and irritability followed by the **'aura'** of a focal neurological event, and then a severe, throbbing, hemicranial headache with photophobia and vomiting. During the headache phase, patients prefer to be in quiet, darkened room and to sleep.

Common migraine: Those with paroxysmal headache (with or without vomiting) but no **'aura'** are said to have migraine without aura (common migraine).

Management

Treatment of an acute attack consists of simple analgesia with aspirin or paracetamol, often combined with an antiemetic such as metoclopramide or domperidone.

DISEASES OF MUSCLES

MYOSITIS

Traumatic myositis ossificans

It is also known as ***'solitary myositis ossificans'*** or ***'localized myositis ossificans'***, ***'Sterner's tumour*** and ***'traumatic myositis circumscripta'***.

Traumatic myositis ossificans is a pseudotumour-like benign disease most frequently found in extremities of the young population. Concerning the head and neck involvement of the temporal muscle, masseter muscle, the buccinator muscle, the platysma muscle and sternomastoid muscle is described. The incidence in head and neck is rare, it is mainly found 80% in extremities.

Traumatic myositis is an unusual condition that occurs in athletes who sustain a blunt injury that causes deep tissue bleeding. This results from repeated injury to a muscle, as in case of rider's bone; or after a severe single injury, accompanied by haemorrhage.

Cases in the cleidofacial skeleton are rare. The masseter and sternomastoid muscles are most commonly affected in this location. Concerning the etiology of myositis ossificans of the masticatory muscles, several causes have been described: tooth extraction associated with involvement of buccinator muscle, and direct pterygoid force with myositis ossificans traumatica of masseter.

The soft tissues that were injured in the traumatic event initially develop haematoma, which is replaced by connective tissue and subsequently develops into osteoid tissue. Localised myositis ossificans is a reactive condition sometimes mistaken microscopically as osteosarcoma.

Clinical features

Oral manifestations

Most commonly involved muscles are masseter and sternocleidomastoid.

Initially painful, these lesions tend to become hard and painless later in their course.

In myositis ossificans of masseter muscles, patients complain of difficulty in opening the mouth, tenderness in masseter muscle and mobility of teeth. Severe trismus occurs after blunt injury of the face.

Microscopically

Section shows a typical zonation composed of fibroblastic proliferation in the centre with transition to an osteoblastic cell population in the intermediate zone and a fully ossified cancellous bone in the periphery. Surrounding or included muscle is sometimes damaged with foci of chronic inflammatory cells and thickened blood vessel.

Radiologically

X-ray shows an ossified lesion with a complete rim of thin peripheral calcification (egg shell calcification). The lesion is separated in its entire length by a fine radiolucent line from the adjacent bone.

Management

Treatment of myositis ossificans consists of: Immobilisation, rest and inflammatory medication.

PROGRESSIVE MYOSITIS OSSIFICANS

Progressive myositis is a specific type of ossificans myositis and it is characterised by formation of bone in the involved muscle.

Progressive myositis ossificans is also known as multicentric myositis ossificans, which results from mutations of GNAS1 gene.

It is a rare, progressive disease, which commences in children and slowly kills the patients.

Macroscopically

The lesion appears as uncapsulated gritty mass replacing the muscle. These masses vary considerably in size and shape and may disappear or become transformed into bony nodules.

Microscopically

Alongside and spreading between the deeply eosinophilic striated muscle fibres there is a sheet of pale edematous moderately cellular connective tissue.

In the connective tissue there is a scattered population of spindle-shaped fibroblast-like cells with elongated nuclei. Within this tissue there are two group of cells, some elongated with abundant cytoplasm and ill-defined margins. The nuclei are round or ovoid and minimally pleomorphic and the chromatin is finely granular. The group of cells has elongated nuclei to become osteocytes and some of them are surrounded by deeply basophilic calcified matrix.

PROLIFERATIVE MYOSITIS

Proliferative myositis is very rare and was first described as a specific entity in 1960 by Kem.

Proliferative myositis can be confused with sarcoma clinically as well as microscopically.

Cause

Although exact etiology of proliferative myositis is unknown, a local traumatic event has been considered to be a predisposing factor. It is a rarely seen intramuscular inflammatory process. Cases have been reported in association with rheumatoid vasculitis, desmoplastic fibroma, application of cast for fracture and chromosomal abnormality.

Clinical features

It has a special predilection for the trunk and upper extremities, though it frequently involves the head and neck muscles, masseter, and tongue.

Children are rarely affected and the typical patient is 45-65 years of age at tumour onset. There is slight female predilection.

Oral manifestations

Proliferative myositis of the oral lesions is a rapidly enlarging, immovable, perhaps tender submucosal mass. The lesion is usually 1.5-5.0 cm in greatest dimension at the time of diagnosis and involves the muscles in a diffuse, infiltrative fashion.

Macroscopically

On gross examination the lesion appears almost scar-like, with poorly circumscribed borders. Cut surface is greyish-white.

Microscopically

The lesion is composed of numerous fibroblastic (perimysium and epimysium) or myofibroblastic spindle cells and variable numbers of large ganglion cells infiltrating between and around muscle fascicles resembling 'checker-board configuration'. There is no evidence of muscle damage. Mitotic figures are infrequent. Typical ganglion cells are present having large round regular nuclei, occasional binucleate and trinucleate cells may be seen. Chromatin is dispersed with prominent nucleoli. Cytoplasm is basophilic to amphophilic. Focal ossification or dystrophic calcification may be observed in some cases, but never is it as pronounced as in heterotopic ossification.

Lesional cells are immunoreactive for vimentin, actin, smooth muscle actin, factor XIIIa, and fibronectin, and are usually not reactive for desmin or myosin.

Radiologically

Proliferative myositis manifests as solid, ill-defined, soft tissue mass causing an expansion in the muscular tissue.

Management

Surgical excision of lesion is the choice of treatment.

FOCAL MYOSITIS

Focal myositis was first described by Heffner et al (1977) as a non-malignant pseudotumour of skeletal muscle, which often presents as a painful soft tissue mass in one limb—most commonly in the lower limb—with no associated systemic pathology.

It is a rare idiopathic form of inflammatory myositis involving single muscle.

Cause

Etiology of focal myositis is unknown. Various theories, including viral infection, degenerating processes, and ischaemic necrosis of muscle have been suggested, but not established.

Clinical features

Affect young and middle-aged adults with no sex predilection. The thigh and lower legs are most common locations but shoulder, arm, back, and even the tongue have all been affected.

It presents as a rapidly enlarging mass with no previous history of trauma. The most common presentation in focal myositis is the development of a localised mass within the muscle, although slow progressive muscle weakness may occur.

Microscopically

There is intense predominantly interstitial foci of muscle fibre destruction and regeneration which resemble muscle infarcts. Endomysial chronic inflammatory cell infiltration is present. The lesion may also have substantial fibrosis.

Management

Surgical removable of lesion is necessary.

SEVERE GENERALISED MUSCULAR DYSTROPHY

Due to lack of muscle tension teeth cannot be kept properly aligned in the arch.

Duchenne muscular dystrophy is a form of muscular dystrophy that is characterised by decreasing muscle mass and progressive loss of muscle function in male children. Distribution of apparently hypertrophied (pseudohypertrophied) and atrophied muscles is characteristic. The calf muscles, glutei, deltoid, serrati, anterior brachio-radialis, and tongue muscles appear large. Muscle fibres show diffuse changes of degeneration.

Cause

The disorder is caused by a mutation in a specific gene within the X chromosome that provides instructions for the formation of dystrophin protein, an important structural component of muscle tissue. Females can be carriers but generally do not experience the symptoms.

Pathology: Up to 1 year the predominant finding is the presence of frequent hyaline and necrotic fibres with adequate regeneration. Ultimately, muscle is replaced by fat and degenerative changes.

Diagnosis

1. A characteristic feature is the elevated creatinine phosphokinase (CPK) enzyme levels in early stages of disease. Affected individuals may have a value as high as 15,000 to 35,000 IU/l (normal 60 IU/l).
2. **DNA test:** The dystrophic genes are composed of 79 exons and DNA testing and analysis can usually identify the specific type of mutation. DNA testing confirms the diagnosis.
3. **Muscle biopsy:** A small sample of muscle tissue is extracted and a dye is applied that reveals the presence of dystrophin. Complete absence of the protein indicates the condition.

MILD RESTRICTED MUSCULAR DYSTROPHY

It is also known as facioscapulohumeral dystrophy of Landouzy-Dejerine. It is an autosomal dominant form of muscular dystrophy that initially affects the skeletal muscles of the face, scapula, and upper arm.

Clinical features

Symptoms may develop in early childhood and are usually noticeable in the teenage years with 95% of affected individuals manifesting disease by age 20 years. Both sexes are equally affected.

Following are the symptoms of the disease:

- Facial muscle weakness, eyelid drooping, inability to whistle or to purse the lips (tapir mouth), decreased facial expression, depressed or angry facial expression, difficulty in pronouncing letters M, B, and P.
- Shoulder weakness (difficulty in working with the arms raised, sloping shoulder)
- Hearing loss
- Abnormal heart rhythm
- Unequal weakening of biceps, triceps, deltoids, and lower arm muscles
- Loss of strength of stomach muscles and eventual progression to the legs
- Foot drop.

Microscopically

Biopsy shows variation in the size of muscle fibres. There is atrophy of muscle fibres with infiltration by connective tissue.

MYOTONIAS

DYSTROPHIC MYOTONIA

It is also ***called Steiner's*** disease. It is a form of muscular dystrophy, which involves the muscles of the jaw and sternomastoid.

It is also known as myotonic dystrophy. It is a chronic, slowly progressive, highly variable inherited multisystemic disease that can manifest at any age from birth to old age. Dystrophic myotonia is a genetic condition which is inherited in an autosomal dominant pattern.

Clinical features

Progressive muscle wasting and weakness, particularly in the lower legs, hands, neck, and face, characterise the disorder. Other signs and symptoms of myotonic dystrophy include clouding of lens of the eye (cataract) and abnormalities of the electrical signals that control the heart beat.

Swan neck: There is ***'swan'*** *neck* appearance with wasting of sternocleidomastoid muscles with weakness of flexion of neck.

On shaking patient's hand, there is a delay in releasing his grip. In addition, often making a fist, he is unable to quickly open it—especially after doing it repetitively. Other features associated with dystrophic myotonia include gynaecomastia, dilated cardiomyopathy, testicular atrophy, thyroid enlargement, dysphagia, and diabetes mellitus.

Oral manifestations

Myopathic facies: Myopathic facies (fish facies) that is triangular in appearance with an expressionless (hatchet face) look. There is wasting of the muscles involving the temporalis and masseter muscles associated with frontal balding and bilateral ptosis. Patient has difficulty in opening his eyes after firm closure.

Due to weakness or myotonia of mouth, tongue, and throat there is difficulty in chewing and swallowing. Orofacial areas are more affected than proximal muscles. Impairment of facial expression, lip function, tongue motility, lip force, wide-open mouth at rest is common, and deviant production of bilabial and dental consonants is a frequent finding.

Recurrent dislocation of the jaw is also reported in this disease.

CONGENITAL MYOTONIA

It is also called Thomson's disease.

Cause

Sequence analysis detects the majority of mutations that cause both autosomal recessive myotonia congenital and autosomal dominant congenita.

The disease is caused by mutations in a gene responsible for shutting of electrical excitation in the muscles, causing muscle fibre membranes to have an unusually exaggerated response to stimulation. Mutation in the CLCN 1 gene causes myotonia congenita.

Clinical features

Myotonia congenital is characterised by muscle stiffness present from childhood; all striated muscle groups including the extrinsic eye muscles, the facial muscles, and the tongue may be involved. Men are more severely affected than women. Stiffness is relieved by repeated contractions of the muscle (the 'warm-up phenomenon'). Muscles are usually hypertrophic. The autosomal recessive form of myotonia congenital is often associated with more severe stiffness of muscles than the autosomal dominant form. Individuals with the autosomal recessive form may be progressive, minor distal weakness brought on by movement after rest.

Age: The age of onset is variable. In autosomal dominant myotonia congenital, onset of symptoms is usually in infancy or early childhood. In the autosomal recessive form, the average age at onset is slightly older.

Early symptoms

Difficulty in swallowing, gagging, stiff movements that improve when they are repeated.

Another characteristic feature is the generalised muscular hypertrophy leading to classic description of a Herculean appearance. This hypertrophy is principally seen in lower limbs, probably as a result of work hypertrophy, since the quadriceps and other muscles are in a continued state of contraction.

There is prolonged contraction of the lids after closure of eyes. Prolonged spasm of the muscles of the face, tongue, larynx, neck, and chest occurs after sneezing.

Possible complications may include aspiration pneumonia; frequent choking or gagging in infants, abdominal muscle weakness and chronic joint problems.

ACQUIRED MYOTONIA

This disorder is often termed Isaac's syndrome.

Clinical features

A rare neuromuscular disorder with onset usually in late childhood or early adulthood, characterised by intermittent or continuous widespread involuntary muscle contractions, fasciculation, hyporeflexia, muscle cramp, muscle weakness; hyperhydrosis, tachycardia, and myokymia. In the limbs, the myotonia and weakness affect the distal muscles more than the proximal ones.

Myotonia of the tongue and face cause a characteristic dysarthria, with slow and imprecise oral-lingual movements. Involvement of pharyngeal or laryngeal muscles may interfere with speech and breathing.

HEMIFACIAL SPASM

First described by Gower's in 1884, hemifacial spasm represents a segmental myoclonus of muscles innervated by the facial nerve.

Causes of hemifacial spasms

A. Idiopathic.

B. Compressive lesions
   - (i) Tumours
   - (ii) Arteriovenous malformation
   - (iii) Paget's disease.

C. Non-compressive lesions
   - (i) Stroke
   - (ii) Multiple sclerosis plaque
   - (iii) Basilar meningitis.

Clinical features

It is more common in women. Left-sided spasms are more common than right spasms. The disorder presents in the fifth or sixth decades of life, almost always unilaterally, although bilateral involvement may occur rarely, in severe cases.

The first symptom is usually an intermittent twitching of the eyelid muscle that can lead to forced closure of the eye. The spasm may then gradually spread to involve the muscles of the lower face, which may cause the mouth to be pulled to one side. Eventually, the spasms involve all the muscles on one side of the face almost continuously.

Diagnosis

It is confirmed by electromyogram.

Management

Treatment usually involves injecting mild doses of highly poisonous botulinum toxin (Botox) into the affected muscles. Surgery is considered when it is believed that the cause of the spasms is a blood vessel that is pressing on the facial nerve.

PARAMYOTONIA

Paramyotonia congenita, also known as paratonic congenita of von Eulenburg, or Eulenburg disease.

It is a rare congenital autosomal dominant neuromuscular disorder characterized by **'paradoxical myotonia'**. The stiffness chiefly affects muscles in the face, neck, arms, and hands. Symptoms can be triggered by exposure to cold.

Cause

The condition is inherited in an autosomal dominant pattern, which means one copy of the altered gene in each cell is sufficient to cause this disorder. In many cases, an affected person has one parent with the condition. Mutation in the gene SCN4A gene causes paramyotonia congenital.

MYASTHENIA GRAVIS

Myasthenia gravis is an organ-specific autoimmune disorder characterised by rapid disorderioration of muscle power and repetitive firing of the presynaptic nerve fibres, corrected by neostigmine (acetylecholinesterase inhibitor). A reduction in the number of Ach results in a characteristic pattern of progressively reduced muscle strength with repeated use of the muscle and recovery of muscle strength following a period of rest.

The prevalence of myasthenia gravis in the United States ranges from 0.5-14.2 cases per 100,000 people.

Etiology

It may be associated with thymus hyperplasia and tumours of thymus (thymoma). Thyroid disorders may be seen in as many as 10% of patients with myasthenia gravis, and symptoms of hypothyroidism or hyperthyroidism may be present.

Clinical features

It may occur at any age, but the peak incidence is in young adults. Women are more affected than men.

Types of myasthenia gravis

Myasthenia gravis is classified according to which skeletal muscles are affected:

Generalised myasthenia gravis: Within a year of onset, approximately 85-90% of patients develop generalised myasthenia gravis, which is characterised by weakness in the trunk, arms, and legs.

Ocular myasthenia gravis: The most common sites of initial involvement are the muscles of the eyelids and the muscles controlling eye movement, manifested by drooping of eyelids (ptosis) and double vision.

Congenital myasthenia gravis: It is an inherited condition caused by genetic defect and transient neonatal, which occurs in infants born to mothers who have myasthenia gravis. Congenital myasthenia gravis develops at or shortly after birth and causes generalised symptoms.

Transient neonatal myasthenia gravis is a temporary condition that develops in 10-20% of infants born to mothers who have myasthenia gravis. Transient neonatal myasthenia gravis is caused by circulation of the mother's antibodies through the placenta and it lasts as long as the mother's antibodies remain in the infant (usually up to a few weeks after birth).

Commonest cause of death is aspiration pneumonia due to respiratory muscle weakness.

Oral manifestations

Dysphagia and regurgitation of food are common. Involvement of other facial and neck muscles commonly causes difficulty in chewing food and holding neck upwards. The involvement of facial muscles results in changes in expression and speech, whereas involvement of the pharyngeal muscles results in progressive difficulty with mastication and deglutition.

Microscopically, lymphocytic infiltration (lymphorrhage) is found in the affected muscles, pancreas, and adrenals. The lymphocytic infiltration is found surrounding small blood vessels in the interstitial tissue of the affected muscle.

Antibodies to acetylecholine receptors (AchR) are common.

Oral manifestations: The oral mucosa may show dark red or bluish erythema.

CONGENITAL FACIAL DISPLEGIA (MOBIUS SYNDROME)

It is named for Paul Julius Mobius, neurologist who first described the syndrome in 1888.

Mobius syndrome is congenital, and most cases are diagnosed during infancy.

Etiology

Mobius syndrome results from the underdevelopment of VI and VII nerves. Occasionally, the cranial nerves V and VIII are affected. Pathological findings are variable and include brain stem nuclear aplasia, and facial nerve aplasia, consistent with a multifactorial etiology.

The majority of patients have other associated deformities, including craniofacial dysmorphisms, congenital abnormalities of the extremities, cleft palate, defect of pectoral muscles, paralysis of the tongue, soft palate and jaw muscles.

Cocaine and prostaglandin abuse is occasionally associated with the occurrence of this syndrome. Most cases are sporadic but autosomal-dominant, recessive and X-linked patterns of inheritance have been described.

Clinical features

Mobius syndrome is an extremely rare congenital neurological disorder, which is characterised by facial paralysis, and inability to move eyes from side to side. Most people with Mobius syndrome are born with complete facial paralysis and cannot close their eyes and form facial expressions. Often, the upper lip is retracted due to muscle shrinkage. Other symptoms include feeding, swallowing and choking problems, excessive drooling, crossed eyes, inability to smile, eye sensitivity, motor delays and hearing problems.

Treatment

There is no specific treatment for Mobius syndrome. Surgery may correct crossed eyes and improve limb and jaw deformities. Physical therapy might be useful in managing congenital orthopedic problems or for postoperative care if orthopedic intervention is required.

Occupational and speech therapy is useful.

ATROPHY OF MUSCLE

Muscle atrophy is defined as a decrease in the mass of the muscle. It can be partial or complete wasting of muscles.

Causes of muscle atrophy include poor nourishment, poor circulation, loss of hormonal support, toxins, loss of nerve supply to the target organ, disease or lack of exercise, or disease intrinsic to the tissue itself.

Disuse atrophy is common. In this the fibres of the affected muscle shrink in size, and, when the disuse is permanent, they are converted into fibrofatty tissue.

Atrophy due to joint diseases is seen in tuberculosis or rheumatoid arthritis. It is partly due to a local toxic action.

HYPERTROPHY OF MUSCLE

Definition: Muscle hypertrophy is the increase of the size of muscle.

Types of muscular atrophy

There are two different types of muscular hypertrophy.

1. Sarcoplasmic
2. Myofibrillar

Sarcoplasmic hypertrophy: During sarcoplasmal hypertrophy, the volume of sarcoplasmic fluid in the muscle cell increases with no accompanying increase in muscular strength.

Myofibrillar hypertrophy: During myofibrillar hypertrophy, actin and myosin contractile protein increases in number and add to muscular strength as well as a small increase in the size of the muscle.

Causes of muscular hypertrophy

1. Power lifters
2. Olympic lifters

Factors, which increase muscular hypertrophy include testosterone, microtrauma, which is tiny damage to the fibres, may play a significant role in hypertrophy.

Bibliography

Singh A, Philpott JM, Patel NN, Mochloulis G: Proliferative myositis arising in tongue. Journal of Laryngology and Otology (2000), 114:12:978-979.

CHAPTER

18

CYSTIC LESIONS OF ORAL CAVITY

CYSTIC LESIONS OF ORAL CAVITY

TABLE 18.1
CLASSIFICATION OF CYSTIC LESIONS OF ORAL CAVITY

I. **Cysts of jaw**
   - A. **Epithelial Developmental**
     - a. **Odontogenic cysts**
       - Primordial cyst
       - Lateral periodontal cyst
       - Calcifying odontogenic cyst
       - Gingival cysts of adults
       - Glandular odontogenic cysts.
       - Dentigerous cyst
       - Odontogenic keratocyst
       - Eruption cyst
       - Botryoid odontogenic cysts
     - b. **Non-odontogenic cyst**
       1. **Non-inflammatory cyst**
          - Globulomaxillary cyst
          - Nasopalatine duct cyst
          - Nasolabial cyst
          - Median mandibular cyst
          - Median palatal cyst
          - Midpalatal raphe cyst of infant.
       2. **Inflammatory cyst**
          - Radicular cyst
          - Inflammatory collateral cyst
          - Residual cyst
          - Paradental cyst.
       3. **Other non-epithelial cysts**
          - Traumatic bone cyst
          - Aneurysmal bone cyst.

Contd.

Contd.

II. Cysts of maxillary antrum

- Benign mucosal cysts of maxillary antrum
- Surgical ciliated cysts of maxilla.

III. Cysts of soft tissue of mouth, face and neck

- Dermoid and epidermoid cyst
- Branchial cleft cyst (lymphoepithelial cyst)
- Anterior median lingual cyst
- Stafne bone cavity
- Mucocele
- Ranula
- Cystic hygroma
- Oral cysts with gastric or intestinal epithelium
- Lymphoepithelial cyst
- Eruption cyst
- Gingival cyst of the newborn
- Gingival cyst of adults
- Thyroglossal duct cyst
- Palatine papilla cyst
- Parasitic cyst, hydatid cyst, cysticercus celluloase, Trichinosis.

EPITHELIAL-LINED CYSTS OF THE JAWS

A. INFLAMMATORY CYSTS

RADICULAR CYST

Radicular cyst is the most common odontogenic cyst. It is also called ***'periapical cyst' 'periodontal cyst'*** or ***'dental root end cyst'***.

Radicular cyst accounts for almost 50% of the jaw cysts.

Etiology

The usual etiology is a tooth that becomes infected, leading to necrosis of the pulp. Toxins exist in the apex of the tooth, leading to periapical inflammation. This inflammation stimulates the Malassez epithelial rests, which are found in the periodontal ligament resulting in the formation of periapical granuloma that may be infected or sterile. Eventually, this epithelium undergoes necrosis caused by a lack of blood supply, and the granuloma becomes a cyst.

Clinical features

A radicular cyst is usually asymptomatic. Occasionally, however, the associated tooth is sensitive to percussion. It is usually associated with caries teeth. Rarely, the lesion may be associated with fistula. They occur in all age groups but are commonly diagnosed during the third and fourth decades.

Sex: It is more common in males than females.

Site: The favourable site of occurrence is the periapical areas of permanent maxillary anterior teeth. Large cysts may involve a complete quadrant with some of teeth occasionally mobile and some of pulps non-vital.

It is always associated with a normally erupted tooth, chronically infected or carious tooth. It is usually painless, unless infected when it becomes painful.

Swelling may be bony hard or due to thinning of bone crepitations may be present.

Microscopically

They are lined by stratified squamous epithelium, the thickness of which varies according to the degree of inflammation present. In rare occasions however, respiratory or other forms of epithelium may be seen. Cyst wall is fibrous and contains chronic inflammatory cells. Metaplasia, calcification, and hyaline bodies (ruston bodies) occasionally may be identified in the epithelium. Deposits of cholesterol crystals may be associated with foreign body giant cells.

Radiologically

It appears as a small 3-4 mm radiolucent area situated at the apex or side of the root.

Complications: Rarely, a festering infection within the cyst can lead to osteomyelitis. Extremely rarely cystic epithelium of cysts may give rise to primary carcinomas of jaw.

Treatment

Treatment consists of endodontic therapy or extraction of associated tooth with curettage of the cyst.

DEVELOPMENTAL CYSTS

B. ODONTOGENIC CYSTS

I. DENTIGEROUS CYST

This cyst is usually associated with non-erupted permanent tooth.

Clinical features

It usually occurs in young adults during the second and third decade. They are common in males as compared to females.

The commonest sites are around unerupted mandibular and maxillary third molars and maxillary canines. It presents as bluish swelling. The swelling consists of a cyst containing the tooth. The cyst grows larger and expands the outer table of the jaw causing eggshell crackling. Some large cysts may lead to facial asymmetry. Sometimes it may be multilocular.

Microscopically

The cyst mainly consists of fibrous tissue lined by non-keratinised stratified squamous epithelium and mucus secreting cells. In few instances, the lining may be keratinised and it may be mistaken as keratocyst or keratin may be produced rarely as due to metaplastic changes. The periepithelial stroma shows islands of odontogenic epithelium. The stroma consists of young fibroblasts cells, which are widely separated by a ground substance rich in mucopolysaccharides and collagen bundles.

Radiologically

The lesion usually appears as a radiolucent well-defined uniocular area surrounding the crown up to its neck. Dentigerous cysts can vary in size. The cyst can be 2 cm in diameter or larger.

Rarely ameloblastoma, squamous carcinoma, and mucoepidermoid carcinoma have been reported to arise from the cyst lining.

Treatment

Treatment of dentigerous cyst consists of enucleation of the cyst with removal of unerupted tooth.

II. LATERAL PERIODONTAL CYST

Lateral odontogenic cyst is a common well-recognised type of developmental odontogenic cyst.

Pathogenesis

Pathogenesis of lateral periodontal cyst is not fully known. There seems to be three possibilities: Reduced enamel epithelium, remnants of dental lamina and cell rests of Malassez. They are not inflammatory, they do not arise from periodontitis, and they are not associated with lateral canals within the tooth structure.

Clinical features

This lesion is more common in adults (5th to 6th decade) and has no sex predilection.

The most common odontogenic cyst is the periodontal cyst. Most often it is observed at the apex of an erupted tooth. The origin of this appears to be cystic degeneration of epithelialised granulomas that have resulted most frequently as sequelae to dental caries and pulpitis.

They are commonly associated with the mandibular area and are occasionally found in the maxillary anterior. Some of them are less than 1 cm in diameter and are located on the cervical margin of the tooth.

Radiological findings

These cysts are always well-demarcated, round or tear-dropped, relatively small and radiolucent area (sometimes radiopaque roof) usually within a sclerotic margin.

Microscopically

The cyst wall is of connective tissue fibres with stratified squamous epithelial lining. It is characterised by a thin lining of epithelium usually 1 to 5 layers thick. The characteristic features of this cyst are the presence of epithelial plaque extending into the lumen. The connective tissue subjacent to the epithelium exhibits a zone of hyalinisation.

Management

Lateral periodontal cyst is treated by surgical enucleation and has no tendency to recur.

III. ERUPTION CYST

Eruption cyst is an uncommon type of dentigerous cyst associated with erupting deciduous or rarely permanent cyst. The cyst develops as a result of separation of the distal follicle from around the crown of an erupting tooth that is within the tissues overlying the alveolar bone. It represents the accumulation of fluid or blood in a dilated follicular space about the crown of an erupting tooth.

Clinical features

It may be unilateral or bilateral, single or multiple, and may be present at birth. They appear bluish and transparent dome-shaped soft tissue lesions overlying on erupting tooth. When the fluid in the cyst is mixed with blood, the cyst is referred to as an eruption haematoma.

Microscopically

Cyst wall is subacutely inflamed and haemorrhagic. It is lined by thin non-keratinising stratified squamous epithelium.

X-ray findings: It may show a soft tissue shadow since the cyst is confined within it and there is no bone involvement.

Management

Eruption cyst and eruption haematomas are usually asymptomatic and resolve with eruption of the tooth. The lesions should not be incised as this may increase the risk of infection.

IV. GINGIVAL CYST

GINGIVAL CYST OF THE NEWBORN

Synonyms: Dental lamina cyst of the newborn, Bohn's nodules.

Gingival cyst of newborn infants (Bohn's nodules) present as minute cystic or nodular formations. They are seen in most neonates.

Site: Gingival cyst of newborn can manifest as few or many white to yellowish round to oval nodes in the maxillary and/or mandibular gingival and alveolar ridge of newborns.

Size: These nodes generally measure 2 to 3 millimetres in their largest diameter, which rupture spontaneously after 2-3 months.

Etiology

These nodes are formed as a result of cystic degeneration of epithelial rests of the dental lamina (rests of Serres). After the dental lamina invaginates to form the dental organ, the epithelial pedicle that connects the dental organ to the surface epithelium is broken down—giving rise to the rests of Serres.

Microscopically

The cyst is lined by odontogenic epithelium, or stratified squamous epithelium, which is covered by a thick layer of keratin. Keratin gives the cysts its yellow colour. The epithelium lacks rete ridges. There is presence of inflammatory cells, dystrophic calcification and hyaline bodies.

Treatment

No treatment is required for these lesions, which usually disappear either by opening onto the surface mucosa or through disruption by erupting teeth.

V. GINGIVAL CYST OF ADULTS

They are rare extraosseous cysts situated in the soft tissue of the labial gingival.

Clinical features

Gingival cyst of adult is a slow-growing lesion, which as a rule does not measure more than one centimetre in diameter. The cyst may even develop in the interdental papilla and in either location, is a painless swelling presenting the normal gingival colour, however, some of them may have a bluish colour.

Microscopically

The gingival cyst of the adult is mostly lined by an odontogenic epithelium, which resembles the reduced enamel epithelium and is formed by a few rows of cells. Many of the epithelial cells exhibit pyknotic nuclei with perinuclear cytoplasmic vacuoles.

Treatment

Treatment is surgical excision of lesion.

VI. KERATINISING AND CALCIFYING ODONTOGENIC CYST

Clinical features

This cyst can occur at any age, but more than 50% are seen in patients less than 40 years of age. Almost 80% of lesions occur within the jaws and 20% in the soft tissue around the jaw.

This is commonly seen in the premolar area of the mandible in association with an unerupted tooth. Lesions range in size from 1 to 8 cm. In the later stages, thinning of the involved bone with egg-shell crackling, loosening of teeth and pathological fracture occurs.

Microscopically

Prominent basal palisading and large masses of keratinised ghost cells characterise the cyst. Some cells may be the clear cell type. The cyst shows various degrees of calcification as it grows. Melanin pigmentation may be occasionally present in cyst layer.

Radiographs show a single or multilocular, well demarcated radiolucency in which specks of radiopacities can be seen.

Treatment

Successful treatment of intraosseous calcifying odontogenic cyst has been accomplished by curettage, enucleation, and conservative surgical excision.

VII. PRIMORDIAL CYST

A primordial cyst is a developmental odontogenic cyst.

Primordial cyst constitutes about 5% of all follicular cysts and 1.5% of all odontogenic cysts. It arises from a tooth germ that, instead of forming a tooth, degenerates into a cyst.

Site: It is commonly seen in the ascending ramus of the mandible and third molar.

Microscopic

Section show a cystic cavity lined by stratified squamous epithelium and a connective tissue wall that usually—but not always—is free of inflammatory cells and that may contain small islands of odontogenic or ameloblastic epithelium. The cells are arranged in a *'picket fence'* or ***'tombstone pattern'*** and no rete peg formation.

VIII. ODONTOGENIC KERATOCYST

This is the third most common odontogenic cyst. It constitutes 11% of jaw cysts. The odontogenic keratocyst (OKC) was first described in 1876 and named by Phillipsen in 1956.

Multiple odontogenic keratocysts of the jaws may be associated in the nevoid basal cell carcinoma syndrome, which has autosomal dominant inheritance.

Clinical features

The majority of patients are in the age ranges of 20-29 and 40-59 years, but cases ranging from 5 to 80 years have been reported.

It is the most aggressive odontogenic cyst of the oral cavity. Odontogenic keratocyst is known for its tendency to invade the adjacent tissues including bone. Anatomically, the mandible is affected more frequently than the maxilla, with 75% of lesion occurs in mandible.

Microscopically

Histologically, these cysts are formed with a stratified squamous epithelium that produces orthokeratin (10%), parakeratin (83%), or both types of keratin (7). No rete ridges are present; therefore, the epithelium often sloughs from the connective tissue. The epithelium is thin, and mitotic activity is frequent. The lumen is filled with a cheese-like material that is not pus but, rather, collected degenerating material.

Radiologically

It can mimic any of the jaw cysts and may appear as a well-marginated inter-radicular periodontal or a multilocular radiolucency.

Treatment

Small keratocysts may be treated with simple enucleation if the entire cyst lining can be removed.

BASAL CELL NAEVUS SYNDROME (GORLIN'S SYNDROME)

It is also known as ***'nevoid basal cell carcinoma'***, ***'Goltiz's' syndrome, 'Hemans Herzberg phacomatosis', 'epitheliomatous multiplex'***.

It is now greatly known as Gorlin syndrome, after the late professor Robert J Gorlin (1923-2006).

Etiology

It is a condition inherited as an autosomal dominant trait and characterised by a predisposition for keratocystic odontogenic tumour (Odontogenic keratocysts) and skin cancers, especially basal cell carcinoma, as well as the presence of a number of abnormalities of tumours in the skeletal, nervous, endocrine and other systems. Recent work in molecular genetics has shown NBCCs to be caused by mutations in the PTCH (patched) gene found on chromosome arm 9q.

Oral abnormalities

Oral changes are:

- Non-vital, discoloured teeth are commonly associated with periodontal cysts.
- Unerupted third molars and maxillary canines beyond the normal age of eruption must be radiographed and the formation of dentigerous cyst excluded.
- Any loosening, change in inclination, divergence of teeth and expansion of bone can all result due to cysts of the jaws.
- Cleft palate and cleft lip occurs in 3-5% of patients.

Cutaneous abnomalities

The most prominent skin lesions in NBCCs are multiple basal cell carcinomas that typically develop by a median age of 20 years. There is presence of palmar and plantar pits.

Skeletal abnormalities

Skeletal abnormalities include polydactyly of the hands or the feet, hallus valgus, pectus excavatum, or pectus carinatum, and syndactly of the second and third fingers. Kyphoscoliosis may also be more common or severe in NBCC syndrome. Sprengel deformity of the shoulder occurs in 5-10% of patients.

Ophthalmologic abnormalities

Ophthalmologic abnormalities include hypertelorism with wide nasal bridge, dystopia canthosum, congenital blindness, and internal strabismus. Congenital blindness is due to corneal opacity and cataract or glaucoma occurring as many as 10-15% of patients.

Neurological abnormalities

Medulloblastoma, a cerebellar tumour of young childhood, may present with neurologic symptoms in a child who is affected. Other neurological abnormalities are mental retardation, calcification of falx cerebri, other parts of dura, agenesis of corpus callosum, and congenital hydrocephalus.

Cardiac lesions

Cardiac findings are less common, but an increased risk of cardiac fibroma may be present. Cardiac fibroma usually presents in children or young adults.

Genitourinary symptoms

Ovarian fibromas are usually asymptomatic, but they may present with pain secondary to torsion. Men may have associated cryptorchidism or gynaecomastia and reduced body hair.

Other tumours, including fibrosarcoma, rhabdomyosarcoma, and meningioma may be increased in frequency in persons with NBCC syndrome.

Diagnosis

Diagnosis of nevoid basal cell carcinoma syndrome is made in the presence of 2 major criteria or 1 minor criterion.

The major criteria consists of:

- More than two basal cell carcinoma or one basal cell carcinoma in patients younger than 20 years
- Odontogenic keratocysts of the jaw
- 3 or more palmar or plantar pits

- Bilamellar calcification of the falx cerebri
- Bifid, fused, on markedly splayed ribs, and
- First-degree relative with naevoid basal cell cyst syndrome
- Minor criteria include:
- Macrocephaly
- Congenital malformation as cleft lip or palate, frontal bossing and coarse facies, and moderate or severe hypertelorism.
- Other skeletal abnormalities, such as Sprengel deformity, marked pectus deformity, and marked syndactyly of the digits.
- Radiological abnormalities, such as bridging of the sella turcica, vertebral anomalies, modelling defects of hands and feet, and ovarian fibroma or medulloblastoma.

IX. GLANDULAR ODONTOGENIC CYST

Gardener described the cyst in 1988.

Clinical features

Over half of the patients are in between 40 and 60 years of age—so has a slight male predilection.

Commonest site is mandible in 87% of cases. It is of slow progressive growth. The patient presents with swelling and pain in 40% of cases.

Microscopically

Histological findings which should be detected are:

- A cystic cavity lined by epithelium of varying thickness with a flat interface between the epithelium and underlying connective tissue
- Variable number of mucus cells in the epithelium
- Eosinophilic cuboidal cells in the superficial layer
- Localised plaque-like thickening of the epithelium
- Little inflammation
- Occasional findings of hyperchromatic basal cells within the cyst.

Radiologically

These cysts may be uniocular or multiocular with a well-defined border. Sometimes it may present with peripheral osteosclerotic border and scalloping, root resorption and displacement of the teeth.

Management

Recurrences after enucleation or curettage are seen in 25% of cases. Marginal resection suggests for larger lesions or involvement of posterior maxilla.

NON-ODONTOGENIC AND FISSURAL CYST

I. NASOPALATINE OR INCISIVE DUCT CYST

Cysts that arise in the nasopalatine canal constitute about 54% of all non-odontogenic cysts and non-epithelial cyst. It occurs in 1% of population.

This is the most common non-odontogenic fissured cyst and arises from the epithelial remnants of the nasopalatine duct.

Clinical features

The nasopalatine duct cyst may develop at any age but is most common in the 4th to 6th decades. Males are more often involved. Presenting symptoms include swelling of the anterior palate, drainage, and pain.

Histologically

Stratified squamous epithelium, respiratory epithelium, or both line the cyst. There is presence of mucous glands and nerves in the connective tissue wall and lymphocytic and plasma cell infiltration of the connective tissue.

Radiographs reveal well-circumscribed radiolucency in or near the midline of anterior maxilla. Some cysts have a pear-shape or heart-shape.

Treatment

Nasopalatine duct cysts are treated by enucleation.

II. NASOALVEOLAR CYST

The nasoalveolar cyst is a developmental cyst probably derived from epithelial remnants of the nasolacrimal duct.

It is also known as nasolabial cyst.

Clinical features

Nasolabial cyst has a strong female predilection (75% occur in women) and is seen usually in blacks and is located at the base of the nostril. The cyst is less than 1-5 cm in greatest diameter but has reached much larger size. It is one of the least common of the non-odontogenic cysts and non-epithelial cysts of the jaws and constitutes only about 2.5% of these lesions.

Physical examination reveals dark-blue mass in anterolateral nasal floor and vestibule after extending into sublabial sulcus. It can cause swelling in lateral aspect of upper lip, may elevate nasal vestibule, and cause nasal flaring and obliteration of nasolabial fold.

Histologically

Various types of epithelial cells may form the lining of the cyst lumen, often including ciliated and goblet cells. Chronic inflammatory cells may be seen in the surrounding fibrovascular stroma.

Treatment

Transoral surgical excision via sublabial approach is preferred. Prognosis is excellent, rare recurrence. If left untreated; long-standing pressure may result in erosion of nasal floor and premaxilla.

III. ANEURYSMAL BONE CYST

In 1942, Jaffe and Lichenstein first classified the aneurysmal bone cyst as a distinct entity.

Age: Aneurysmal bone cyst may occur in patients aged 10 to 30 years, with a peak incidence in those aged 16 years. About 75% of patients are younger than 20 years.

Sex: Females have an increased incidence.

Sites: Aneurysmal cysts are more likely to occur in the mandible than the maxilla. It is common in the metaphysis of bone. The molar region, ramus, angle, symphysis and condyle are the commonest sites for an aneurysmal bone cyst to occur.

Macroscopically

Within the thin bony shell the cyst consists of cavernous blood-filled spaces separated by brownish spongy meshwork of vascular fibrous trabeculae. Osteoid or bony strands reinforce the larger spaces.

Microscopically

Conventional (95%): **Osteolytic lesion:** Expansive with vascular lagoons of variable sizes, separated by connective tissue that includes bone trabeculae, osteoid tissue, and multinucleated giant cells. The giant cells are smaller and less evenly distributed than in a true giant cell tumour—especially around areas of vascular spaces and haemorrhage.

Solid (5%): Solid mass without a cystic compound of regular density contains multiple haemorrhagic foci. It has a great fibroblastic, osteoclastic, and osteoblastic compound.

Radiological features include cystic bone expansion. Honey comb or soap-bubble appearance. There may be destruction of bone cortex and periosteal reaction.

Etiology

Trauma is considered an initiating factor in the pathogenesis of some cysts in well-documented cases involving acute fracture.

Treatment

Treatment is intralesional curettage. Recurrence is not common. Other surgical options include en block resection or wide excision, selective arterial embolisation, and curettage with locally adjuvalents such as liquid nitrogen or phenols.

IV. STAFNE'S BONE CYST

Stafne first recognised Stafne bone cyst in 1942.

The incidence of occurrence has been reported as 0.1-1.3% in various studies.

It is also called static bone cyst or submandibular salivary gland depression.

Stafne bone cyst is an unusual form of slightly aberrant salivary gland tissue wherein a developmental inclusion of glandular tissue is found within, or, more commonly—adjacent to the lingual surface of the body of the mandible within a deep and well-circumscribed depression.

Etiology

Stafne's bone cavities are presumed to form by the remodelling of the mandibular cortex around an extension of salivary tissues.

Radiologically

The lesion is well-circumscribed, corticated and radiolucency situated; periapical to the second or third mandibular molar. The defect is not in continuity with tips, rather it is located below the inferior alveolar canal.

Complication

A complication occasionally reported in the literature is the development of a true salivary gland neoplasm in the tissue associated with one of the cortical defects.

Treatment

No treatment is required.

V. GLOBULOMAXILLARY CYST

Globulomaxillary cyst was described by Thoma as a developmental cyst. The cyst was considered to be an inclusion or developmental cyst that arises from entrapped non-odontogenic epithelium in the globulomaxillary suture.

It is described as intraosseous and located between the maxillary lateral incisor and canine.

Clinical features

As the cyst enlarges, it expands the buccal cortical plate between maxillary lateral incisors and canines.

Microscopically

It shows lining of stratified squamous epithelium. Sometimes it is lined by either cuboidal or columnar epithelium.

Radiologically

X-ray shows characteristic pear-shaped radiolucency causing displacement of the roots of vital maxillary lateral and cuspid teeth is characteristic of globulomaxillary cyst. The adjoining teeth are vital. Large radiolucency between the lateral incisor and cuspid tends to cause divergence of the roots.

Treatment

Complete removal is needed. The prognosis is good, and the recurrence rate is low with complete removal.

VI. MUCOCELE

Partial or total excretory duct obstruction is involved in the pathogenesis of ranulas in some instances. The duct may be occluded by a sialolith, congenital malformation, stenosis, periductal fibrosis, and agenesis, or even tumour.

Mucoceles are formed because of a traumatic rupture of the excretory ducts of a salivary gland, which leads to periductal scarring and subsequent accumulation of saliva in the tissues.

Clinical features

Clinical features associated with mucoceles include a non-tender, mobile, dome-shaped enlargement with intact epithelium that lies over it. Superficial lesions take on a bluish to translucent hue, whereas deep lesions have normal mucosal colouration. Bleeding into the swelling may impart a bright red and vascular appearance. Mucosal lining is intact, however, repeated sucking on the lesion may result in a white, rough, keratotic surface.

Mucoceles are usually seen before 50 years of age with equal gender predilection. Lower lip, buccal mucosa, palate, tongue, floor of the mouth, retromolar area and maxillary sinus are the commonest sites.

Patients may complain of painless swelling which is frequently recurrent.

The swelling is round or oval and smooth. It is usually less than 1.5 cm.

Microscopically

There is pooling of mucus in soft tissues, surrounded by granulation tissue and fibrous tissue.

Treatment

Treatment is enucleation or surgical removal.

VII. RANULA

The word ranula is derived from the resemblance of the swelling to the belly of the frog Rana Hexadactyla.

Ranula is a large mucocele arising from the sublingual salivary glands located on the floor of the mouth called glands of Blandin and Nuhn. Ranulas may be either mucous extravasations phenomenon or mucus retention cysts, and most commonly associated with sublingual salivary ducts.

Common cause of ranula formation is trauma. Other causes include an obstructed salivary gland or ductal aneurysm. A sarcoid-associated ranula also has been reported.

Clinical features

The lesion most commonly presents as a painless, slow-growing, soft and movable mass located in the floor of the mouth.

The ranula is a large soft, mucus-containing swelling in the floor of the mouth.

Microscopically

Flattened layer of modified duct epithelium, which may be cuboidal or columnar, usually lines ranulae or there may be squamous metaplasia. There is frequently an inflammatory infiltration in the walls and the cyst may be multilocular.

Complications

1. Rupture of the cyst decreases the size but it can reappear at a later date.
2. When the swelling is big, the tongue is pushed upwards and may cause difficulty in speech or swallowing.

Treatment

Ranulas are treated surgically.

VIII. PLUNGING RANULA

The plunging ranula is a cyst containing extravasated saliva originating from the sublingual gland. If the ranula extends behind the posterior border of the mylohyoid it forms a plunging ranula which manifest as a lateral neck swelling.

Plunging ranulas generally appear in conjunction with an oral ranula. Rarely, they can arise independently of the oral component.

Clinical features

The plunging ranula is asymptomatic, continuously enlarging mass that may fluctuate in size. The mass is fluctuant, freely movable, and non-tender.

In some instances, detecting salivary gland herniation of a portion of sublingual gland through the myolohyoid muscle into the neck may be possible. Complications of plunging ranula includes infection, bursting, repeated trauma, a big ranula may cause difficulty in speech and eating.

IX. EPIDERMOID CYST

An epidermoid cyst may occur in the floor of the mouth, the lips and the cheek mucosa. Just a few cases of lingual involvement have been reported.

An epidermoid cyst may result from traumatic implantation of epithelial cells into surface epithelium.

Clinical features

In the oral cavity these cysts occur most frequently in the area of the floor of the mouth and may also occur on the tongue, lips, buccal mucosa or the interior of the bone. Plunging ranula is brilliantly translucent cyst; therefore transillumination test is positive.

Microscopic examination of epidermoid cyst reveals a cavity lined by stratified squamous epithelium resembling epidermis. A well-developed granular layer is seen, and the lumen is filled with degenerating orthokeratin. Not infrequently, the epithelium lining will be disrupted, when this occurs, a prominent granulomatous inflammatory reaction—including multinucleated giant cells—can be present in cyst wall because the exposed keratin is recognised as foreign material.

X. DERMOID CYST

Dermoid cysts of the floor of the mouth are dysembryogenetic lesions derived from entrapment and subsequent growth of epithelial cells during the midline fusion between the first and second branchial arches in the third and fourth embryonic week.

Acquired form is derived from iatrogenic or traumatic inclusion of epithelium and skin appendages.

Clinical features

Sites: Dermoid cysts develop in the floor of the mouth and base of the tongue along the midline and present as a submental swelling and elevate floor of the mouth.

It is a midline cyst yet a few dermoid cysts are seen to be of lateral variety. These lateral cysts are derived from the branchial cleft, so the types are:

1. Median variety
   a. Suprahyoid variety
   b. Infrahyoid variety.
2. Lateral variety
   a. Suprahyoid variety
   b. Inframylohyoid variety.

Median variety: Patients usually complains of swelling under the tongue in the floor of the mouth or just below the point of the chin.

Inframylohyoid variety or cervical variety: It is a swelling in the submental region and gives rise to a 'double chin' appearance.

Suprahyoid variety: It is an opaque cystic swelling in the floor of the mouth on one side or the other.

Most dermoid cysts on the floor of the mouth are in individuals aged 10-30 years. Only a few cases describe oral dermoid in newborn or children. The size is small, but the cyst expands progressively and slowly and, finally, may reach several centimetres in diameter. Clinically, it is a painless elevated swelling with normal or slightly reddish colour and characteristic dough-like consistency on palpation. The lesion is not translucent.

Macroscopically

It is a freely movable well-circumscribed mass. The cut section reveals cheesy or liquid material.

Microscopically

The cyst wall is lined by keratinising stratified epithelium and contains skin appendages.

Treatment of dermoid cysts of the floor of the mouth is surgical and can be done by an intraoral or extraoral route according to the localisation and the size of the mass.

XI. THYROGLOSSAL DUCT CYST

Thyroglossal duct cysts are remnants of the embryonic thyroglossal duct that may occur anywhere from the tongue to the thyroid gland. Thyroglossal cyst is a congenital defect. Thyroglossal cyst arises out of remnants of the thyroglossal tract or duct-connecting thyroid to the tongue.

According to frequency, its position may be:

a. Sublingual (below the hyoid bone)
b. In the region of the hyoid cartilage (may be deviated to the left side)
c. Suprahyoid
d. At the level of the cricoid cartilage
e. In the floor of the mouth
f. Beneath the foramen caecum.

Clinical features

In oral cavity it is present in the region of foramen caecum on the tongue and floor of the mouth.

Thyrogolssal cysts are associated with an increased incidence of ectopic thyroid tissue. Occasionally, lingual thyroid can be seen as a flattened strawberry-like lump at the base of the tongue.

It is seen in the first decade of life.

Symptoms of thyroglossal duct cyst include:

- A small, soft, round, palpable mass in the midline or slightly off the midline, between the isthmus of the thyroid and hyoid bone or just above the hyoid bone.
- Thyroglossal duct cyst moves upward with protrusion of the tongue. This occurs because it is attached to the thyroglossal tract that attaches to the larynx by the peritracheal fascia.
- There is tenderness, redness, and swelling of the mass, if infected.
- A small opening in the skin near the mass, with drainage of mucous from the cyst.
- Infected cyst causes difficulty in swallowing, and breathing, and fever.
- Lingual thyroglossal cyst may cause feeding problems and airway obstruction in neonates.
- As the cyst enlarges it expands the buccal cortical plate between maxillary lateral incisors and canines.

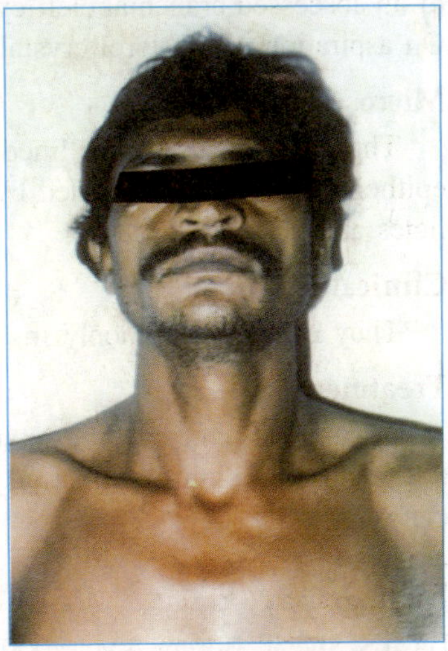

Fig.18.1: Showing cystic swelling in neck (Thyroglossal cyst)

Complications

Infection is probably the most common complication. Papillary carcinoma of thyroid occurs in 1% to 2% of patients.

Microscopically

Well-defined cysts with an epithelial lining composed of either squamous or respiratory epithelium. There are sometimes islands of thyroid tissue lying in the walls of the cysts. Cysts are filled with mucoid or mucopurulent material, depending on whether the cyst has been infected.

Treatment

Antibiotics are indicated if there is infection. Surgical excision serves as a radical cure for lingual thyroglossal duct cyst.

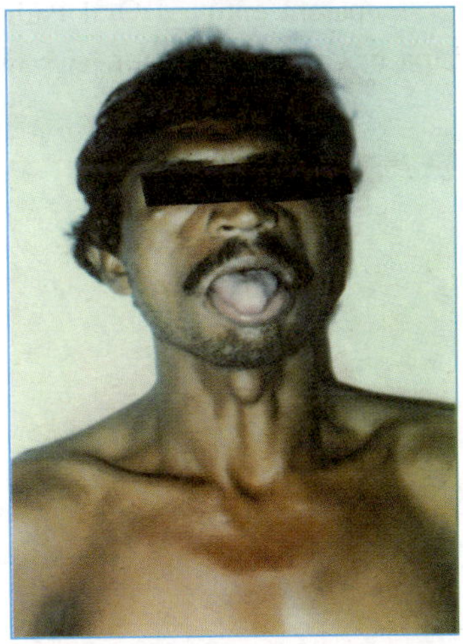

Fig.18.2: Showing cystic swelling in neck, moves with deglutition (Thyroglossal cyst)

XII. BRANCHIAL CYST NECK

It is also called lymphoepithelial cyst or branchial cleft cyst.

In embryonic life, the second branchial arch migrates over the third and fourth branchial arch. The resulting cleft is the cervical sinus and accumulation of secretions leads to the formation of a branchial cyst. Failure of fusion of the second arch with the sixth arch results in branchial fistulas.

These are congenital cysts that appear from non-closure of branchial clefts. Branchial cysts are thought to develop from cystic degeneration of epithelium enclosed in cervical lymph nodes, and cyst becomes apparent in 3rd decades.

Clinical features

The branchial cysts occur as smooth, ovoid, thin-walled cystic structures deep to the sternomastoid, near the bifurcation of the carotid artery. Lateral branchial cysts are located in the anterolateral part of neck and most commonly of mandible, anterior to sternomastoid muscle. The cysts usually measure less than 2 cm in diameter. Some cysts are between 5 to 10 cm.

Many branchial cysts are asymptomatic. The lump is not freely mobile as it is deep to sternomastoid. Overlying skin is normal, though, if infected, may be red and angry-looking. They may become tender, enlarged or inflamed, or they may develop abscesses, especially during periods of upper respiratory tract infection, due to lymphoid tissue located beneath the epithelium. Spontaneous rupture of an abscessed branchial cleft cyst may result in purulent draining sinus to the skin or the pharynx. On aspiration, cholesterol crystals can be demonstrated in the aspirated fluid.

Microscopically

These are cystic lesions lined by stratified squamous or pseudostratified squamous or columnar epithelium and are surrounded by abundant lymphoid tissue, sometimes with reactive germinal follicles and germinal centers.

Clinical features

They occur uncommonly in early childhood.

Treatment

Treatment is conservative, or surgical excision. As complete surgical excision may be difficult (due to the close proximity of internal jugular vein and carotid vessels that lie deep to the swelling), they can recur.

Bibliography

Basu S, Shet T, Borges AM: (2009) Outcome of papillary carcinoma thyroglossal with local infiltration of soft tissue. Indian Journal of Cancer: Volume 46(2) 170-172.

Gardener DG, Kessler H, Morency R, Schaffner D: (1988). The glandular odontogenic cyst: An apparent entity. J Oral Pathology 17:359-366

Lipa b: Cystic lesions of jaws in children. Ind Journal Pedia Otorhinolaryngol 2002; 62:25-29.

CHAPTER

19

BENIGN TUMOURS OF ORAL CAVITY

INTRODUCTION

Neoplasm or tumour is an abnormal mass of new growth characterised by purposeless, progressive, uncoordinated, and autonomous proliferation of cells, which persists after the stimulus—which initiated it—has been withdrawn.

Neoplasms are broadly divided into two categories—benign and malignant.

Characteristics of benign tumours

1. **Rate of growth:** Benign tumours grow slowly and, after reaching a size, may remain stationary.
2. **Size of tumour:** Many benign tumours become very large.
3. **Shape:** Benign tumours are generally spherical and ovoid in shape. They are well- capsulated.
4. Benign tumours do not have the capacity to metastasise.
5. Recurrence of benign tumour is not common.
6. Benign neoplasms are usually fully differentiated, e.g., they closely resemble normal tissue—both histologically and cytologically.
7. As benign tumour grows, it causes compression of adjacent tissues.

TABLE 19.1
CLASSIFICATION OF BENIGN TUMOURS AND TUMOUR-LIKE LESIONS OF THE ORAL SOFT TISSUES

I. **Epithelial tumours**

- Squamous papilloma
- Verrucous xanthoma
- Squamous acanthoma
- Nevus

Contd.

Contd.

II. Mesenchymal tumours

A. Fibrous connective tissue
- Fibroma
- Fibrous hyperplasia
- Fibrous histiocytoma
- Fibrous epulis
- Giant cell fibroma
- Desmoplastic fibroma

B. Myxomatous tissue
- Myxoma
- Myxofibroma

C. Vascular tissue
- Haemangioma
- Hereditary haemorrhagic telangiectasia
- Glomus tumour
- Lymphangioma
- Arteriovenous fistula

D. Muscle tissue
- Leiomyoma
- Granular cell myoblastoma
- Rhabdomyoma

E. Nerve tissue
- Neurofibroma
- Schwannoma
- Traumatic neuroma
- Ganglioneuroma

F. Adipose tissue
- Lipoma
- Angiolipoma

G. Bone
- Osteoma
- Osteoblastoma
- Osteoid osteoma
- Osteochondroma

H. Cartilage tissue
- Chondroma
- Chondroblastoma
- Mesenchymoma
- Chondromyxoid fibroma
- Lymphoid patches
- Plasmacytoma

TUMOUR LIKE-LESIONS

The **'Epulis'** is an old term, which means **'upon the gum'**. So **'epulis'** is a swelling situated on the gum. It arises from the alveolar margin of the jaw. It can originate from the bone, periosteum, or the mucous membrane.

EPULIS

FIBROUS EPULIS

1. It is the commonest type of epulis.

Clinical features

- **Site:** It arises from periosteum, at the neck of an incisor or premolar tooth. As it grows, it separates the teeth and ultimately loosens them.
- It is more common in females, in the ratio of 4 : 1.
- It is a firm nodule at the junction of the gum and tooth.
- It becomes polypoid in shape.
- It is a slow-growing tumour.
- It is often seen in relation to the incisor or premolar tooth.
- It is not tender.

- The adjacent tooth may be slightly separated and be loosened.
- Draining lymph nodes are not enlarged.
- Rarely, a soft bluish-red, bleeding and rapidly growing fibrosarcomatous epulis occurs.

Microscopically: It is fibroma and is composed of fusiform cells with many new blood vessels.

Management

Excision of lesions with neighbouring normal tissue is the treatment of choice.

GRANULOMATOUS EPULIS

Clinical features

- The mass looks bright red.
- It is soft and firm in feel.
- It easily bleeds on touch, as it is a mass of granulation tissue.
- It is often associated with carious teeth, so it is found in those who do not maintain oral hygiene.

2. GIANT CELL EPULIS

It is a giant cell reparative granuloma rather than a neoplasm.

Jaffe introduced the term giant cell reparative granuloma in 1953 to describe an apparently intraosseous lesion of mandible and maxilla following trauma-induced intraosseous haemorrhage and containing prominent giant cells.

Two forms of giant cell reparative granuloma are described:

1. **Central:** Arising from bone.
2. **Peripheral:** Arising from the soft tissue of maxilla and mandible, involving gingival and alveolar mucosa.

CENTRAL GIANT CELL GRANULOMA

Central giant cell granuloma is a benign intraosseous lesion found in the anterior of maxilla and mandible in younger age people (before age 20).

Cause

Chronic trauma plays a major role in the etiology of this lesion, which occurs on anterior gingiva. Marked growth of the lesion associated with pregnancy has been described, presumably related to hormonal stimulation.

Clinically

Age: It is a disease of the young, presenting as a painless swelling in the anterior jaw.

Site: Commonest site is anterior part of mandible between the second premolar and second molar with extension across the midline.

Sex: Females are affected more frequently (2 : 1 ratio) than males.

Microscopically: It is composed of osteolytic-like multinucleated giant cells. The distribution of giant cells is patchy, usually associated with areas of haemorrhage. Stroma is highly cellular and vascular. Often, new bone formation is seen. Proliferated cells include fibroblasts, myofibrils, and histiocytes.

Radiographically: Appearing as a lytic expansile lesion with a characteristic tendency of resorbing the root tips of adjacent unerupted teeth.

Treatment

The treatment of central giant cell granuloma is curettage.

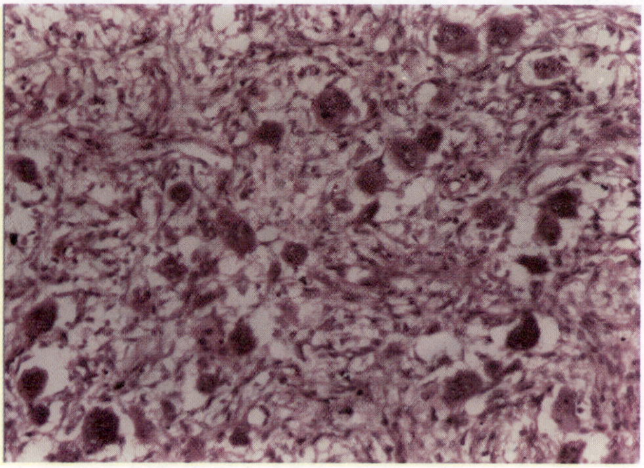

Fig.19.1: Showing multinucleated giant cells in and fibrous vascular stroma

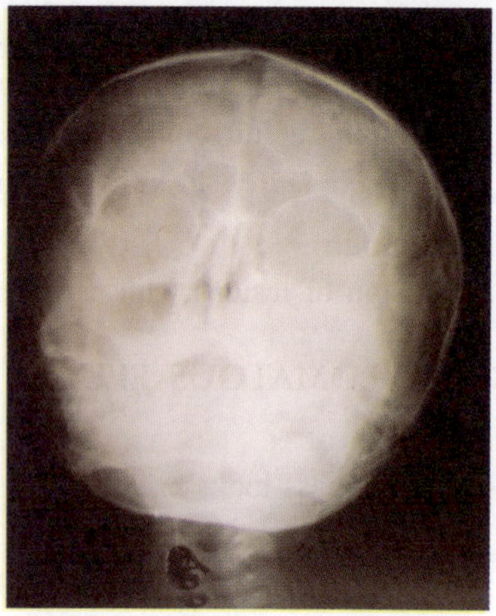

Fig.19.2: Shows X-ray findings in case of reparative granuloma in right maxilla

PERIPHERAL GIANT CELL GRANULOMA

It is the second-most common growth of gingival followed by the common pyogenic granuloma.

Clinical findings

Age: Vast majority of lesions occur after the age of 20 years, 40% in the fourth and fifth decades. It is more common in females.

Clinical examination shows a dusky purple, sessile or pedunculated, smooth-surfaced, dome-shaped papule or nodule.

Size: Most lesions are less than 1.5 cm in diameter, though, infrequently, a peripheral giant cell granuloma may grow as 5 cm in greatest dimension. In 50% of cases, ulcerations are present.

Site: The lesion is always located on the alveolar mucosa or the gingival, and 70% are found in the anterior segments of the jaws, such as in the premolar, canines, and incisor regions. It appears on the gingival or on an edentulous (without teeth) alveolar margin.

Underlying alveolar bone can be destroyed, leaving a unique appearance referred to as **'cupping resorption'** or **'saucerisation'**.

Microscopically

Giant cell granuloma consists of plump spindle or ovoid mononuclear cells. Interspersed within this tissue are plenty of benign multinucleated giant cells. The giant cells are large and round or small and irregular; they vary in size and shape. There is evidence that these giant cells represent osteoclasts, others suggest more like macrophages. Areas of necrosis, haemorrhage, lipid-laden macrophages and cholesterol are sometimes seen.

Radiologically: It appears as multilocular radiolucencies of bone.

Cause

The cause of peripheral giant cell granuloma is unknown, although local irritation due to dental plaque or calculus, periodontal disease, poor dental restorations, ill-fitting dental appliances, or dental extractions have been suggested to contribute to the development of the lesion.

Recent reports have described the development of the peripheral giant cell granuloma in association with dental implant.

Treatment

Treatment usually involves surgical removal of the lesion down to the bone. If there are any adjacent teeth, they are cleaned thoroughly to remove any possible source of irritation. Recurrence is common in 10% of cases.

Congenital epulis of newborn

Epulis is a rare tumour of the newborn, also known as granular cell tumour of the newborn, or Neumann's tumour.

Clinical features

Site: Tumour arises from the mucosa of the gingival, most commonly from the anterior part of the maxillary gingival, anterior part of the maxillary alveolar ridge, and is typically seen as a mass protruding out of the newborn child's mouth, which may interfere with respiration or feeding.

Sex: The tumour has a marked female preponderance.

Macroscopically: The size varies from several millimeters to 7.5 cm.

Microscopically: The tumour is composed of diffuse sheets and clusters of polygonal cells containing small round to oval nuclei and abundant coarsely granular cytoplasm.

The tumour cells are positive for vimentin, and negative for S100-protein, actin, desmin, laminin, keratin, estrogen, and progesterone receptors.

Electron microscopic examination showed granular cells containing heterogeneous electron-dense granules, lysosomes, and cytoplasmic lipid droplets.

PYOGENIC GRANULOMA

Synonyms: Lobular capillary haemangioma or granuloma pyogenicum. Pyogenic granuloma was originally described in 1897 by two French surgeons, Poncet and Dor, who named this lesion olyomycosis hominis.

Clinical features

Females are affected more than males.

Sites: It mostly involves anterior gingival but sometimes the other sites such as tongue, buccal mucosa, or lips, palate and frenum.

Age: Pyogenic granuloma is rare in children younger than 6 months. The mean age of presentation is 6.7 years. It is commonly seen in between 11 to 40 years.

Causes

The cause of the typical pyogenic granuloma is not known. Trauma, hormonal influences, Bartonella species seropositivity, viral oncogens, underlying microscopic arteriovenous malformations, production of angiogenetic factors, and cytogenetic clonal deletion abnormalities have been implicated while trauma was long considered as primary cause.

Pyogenic granuloma often arises in pregnancy—particularly on the gingival or elsewhere in the oral mucosa—and then is termed as **'pregnancy tumour'**.

Pyogenic granulomas are most often seen in people taking certain oral retinoid medications, including isotretinoin (accutane) or acitretin.

It is seen in people taking protease inhibitors such as indinavin.

It is common in people on chemotherapy.

Visual appearance

1. Solitary, red, purple or yellow papule or nodule arising from normal mucosa. Usually it is soft, smooth, and reddish to purple mass, which bleeds on touch.

2. Size varies from a few millimetres to several centimetres.
3. Polypoid appearance—often develops a stalk or collarets of scale at the base.
4. Friable lesion—often seen to be bleeding, crusted or ulcerated.

Microscopically: Early lesions resemble granulation tissue (numerous capillaries and venules) with plump endothelial cells arrayed radially towards the surface amidst oedematous stroma containing a mixed inflammatory infiltrate.

Prognosis

1. Pyogenic granulomas are benign lesions.
2. Untreated lesions with atrophy eventually but only a minority spontaneously involutes within six months.
3. Recurrence rates following treatment can be quite high—4-5.5%—regardless of treatment modality.
4. Pregnancy tumour tends to regress spontaneously following childbirth—so treatment should be postponed accordingly.

Management

Surgical excision, but many of these lesions regress spontaneously.

PALATAL AND MANDIBULAR TORI

Tori are benign, non-neoplastic, bony protuberances that arise from the cortical plate. They are sometimes mistaken for malignancies. These exostoses are considered developmental anomalies, although they usually do not appear until adulthood. A torus located along the midline of the hard palate is called a palatal torus, or torus palatinus and a torus located along the lingual aspect of the mandible is called mandibular torus, or torus mandibularis.

Palatal tori

Incidence: Palatal tori are reported to 20 to 35% of the United State population with similar findings between blacks and whites. Palatal tori are more common in Asian and Inuit populations. The prevalence of palatal tori forms 9 - 60% and are more common than bony growths occurring on the mandible, known as torus mandibularis.

Age: Palatal tori are twice common in females.

Site: Palatal tori are a bony growth on the palate and are usually present on the midline of the hard palate.

Clinical features

Most palatal tori are less than 2 cm in diameter, but their size can change throughout life. Sometimes the tori are categorised by their appearances:

1. Arising as a broad base and smooth surface, flat tori are located on the midline of the palate and extend symmetrically to either side.
2. Spindle tori have a ridge located at their midline.
3. Nodular tori have multiple bony growths—each has its own base.
4. Lobular tori have multiple bony growths with a common base.

Causes

Although some research suggest palatal tori to be an autosomal dominant trait, they are more common in early adult life and can increase in size. In some older people, the size of the tori may decrease due to bone resorption.

Microscopically: It is usually composed of compact bone or cancellous bone surrounded by a capsule of compact bone.

Mandibular tori

Mandibular tori are common in Asians and Inuit populations, and slightly more common in males.

Cause

A definite genetic basis has been established for the trait. It is inherited as an autosomal dominant trait with 100% penetrance in female and 70% penetrance in males. Masticatory stress is reported as an essential factor underlying the formation.

Clinical features

There is no gender predilection.

It can exist as a single bump or as a cluster of bone bumps like an arrangement of grapes and is often located on the inside of the premolar area. Torus mandibularis refers to an exostosis on the lingual side of the mandible. It may be single-or multilobed. The overlying epithelium may be hypertrophic or blanched.

Microscopically: The tumour shows a dense mass of cortical lamellated bone.

Treatment

The bone bumps are harmless and do not need treatment till removable dentures have to be made.

EPITHELIAL TUMOURS

SQUAMOUS CELL PAPILLOMA

The papilloma is a benign hyperplastic lesion of stratified squamous epithelium.

Cause

Squamous papilloma is caused by HPV-6 and HPV-11.

Clinical features

The benign epithelial neoplasm constitutes about 2% of all oral biopsy specimens. This is most commonly seen during the 3rd and 4th decades of life. The mean age of oral papilloma is about 35 years. The hard and soft palate and uvula are the most common sites but the lesion can occur anywhere in the oral mucosa (tongue, gingival, buccal mucosa, lips, cheek, and larynx).

Clinically, the oral papilloma is a white—sometimes pink—lesion, pedunculated, cauliflower-like growth. Lesions within the oral cavity are soft; whereas those on the exposed areas of the lips are usually rough and scaly. The lesion is usually a single lesion (not more than 0.5 cm in size).

Microscopically

Cauliflower-like lesion that has a narrow stalk and formed by many finger-like projections. The tumour consists of a central core of connective tissue, containing blood vessels and inflammatory cells reaching near about the surface and covered by stratified squamous epithelium. The epithelium shows a thick surface keratin (usually parakeratin). Superficial layer of squamous epithelium shows presence of koilocytes.

Management

Surgical excision including the base of the lesion is the treatment for squamous papilloma.

VERRUCIFORM XANTHOMA

It is also known as histiocytosis Y.

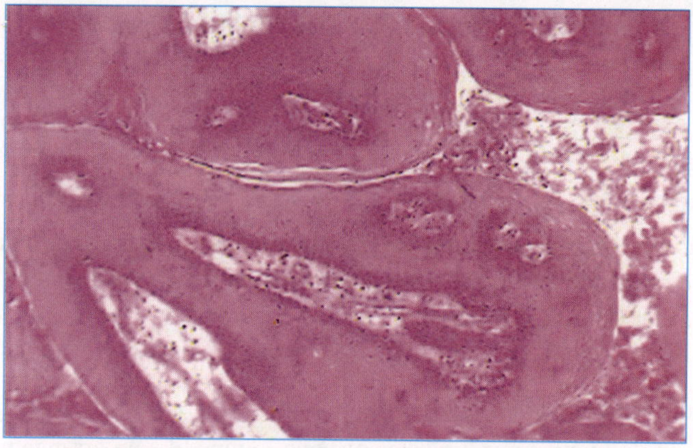

Fig.19.3: Shows finger-like projections with central core (squamous papilloma)

Etiology

Human papilloma virus 6 was detected in a verrucous xanthoma by electron microscopy, immunochemistry, and polymerase chain reaction.

Clinical features

Verrucous xanthoma is an uncommon lesion that occurs on the oral mucosa of middle-aged persons (mean age 40-51 years). It is more common in females. It can occur at any site and is most frequently seen on the gingival, or alveolar ridge, followed by the bucccal mucosa, palate, floor of the mouth, lip, and lower mucobuccal fold.

The lesion may appear as verrucous, papillary, or flat-to-lichenoid process varying from 0.2-2 cm in diameter. Depending on degree of the keratinisation, the xanthoma may appear grey to reddish-pink.

Microscopically: Verruciform xanthoma is a benign lesion of the oral mucosa, histologically characterised by the presence of numerous foam cells in the connective tissue papillae.

Management

Treatment of choice for verrucous xanthoma is surgical excision and recurrence is rare.

NEVI

In 1943, Field and Ackerman reported the first documented case of an intraoral nevus. Oral nevus is considered to be a developmental anomaly or hamartomas rather than a neoplasm.

Nevi are benign proliferations of nevus cells located either entirely within the epithelium, in both the epithelium and underlying stroma, or in the subepithelial stroma alone.

Oral nevi are classified into intramucosal nevus, compound nevus, junctional nevus, halo nevus, blue nevus and spitz nevus.

Nevi may be classified into congenital or acquired:

Congenital nevi of the oral cavity are rare. Their architecture is quite compact and pigment is synthesised even in the depth of the lesion.

Lesions show large and deep aggregates of melanocytes organised in sheets. Neither mitoses nor cellular pleomorphism are present but only high cellular density of the lesion. The lesion is large—up to 3 centimetres can be present.

Oral nevi are reported more frequently in whites, in whom 55% of reported oral nevi occurred.

Intramucosal nevus

The intraoral nevus is usually intramucosal nevus. The lesion is usually 4-6 mm in greatest diameter; the most common sites of oral involvement are hard palate, buccal mucosa, and gingival.

The oral intramucosal nevus presents as an uncapsulated proliferation of nevus cells within the subepithelial stroma. Lesional cells are often clustered together and are usually ovoid and uniform in size. Most superficial cells are usually epitheloid and frequently contain intracellular melanin, while nevus cells of the midportion of the nodule have less cytoplasm, are seldom pigmented and appear much like lymphocytes. Deeper nevus cells appear elongated and spindle-shaped, much like Schwann cells and fibroblasts.

Junctional nevus

Junctional nevus is extremely rare in oral cavity. It accounts for proximately 4% of reported intraoral nevi. They are most commonly found in children. Junctional nevi are flat or slightly raised, brown-tan papules. This common condition develops on hair bearing and glabrous skin. Nevi of palms, soles, genitalia and mucosa are usually junctional nevi. As they enlarge, they become slightly raised and can evolve into an intradermal or a compound nevus or a malignant change.

Microscopically, it is characterised by nests of nevus cells along the basal layer of the epithelium. The nevi cells are cuboidal, oval, or spindle shaped. Cytoplasm is distinctly outlined. Nuclei are large round or oval. Some of these cells drop off into underlying connective tissue, showing junctional activity.

Compound nevi

These are found in adolescents and are usually benign. This is the commonest type of pigmented nevus in late childhood. It is rare in oral cavity, representing about 6-8.5% of all oral nevi. It is located on the buccal mucosa, the palate and the gingival.

Compound nevi are slightly to markedly raised pigmented papule. The surface may be smooth or slightly papillomatous. Size varies from a few millimetres to 1cm in diameter.

Microscopically: Compound nevi show junctional activity in the overlying epithelium. In the subepithelial tissue there are loose aggregates of rounded inactive cells, some of which contain granules of melanin pigment. Compound nevi may be transformed into malignant melanoma.

Blue nevus

Tieche, a student of Jadassohn, first described the common blue nevus in 1906.

Blue common nevus is the second-most common type found in oral cavity. Blue nevi account for 25-36% of all oral nevi. Blue nevus is usually seen in females in their fourth decade of life. It is typically found on the hard or soft palate, it presents as flat to slightly elevated, smooth surfaced macular or dome shaped, or plaque that is blue-black lesion less than 1 cm in diameter.

Microscopically: Biopsy from lesion shows submucosal aggregation of elongated, slender melanocytes with intracellular melanin deposition and branching dendritic extensions. These cells usually align themselves parallel to the surface epithelium and may be quite deep within the subepithelial stroma.

Halo nevus

The oral halo nevus appears as a central pigmented papule or macule with a surrounding zone of pallor which may be as much as 1.5 cm in diameter.

Treatment

No treatment is required for any of the histologic subtypes of the oral mucosal nevus. However, surgical excision is recommended when the nevus is located at a site of chronic irritation or exhibits any change in its appearance.

FIBROMA

Fibroma is a benign tumour mainly composed of connective tissue.

This lesion is quite rare; the prevalence in Sweden is 3.25% of the population.

Cause

Oral fibromas form as a result of irritation or masticatory trauma, especially along the buccal occlusal line.

Clinical features

The fibromas can occur in any age group but are common in the fourth to sixth decades of life and equally in males and females. They are usually painless, but if they are in a position where they can be bitten or injured, there may be pain, discomfort and bleeding.

The fibroma is asymptomatic and can be located at all sites of the oral and oropharyngeal mucosa. It is common in gingival, lips, and buccal mucosa along the occlusal plane of maxillary and mandibular arch.

The fibroma is usually manifested as solid, well-demarcated, rounded structure covered by ordinary mucosa. It is hard or soft, pale or reddish, depending on the density of collagen and abundance of vascularity.

Microscopic section reveals a tumour consisting of fibroblasts and collagen fibres in varying proportion underlying a stratified squamous epithelium. The epithelium may be hyperkeratotic, either hyperplastic or atrophic or even ulcerated.

Management

Treatment of choice is surgical excision.

FIBROUS HISTIOCYTOMA

It is also known as fibroxanthoma. It may occur on the sun-exposed skin but rarely arises in the oral cavity.

Clinical features

- Both sexes are affected, between 8 and 70 years old.
- Buccal mucosa is the most common site of involvement, followed by the tongue, the lower lip, palate and gingival.
- Clinically it appears painless, mobile, and firm tumour covered by normal epithelium, which may be ulcerated.
- Size of the tumour ranges between 0.5 and 2 cm.
- There is displacement of regional teeth.

Microscopically

Surgical specimen consists of uniform spindle-shaped cells arranged in a storiform pattern. It is mainly composed of a mixture of fibroblast and histiocytes. Lipid laden macrophages and multinucleated giant cells are also commonly seen in certain tumours. There is no evidence of cellular atypia or mitotic figures.

Immunohistochemically, the tumour cells are negative for the actin (HHF-35) and CD34. The cells are positive for CD68, ALPHA-1 anti-chymotrypsin, ALPHA-1-antitrypsin, and vimentin.

Fibrous histiocytomas have cytogenitic abnormalities that give rise to a fusion gene derived from platelet derived growth factor β (PDGF-β) and collagen type 1α (COL1A1). This fusion gene is believed to give rise to an autocrine loop of PDGF-β.

Treatment

Wide local excision is the treatment of choice in these cases.

Involved teeth should be extracted.

MYXOMA

Myxoma is an uncommon tumour of the primitive mesenchyme.

Clinical features

Myxoma is the most common primary tumour of the heart but can occur in oral cavity, striated muscle, subcutaneously, genitourinary tract and retroperitoneal area.

Intraorally, it occurs on the buccal mucosa, tongue and retromolar area.

Microscopically: The tumour shows features of myxomatous tissue containing a homogeneous intercellular matrix and branching or stellate myxomatous cell, irregular in shape with deeply stained nuclei and long fibrillary processes.

The myxomas are not encapsulated and tend to infiltrate the surrounding tissue.

Nerve sheath myxoma is a benign peripheral nerve sheath tumour that rarely occurs in oral cavity.

Osseous myxomas are rare, slowly growing, locally invasive, benign tumours that generally arise in second and third decades of life. It is reported in maxilla.

BLOOD VESSELS AND LYMPHATICS

HAEMANGIOMA

Haemangiomas of the oral cavity are often present at birth or shortly thereafter. Most haemangiomas appear within a week or two after birth. They are tumours of infancy and childhood and constitute 7% of all benign tumours.

They have a strong preference for occurrence in the tongue, lips and floor of the mouth. Intramuscular haemangiomas in the oral region are most commonly seen in the masseter, comprising 5% of all intramuscular haemangioma.

Clinically

The tumour appears as a flat or raised reddish-blue lesion and is generally solitary. Cavernous haemangiomas are blue, soft, spongy masses that are not capsulated. Although haemangiomas of tongue are asymptomatic, they could sometimes cause significant bleeding, pain, or difficulty in chewing, speaking, and even swallowing.

Haemangiomas are classified on the basis of their histological appearance as capillary, mixed, cavernous, or a sclerosing variety that tends to undergo fibrosis.

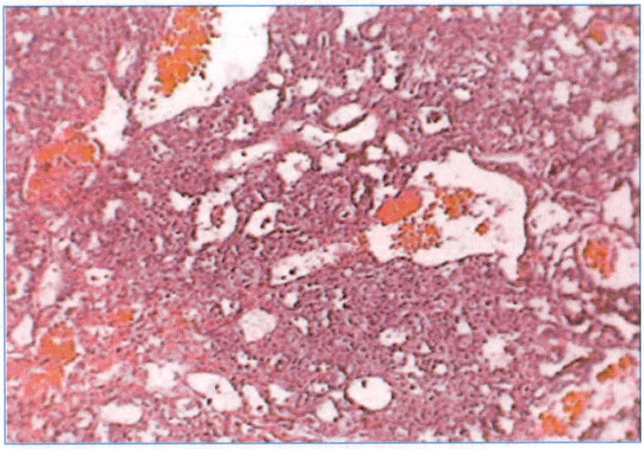

Fig.19.4: Capillary haemangioma

Capillary haemangioma

The tumour is composed of tuft of proliferating thin-walled capillaries. It consists of network of newly formed blood vessels filled with blood. Endothelial cells lining the blood vessels are large and swollen. Endothelial proliferation is marked, may produce solid buds of cells, become several layers deep occluding the lumen. Majority of capillary haemangioma regress spontaneously.

Cavernous haemangioma

It has the structure of erectile tissue, being composed of large spaces. Blood spaces are separated from one another by scanty connective tissue stroma. The thin-walled caverns (blood spaces) or sinusoids are limited by flattened endothelium and freely communicate with one another. Thrombosis is fairly common in blood spaces.

When haemangiomas undergo regression, extensive sclerosis can occur, sometimes followed by calcification, such concretions are called phleboliths.

Occasionally, mature bone may be seen.

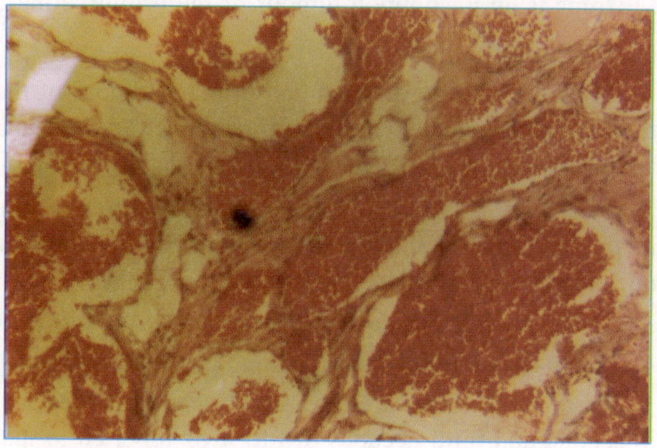

Fig.19.5: Showing large vascular spaces separated by scanty connective tissue

Cause

The causes of vasoformative tumours are unknown. One hypothesis postulates that placental cells, such as the trophoblast, may be the cell of origin for haemangiomas. Therefore, haemanigomas may arise secondary to some event in utero. One study found placenta associated vascular antigens to be expressed by haemangiomas but not by other vascular malformation.

LYMPHANGIOMA

Lymphangiomas and cystic hygromas are rare benign hamartomatous lesions of lymphatic systems.

Whites appear to be affected more often than people of other races.

These are tumours consisting of well-formed lymph spaces lined by endothelium and supported by fibrous stroma.

Cause

Lymphangioma are the result of sequestration of lymphatic tissue that has retained its potential for growth and do not communicate with other lymphatic tissue. Embryologically, it is derived from five primitive buds developing from the venous system which include paired jugular sacs, paired posterior sacs and single retroperitoneal sac.

Types

Some authorities prefer to subclassify lymphangiomas into four categories:

1. Lymphangioma simplex (lymphangioma circumscripta, capillary lymphangioma) composed of small thin-walled capillaries.
2. Cavernous lymphangioma composed of dilated lymphatic vessels with surrounding adventitia.
3. Cystic lymphangioma.
4. Benign lymphoepithelioma (acquired progressive lymphangioma) consisting of huge, macroscopic lymphatic channels appear to be dissecting through dense collagenic bundles.

Clinical features

Oral mucosal lymphangiomas almost always becomes apparent prior to third year of life, half of all cases are congenital.

Site: In the mouth lymphangiomas are seen most frequently on the tongue, lip, buccal mucosa and cheek. Of lymphatic malformations of the oral cavity, 40-50% involve the tongue, which is preferred site of intraoral involvement. Patients tend to have speech disturbances, poor oral hygiene, and bleeding from the tongue associated with oral trauma.

Dilatation and diffuse growth of vessels may give rise to macroglossia. The lesion of the tongue is usually superficial and appears in clusters with surface simulating frog eggs.

Microscopically: The tumour consists of anastomosising spaces lined by flat or conical epithelium filled with clear fluid containing a few lymphocytes. The stroma is composed of fibrous tissue. Lymphatic vessels are seen below squamous epithelium with extension into deeper connective tissue and muscles.

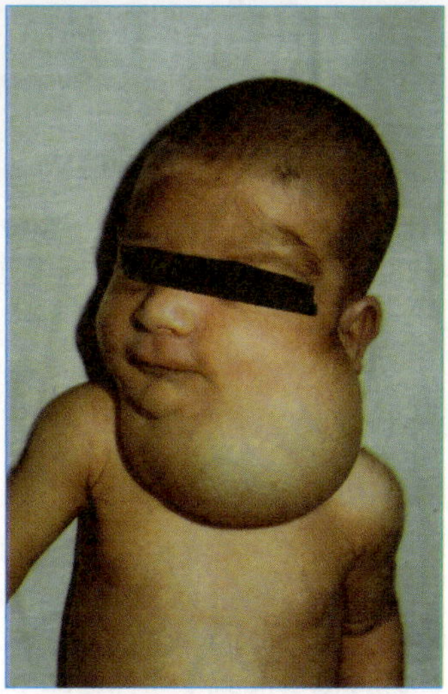

Fig.19.6: Showing swelling in neck. A case of cystic hygroma

Management

The various treatment modalities for lymphangiomas are surgical excision, radiation therapy, cryotherapy, electrocautery, sclerotherapy, steroid administration, embolisation and ligation.

NEURAL TISSUE

GRANULAR CELL MYOBLASTOMA

It is also known as 'Abrikosov's tumour', 'myoblastic myoma', 'granular cell tumour' or 'granular cell Schwannoma'.

Clinical features

Granular cell myoblastoma is a nerve sheath tumour occasionally seen on the lateral and dorsal surfaces of the tongue, lips, vocal cord and floor of the mouth. Other sites are skin, breast, and subcutaneous tissues. It is usually presents as a raised, domed nodule or an even more raised polyp, smoothed surface, non-ulcerated growth of the mucus membrane. Its size is variable, from a few millimetres up to a few centimetres.

Microscopic appearance

The tumour consists of large polyhedral cells with acidophilic granular cytoplasm. The size of the cell varies from 20 to 40 microns in diameter. No signs of cellular or nuclear pleomorphism or any mitotic activity exist. In about 50% of cases the overlying epithelium shows pseudoepitheliomatous hyperplasia. Ultra-structurally, the small pyknotic granules represent lysosomal structure. The granules are PAS positive and Sudan B-positive.

Histogenesis of granular cell myoblastoma is not settled; the three important views are (i) Myogenous origin, (ii) origin from Schwann cells, and (iii) origin from fibroblasts of peripheral nerves.

NEUROFIBROMA

Neurofibromas are non-capsulated focal or diffuse proliferations of Schwann cells and fibroblasts of nerve sheaths.

The neurofibroma is asymptomatic and rarely occurs as a single lesion. Most often neurofibromas are part of von-Recklinghausen's disease. Quite often the tongue is involved, in some cases resulting in unilateral macroglossia. Other sites include mandibular canal, buccal mucosa, and alveolar ridge.

Microscopic appearance: Neurofibromas consists of proliferating spindle-shaped Schwann cells and sparse or abundant collagenous tissue arranged haphazardly around nerve fibres. The structure is loose-textured and oedematous, and palisading is usually absent. Distorted fibrils of the affected nerve may be found scattered in the tumour tissue.

TRAUMATIC NEUROMA

It is also known as ***'pseudoneuroma'*** or ***'amputation neuroma'***.

A traumatic neuroma is a reactive hyperplasia caused by injury of a nerve due to fracture, dissection, removal of cyst, nerve avulsion for neuralgia or even extraction of teeth. .

Clinically: Traumatic neuromas may occur anywhere in the oral cavity. Most common sites are region of the mental foramen, lips, tongue and within the jaw. They are seen in middle-aged adults.

The lesions usually present as movable nodules in the oral mucosa that may be painful.

Microscopically: In this type of neuroma, small bundles of axons appear randomly oriented; organised layers containing Schwann cell, fibroblasts, and perineural cells, however, surround each.

NEUROFIBROMATOSIS

It is also known as von Recklinghausen's disease of the skin or **'Fibroma Molluscum'**.

The incidence is estimated in 1 in 300 live births. It is an autosomal dominant inherited disorder affecting the ectodermal tissues. The inheritance is autosomal dominant; the gene locus is 17Q 11.2. The pathogenesis is believed defect in neurofibrin gene. Neurofibrin is a suppressor of products of photooncogenes, and its loss leads to tumour progression. Neurofibromatosis MF2 is caused by mutation in a gene on chromosome 22, which codes for a protein that has been termed schannomin or mertin by different workers.

Associated lesions include pigmented skin areas (café-au-lait—milk-coffee—spots), hamartomas of the iris, skeletal deformities and numerous other abnormalities.

SCHWANNOMA

Schwannoma is a benign neoplasm composed of Schwann's cells of the nerve fibres. Tongue, palate, cheek mucosa, lip and gingival are the most frequent locations in the oral cavity. Schwannoma may occur on any cranial or spinal nerve. They are most frequently located on acoustic nerve and on the dorsal root of spinal nerve.

Lingual Schwannomas are usually benign, slow-growing, solitary, grey, firm and encapsulated tumour, sometimes cystic lesions are seen.

Microscopically: The tumour is composed of spindle cells considered to be Schwann cells.

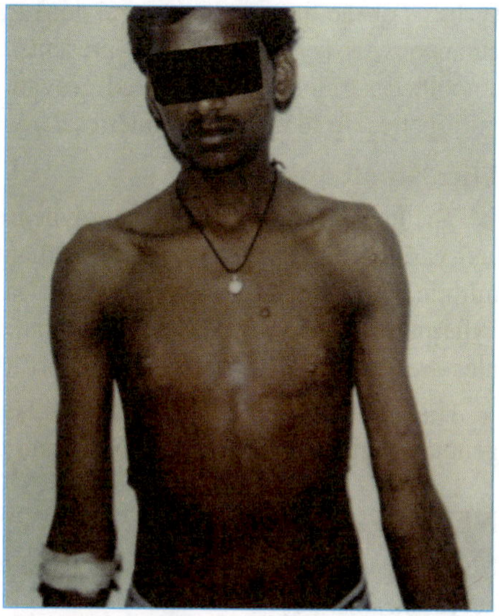

Fig.19.7: A case of von Recklinghausen's disease

Two main patterns are seen

1. Antony A tissue, in which there is a dense accumulation of elongated cells often with nuclear pallisading. Fascicular tissue presents a solid complex appearance almost like an exaggerated tactile corpuscle, known as Verocay body.
2. Antony B tissue, where cells are less densely arranged in a loose myxoid matrix, within which xanthoma cells may be present. These tumours contain hyalinised blood vessels and may show evidence of previous haemorrhage. Nerve fibres can usually be found streched over the capsule but not within the tumour. In exceptional cases melanin pigmentation is found.

   Immunohistochemistry shows a strong positive reaction for S100 protein and Leu 7.

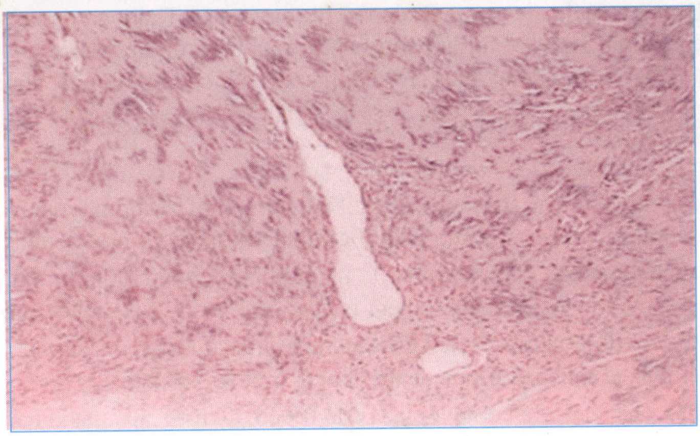

Fig.19.8: Showing microscopic appearance of schwannoma

ADIPOSE TISSUE

LIPOMA

Lipoma is a very common benign tumour of adipose tissue, but its presence in the oral and oropharyngeal region is relatively uncommon, with a prevalence rate of only 1/5,000 adults. They occur commonly in subcutaneous tissues, the neck, back, breast, abdominal wall, forehead and buttocks.

Incidence of lipoma in the oral cavity is between approximately 1.0% and 4.5% of all oral lesions.

Age and Sex: Most of the cases affected are adults from 40 to 60 years of age but can be found in children. Solitary lipomas are seen predominantly in women and multiple lipomas occur more in men.

Sites: Oral lipomas occur at various sites including the major salivary glands, buccal mucosa, lip, tongue, palate, vestibule, and floor of the mouth.

Etiology

Possible aetiological factors in aetiology of lipoma are:

1. Lipoblastic embryonic cell nest in origin
2. Metaphase of muscle cells
3. Fatty degeneration
4. Hereditary
5. Hormonal cause
6. Trauma
7. Infection
8. Chronic irritation
9. Infarction.

Macroscopically: The lesion may be pedunculated or sessile and occasional cases show surface bosselation. Once present, a mucosal oral lipoma may increase to 5-6 cm over a period of years, but most cases are less than 3 cm in greatest dimension at diagnosis. The tumour is soft, elastic, well-circumscribed or lobulated, encapsulated and easily shelled out. Cut surface is pale yellow and greasy to touch.

Microscopically: The lipoma is composed predominantly of mature adipocytes, possibly admixed with collagenic streaks, and is often well-demarcated from the surrounding connective tissues. Fat cells showing unstained empty areas with nuclei are pushed to one side of the cells. The cells are irregular in size. Blood vessels are seen within the fibrous septa. There are areas of calcification and myxomatous degeneration. Signs of inflammation infiltration of inflammatory cells occur sometimes. Based on morphological features, lipomas are sub-classified into fibrolipoma, angiolipoma, myolipoma, and pleomorphic lipoma.

RHABDOMYOMA

Rhabdomyoma is a lesion of striated muscle. Two types of rhabdomyomas are neoplastic and hamartoma. The neoplastic variety is sub-classified into adult, fetal, and genital.

Adult form of rhabdomyoma occurs primarily in middle-aged and older individuals, usually (70% of cases) in males. Common site of involvement is head and neck. It is slowly growing and painless.

Site: Within the oral floor is most often affected pharyngeal lesions occurs most frequently in the base of the tongue, buccal mucosa, floor of the mouth and soft palate.

Microscopically: The adult rhabdomyoma is composed of an encapsulated mass of large, uniform polygonal cells with granular eosinophilic cytoplasm. Vacuoles beneath the cell membrane often give the cytoplasm a stellate or **'spider web'** appearance. Cells with cross- striations can be found in almost all cases. A fibrous stroma is present and mitotic activity is extremely low. Many cases demonstrate occasional degeneration vacuoles or clear spaces between the tumour cells.

Immunohistochemical examination of the tumour cells show positive immunostaining for myoglobin, desmin, and striated muscle actin, but negative for smooth muscle actin.

Electron microscopy shows many glycogen granules and mitochondria in the tumour cells.

Fetal type usually occurs in newborns and young children but the lesion have been reported in patients as old as 50 years.

LEIOMYOMA

Leiomyoma is a benign tumour of soft tissue. Common sites of leiomyoma are uterus, gastrointestinal tract, skin and subcutaneous tissues.

It is extremely rare tumour of the oral cavity.

Site: The lesions are usually in the tongue and cheek.

The tumour occurs in patients between 40 and 60 years of age, and in females twice as frequently as in males. They are small and grow slowly.

Macroscopically: Leiomyoma may be single or multiple of various size, dense solid growths, often becoming soft due to cystic degeneration.

Microscopically: The tumour is composed of spindle-shaped cells with cigar-shaped nuclei and eosinophilic cytoplasm. The cells are arranged in whorls and parallel bundles.

BONE

OSTEOMA

Osteoma is a hamartoma containing only osseous tissue.

Clinical features

It usually develops in membranous bones such as calvarium, frontal sinus, and mandible.

Microscopically: It is composed of dense, mature, predominantly mature bone. Prominent osteoblastic activity is seen.

Radiology: An ivory-like dense sclerotic mass—less than 1 cm—attached to cortex with sharply demarcated margin is seen.

Patients with Gardener's syndrome (intestinal polyposis and soft tissue tumours) may have multiple osteomas and other abnormalities.

OSTEOID OSTEOMA

The termed osteoid osteoma was introduced by Jaffe (1935) to describe a type of benign osteoblastic lesion. Osteoid osteoma are benign osteogenic lesions characterised by proliferation of either cancellous or compact bone and can be central, peripheral or extraskeletal.

Types

1. **Endosteal:** The tumour arises in medullary bone.
2. **Periosteal:** The tumour arises on the bone surface as a polypoidal or sessile mass.

Clinical features

This benign tumour is common in limbs, hands and feet, vertebrae and skull. Very few cases of osteoid osteoma occurring in the jaws (mandible) have been reported. The most common locations being the posterior lingual surface and the mandible angle area.

Osteoid osteoma is a benign tumour that is found more frequently in patients between 10 and 30 years of age and exhibits a 2 : 1 male: female ratio.

Macroscopically: The tumour is characterised by its small size (usually less than 1 cm), its clearly demarcated outlines and by the usual presence of surrounding zone of reactive bone. The nidus is usually gritty and dark red, representing the partially mineralised woven bone and rich capillary vascular supply, respectively.

Microscopically: The tumour consists of a well-vascularised nidus made up of osteoid trabeculae with fibrovascular intratrabecular tissue.

Radiologically: The nidus may be radiolucent with dense centre due to calcific deposits.

OSTEOBLASTOMA

It is also called giant osteoid osteoma.

Clinical features

Tumour is more common in males. Commonest age group is 2nd and 3rd decades of life.

Osteoblastomas arise most often in the vertebral column, although they may occur in other sites as well. It is rare in jaws and, if it occurs there, it is found more commonly in mandible.

It is characterised by its larger size (usually more than 1cm) and by the usual absence of any surrounding zone of reactive bone.

Microscopically: The intervening stroma is made up of vascular connective tissue instead of normal marrow elements and contains a large number of giant cells.

Radiologically: There is central radiolucent area and surrounding osseous sclerosis more than 1.5 cm in diameter. There may be multiple small calcifications and a peripheral sclerotic bone.

OSTEOCHONDROMA

Osteochondroma is one of the most common benign tumours of bone, accounting for approximately 35% of benign tumours.

Clinical features

The most common sites for osteochondroma are at the growing ends of bone, including the distal femur, proximal tibia, and proximal humerus. Osteochondroma of the tongue represents a very rare benign tumour at this site. The average age of the patient at onset is approximately 10 years: in large majority of the cases, the tumour appears before patient is 20 years old.

Macroscopically: Osteochondroma vary in size, and larger lesions may project outward.

Microscopically: The histology shows a well-circumscribed lesion of mature lamellar bone or cartilage or a mixture of those tissues.

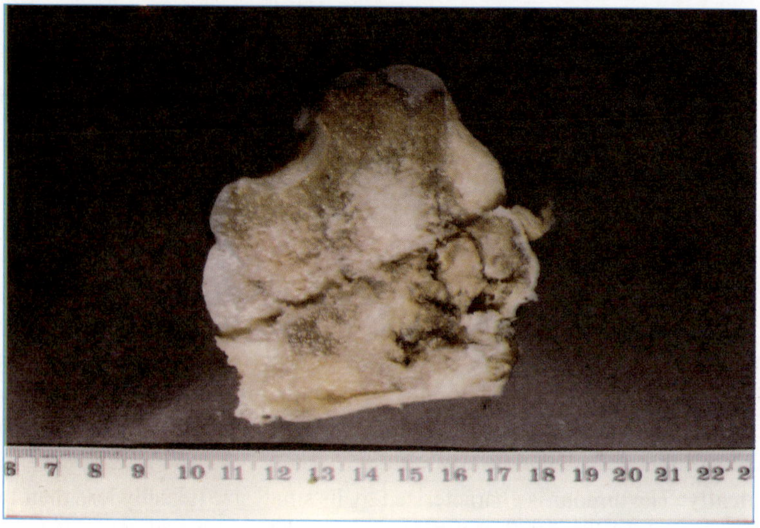

Fig.19.9: Showing gross appearance of osteochondroma

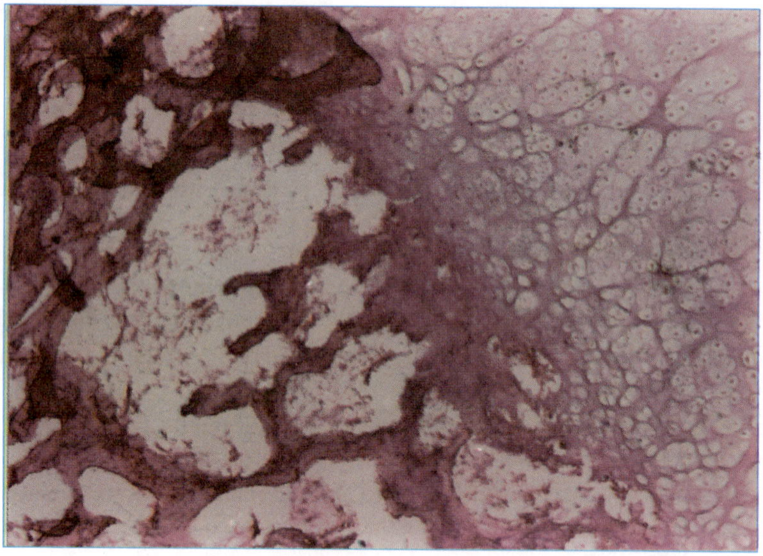

Fig.19.10: Showing osteoid tissue and cartilaginous cap

CARTILAGE

CHONDROMA

Chondroma is a cartilaginous tumour most commonly found in small bones of hands and feet. It may arise from maxilla and mandible.

Clinical features

Maximum age incidence is between 20 to 30 years. Occasionally, chondromata are complicated by pathological fractures or pain from bone-weakening.

Macroscopically: The tumour may be single or multiple. An enchondroma shows lobules of bluish-grey cartilage which is often more gelatinous than normal. The mass is surrounded by thin shell of bone.

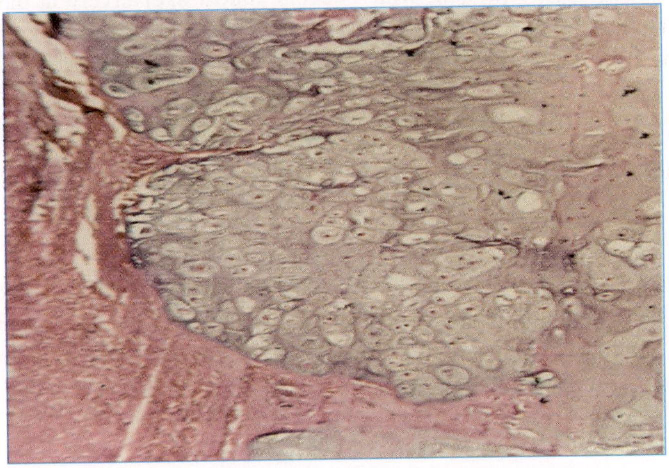

Fig.19.11: Show cartilaginous tissue in lobules separated by fibrous septa (chondroma)

Microscopically: Chondroma consists of mainly hyaline cartilage incompletely divided into lobules by fibrous septa carrying blood vessels. Cartilage cells lie in lacunae singly, in pairs, quartlets, or groups. Intercellular matrix may be mucinous or show elastic fibres.

Cytological atypia may be encountered in chondromas associated with Ollier's disease and Maffuci's syndrome (multiple haemangiomas). Chondrosarcomas develop in one-third of patients with multiple chondroma syndrome.

CHONDROMYXOID FIBROMA

It is a rare benign tumour of cartilage which rarely occurs in mandible. Jafee and Lichtenstein described it in 1948.

Clinical features

It occurs in young persons under the age of 20 years. Pain and soft tissue swelling are the common presenting complaints (approximately 85% and 65%, respectively). Pathologic fracture is observed in some patients with painful tumours.

Macroscopically

The lesion is solid, yellowish white or greyish white, replacing bone and thins out cortex. Their appearance mimics fibrous tissue or hyaline cartilage. Some tumours show haemorrhage and cystic degeneration.

Microscopically: The tumour is composed of mixed elements of fibrous tissues in varying proportions. The lobulated tumour has a significant degree of peripheral lobular hypercellularity, focal spotty calcification, cartilage, a few reactive osteoclastic giant cells as well as haemorrhagic area.

X-ray demonstrates an eccentric geographic lucency that is well-delineated from the adjacent bone by a rim of sclerosis.

CHONDROBLASTOMA

It is also known as 'Codman's tumour'.

Clinical features

Most patients of chondroblastoma are between 10 to 20 years old when the tumour is discovered. There is male preponderance over the female, usually in the ratio of 2 : 1. Chondroblastoma is an uncommon benign chondrogenic tumour, which occurs almost exclusively in the epiphysis of long bones, especially the upper tibia and humerus. There are some reports available in the literature that the tumour can arise from the condyle of mandible.

Macroscopically

It is well-defined and about 80% of chondroblastomas are 1 to 7 cm across. Cystic changes may simulate those of aneurysmal bone cyst, especially when the tumour occurs in the patella, talus or calcaneum.

Microscopically

Chondroblastomas consists of chondroblasts, which are round or oval primitive cells of epiphyseal cartilage plate that contain dense eosinophilic cytoplasm. The shape of chondroblast is usually polyhedral, although spindle element can also be present. Scattered among the tumour cells are large multinucleated cells with 5 to 40 nuclei. A distinctive microscopic change is the presence of small zones of focal calcification. These zones range from a network of thin lines (chicken wire) to obvious deposits surrounded by giant cells. Cytologic atypia is rare.

Cytogenetically, recurrent anomalies of 6_q25 have been found. The most characteristic of these consists of the pericentrometric inversion inv (6) (P25_q 23).

PLASMACYTOMA

Plasmacytoma usually arise in marrow and rarely in lymph nodes.

Extramedullary plasmacytomas are most common in palate, paranasal sinuses, nasopharynx, oropharynx and upper respiratory tract. Solitary plasma cell tumours occur occasionally in the soft tissues.

Microscopically: The stratified squamous epithelium of the palatal mucosa is intact. It is stretched over an extremely vascular and extensively vacuolated sheet of moderate neoplastic cells. Cytoplasm is abundant, and the nuclei are round and of moderate size. Within the nuclei, the chromatin is distributed as granules, which are arranged in a coarse clock-face or cartwheel appearance.

Bibliography

Ibrahim A Al-Hoquail, Taseen A Bhatt: Keratoacanthoma an unusual presentation: Baharin Medical Bulletin, Vol. 31, No 1 March 2009.

Neville, Brad et al: Oral and Maxillofacial Pathology. Second edition. 2002.

Showkat SA, Mohmmad Latef, Asif A Wani, Ahafquat A. Lone, Kanwajeet Singh: Clinicopathological profile of cervicofacial masses in pediatric patients. Indian J Otolaryngol Head and Neck Surgery 2009 61: 141-146.

Trivedi C, Baldwin D, Warnakulasurriya S, Johnson N, Peters T, Copper content in areca catechu (betel nut) products and oral submucus fibrosis. Lancet 1997: 349: 1447.

CHAPTER

20

PREMALIGNANT LESIONS AND CONDITIONS

INTRODUCTION

Oral premalignant lesions: Which show histologically detectable mucosal changes. Premalignant lesions include leukoplakia, palatal changes associated with smoking.

Premalignant lesions and conditions of the oral, oropharyngeal and laryngeal mucosa:

Premalignant conditions: More widespread or systemic disorders affecting oral mucosa where cancer is statistically more likely to develop although the site is unpredictable.

Premalignant conditions include sideropenic atrophy and dysphagia caused by iron deficiency.

TABLE 20.1 CLASSIFICATION OF PREMALIGNANT LESIONS AND CONDITIONS
A. Precancerous lesions
❑ 1. Proliferative verrucous leukoplakia
❑ 2. Erythroleukoplakia
❑ 3. Granular leukoplakia
❑ 4. Smooth, thick leukoplakia
❑ 5. Smooth and thin leukoplakia
❑ 6. Erythroplakia
❑ 7. Verrucous hyperplasia
• Nicotine palatinus in reverse smokers
• Carcinoma in situ
B. Precancerous conditions
• Sideropenic dysphagia

Contd.

Contd.

- Lichen planus
- Syphilitic leukoplakia
- Oral submucus fibrosis
- Discoid lupus erythematosus
- Laryngeal keratosis
- Actinic keratosis
- Smooth red tongue of Plummer-Vinson syndrome
- Smokeless tobacco keratosis

TABLE 20.2
CLASSIFICATION OF CONDITIONS ASSOCIATED WITH MALIGNANT TRANSFORMATION

High-risk lesions
- Erythroplakia
- Speckled leukoplakia
- Chronic hyperplastic candidiasis

Medium-risk lesions
- Oral submucus fibrosis
- Syphilitic glossitis
- Sideropenic dysphagia (Peterson-Kelly syndrome)

Low-risk/equivocal-risk lesions
- Oral lichen planus
- Discoid lupus erythematosus
- Dyskeratosis congenita

LEUKOPLAKIA

The word comes from Greek *leukos* (white) and means white plaque. A condition characterised by a whitish patch that develops inside mouth or throat. Occasionally they are warty, with cracks and fissures.

Causes

No aetiologic factor can be identified for most persistent oral leukoplakias (idiopathic leukoplakia)

Known causes of leukoplakia include:

- Trauma (e.g., chronic trauma from a sharp or broken tooth, ill-fitting denture or mastication may cause leukoplakia.
- **Actinic radiation:**
- **Tobacco use:** Chewing tobacco is probably worse than smoking.
- **Alcohol:** The use of alcohol has been suggested as a possible etiology.
- Because alcohol may irritate the mucosa. Persons who habitually consume considerable quantities of alcohol usually also smoke inveterately; therefore, establishing the effects of alcohol alone is difficult.
- **Infections (e.g., candidiasis, syphilis, Epstein-Barr virus infection):** Epstein Barr virus infection causes a separate and distinct non-premalignant lesion termed hairy leukoplakia.

- **Candidiasis:** Chronic hyperplastic candidiasis (candidial leukoplakia) is considered a premalignant lesion of oral mucosa, occurring as speckled or homogeneous white lesions (leukoplakia). If the lesions are untreated, a proportion may become dysplastic and progress to carcinoma.
- **Chemicals (e.g., senguina):** Accidental contact with agricultural compounds cause severe and extensive erosion of the tongue and lips and causes leukoplakia.
- **Immune defects:** Leukoplakias appear to be more common in transplant patients.

Incidence: Leukoplakic lesions are found in approximately 3% of the world population.

Sex: Oral leukoplakia is more common in men, with a male-to-female ratio of 2 : 1.

Age: Most cases of oral leukoplakia occur in persons in their fifth to seventh decade of life. Approximately 80% of patients are older than 40 years.

Sites: The most common sites are the buccal mucosa, alveolar mucosa, and lower lip; however, lesions in the floor of mouth, lateral tongue, and lower lip are most likely to show dysplastic or malignant changes.

TABLE 20.3
CLASSIFICATION OF LEUKOPLAKIA

- According to clinical description
- Early and thin leukoplakia
- Homogeneous leukoplakia
- Granular and nodular leukoplakia
- Verrucous leukoplakia
- Proliferative verrucous leukoplakia
- Erythroleukoplakia
- Syphilitic leukoplakia

Types of leukoplakia

1. Early and thin leukoplakia appears as a slightly elevated greyish-white plaque—may be either well-defined or may gradually blend into surrounding normal mucosa. The lesion may be translucent, fissured or wrinkled, soft and flat.
2. **Homogenous leukoplakia:** It is also called leukoplakia simplex. The lesion shows characteristic raised plaque or comprise of group of plaques, which may be uniformly flat and thicker than the early lesions. The lesions are usually white in colour but may be yellowish-white or yellow. The lesions are mostly associated with the oral use of snuff. The thick or homogeneous leukoplakia may become dysplastic—even invasive—with surface change over time. Multiple circular or oval patches of non-blanching redness or erythroplakia begin appearing in scattered area.
3. **Granular or nodular leukoplakia:** It is also called 'leukoplakia erosive' or 'speckled leukoplakia'. Some leukoplakias develop surface irregularities and are referred to as granular or nodular leukoplakia. It has high malignant potential.
4. **Verrucous leukoplakia:** It is called 'leukoplakia verrucosa'—occasionally pointed projections develop on the surface and may be so numerous that the resulting lesions are called verrucous leukoplakia.
5. **Proliferative verrucous leukoplakia** is an uncommon form of proliferative multifocal leukoplakia with a high rate of malignant transformation to either squamous cell cancer or verrucous carcinoma and a high probability of recurrence.

The etiology of proliferative verrucous leukoplakia is unknown. An association with human papilloma virus (HPV) infection—particularly strains 16 and 18 have been implicated in some cases.

Microscopically: There is hyperkeratosis with dysplastic changes in advanced lesions.

6. **Erythroleukoplakia:** It is also known as speckled leukoplakia. This is variation of leukoplakia arising on an erythematous base. It has the highest rate of transformation.
7. **Syphilitic leukoplakia:** Syphilitic leukoplakia would appear to be homogeneous white patch affecting large areas of the dorsum of the tongue. The association between tertiary syphilis and oral squamous cell carcinoma—particularly of the tongue—has been suggested for many years.

The clinical criteria demonstrate particularly high risks of malignant change as:

1. Verrucous type is considered high risk.
2. Erosion or ulceration within the lesion is highly suggestive of malignancy.
3. The presence of a nodule indicates malignant potential.
4. A lesion that is hard in its periphery is predictive of malignant change.
5. Oral leukoplakia of the anterior floor of the mouth and under surface of the tongue is strongly associated with malignant potential.

Clinically, appearance varies from non-palpable, faintly translucent-white areas to thick, fissured papillomatous, indurated lesions. They may feel rough and leathery. Colour of leukoplakia may be white, grey, yellowish-white, or brownish-grey. The lesions may be macular or plaque like and cannot be wiped-off.

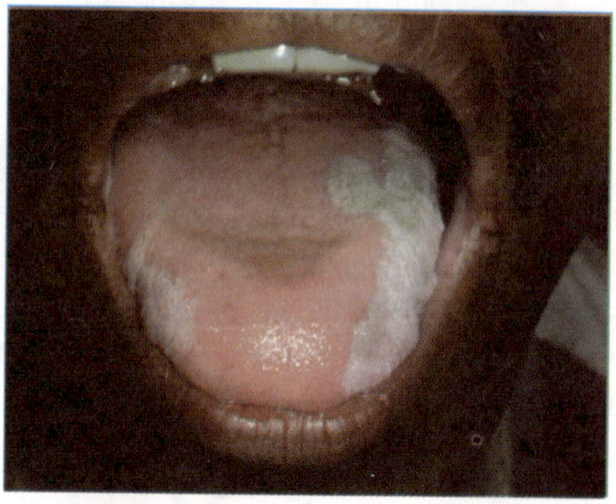

Fig.20.1: Shows leukoplakia tongue

Microscopically

Leukoplakia demonstrates a thickened surface layer of parakeratin, sometimes orthokeratisation, basilar cells and keratinocytes in the lower portions of the epithelium usually show evidence of dysplasia, besides a mild basilar hyperplasia but about 10% of cases will be dysplastic and have an increased risk of malignant transformation.

ERYTHROPLAKIA

A condition characterised by a red, raised patch that develops inside mouth. Leukoplakia may vary from a small, circumscribed white plaque to an extensive lesion involving wide areas of the oral mucosa.

Age and sex: It is mostly found in elderly men around the ages of 65-74.

Sites: The most common areas in the mouth where erythroplakia is found are the floor of the mouth, tongue, lip, and the soft palate.

Clinically: It appears as a red macule or plaque with demarcated borders. The texture is characterised as soft and velvety. An adjacent area of laukoplakia may be found along with erythroplakia. The typical oral lesion is less than 1.5 cm in greatest diameter, but many examples larger than 4 cm have been seen.

Histological features

1. There is an absence of keratin production.
2. Reduced amount of epithelial cells. The viable cell layers of the epithelium may show acanthosis or atrophy.

3. There is dilatation and engorgement of the subepithelial microvascular system.
4. There is severe epithelial dysplasia, carcinoma in situ or invasive carcinoma in 90% of cases.
5. Variable inflammatory infiltrate is present.

The most frequent causes of leukoplakia and erythroplakia are smoking or chewing tobacco, spirits, spices, syphilis, sharp teeth, sepsis and vitamin deficiency.

CHRONIC HYPERPLASTIC CANDIDIASIS

Chronic hyperplastic candidiasis produces dense plaques of leukoplakia, particularly around the commissures of the mouth. The lesions occasionally extend on to the vermilion and even the facial skin. These lesions have a high incidence of malignant transformation, thought to be the result of invasion of the lesion by candida albicans. A small percentage of patients have an associated immunological defect, which encourages the invasion of c. albicans, rendering the patient susceptible to malignant transformation. Chronic hyperplastic candidiasis (candidial leukoplakia) is a chronic discrete, raised, lesion that may vary from a small, palpable, translucent or whitish area to a large, dense, opaque plaque that is hard and rough to touch (plaque-like).

Early symptoms include burning in the mouth, vesicular eruptions ulceration of the mucosa, and recurrent attacks of stomatitis. Disturbances of speech and mastication occur later.

SUBMUCUS FIBROSIS

Joshi first described the condition in India in 1959. Oral submucus fibrosis is a tropical disease occurring mainly in the Indian subcontinent. It is also reported from Pakistan, Taiwan, Sri Lanka, Nepal, and Thailand due to the common habit of betel nut chewing. Oral submucus fibrosis (OSMF) is a chronic disease of oral mucosa characterised by inflammation and progressive fibrosis followed by stiffening of an otherwise yielding mucosa resulting in difficulty in opening the mouth. Diffuse, dense white patches in the oral cavity—and occasionally in pharynx—characterise it.

Etiology

1. In India, submucus fibrosis or lock-jaw is caused by gutka chewing in school children.
2. Socioeconomic status has been associated with higher risk of precancerous lesions like leukoplakia, erythroplakia, and submucus fibrosis. This is related to education, diet, life-style and access to medical care.
3. Chewing areca nut alone, or as a component of betel quid, is widespread in the Indian subcontinent. Areca nut chewing is also causally linked to oral submucus fibrosis. Areca nut has a high copper content (302nmol/g), a substantial amount of which is released into saliva while chewing. The role of copper in submucus fibrosis is not clearly understood although it is known that the copper dependent enzyme, lysyloxidase, secreted by the fibroblasts, facilitates the cross-linking of collagen, thereby inhibiting its degradation.
4. **Tobacco chewing:** It is a major risk factor in submucus fibrosis as it is in lesions of leukoplakia and erythroplakia. Tobacco smoking alone is not associated with oral submucus fibrosis.
5. **Areca nuts:** Areca nuts are chewed alone with tobacco or in the form of pan (containing lime, catechu, and other ingredients on a betel leaf). Betel quid without tobacco also increases the risk of precancerous lesions, but causes higher risk for oral submucus fibrosis relative to leukoplakia, erythroplakia or multiple precancerous lesions. International agency for research on cancer has classified betel quid without tobacco also as a carcinogen for humans. Research strongly indicates that oral submucus fibrosis is significantly associated with the use of pan-masala areca nut, with or without concurrent alcohol use.

Areca nut is found to contain different types of alkaloids like arecoline, arecadine, guvacoline, guvacine and isovacine.

6. **Alcohol:** It is observed that drinking increases the risk of leukoplakia by 1.5 fold, OSF by 2-fold and that of erythroplakia 3-fold.
7. **Nutritional:** Deficiency of vitamins and micronutrients has been suggested in the etiology of OSF. Therapy of OSF with vitamin A, zinc, and antioxidants has shown some beneficial effect. Lesser intake of fruits and vegetables has been associated with oral premalignant lesion.
8. **Immune process:** OSF is considered a cell mediated immune reaction to arecoline in areca nuts. It may reflect a localised collagen disorder or an autoimmune process in the oral cavity. Serum immunoglobulin levels of IgA, IgG and IgM are raised significantly in oral submucus fibrosis. Circulating autoantibodies are also present in some cases of oral submucus fibrosis.
9. **Genetic susceptibility:** The familial occurrence of oral submucus fibrosis has also been reported.
10. Excessive consumption of chillies (capsicum annum and capsicum frutescence) has been thought to play an etiological role in oral submucus fibrosis. Chillies contain an active ingredient called 'capsicin' that produces allergic reactions in the oral mucosa. It is the vanillymide of 8-methyle-6-nonenic acids, which is the active irritant of the chillies.
11. Psychological stress:
12. Defective iron metabolism
13. Bacterial infections.

Clinical features

Females are more affected than males and the disease is commonest in the age group of 30-50 years.

Sites: Changes of submucus fibrosis are most marked over (i) soft palate (ii) faucial pillars, and (iii) buccal mucosa.

Symptoms: Patient often presents with:

1. Intolerance to chillies and spicy food.
2. Soreness of mouth with constant burning sensation; worsened during meals, particularly of pungent spicy type.
3. Repeated vesicular eruption on the palate and pillars.
4. Difficulty to open the mouth fully.
5. Difficulty to protrude the tongue.

Various stages of the disease

1. **Prodromal stage:** In this stage, the patient complains of soreness, and intolerance to spices and salts. The ulcers and blisters are not seen.
2. **Stage II.** In this stage, the patient has sense of stiffness inside the mouth and some difficulty in opening the mouth. There is pallor over the soft palate and fauces.
3. **Advanced stage:** The patient has marked trismus and difficulty in protrusion of the tongue. The incisor bite is reduced from the normal 4.5 cm to 2.5 cm. The mucosa of the oral cavity and oropharynx looks pale and rigid. The vestibule of mouth is obliterated and the patient cannot puff out the cheek. The anterior faucial pillars are markedly fibrosed with marked limitation of movement of the soft palate. The uvula looks like a rudimentary bud.

Microscopically

The overlying epithelium may be either atrophic or hyperplastic and there is often hyperkeratosis. There is variable degree of cellular atypia, nuclear pleomorphism, marked irregular epithelial hyperplasia and intercellular edema. There is deposition of fibrous and hyaline tissue in the submucosa of the oral cavity. Stromal blood vessels are dilated and congested. Degeneration of the muscle fibres and chronic inflammatory cell infiltration in the connective tissue is seen.

Complications of submucus fibrosis:

1. Oral dysplasia
2. **Squamous cell carcinoma:** The risk of developing oral carcinoma is 7.6% over a 10-year period. 30% of oral cancers have been associated with submucous fibrosis.

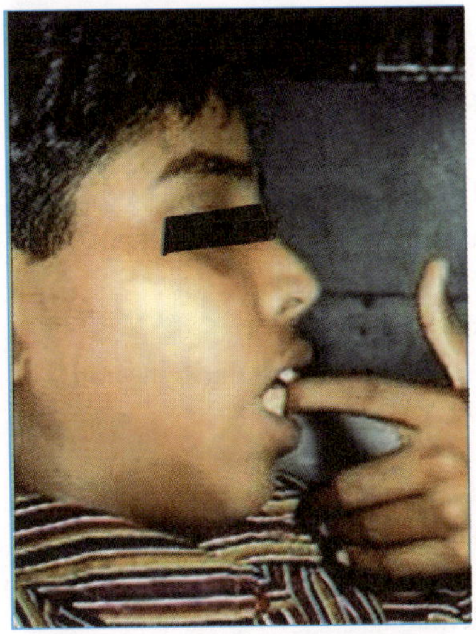

Fig.20.2: A case of submucus fibrosis. Child is unable to open his mouth more than 1 finger

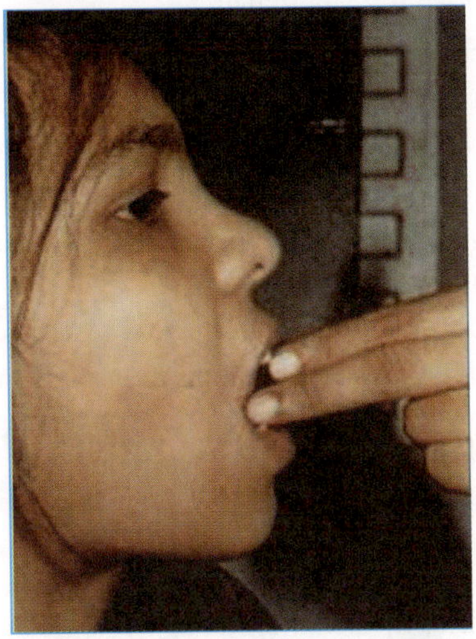

Fig.20.3: Showing a case of submucus fibrosis. Child is unable to open mouth

NICOTINE REVERSE SMOKER'S PALATE

Thoma named the lesion stomatitis nicotine because it is almost always observed in individuals who smoke tobacco.

A large study in Saudi Arabia showed that 29.6% of all smokers had nicotine stomatitis and 60% of pipe smokers had this lesion.

In some South Americans and Southeast Asian cultures hand-rolled cigars are smoked with the lit end held within the mouth. This 'reverse smoking' habit produces a similar but more pronounced palatal keratosis, called reverse smoker's palate, which is definitely a premalignant lesion. The concentrated heat stream of smoke from tobacco and not the chemicals in tobacco smoke irritate the mucosa resulting in nicotine stomatitis.

Clinical features

- The lesion occurs in males, frequently older than 40-45 years.
- Lesions are exclusively found on palatal mucosa. It is limited to posterior hard palate and often to adjacent soft palate.
- They have a white cobblestone appearance, of with a red spot in the centre of cobblestone. The lesions cannot be wiped-off and can have some fissuring and dried mud appearance from excess keratin production by cells.
- The palate may appear grey and white, and may contain many papules that are slightly elevated.

Microscopically

Histologically, epithelial cells of the palate exhibit signs of hyperkeratosis and acanthosis. There may be metaplasia of excretory ducts, which results in visible papules if the ducts become hyperplastic.

EPITHELIAL DYSPLASIA

Lesions characterised by disordered cell maturation and proliferation associated with increased risk of progression to malignancy.

Microscopically

1. Irregular hyperplasia of cells with basal cell morphology
2. Rete ridges show a drop-shaped configuration
3. Loss of both polarity of cells and stratification of the epithelium
4. Nuclear changes, such as increased nuclear cytoplasmic ratio, hyperchromatism, and pleomorphism
5. Mitoses in the upper layers of epithelium, abnormal mitoses
6. Individual cell keratinisation often in deep layers and loss of cellular cohesion.

ACTINIC CHEILOSIS

Actinic cheilitis, sometimes known as *'farmer's lip'* or *'sailor's lip'*.

Actinic cheilosis is a diffuse degenerative change of the lower lip as a result of sun damage. Lifetime occupational sun exposure increases the risk. Other factors may also play a role including tobacco use, lip irritation, poor hygiene, and ill-fitting dentures.

This is precancerous with an estimated 6-10% risk of cancer development.

Clinical features

It occurs primarily in men and does not present until after 50 years of age, but the cause is often extreme sun exposure during the teen years and young adult life.

Most common features of actinic cheilitis are dryness and cracking of the lips, thinned skin and scaly patches.

The lip becomes puffy and blotchy red and pale pink, with occasional white plaques and chronic ulcers. Other less common features include loss of demarcation between the vermilion border of the lip and adjacent skin, prominent folds and lip lines, white thickened patches and discoloured skin with pale and yellow areas.

Microscopically

There is epithelial hyperkeratosis, parakeratosis with dysplastic changes ranging from atypia to carcinoma in situ. Epithelium is flattened or atrophic, beneath which is a band of inflammatory infiltrate. In more severe cases there is nuclear atypia and mitoses, and some develop into invasive squamous cell carcinoma. The collagen and elastic fibres generally show basophilic degeneration of collagen along with an infiltration of lymphocytes, and plasma cells scattered in the upper dermis suggest actinic damage.

Management

Treatment options include 5-fluorouracil, imiquimod, scalpel vermillonectomy, chemical peel, electrosurgery, and carbon dioxide laser vaporisation.

5-fluorouracil has been shown to be effective therapy for diffuse but minor actinic cheilitis.

More extensive or recurring areas of actinic cheilitis may be treated with either a shave vermillectomy or a carbon dioxide laser.

PLUMMER-VINSON SYNDROME

The most used name is Plummer-Vinson syndrome, named after Henry Stanley Plummer and Porter Paisely Vinson.

The association of anaemia, glossitis and dysphagia is known as the Plummer-Vinson syndrome; it may predispose to the later development of post-cricoid carcinoma of oesophagus.

There is a well-known relationship between sideropaenia (iron deficiency in the absence of anaemia) and the development of oral cancer. Sideropaenia is common in women in Scandinavian women and leads to epithelial atrophy, which renders the oral mucosa vulnerable to irritation from topical carcinogens. Correction of sideropaenia with iron supplements reduces the epithelial atrophy and risk of malignant transformation.

Clinical features

Most of the patients are white middle-aged women, in the fourth to seventh decade of life, but the syndrome has been described in children and adolescent.

In severe iron deficiency, minority of patients suffers from dysphagia (difficulty in swallowing), which may be due to folding of lax mucosa in the upper oesophagus. There is throat pain and burning during swallowing. Tongue is smooth, red, painful and atrophy of lingual papillae. Haematological findings include sideroblastic anaemia and microcytic hypochromic anaemia. Other findings include spoon-shaped fingernails, fatigue, pallor, angular stomatitis and gastritis.

Microscopically

The oesophageal webs appear smooth, thin and grey with eccentric or central lumen. They are characterised by one or more thin horizontal membrane consisting of squamous epithelium and submucosa. Sometimes, chronic inflammatory cells may be observed in the submucosa. The webs typically occur in the proximal part of the oesophagus. They usually protrude from the anterior wall, extending laterally but not to the posterior wall, which means that they rarely encircle the lumen.

SYPHILITIC GLOSSITIS

Syphilitic glossitis or sclerosis is seen in the central part of the tongue and there exists two varieties: One superficial, the other deep—reaching the muscle. The superficial type presents as a glassy or glossed tongue with hard, depapillated red and white islets that sometimes fissurate or have sulci running through, and generally, are accompanied by leukoplakia-type plaques. It is a precancerous lesion.

The furrows of syphilitic glossitis are mainly longitudinal and deeper than congenital type. The intervening epithelium is desquamated.

The syphilitic infection produces an interstitial glossitis with an endarteritis that results in atrophy of the overlying epithelium appears to be more vulnerable to those irritants that cause leukoplakia or oral cancer. Squamous cell carcinomas may arise in syphilitic glossitis, even in absence of leukoplakia.

Microscopically

There is atrophy of filiform and fungiform papillae and dorsum of tongue becomes smooth and atrophic. Vasculitis ending in endarteritis is the process underlying these changes.

LICNEN PLANUS

Lichen planus is a common mucocutaneous disease. It is a chronic autoimmune inflammatory condition affecting the lining of the mouth. The condition can affect either the skin or mucosa or both. About half of the patients with skin lesions have oral lesions, whereas about 25% present with oral lesions alone. Oral lichen planus is a chronic disease—can persist in some patients for a long time in contrast to cutaneous lichen planus—the oral form may persist for up to 25 years. Oral lesions may coexist with lesions of genital mucous membranes or with lesions of cutaneous lichen planus.

Definition: Oral lichen planus is a chronic autoimmune inflammatory condition affecting the lining of mouth.

It was first described by Erasmus Wilson in 1869 and is thought to affect 0.5-1% of the world's population. Overall prevalence of oral lichen planus among Indians was 1.5%.

Sites: Lesions of oral lichen planus are typically bilateral. Any location in the oral cavity may be involved, with the most common site being the posterior buccal mucosa. Other common locations cited for oral lichen planus include tongue, gingival, retromolar/tuberosity area, vestibule, palate, floor of the mouth, and lip.

Clinical forms of lichen planus

1. **Reticular form:** This is the most common type. It consists of slightly raised slender whitish pattern (Honiton lace or Whickham's striae) or in an annular arrangement. This include network, which is often interspersed with papules or rings.
2. **Papular form:** Minute white papules (0.5mm) may be seen. They gradually enlarge and coalesce to form either a reticular, annular or plaque pattern. It is rarely seen and, being small, it is possible to overlook them during a routine oral examination.
3. **Plaque-like oral lichen planus:** The plaque like form may range from a slightly elevated and smooth to a slightly irregular form and may be multifocal. The primary sites are over the dorsum of the tongue and the buccal mucosa. The plaque form may be difficult to distinguish from leukoplakia, but in oral lichen planus there is usually no change in the flexibility of the affected mucosa. Another distinguishing feature may be the presence of a reticular periphery. Plaque-like oral lichen planus resolves in only 7% of cases. This form is significantly more common among tobacco smokers and HIV positive patients.
4. **Atrophic form:** The atrophic type is diffuse, red and there are usually white striae in the lesion. Such striae that radiate peripherally are usually evident at the margins of the atrophic zones of the lesion. The gingival tends to show patchy distribution over all the four quadrants in a relatively symmetrical pattern.

   Histologically, it shows thin epithelium and loss of rete ridges.
5. **Erosive (ulcerative) form:** These are characteristically occurring on the feet as ulcerative or bullous lesions, mucosal lesions, and alopecia.
6. **Bullous form:** This form of oral lichen planus is quite rare. The intraoral bullae rupture soon after they appear, resulting in classic appearance of erosive lichen planus. The most common site is buccal mucosa especially into posterior and lateral margins of tongue.
7. **Annular form:** Lichen planus papules that are purely annular are rare. Amular lesions with an atrophic center can be found in the buccal mucosa.

Causes

The etiology of oral lichen planus is unclear, though there is clear evidence of T lymphocyte attack on the stratified epithelium.

Risk factors

1. **Sex:** Lichen planus affects women more than men (at a ratio of 3 : 2).
2. **Age:** Oral lichen planus predominantly occurs in adults older than 40 years, although younger adults and children can be affected.

3. **Medication:** Oral mucoid lichenoid lesions may occur after the administration of systemic drugs, sulphonyl ureas, antimalarials, betablockers, and some angiotensin-converting enzyme inhibitors. The period between commencement of the drug therapy and the critical appearance of old lichen planus-like disease varies.
4. **Allergies:** Reactions to amalgam, or gold, or occasionally other dental materials may cause lichen planus.
5. **Medical conditions:** Certain medical conditions including other immune disorders are associated with oral lichen planus. These may include lichen planus of the skin, liver disease, graft versus host disease, primary sclerosing cholangitis, Lupus erythematosus, primary biliary cirrhosis, Sjogren's syndrome, ulcerative colitis, alopecia areata, and myasthenia gravis.
6. **Dental issues:** Sharp edges on teeth, dental restorations ill-fitting dental prostheses, some periodontal surgical procedures, and oral habits such as lip and cheek chewing may raise the risk of oral lichen planus.
7. **Smoking and tobacco chewing:** It was highest (3.1%) in those people with mixed oral habits and lowest (0.3%) in non-users of tobacco. The annual age-adjusted incidence rate was 2.1 and 2.5 per 1,000 among men and women, respectively. It was highest (8.2 per 1,000) among men who smoked as well as chewed tobacco; among women it was highest (4.5 per 1,000) in chewers. The relative risk for oral lichen planus was highest (13.7%) among those who smoked and chew tobacco.
8. **Psychological issues:** A relationship of lichen planus with stress is quoted and neurogenic basis is suggested. Observation mostly in nervous and highly stressed persons is associated emotions, upset, overwork and some form of mental strain.
9. **Immunology:** The cause is unknown but an immune pathogenesis is suspected, as there is an association with some autoimmune diseases such as myasthenia gravis, thymoma, alopecia areata, dermatomyositis, primary biliary cirrhosis, ulcerative colitis. and graft versus host reaction. Oral lichen planus is a T-cell-mediated autoimmune disease in which cytotoxic CD8 + T cells trigger the apoptosis of oral epithelial cells. The lesional CD8 + T cells being more cytotoxic—may produce lymphokines, interferon, and tumour necrosis factor.
10. **Infections:**
11. Triad of diseases lichen planus, diabetes mellitus and vascular hypertension was described by Grinspan and known as Grinspan's syndrome.

Investigations

Histological examination of lesional tissue is the most relevant investigation in cases of oral lichen planus.

Histologic findings

Histological examination of lesional tissue is the most relevant.

Histological findings are:

1. The epithelium shows hyperparakeratosis with thickening or thinning of granular cell layer.
2. Development of saw-tooth appearance of the rete pegs.
3. Liquefaction degeneration of the basal layer.
4. Band-like subepithelial mononuclear infiltrate consisting of T cells and histiocytes, increased numbers of intraepithelial T cells and degenerating basal keratocytes that form colloid (civatte, hyaline, cytoid) bodies, which appear as homogeneous eosinophilic globules.

Electron microscopy: In oral lichen planus electron microscopy is used principally as a research tool. The ultrastructure of the colloid bodies suggests that they are apoptotic keratocytes, and recent studies using the end labelling method revealed DNA fragmentation in these cells. Electron microscopy shows breaks, branches, and duplications of the epithelial basement membrane in oral lichen planus.

Immunofluorescence shows heavy deposits of fibrin at the dermal-epidermal junction. Deposits of IgM, and, less frequently, IgG, IgA and C3, are also found in the colloid bodies.

Complications

High risk factors for malignant transformation include smoking, excessive alcohol intake, atrophic, ulcerative or erosive clinical types, presence of erythroplakic lesions and sites involving the tongue, gingival, or buccal mucosa. The malignant transformation of oral erosive and atrophic lesions has been described as 0.3 percent to 12.5 percent. The development of squamous cell carcinoma may occur in areas directly affected by lichen planus, as well as other areas of the oral mucosa. However, it is not established if atrophic and erosive forms of lichen planus have an intrinsic potential for malignant transformation or if the disorder facilitates the development of oral mucosa squamous cell carcinoma of exogenous carcinogen.

LUPUS ERYTHEMATOSUS

Types

- **Discoid lupus erythematosus:** When the lesions are confined to skin and mucosa.
- **Systemic lupus erythematosus:** When multiple organs are involved.

Etiology

- Genetic predisposition
- Immunological abnormality
- Autoimmune disease
- Deposition of antigen
- Endocrine
- Biochemical increase.

DISCOID LUPUS ERYTHEMATOSUS

Microscopically

There is basal cell vacuolar degeneration in the epidermis, loss of rete pegs, and aggregates of lymphocytes mainly in a perivascular/peri-adnexal distribution, but also in a lichenoid pattern. Hair follicles show prominent changes in DLE and subacute cutaneous lupus erythematosus (SCLE). There is follicular plugging due to hyperkeratosis into the empty follicle, atrophic epithelium and loss of hair shafts.

Clinical features

Systemic lupus erythematosus (SLE) is a chronic multisystem disease of autoimmune origin. SLE is predominantly a disease of women with a female to male ratio of 9 : 1. It can develop at any age but has peak incidence in between 15–35 years. The name comes from the Latin (*lupus*) for wolfs because the flushing of the cheeks sometimes resembles the malar flush of a wolfs.

Oral lesions of systemic lupus erythematosus develop in 20–50% of patients. The oral mucosa may be involved either prior to or following the development of skin lesions, or even in the absence of skin manifestations.

Systemic lupus erythematosus can and does manifest itself intraorally in the form of ulcerations, erythema (red lesions) and keratosis (thickened dermal layer). Intraoral lesion is composed of a central depressed red atrophic area surrounded by 2 to 4 mm elevated keratotic zone that dissolves into small white lines. The vermilion border of the lip, the inner cheek, gums, and roof of the mouth are areas often affected.

Oral ulcerations are generally painless and often involve the palate.

Purpuric lesions such as ecchymoses and petechiae may also occur.

Diagnosis

Antinuclear antibodies (ANAs) are directed against several nuclear antigens. A screening test for ANA is standard in assessing SLE because it is positive in close to 100 percent of patients with active SLE. Several techniques are used to detect ANAs. The most commonly used method is indirect immunofluorescence, which detects a variety of nuclear antigens including DNA, RNA, and proteins. Four basic patterns are recognised:

1. Nuclear pattern (Anti-Ro, SSA) and anti-La refers to the presence of a few discrete spots of fluorescence within the nucleus. This indicates the presence of antibodies to nuclear RNA. Anti-Ro is found in 30 percent of SLE patients and highly associated with photosensitivity.
2. Homogeneous or diffuse nuclear staining antibodies to deoxyribonucleoprotein, histone, and, occasionally, DNA staining.
3. Peripheral or rim staining indicates the presence of antibodies to double-stranded DNA.
4. Speckled pattern indicates the presence of non-DNA nuclear constituents. These are called extractable nuclear antigens, e.g., Smith (SM) antigen and SS-A and SS-B reactive antigen. Anti Sm is an immunoglobulin specific against Sm—a ribonucleoprotein found in the cell nucleus.

LE bodies: In tissues, nuclei of damaged cells react with ANAs, lose their chromatin pattern, and become homogeneous, to produce so-called LE bodies. Related to this phenomenon is the LE cell, which is readily seen in vitro. Basically, LE cell is phagocyte leukocyte (neutrophil or macrophage) that has engulfed the denatured nucleus of an injured cell.

Direct and indirect immunofluorescence of this lesion shows granular staining.

SMOKELESS TOBACCO KERATOSIS

The term smokeless tobacco is also known as dip, plug, chew, or spit tobacco (coarse cut) and snuff (fine cut). Snuff may be used in a dry form, which is inhaled nasally, or in the commonly used moist form, which is placed in the oral cavity.

White patches called leukoplakia or more specifically, smokeless tobacco keratosis, may be found in the mouth on the gums, cheeks, or, whatever tobacco contact is most frequent. Early changes may be reversible if caught soon enough and smokeless tobacco use is stopped.

Smokeless tobacco keratosis is the clinical diagnostic term used for the white keratotic plaque, which develops on oral mucosa in the area of chronic placement of chewing tobacco or snuff. The lesion is a precancerous, i.e., it carries a higher normal risk of malignant transformation.

DYSKERATOSIS CONGENITA (DC)

It is also known as Hoyeraal-Haeidarsson syndrome, Zinsser-Cole-Engman syndrome.

Dyskeratosis congenita is caused by mutated gene DKC 1, located on the X chromosome and most of the cases are inherited as an X-linked recessive disorder.

Clinical features

X-linked recessive form constitutes more than 80% of cases and 91% of DC patients are males. The symptoms usually appear when patients are between 5 and 10 years old, although they may occur at birth or 60 years of age.

The typical symptoms of dyskeratosis congenita involve the skin, nails, mucus membranes as well as bone marrow failure.

Skin shows reticulate hyperpigmentation, affecting the flexures, particularly neck, axillae, and inner upper thighs.

Microscopically

Skin biopsy specimens from the areas of reticulated pigmentation typically show non-specific changes, including mild hyperkeratosis, epidermal atrophy, telangiectasia of the superficial blood vessels, and melanophages in the papillary dermis. There is mild basal layer vacuolisation and lymphocytic infiltrate in the upper dermis.

Nails: Nails show progressive nail dystrophy with longitudinal ridging.

Bone marrow failure: Bone marrow failure causes anaemia, leukopaenia, thrombocytopaenia, aplastic anaemia, and myelodysplastic syndrome. Cancers associated with DC include carcinoma of oesophagus, stomach, colon and rectum, and leukaemia.

Other features of DC include dental caries, small sella turcica, dysphagia, sparse eyebrows, alopecia, mental retardation, pulmonary disease and genitourinary, skeletal and gastrointestinal abnormality.

Oral manifestations

Oral lesions consist of aggregates or recurrent blisters that rupture leaving a raw ulcerated surface—mainly on the lateral border of tongue and buccal mucosa. Atrophy of the buccal mucosa is the result of repeated episodes.

White patches (leukoplakia) on the insides of cheeks, tongue, and upper throat; these patches may become malignant later on. Other oral manifestations include rapidly progressing periodontal disease, hypodontia, increased dental caries, thin enamel structure, intraoral brown pigmentation traurodontism and blurred roots.

Prognosis

Major part of patients die before 20 years—mainly from infectious complications of immune deficiency.

Bibliography

Chaturvedi P: Gutka or areca nut chewer's syndrome. Indian Journal of Cancer April 2009 Volume 46 (2) 170-172

Kahn Micheal : Basic Oral and Maxillofacial Pathology. Volume 1. 2001

Norman S, Williams, Cristopher J K, Bulstrode P, Roman O'Connell: Bailey and Love's Short Practice of Surgery. Twenty-fifth Edition: Hodder Armold 2008.

Stephen J. Macphee, Maxine A. Papadakis Current Medical Diagnosis and Treatment 2008. Lange 47th edition.

CHAPTER

21

MALIGNANT TUMOURS OF ORAL CAVITY

CHARACTERISTICS OF MALIGNANT TUMOURS

Characteristics of malignant tumours are described under the following heads:

1. **Rate of growth:** Malignant tumours grow much faster and progressively by a process of infiltration. The rate at which the tumour enlarges depends on three factors—the rate at which the tumour cells divide, the rate at which the tumour cells are destroyed, and the behaviour of the non-neoplastic elements within the tumour.
2. **Differentiation—Structural:** Malignant tumours are characterised by a wide range of parenchymal cell differentiation, from surprising well-differentiated to completely undifferentiated cells. When constituent cells closely resemble the tissue of origin, the tumour is termed well-differentiated.

   When tumour cells show only a passing resemblance to the tissue of origin, the neoplasm is termed as poorly differentiated malignant neoplasm.

   When the failure of differentiation, it is not possible to identify the cell of origin, on morphological observation the growth is termed anaplastic malignant neoplasm. Lack of differentiation is a hallmark of malignancy.
3. **Anaplasia Cellular features of anaplasia**
   a. **Cellular pleomorphism:** Increase variation in the shape and size of the cell.
   b. **Nuclear pleomorphism:** Increase nuclear variation in the shape and size of nuclei.
   c. **Hyperchromatism:** The nuclei are hyperchromatic and large. There is increase in the density of staining of nuclei, due to increase in amount of nucleoprotein. When measured precisely by flow cytometry, the DNA content of malignant cells correlates well with degree of malignancy in multiple myeloma.

d. **Nuclear-cytoplasmic ratio:** Increase in size of nuclei relative to the size of the cytoplasm, nuclear-cytoplasmic ratio may approach 1 : 1 instead of 1 : 6.

e. **Mitosis:** Mitotic figures are numerous and distinctly atypical. Mitotic figures are more important in malignant tumours as tripolar, quadripolar and multipolar spindle.

f. **Chromatin:** Coarse and clumped chromatin and increase chromosomal number (aneuploidy).

g. **Nuclear membrane:** Irregular.

h. **Nucleoli:** Macro and multiple nucleoli are present.

i. **Giant cells:** Large multinucleated tumour giant cells with several nucleoli may be present.

4. **Loss of polarity:** Epithelial cells arranged in sheets show a normal alignment to their neighbors. This normal arrangement is lost in a malignant growth with the result that cells are in chaotic fashion and present a jumbled up arrangement in relation to the surface and to each other. Tumour cells lose their basal polarity, so that the nuclei tend to lie away from the basement membrane.
5. **Rupture of basement membrane:** This is the most important marker to indicate that a particular tumour is malignant.
6. **Functional:** Well-differentiated squamous cell carcinomas elaborate keratin. There may be qualitative and quantitative abnormality of the cellular function in some anaplastic tumour, e.g., multiple myeloma producing immunoglobulin in large quantity.
7. **Invasion:** Cancer grows by progressive infiltration, invasion, destruction and penetration of the surrounding tissue. They are non-capsulated and cannot be demarcated from surrounding tissue.
8. **Metastasis:** The cells from primary malignant neoplasm can become detached, move to a different part of body and grow as a separate mass of tumour—this process is known as metastasis. The term metastasis denotes the development of secondary implant. Metastasis is discontinuous with primary tumour possibly in some remote tissue. Basal cell carcinoma of the skin and most primary tumours of central nervous system are highly invasive in their primary sites of origin but rarely metastasise.
9. **Chromosomal abnormalities:** The chromosomal abnormalities are marked in malignant tumours. Most malignant tumours show DNA aneuploidy. One of the most important examples of a consistent chromosomal abnormality in human malignancy is the presence of Philadelphia chromosome in 90% of chronic myeloid leukaemia. Other tumours showing chromosomal abnormalities are Burkitt's lymphoma, acute lymphoid leukaemia, multiple myeloma, retinoblastoma, and oat cell carcinoma of lung.

TABLE 21.1
CLASSIFICATION OF MALIGNANT TUMOURS OF ORAL CAVITY

I. *Epithelial tumours*

A. Surface epithelium

- Keratoacanthoma
- Malignant melanoma
- Transitional cell carcinoma
- Spindle cell carcinoma
- Carcinomatous epulis
- Squamous cell carcinoma (primary and metastatic)
- Basal cell carcinoma
- Verrucous carcinoma
- Primary intraalveolar carcinoma

Contd.

Contd.

B. Glandular epithelium	
❖ Malignant pleomorphic adenoma	❖ Mucoepidermoid carcinoma
❖ Adenocarcinoma	
II. Connective tissue	
A. Fibrous tissue	
❖ Fibrosarcoma	❖ Malignant fibrous histiocytoma
B. Adipose tissue	
❖ Liposarcoma	
C. Muscle tissue	
❖ Rhabdomyosarcoma	❖ Leiomyosarcoma
❖ Malignant granular cell tumour	
D. Vascular	
❖ Haemangioendothelioma	❖ Kaposi's sarcoma
❖ Ewing's tumour	
E. Osteogenic	
❖ Osteogenic sarcoma	❖ Multiple myeloma
❖ Osteochondrosarcoma	
F. Cartilage	
❖ Chondrosarcoma	
G. Neural tissue	
❖ Neurosarcoma	❖ Neurofibrosarcoma
❖ Neuroblastoma	❖ Ganglioneuroma
H. Lymphoid tissue	
❖ Hodgkin's lymphoma	❖ Non-Hodgkin's lymphoma
❖ Primary reticulum cell sarcoma	❖ Burkitt's lymphoma

KERATOACANTHOMA

It is also known as 'self-healing carcinoma', 'molluscum sebaceum'.

Jonathan Hutchinson first described Keratoacanthomas in 1889 as crateriform ulcers of the face.

In the past it was regarded as benign, but some of these tumours have been seen to transfer into squamous cell carcinoma. Keratoacanthoma is now regarded and treated by many as malignant tumour. It is a cancer that resembles a benign neoplasm (pseudobenignity).

Keratoacanthoma is reported in Japanese, Filipino, Americans and Hawaiian population. It is less common in darker skinned individuals. Annual incidence is 104 per 100,000.

Classification

Keratoacanthoma may be divided into the following types:

- Giant keratoacanthoma.
- Keratoacanthoma centrifugam marginatum.
- Multiple keratoacanthoma (Multiple keratoacanthomas of the Feruson-Smith type).
- Generalised keratoacanthoma.
- Subungual keratoacanthoma.

Clinical features

Site: Keratoacanthoma is a neoplasm-like swelling that occurs on the skin and may involve the vermilion border. It has been reported to occur intraorally but rarely does so—on the lower lip.

Keratoacanthoma appears between the ages of 12 and 80 years. Males are more often affected.

It appears clinically as a painless, crater-forming tumour. On examination it is firm, bud-mulberry shaped, non-tender, well-demarcated, dome-shaped, sessile nodule, solitary and rarely multiple. Spontaneous healing over a period of two to four months may be observed, but surgical excision remains the treatment of choice.

Microscopically: The lesion demonstrates a cup-shaped invagination of squamous epithelium with abundant cytoplasm surrounding a central crater of parakeratotic material.

Etiology

The etiology of the lesion is uncertain, but UV light, viruses, chemical carcinogens, and immunosuppressive drugs have been suggested as contributing factors.

1. Keratoacanthoma of oral cavity and lips in the Middle East is known to occur in smokers of **'Shisha'** and **'Goza'** which contains a mixture of crude tobacco fermented with molasses and fruits.
2. Chemical carcinogens have been implicated as pathologic factors in the tumour. Industrial workers exposed to pitch and tar has been well-established.
3. Finally, research has identified that up to one-third of keratoacanthomas harbor chromosomal aberrations. Recurrent aberrations include gains on 8q, 1p, and 9q with deletions on 3p, 9p, 19p and 19q.
4. There may be seasonal presentation of keratoacanthoma that suggests ultraviolet radiation has an acute effect on the development of keratoacanthoma.
5. Keratoacanthoma may develop at the site of previous trauma.
6. Viral etiology is uncertain, as human papilloma virus-DNA sequences were not detected in lesions by polymerase chain reaction.
7. The keratoacanthoma may serve as a marker for the important autosomal dominant familial cancer syndrome, the Muir-Torre syndrome, as a result of a defective DNA mismatched repair gene.

Treatment

1. **Liquid nitrogen freezing:** If keratoacanthoma is small it may be treated by freezing with liquid nitrogen with a spray or on cotton wool swab.
2. **Curettage and Cautery:** It is sometimes used for thicker lesions. A little anesthetic is injected around the base of the lesion and it is then scraped out with a sharp spoon. The base of keratoacanthoma is cauterised with an instrument similar to a soldering iron.
3. **Excision** is another common method of removing keratoacanthomas. After local anesthetic, the affected area is cut out in an ellipse ensuring complete removal. Rarely Moh's microscopic controlled surgery may be required for larger keratoacanthomas, especially if they have recurred.
4. **Radiotherapy:** Sometimes a large keratoacanthoma is treated by radiotherapy. Several visits over a period of days are usually required. The treatment is quite painless. A scab then forms and drops off after several weeks.

SQUAMOUS CELL CARCINOMA

Oral and pharyngeal cancer represents 3% to 5% of all forms of cancer. The cancers of the oral cavity represent 2% of all cancers diagnosed annually in the United States. In India, nearly 48% of all cancers are located in oral cavity.

Common sites of oral cancers are the floor of the mouth, the sides and undersurface of tongue, the back of the throat and the lips.

90% of oral cancers are of a type called squamous cell carcinoma.

Risk factors

1. **Genetic factors:** Genetic factors involved in the development of cancer include:
   a. **Hereditary predisposition:** An individual with a hereditary predisposition for cancer is a person with an increased likelihood of developing cancer due to inherited genes. These inherited genes make body cells more sensitive to environmental factors, such as sunlight, tobacco, and, therefore, change normal cells into cancer cells. Lip cancer is amongst the sites which show strongest cancer clustering in families.

   b. **Oncogenes:** Cancers can be derived from mutations in genes that change cell growth patterns. These genes are called oncogenes. Such a mutation in an oncogene can convert ordinary body cells into cancer cells. Cancers caused by oncogenes are not inherited. Several oncogenes have been associated with oral cancers. Chromosomal abnormalities detected in tumour cells that might have a role in the primary pathogenesis of the tumour are del 18q, 10p, 8p, and 3p, point of mutations in the TP53 gene and amplification of the INT-2 and BCL-2 oncogenes.

   c. **Tumour suppressor genes:** Normal tumour suppressor genes are anti-cancerous genes that slow down or stop growth of normal body cells. Mutations of tumour suppressor genes can also cause the development of oral and pharyngeal cancers.

2. **Tobacco:** Tobacco is a known carcinogen, which means that it is known to damage cellular DNA. Thus the tobacco causes malignant mutations in the cellular DNA. 90% of people with oral cancers use tobacco by smoking cigarettes, cigars, and pipes, chewing tobacco and dipping snuff. Tobacco can damage cells in the lining of the oral cavity and oropharynx, causing abnormal cells to grow more rapidly to repair the damage. Smoking is strongly associated with soft palatal cancer than anterior sites.

   Khaini cancer: It is a squamous cell carcinoma of the lower lip encountered in people of Uttar Pradesh and Bihar. Khaini is a mixture of freshly powdered tobacco and slaked lime and the mixture is kept for hours in the gingivolabial sulcus and sucked.

   Carcinoma of base of tongue and tonsil has an excessive frequency in Gujarati Hindus who are particularly habituated to smoking bidis and chewing tobacco.

3. **Alcohol:** The majority of patients with oral cancer (75 to 80%) use alcohol frequently. Paired with tobacco use, patients who drink and smoke increase their risk of developing oral cancer even more. Researchers have found that alcohol increases the penetration of DNA-damaging chemicals in the lining of the oral cavity and oropharynx.

4. **Chronic irritation:** Chronic irritation to the lining of the mouth, due to poorly fitting dentures or other reasons may increase a person's risk for oral cancer. Other factors include chronic cheek biting, irregular teeth may act as co-carcinogen and may promote transformation of epithelial cells.

5. **Physical agents: Chutta cancer:** Squamous cell carcinoma of the hard palate prevailing in Andhra Pradesh is associated with the habit of smoking chutta (a cigar) with burning end inside the mouth.

6. **Age and sex:** The large majority of squamous cell carcinoma victims are over the age of 45. The disease affects males more frequently than females, with a male to female ratio of 2 : 1.

7. **Human papilloma virus:** The human papilloma virus is transferred from person to person by vigorous physical contact, especially oral sexual contact. The presence of HPV may be the

major risk factor in the development of oral cancer in patients who are not heavy smokers and drinkers.

8. **Immunodeficiency:** People taking immunosuppressive drugs for certain conditions—such as organ and bone marrow transplantation—may be at increased risk. HIV/AIDS patients are at increased risk of oral cancer.
9. **Excessive exposure to ultraviolet light:** Sunlight has been implicated as a major contributor to the development of lip cancer. Since lip lacks a pigmented layer for protection, it is susceptible to actinic changes.
10. **Certain occupational exposures:** There are no occupational exposures that have been strongly and consistently implicated as causes of oral cavity cancer. However, several exposures, occupations and industries have been inconsistently associated with increased risk. These include polycyclic aromatic hydrocarbons (PAHS), solvents, formaldehyde, phenoxyacetic acid and ionising radiation, working as a wood-worker; wood product worker and carpet installer, outdoor work and work in the pulp mill industry.
11. **Betel nut:** Cancer of mucosa of cheek and the adjacent gingival groove is common in Southwestern coastal region of India and Sri Lanka and attributed to the custom of chewing pan. Betel leaves are carcinogenic.
12. **Lack of fruits and vegetables:** Research has suggested that fruits and vegetables which contain antioxidants that can 'trap' harmful molecules can decrease the risk for oral cancer. Thus, it is speculated that persons with a low intake of these types of foods are at an increased risk for oral cancer.
13. **Syphilis:** Inadequately treated or untreated syphilitic leukoplakia may undergo malignant transformation.
14. **Precancerous intraoral lesion** can be responsible for oral malignancy. They include lichen planus, candidiasis, leukoplakia, median rhomboid glossitis, Plummer-Vinson syndrome, oral submucus fibrosis, oral melanosis and discoid lupus erythematosus.

Macroscopically, these tumours appear ulcerative or exophytic. There may be tethering of tongue by infiltration of the tumour. The tongue and floor of mouth are the common sites of oral carcinoma.

Microscopically

Well-differentiated squamous cell carcinoma is composed of malignant epithelial island which resembles normal stratified squamous epithelium, except that they are invading the underlying tissues and show aberrant abnormal keratinisation; there is often a prominent keratin formation in the infiltrating islands, usually strong host response lymphocytes in the stroma, the tumour may be, frankly, deeply invasive.

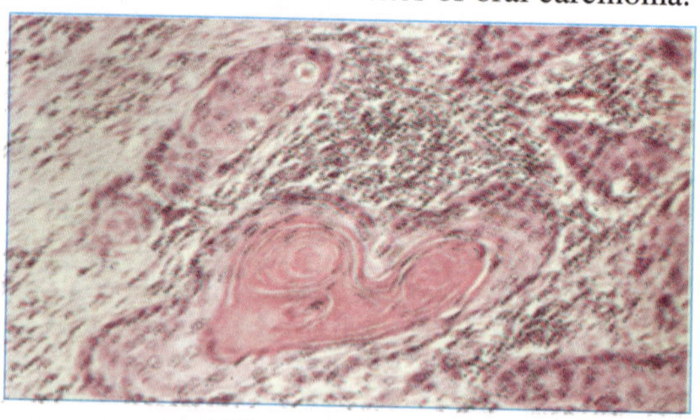

Fig.21.1: Well-differentiated squamous cell carcinoma showing epithelial pearls

Poorly differentiated squamous cell carcinoma is associated with poorer prognosis, keratin formation is minimal, malignant cells do not exhibit distinction between basal and parabasal population, mitoses are more frequent, and host response is usually less conspicuous than in better-differentiated carcinoma.

Spread

Lymphatic: Cervical lymph nodes.

Distant spread: Lungs and bones.

Perineural spread—through the trigeminal nerve to the brain.

VERRUCOUS CARCINOMA

It is a type of squamous cell carcinoma that makes up less than 5% of all oral cavity tumours. It is a low-grade cancer that rarely spreads to other parts of the body but can deeply spread into the surrounding tissue.

Sex: It is more common in males than females.

Age: It is more common above the age of 55 years.

Site: Common sites are mandibular vestibules, buccal mucosa, hard palate and gingival. These are the common sites of tobacco placement.

Etiology: Risk factors are chewing tobacco and use of snuff.

Clinical features: The tumour is white, may be pink. It is a diffuse, painless, thick mass with papillary projections.

Histologically: Verrucous carcinoma is made up of a papillary exophytic and deeply invasive endophytic growth with glassy well-differentiated squamous cells showing minimal atypia. There is abundant keratin and wide and bulbous rete pegs.

CARCINOMATOUS EPULIS

It is the carcinoma of the alveolus and is epidermoid in origin. Usually ulcerative, ulceroproliferative, or fungating in nature, it may invade the bone and involve regional lymph nodes.

SPINDLE CELL CARCINOMA

Spindle cell carcinoma (SPCC) is also known as ***'sarcomatoid carcinoma'***, ***'Lane tumour'*** ***'carcinosarcoma'***, or ***'pseudosarcoma'***. It is a rare neoplasm of head and neck.

Clinical features

The mean age at diagnosis of spindle cell carcinoma is 57 years (range 29 to 93 years). There is equal frequency in male and females. Many cases end up with pronounced parasthesia as the lesion increases in size involving the nerves in the affected region. It was also commented that lower lip lesions have a special propensity to travel along the nerves through mental foramen and into the mandibular canal.

Sites: The neoplasm occurs predominantly in the upper aerodigestive tract, especially the larynx, oral cavity, and oesophagus. In the oral cavity lower lip, lateral posterior tongue and alveolar ridges are common sites, but other areas may be involved.

The spindle cell carcinoma typically appears as pedunculated, polypoid mass, but may occasionally appear as sessile, nodular or fungating mass. Surface ulceration is common.

Microscopically

It is a rare, highly malignant variant of squamous cell carcinoma (SCC); which shows proliferation of conventional squamous cell carcinoma component and malignant spindle cell with sarcomatous appearance.

Spindle cells are elongated with central elongated nuclei. These are arranged in entangled fascicles intertwining bundles. The degree of hyperchromasia, enlarged nuclear cytoplasmic ratio, mitoses, and pleomorphism are strongly suggestive of a leiomyoma or a fibrosarcoma.

Immunohistochemistry reveals that the tumour stains positively with EMA, cytokeratin, and vimentin.

Cervical lymph nodes are invariably involved and may appear indurated and immobile.

Treatment

Surgical removal of tumour with or without radical neck dissection and radiation therapy is used.

BASELOID SQUAMOUS CELL CARCINOMA

This neoplasm tends to occur in persons 40-85 years of age.

Baseloid squamous cell carcinoma is less common than conventional squamous cell carcinoma of the head and neck. It is considerably more aggressive than unqualified squamous cell carcinoma, with a tendency to involve the tongue base, supraglottic, larynx, the pyriform sinuses, oesophagus, and lungs.

Baseloid squamous cell carcinoma is more common in elderly males. Almost 80% of patients have cervical metastases at the time of diagnosis of these high-grade tumours.

Almost all baseloid squamous cell carcinoma have regions of conventional squamous cell carcinoma. In addition, they have a follicular, or lobular pattern of invasion, with peripheral slightly elongated, palisaded cells surrounding each lobules. The lobules often contain central comedo necrosis, with visible necrotic material. At other times the central material completely *'drops out'*—giving a pseudoglandular pattern appearance. Epithelium overlying the tumour may exhibit dysplasia or carcinoma in situ.

Special stains and immunochemistry show predominant expression of keratins 14 and 19 at the periphery.

CARCINOMA TONGUE

Squamous cell carcinoma is by far the commonest malignancy of the tongue.

Etiology

There is an association between lingual cancer and syphilis. Among chewers of betel nut, cancer of tongue is a well-recognised hazard and the incidence of this neoplasm is high in the Indian subcontinent. The excessive use of tobacco, taken as snuff, chewed, smoked in pipes or as cigars or cigarettes and the immoderate consumption of alcohol have also been implicated as predisposing agents. It is usually preceded by precancerous or irritating conditions like chronic ulcer, leukoplakia, and fissures in the tongue.

Clinical features

Clinical features of carcinoma tongue include:

- It is commonly seen in the fifth or sixth decade of life. In younger individuals, there is smaller sex bias; in some series females have outnumbered males
- Persistent soreness
- Mouth or tongue pain: Lingual pain is due to infection and ulceration of the tongue
- Abnormal growths in the mouth or on the tongue
- Solid lumps on cheek
- Difficulty in chewing, swallowing (dysphagia) and speaking
- A white or red patch on the tongue that will not go away
- Unexplained bleeding from the tongue
- Pain in ear
- Change in the sound of voice
- Alterations in the way that dentures fit inside the mouth
- Foetor oris is due to infected necrotic growth.

Sites

In about 75% of cases, lingual cancer affects the anterior two-thirds of the tongue, the remainder appearing at the base of the tongue. Most lingual cancers in Western countries arise along or near the edge of the anterior two-third of the tongue and are sometimes related to a patch of dyskeratotic leukoplakia. Less frequently, the growth develops on the under surface of the mobile portion of the lingula. Carcinoma of the dorsum of the tongue is more common and the tip of the tongue is a very infrequent site of origin.

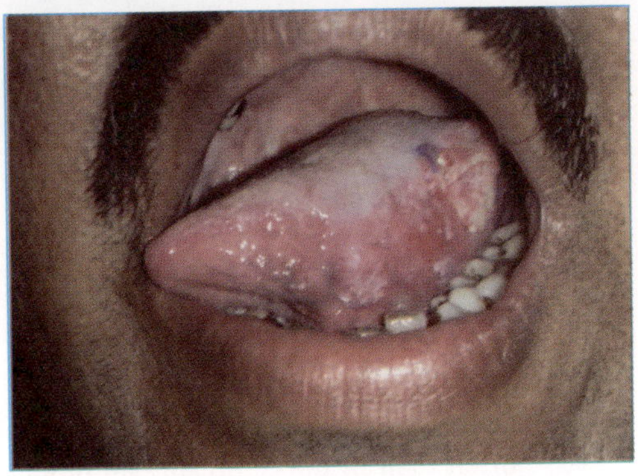

Fig.21.2: Showing ulcerative carcinoma tongue lateral border

Pathological types

1. Lingual carcinoma may appear as an exophytic growth, or a proliferative growth (verrucous carcinoma).
2. A painful non-healing ulcer usually on the lateral surface of tongue.

   The ulcer is usually single, occurring at the margin or near the circumvallate papillae but may be multiple, when superimposed on chronic superficial glossitis. A malignant ulcer of tongue is hard, indurated with a round or everted edge and shows excessive necrosis and sloughing of the floor. Early carcinomas are smaller than 1 cm and may be detected during routine clinical examination.
3. An infiltrative lesion slowly involves the adjacent structures like tongue, mandible, floor of the mouth, skin etc.

   In many cases, cervical lymphadenitis may be present.

Microscopically

Microscopically, the majority of carcinomas arising at front of tongue are squamous cell tumours of varying degrees of cornification and differentiation. Some invasive cancers are well-differentiated variants; others show undifferentiated and an occasional carcinoma consists of predominantly of clear cells filled with glycogen.

Spread

Local invasion may affect floor of the mouth.

Lymphatic spread: Spread through lymphatics is early. Rapid spread of carcinoma of the tongue is due to more than one factor, e.g., (1) extremely rich lymphatic drainage of the tongue, (2) frequent muscular movements, and (3) high grade malignancy of the tumour.

The spread takes place into the submental and submaxillary lymph nodes, superior and inferior deep cervical nodes and even to the supraclavicular nodes. The tumours of the posterior third—the upper deep cervical group of lymph nodes of both the sides of the neck—may be involved.

Haematogenous spread to the lung, liver, skeleton, adrenal and kidney occurs late.

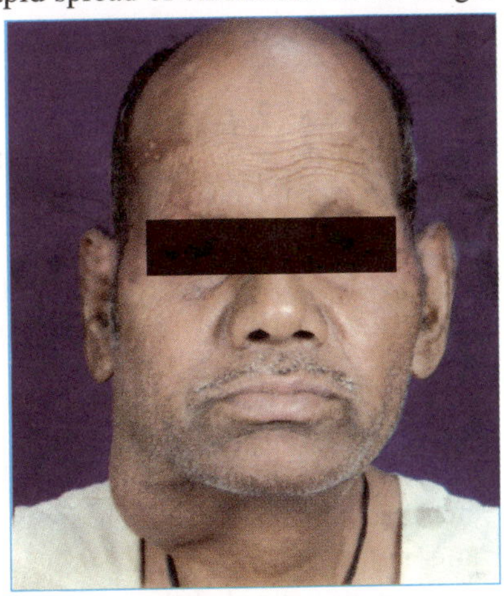

Fig.21.3: Showing metastasis in submandibular lymph node from a case of carcinoma tongue

Treatment

Surgery, radiotherapy, and chemotherapy are the methods of choice.

Two common chemotherapy drugs are used to treat carcinoma tongue. They are cisplatin, 5 flurouracil. Other drugs used less often include carboplatin, bleomycin, and methotrexate.

Recurrences usually occur within 24 months, the majority occurs within first 12 months following primary treatment.

CARCINOMA LIP

Lip malignancies are mostly related to actinic exposure (a pigmented layer is lacking in Caucasian races), although chronic irritation (pipe smokers—heat, smokeless tobacco) may also play a role. Since it is common in agriculturists, who are constantly exposed to sunlight, it is called as '*Countryman's lip*'. It is also seen in sailors, betel-nut chewers, and powdered tobacco users.

Clinical features

1. Carcinoma of the lower lip develops nearly always in males and does so at least 12 times more often than in upper lip. In carcinoma of upper lip the incidence is higher in females than in males.
2. The lesion is common between the ages of 25 to 50 years.
3. Patient complains sore on the lip that does not heal. It begins as a patch of senile keratosis that develops into indurated nodules or wart-like thickening on the mucous membrane or vermilion border.
4. There is presence of lump or thickening on the lips with bleeding, pain or numbness.
5. The tumour often appears clinically as intractable ulcerations on the vermilion border of the lip but may also consist of large exophytic lesions.

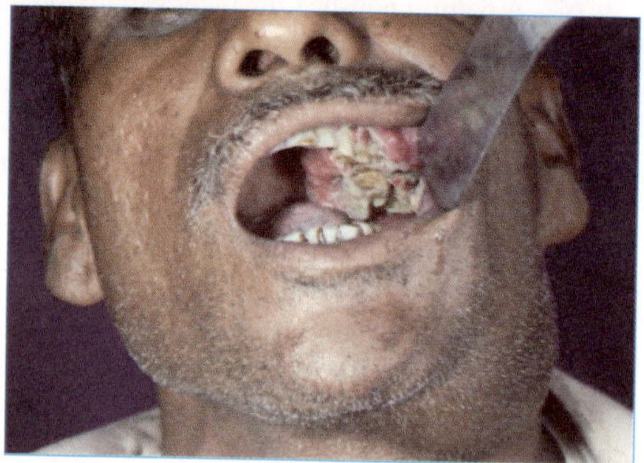

Fig.21.4: Carcinoma left buccal mucosa with ipsilateral secondary in neck

Microscopically

Carcinoma of the lip can occur in three variants: Squamous cell, spindle cell, and baseloid squamous cell. Most of the carcinomas of lip are well-differentiated squamous cell tumours and only a few show a poorly differentiated structure.

Spread

Local spread: A carcinoma lip spreads directly and may eventually involve gum and other adjacent structures.

Lymph node metastasis develops late. Submental and submandibular nodes are the first to be involved; other deep cervical nodes may also get involved later.

Haematogenous spread: Distant metastases to the lung, pancreas, and brain have been reported.

Management

In early cases—especially of well-differentiated carcinomas—the prognosis is favourable after radiotherapy or a local surgical removal of the tumour, provided the growth is small and metastasis to regional lymph nodes has not taken place.

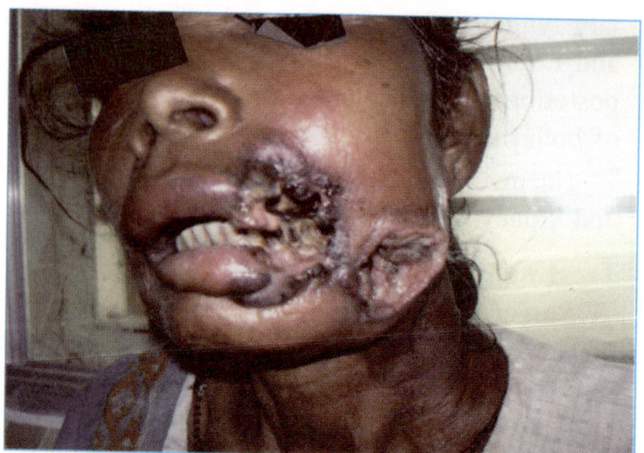

Fig.21.5: Showing carcinoma lip infiltration into cheek

CARCINOMA OF SOFT AND HARD PALATE

In the United States, approximately 25% of all squamous cell carcinomas of the palate occur on the hard palate and 75% on the soft palate.

It is a common lesion in India and is seen equally often on the hard and soft palate. Squamous cell carcinoma of the hard palate is prevailing in Andhra Pradesh—associated with the habit of smoking chutta (a cigar) with burning end inside the mouth. Other factors, including ill-fitting dentures, poor oral hygiene, mechanical irritation, and mouthwash are implicated in palatal carcinoma.

Epidermoid carcinoma of the palate is infrequent and usually occurs on soft palate.

Clinically

Squamous cell carcinomas of the soft palate is two to three times more common in men and tends to occur in older individuals with a mean age of about 60 years.

Patients are asymptomatic in early stages, but they may experience pain in advanced stages. A palate mass, bleeding, a foul odour, ill-fitting dentures in edentulous patients or loose teeth may be presenting symptoms for patients with hard palate cancer. In patients with advanced stage of soft palate cancers, velopharyngeal insufficiency, altered speech, difficulty in swallowing, referred otolgia, trismus, or a neck mass may be present.

Squamous cell carcinoma of the soft palate may present as an exophytic growth, an ulcer, a slightly elevated plaque, or as a diffuse area of erythroplakia with poorly defined margins and multiple superficial ulcers.

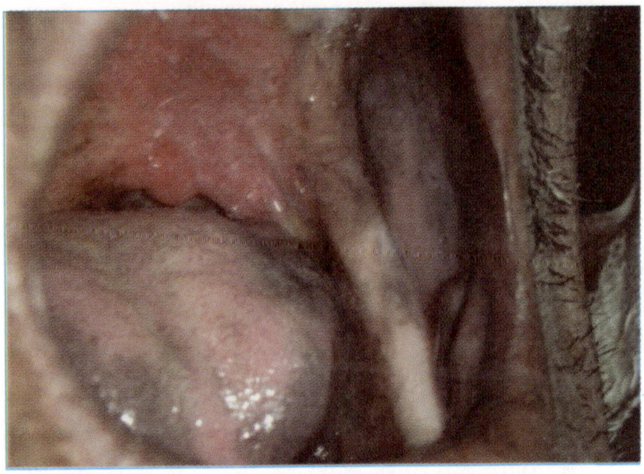

Fig.21.6: Showing ulcerated growth soft palate

Microscopically

The squamous cell carcinoma represents 95% of malignant tumours of soft palate.

Adenocarcinoma of the palate arises in the small collections of salivary tissue, which are normally to be found in the palate as elsewhere in the mucosa of the mouth. Occasionally, a papillary adenocarcinoma and baseloid squamous cell carcinoma may occur.

Spread

Carcinoma of hard palate occurs by direct extension in the underlying bone. Metastases may develop in regional lymph nodes.

Management

Carcinoma of soft palate is treated with radiotherapy, but if tumour proves radio-resistant or recurs, radical excision of soft palate is carried out. A small carcinoma (less than 2.5 cm in diameter) of the hard palate is given preoperative radiotherapy. When complete regression of tumour does not occur—wide surgical excision including the underlying bone involvement, so a partial resection of the maxilla including the whole tumour area is preferred.

CARCINOMA OF BUCCAL MUCOSA

Carcinoma of buccal mucosa is relatively uncommon in North America, compared with other cavity cancers such as carcinomas of tongue or floor of the mouth. Squamous cell carcinoma of buccal mucosa accounts for 5 to 10% of all cancers of the oral cavity in North America and Western Europe. In India, over 90% of patients with buccal mucosa carcinoma have a history of using betel nut.

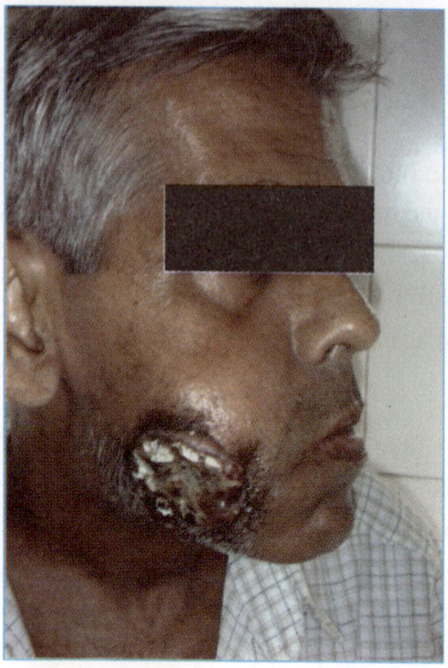

Fig.21.7: Showing ulcerated growth arising from buccal mucosa

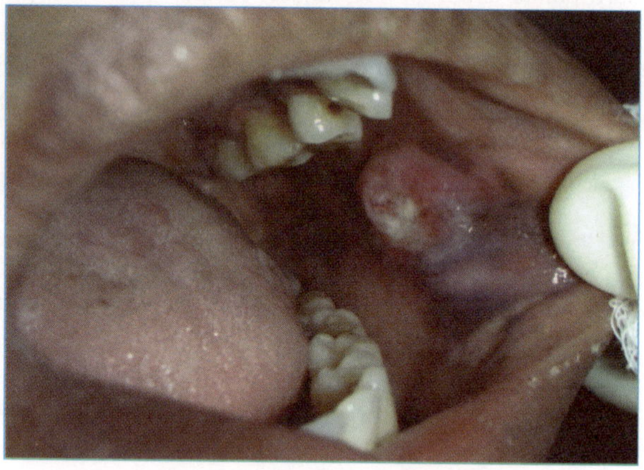

Fig.21.8: Shows malignant lesion arising from left buccal mucosa

Clinical features

1. Most cases occur in sixth and seventh decades of life, with over 90% developing after the age of 40 years. Tumours in younger individuals under the age of 40 years show a less marked sex bias and are of poorer prognosis.
2. In India, buccal mucosa carcinoma is the most common cancer in men and the third-most common cancer in women. It occurs more often in men, with a male female ratio of 3-4 : 1.
3. A patchy type of leukoplakia is often related to carcinoma of buccal mucosa and, not uncommonly, the growth appears to arise from these lesions.
4. The tumours are usually soft growths that thicken in the submucosa beneath an innocent-appearing surface. The nodule in the submucosa, however, consists of infiltrating cords of malignant squamous cells and, as it enlarges, it suffers ulcerations.
5. Carcinoma may be present as an area of leukoplakia—an erthyematous patch or papillomatous, exophytic, ulcerative, infiltrative. Buccal mucosa is also the most common site for verrucous carcinoma, which is a white papillary growth with considerable keratinisation.

Microscopically

Microscopically it is a well-differentiated squamous cell carcinoma comprising of bulbous masses of squamous cells, often with nests of keratinised epithelium. Other patterns include anaplastic carcinoma, verrucous carcinoma, spindle cell carcinoma, adenoid cystic carcinoma, and mucoepidermoid carcinoma.

Spread

Tumour may spread radially from its site of origin and involve angle of the mouth and lip anteriorly, retromolar trigone and medial pterygoid posteriorly, upper gingivobuccal sulcus and maxilla superiorly, lower gingivobuccal sulcus and alveolar ridge and gums inferiorly. Submandibular salivary gland may become involved. Verrucous carcinomas spread superficially and extend into the subjacent tissues, including bone, but seldom metastasise.

Distant metastasis to the lung and brain is also seen.

CANCER OF FLOOR OF MOUTH

Cancer of floor of mouth accounts for 5% of all cancers in the United States, it accounts for 50% of all cancers in India.

Clinical features

Carcinoma of floor of mouth occurs predominantly in males. It is situated on either side of the midline.

Most common presentation of cancer of the floor of the mouth is a painless inflamed superficial ulcer with poorly defined margins or, sometimes, papillomatous area. Preexistent leukoplakia can be observed in adjacent tissues in approximately 20% of cases.

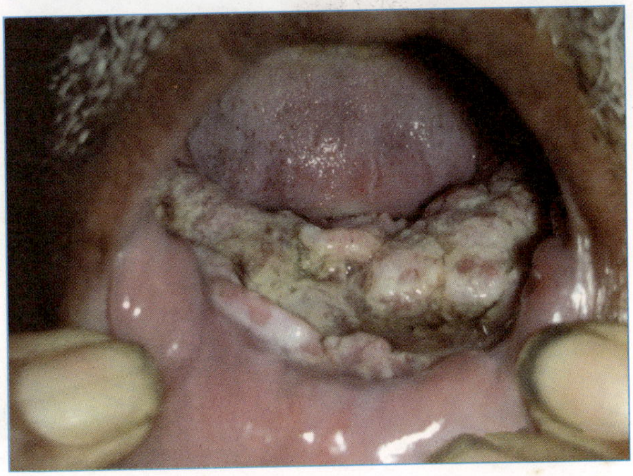

Fig.21.9: Shows exophytic growth arising from floor of mouth

Spread

Primary tumour of floor of the mouth is often silent until assuming significant dimension. Extension onto the ventral surface of the tongue may result in restriction of motion and dysarthria. Lingual nerve is at a risk for direct involvement and perineural spread of disease.

Distant metastases have been found in the liver, lung, kidney, adrenal and brain.

CARCINOMA MAXILLARY SINUS

They are more common in Asia and Africa than in United States.

Squamous cell carcinoma and adenocarcinoma of maxillary sinus are associated with exposure to nickel dust, mustard gas, thorotrast, isopropyl oil, chromium, or dichlorodiethyl sulphide—this is well-established.

Clinical features

The disease mainly affects men in their sixth and seventh decade of life. The disease has predilection for males. M : F ratio 3 : 1 with age range 38-89 years (mean 64 years).

Early symptoms

1. Most common symptoms are pain followed by oral symptoms, and facial swelling. Pain increases on bending forwards and coughing. Pain is due to cranial neuropathy.
2. Nasal obstruction and epistaxis may also be seen.
3. Ipsilateral epiphora (watering of the eye may be present).
4. Rhinorrhoea
5. In the early stages there is mass or small ulcer.

Delayed symptoms

1. Inferior spread causes expansion of the fitting of dentures, ulceration of gingival and swelling of hard palate.
2. When medial wall is involved, nasal obstruction and epiphora occurs due to obstruction of the lacrimal duct. Bleeding from nose can also occur if there is ulceration.
3. Anterior spread causes swelling of cheek and, later, invasion of the facial skin.
4. Superior spread invades the orbit causing proptosis, diplopia, ocular pain, and epiphora.

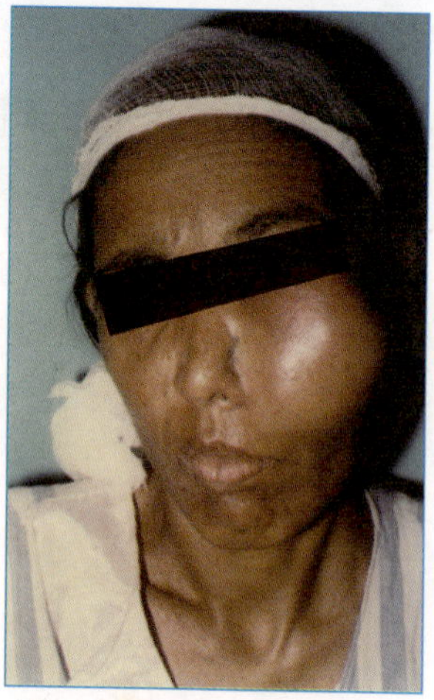

Fig.21.10: Showing growth over maxilla (carcinoma maxillary antrum).

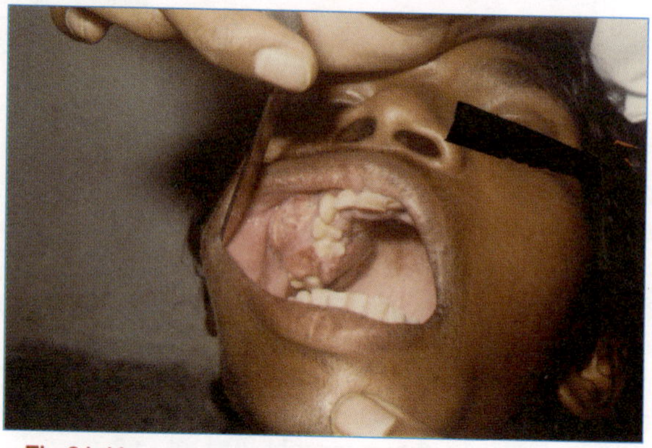

Fig.21.11: Showing carcinoma maxilla in 16-year male infiltrating into oral cavity

5. Posteriorly, the spread occurs to the pterygopalatine fossa and infratemporal fossa resulting in trismus because of involvement of the pterygoids.
6. In advanced disease, large ulceration, necrosis, heaped edges, and bone and soft tissue invasion may be observed.

The tumour metastasises to cervical or submandibular lymph nodes at the time of diagnosis.

Microscopically

Microscopic examination reveals a solid tumour mass invading adjacent bone structures composed of spindle and round epithelial cells arranged in sheets, ribbons, and individual squamous, polyhedral cells with various degrees of keratinisation. There is cellular pleomorphism, nuclear hyperchromatism, mitoses, macronucleoli and altered nuclear cytoplasmic ratio. Several variants of squamous cell carcinoma of paranasal sinuses include verrucous carcinoma, baseloid squamous cell carcinoma, spindle cell carcinoma and transitional cell carcinoma. Other histological varieties include adenocarcinoma of salivary gland origin; mucoepidermoid carcinomas are reported in maxillary sinus.

Immunohistochemical analysis shows positivity for cytokeratin and negative for actin, human epithelial membrane desmin, HMB-45 and S-100.

Management

The optimum management of carcinoma arising in the maxillary sinus remains undefined. Therapeutic approaches include surgery, radiation, and systemic local and topical chemotherapy in a variety of combination and sequences.

MALIGNANT MELANOMA

Melanoma represents 5 to 21% of all skin malignancies. It is predominantly a disease of Caucasian, particularly those of English, Scottish or Irish descents who are exposed to tropical sun.

Approximately 1% of malignant melanomas arise in the oral mucosa.

Etiology

1. Sunlight is very important etiological factor in cutaneous melanomas. Epidemiological studies suggest that exposure to ultraviolet radiation (UVA and UVB) is one of the major contributions to the development of melanoma.

2. **Molecular genetics:** A family history of melanoma greatly increases a person's risk because mutations in CDKN2A, CDK4.

Racial predisposition: Cutaneous phenotype such as fair skin (skin types I to III), blond hair colour, and freckling—all those are racial and also correlate with occurrence of melanoma.

Precursor lesions: Some pigmented lesions have a high risk of malignant transformation e.g., dysplastic naevus syndrome, congenital giant melanocyte nevi.

Age: The patients are usually above the age of 40 years. Most of the cases occur between fourth and seventh decade of life. Oral malignant melanoma is rare before the age of 20 years.

Sites: The most frequent site of occurrence is the hard palate followed by the maxillary gingival. Other oral sites include the mandibular, gingival, buccal mucosa, and floor of the mouth.

Types

There are four main clinical variants of melanoma:

- Superficial spreading melanoma
- Lentigo maligna melanoma
- Nodular melanoma
- Acral lentiginous melanoma

1. **Superficial spreading melanoma:** Most common subtype, accounting for 70 to 80% of all melanomas arising in a pre-existing lesion. They are common on the trunk in men and on the legs in women. The lesion tends to be larger than 6 mm in diameter, flat, asymmetric, with varying colouration. Invasive malignant melanoma generally develops from superficial melanoma in situ in 5 to 10 years.

   Microscopically, it is characterised by presence of buckshot (pagetoid) scatter of atypical melanocytes within the epidermis.
2. **Nodular malignant melanoma:** It accounts for 10% of melanomas. It arises more commonly on the head, neck, or trunk of patients in sixth decade or later. Lesions tend to be raised, brown, to black, and rapidly appearing, growing papules, they may suggest a vascular lesion and may have focal haemorrhage. The melanoma cells contain large nuclei with irregular contours; chromatin is clumped at the periphery of the nuclear membrane and prominent red (eosinophilic) nucleoli.
3. **Lentigo maligna melanoma (Hutchinson's freckle):** Lentigo maligna melanoma represents 5% to 10% of all cases of melanoma. It occurs on the damaged skin of face in elderly people. It arises from a brown macular lesion called lentigo maligna or Hutchinson's freckle. The lesion is brown with some variation in epidermal pigment density. It has got predilection for exposed parts. As the disease advances, invasion and metastasis are frequent.

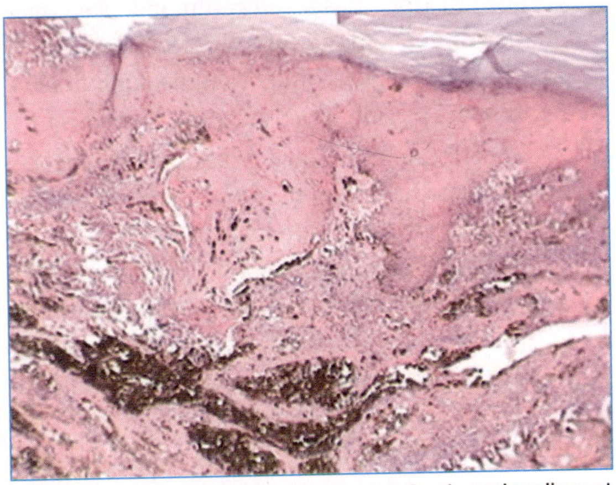

Fig.21.12: Shows hyperkeratosis acanthosis and malignant cells containing brown coloured melanin pigment

Microscopically

The basal layer of the epidermis is replaced by melanoma cells, which are large, pleomorphic, with nuclear chromatin irregularly condensed around periphery of the nucleus, prominent eosinophilic nucleolus. Most of the spindle-shaped melanoma cells are junctional in location and the lesion has prominent solar elastosis, with markedly atrophic epidermis. The melanoma cells spread laterally and in all layers of epidermis.

4. **Acral lentiginous melanoma:** It is more common in males than the female patients and usually found in older individuals. These lesions are the commonest form of malignant melanoma in Japan. Common sites are soles, palms, and mucosal surfaces. It is not related to the sun exposure, grows slowly, has prolonged radial growth phase and seldom metastasise.

Clinically

Clinical presentation of a malignant melanoma is usually brown-black coloured swelling with or without ulceration. Oral melanomas are generally painless. It may represent as a rapidly enlarging mass associated with ulceration, bleeding, pain, and bone destruction. The lesion may have a nodular or papillary surface. Occasionally, there is no distinct melanin pigmentation, being referred to as an amelanotic melanoma.

In cases of amelanotic melanoma tumour marker such as GP100 HMB45 and S100 protein may be helpful to identify the nature of the tumour.

Causes

Possible etiologic factors for melanoma are mechanical trauma, ill-fitting dentures, oral habits, self-medication and exposure to formaldehyde.

Mode of spread

Melanoma is notorious for its unpredictable and widespread metastasis. Metastatic spread to bone, usually vertebrae, is a frequent finding in terminal disease and may be accompanied by multiple metastases to the lymph nodes, central nervous system, lungs, and liver.

Regression of melanoma is a well-recognised phenomenon and may account for many cases of metastatic melanoma with occult primaries.

BASAL CELL CARCINOMA (RODENT ULCER)

Basal cell carcinoma is believed to arise from the pleuripotential stem cell compartments of the basal layer of epidermis as well as follicular structures.

Basal cell carcinoma is the most common form of skin cancer in human and prevalent in India, Australia and New Zealand.

Etiology

1. **Complexion:** Basal cell carcinoma is a common skin neoplasm, usually occurring in the sun exposed areas of light skinned individuals over the age of 40 years
2. **Genetic aspects:** There is increasing evidence that genetic factors play a role in the susceptibility of some individuals to basal cell carcinoma. Mutation in the PATCHED gene (Ptc, PTCH), which is known to be responsible for the nevoid basal cell carcinoma syndrome, has also been reported in sporadic cases of basal cell carcinoma.

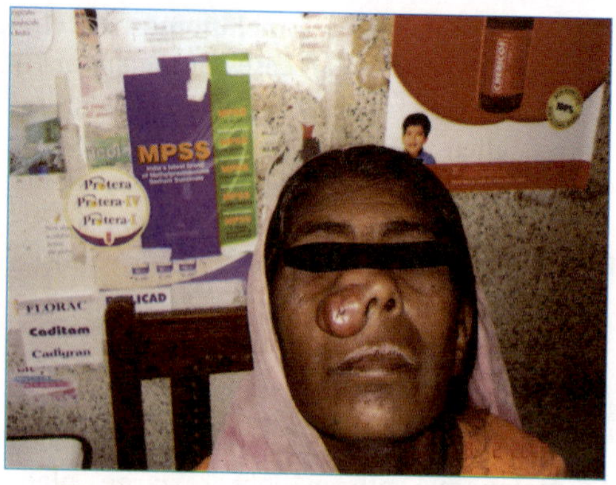

Fig.21.13: A case of basal cell carcinoma

3. **Ultraviolet rays:** UV induced mutations in the TP53 tumour suppressor gene, which resides on chromosome arm 17_p, have been implicated in some cases of basal cell carcinoma in addition to data support mutation of a tumour suppressor gene on band 9Q 22 as causing basal cell naevus syndrome, an autosomal dominant condition characterised by early and continued appearance of many basal cell carcinoma.

4. **Immunosuppression:** Immunosuppression is associated with a modest increase in the risk of basal cell carcinoma.
5. **Arsenic exposure:** Chronic exposure to arsenic is associated with basal cell carcinoma.

Clinically

Males are affected more than females. It may occur at any age but is more common after age 40. The male-to-female ratio is approximately 3 : 2.

Sites: It occurs exclusively on hairy skin, the most common location (90%) being the face, usually above an imaginary line drawn between the tragus of the ear and angle of the mouth.

Clinically, these tumours present as pearly papules, often containing prominent, dilated subepidermal blood vessels (telangiectasia). It begins as a small, pearly subcutaneous nodule, which slowly increases in size and forms an intractable ulcer with rolled out margins and mouse-eaten appearance. A typical basal cell carcinoma develops as a slightly elevated or hemispherical nodule covered by a smooth or, sometimes, horny epidermis. It is malignant and locally invasive and extremely destructive but never metastasises. The tumour is likely to destroy deeper structures including cartilage and bone.

Microscopically

The tumour arises from basal cells of epidermis. A basal cell carcinoma consists of islands of small dark cells, resembling the basal cells of the epidermis. The cell masses show considerable variation in shape and size. The cell masses accumulate in the dermis and are characteristically bordered by a single layer of cells with their nuclei arranged in palisading row. The nuclei are deeply basophilic and surrounded by a small rim of cytoplasm. The tumour may have solid, cystic, adenoid, keratotic, pigmented, infiltrating and sclerosing (morphea-like pattern) type. The cellular masses are separated by a variable amount of loose fibroblastic stroma. An ulcerated part is covered by fibrin, polymorphs, lymphocytes and plasma cells and fibrous overgrowth are noted throughout the deeper regions.

Histological types of basal cell carcinoma

Adenoid basal cell carcinoma: It represents neoplasm, which mimics glandular formation. Elongated or stellate cells sometimes form sinuses ribbon-like strands, acinar, cylindrical or lace like patterns.

Cystic basal cell carcinoma: Cystic spaces and cavities within the tumour masses usually contain a colourless fluid or rarely, mucoid substance.

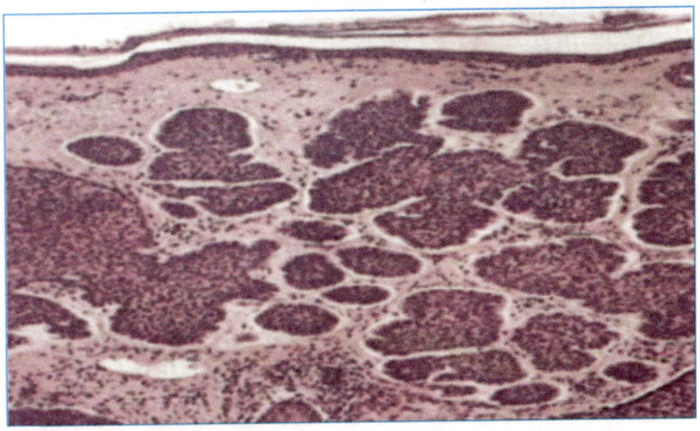

Fig.21.14: Microscopic appearance of basal cell carcinoma

Keratotic basal cell carcinoma: Foci of flattened squamous cells arranged in concentric layers are present in certain basal cell carcinoma. These structures may be numerous and frequently develop into horny pearls with keratin in their centre.

Solid or primordial basal cell carcinoma

Superficial basal cell carcinoma: The lesion originates in a multifocal manner from the basal layer of the epidermis and occasionally from the basal cells of the upper portion of the hair follicles. The condition manifests on covered portion of the body as isolated, psoriasiform plaques, which enlarge slowly and irregularly by a centrifugal process of origin and spread.

Pigmented basal cell carcinoma: In the pigmented basal cell carcinoma (melanotic rodent ulcer) the tumour contains melanin in such amount that clinically it may be mistaken for a melanoma.

Morpheaform and infiltrating basal cell carcinoma: In the morphoeic type narrow cellular strands run widely in the dermis. The stroma of the dermis is condensed and may be hyalinised.

Management

The tumour is radiocurable and radiotherapy is the method of choice.

TRANSITIONAL CELL CARCINOMA

Transitional cell carcinoma may occasionally be seen in oral cavity.

Microscopically

Transitional cell carcinomas are diffusely growing tumours devoid of epidermoid characters and in which lymphocytes are usually absent or present in minimal numbers. These growths consist of more or less uniform closely packed small round or polyhedral cells lacking intercellular bridges and arranged in solid groups, masses, sheets or anatomising columns. The cells have a relatively large nucleus set in a scanty cytoplasm.

FIBROSARCOMA

Fibrosarcoma is a malignant mesenchymal neoplasm of fibroblasts that rarely affects the oral cavity and can cause local recurrences or metastases.

Clinical features

It generally affects the sexes equally with the highest incidence in patients between 20 and 40 years of age. It is commonly seen in children, teenagers and young adults. In oral cavity it is seen in palate, tongue, cheek, maxillary sinus, pharynx, lip, periosteum of maxilla and mandible.

The tumour is slow-growing in the beginning, later on grows rapidly and destroys underlying bone. The tumour is an uncapsulated, painless, firm—sometimes lobulated mass—with surface ulceration.

Microscopically

Well-differentiated forms are cellular with marked cellular atypia and mitotic activity. The matrix is sparse.

The tumour consists of spindle-shaped cells; nucleus is hyperchromatic and show abnormal mitosis. The cells are arranged in herring bone pattern. The blood vessels are wide and thin-walled; they are embryonic which may contain malignant cells.

Treatment

Radical surgical removal of tumour including affected bone.

5 years' survival in 50% of cases.

MALIGNANT FIBROUS HISTIOCYTOMA

Malignant fibrous histiocytoma (MFH), described by O'Brien and Stout in 1964, is the most common soft tissue sarcoma of late adult life.

Types

Six subtypes have been described

1. Storiform
2. Pleomorphic
3. Myxoid
4. Giant cell
5. Inflammatory
6. Angiomatoid.

Clinical features

Malignant fibrous histiocytoma occurs more commonly in white patients than patients of African or Asian descent.

Male female ratio is approximately 2 : 1.

Malignant fibrous histiocytoma tumours are pink, firm, occasionally ulcerated, subepithelial masses that may be painful.

Microscopically

On microscopic examination histiocytomas exhibit fibroblastic and histiocytic characteristic. There is variety of growth patterns, the most characteristic being the presence of swirled fascicles of spindle-shaped cells with associated vascularity and polygonal cells or giant cells.

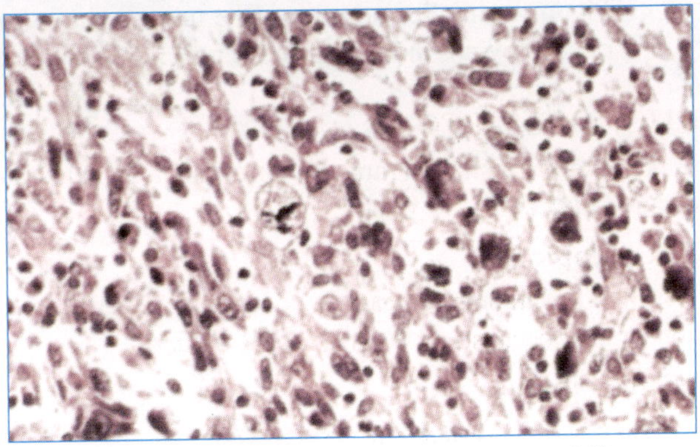

Fig.21.15: Showing microscopic appearances of fibrous histiocytoma

Treatment

Treatment is by radical surgical excision. Recurrence and metastasis occur in about 40% of cases and death may cause.

LIPOSARCOMA

Liposarcoma is a malignant neoplasm of adipocytes.

They can develop in the thigh, behind the knee, and inside the back of the abdomen. Rare instances have been described in the spermatic cord, breast, vulva and bones.

In oral cavity it is seen in buccal mucosa and tongue.

Clinical features

They occur mostly in adults between 50 and 60 years of age. Liposarcoma occurs slightly more frequently in men than females.

Microscopically

Liposarcoma occurs in four main biologic forms (i) well-differentiated liposarcoma (ii) myxoid (iii) round cell (iv) pleomorphic liposarcoma.

1. Well-differentiated liposarcoma, the most common type, is characterised by a delicate plexiform capillary network associated with both primitive mesenchyme-like cells and variable number of lipoblasts.
2. Myxoid liposarcoma is characterised by a delicate plexiform capillary network that is associated with both primitive mesenchyme like cells and variable number of lipoblasts. The stroma contains a large proportion of myxoid ground substance.
3. Round cell type of tumour is composed of small round cells that have a distinct acidophilic cytoplasm and dark round nuclei. Occasionally lipoblasts are present.

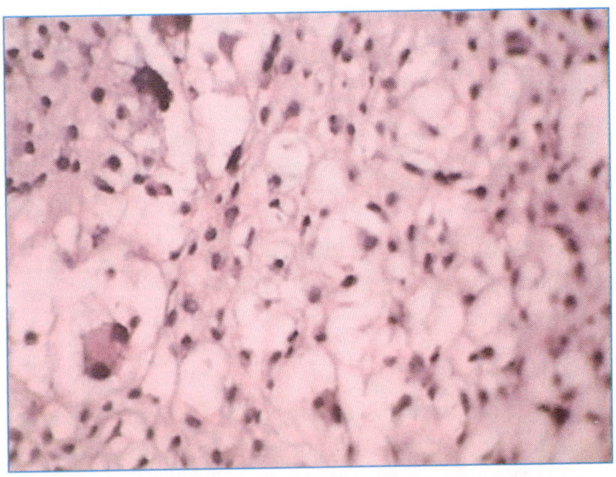

Fig.21.16: Microscopic appearance of liposarcoma

4. **Pleomorphic liposarcoma:** The tumour shows presence of large giant cells and high mitotic rate. They are more aggressive and liable to metastasise.

CHONDROSARCOMA

Chondrosarcoma is a rare tumour of the jaws. It has a slight preference for the maxilla, and usually occurs between 25-50 years.

Macroscopically

Chondrosarcoma appears as a large destructive mass with a characteristic translucent whitish appearance because of the chondroid matrix.

Microscopically

Microscopic variants of chondrosarcoma are:

Clear cell chondrosarcoma: Tumour cells having ground glass appearance characterise it.

Myxoid chondrosarcoma: A prominent myxoid background with trapped tumour cells characterises it.

Mesenchymal chondrosarcoma: There are small round, oval to spindle shaped neoplastic cells with irregular clumping of chromatin and small nucleoli.

Radiologically: X-rays will show expansible lesion, thickening of cortex, and endosteal scalloping. Soft tissue mass may be seen along with characteristic punctate calcification within the bone.

OSTEOGENIC SARCOMA

The osteogenic sarcoma is a malignant tumour of bone, and about 6.5 per cent of reported cases have occurred in the jaw.

Age: It is common in age group between 20–30 years.

The lesion more commonly affects males (twice as frequently as females), and mandible is involved more often than the maxilla.

Signs and symptoms:

- Swelling of bone
- Destruction of bone
- Loosening of teeth
- Intraoral ulceration of mucus membrane
- Vague pain and paresthesia
- Spontaneous pathological fractures may occur
- The mucosa and skin covering the lesion may appear erythematous.

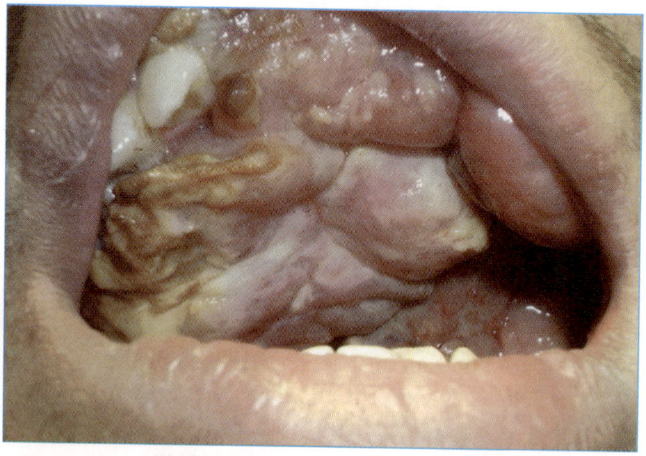

Fig. 21.17: Showing growth palate in a 20-year male (Osteogenic sarcoma)

X-ray shows bone destruction or new bone formation and characteristic sunray appearance.

Microscopically

The tumour cells vary in size. They are spindle-shaped oval or polyhedral cells, with hyperchromatic nuclei. The malignant cells form new bone, which is the most characteristic feature of osteosarcoma. Binucleated or multinucleated giant cells with bizarre hyperchromatic nuclei and mitosis are present. Areas of hyaline tissue, fibrous tissue, cartilage, osteoid and myxomatous tissue are present in tumour stroma.

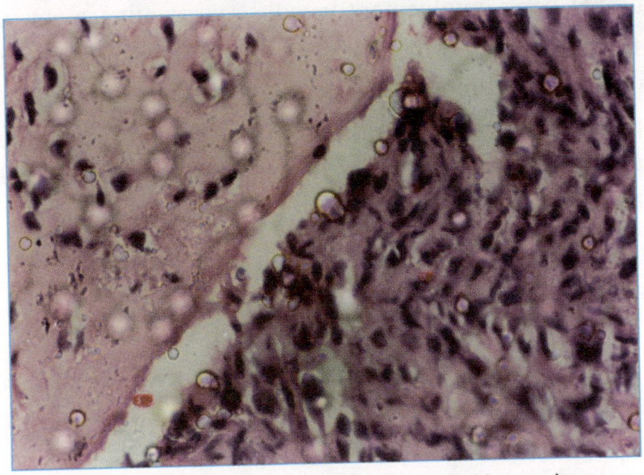

Fig.21.18: Shows sarcomatous tumour with new bone formation and chondromatous element (osteogenic sarcoma)

EWING'S TUMOUR

James Ewing first described Ewing's sarcoma, a highly malignant primary bone tumour, in 1921. Ewing's sarcoma is the common name of primitive neuroectodermal tumour (PNCT).

Clinical features

Age and Sex incidence: The peak incidence is between ages 10 and 20. It is less common in children under 5 years or in adults over 30. Males are slightly more often affected.

Microscopic appearance

The tumour is made up of sheets of uniform round small cells with round nuclei having small nucleoli and ill-defined cell outline resembling lymphocytes. The cells are arranged in syncytial sheets without a lobular arrangement but divided by broad strands of collagen. Tumour cells ring a central clearing, creating a pseudorosette. One of the diagnostic features is the intracytoplasmic glycogen present in these cells that stains with periodic acid–Schiff (PAS) reaction.

Chromosomal abnormality: Ewing's sarcoma is the result of a translocation between 11 and 22, which fuses the EWS gene of chromosome 22 to the FL11 gene of chromosome 11. The fusion gene protein product is termed CD99. There is also cytogenetic translocation abnormality (q24; q12).

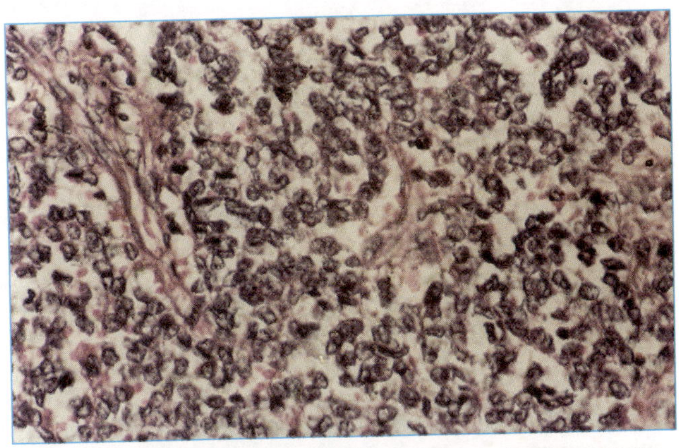

Fig.21.19: Microphotograph of Ewing's tumour showing monotonous small tumour cells separated by fibrous septa

Imaging findings

X-rays: On conventional radiograph, the most common osseous presentation is a permeative lytic lesion with periosteal reaction. The classic description of lamellated or '*onion skin*' type of periosteal reaction is often associated with this lesion. Ewing's sarcoma is typically located in the medullary cavity and produces expansion of the affected diaphysis, often extending into the adjacent soft tissue. About 10 % presents with multiple bone involvement usually representing metastasis.

MRI will show the full bony and soft tissue extent. Contrast enhanced MRI may help to determine the amount of necrosis within the tumour, thus determining response to treatment prior to surgery.

Cell of origin: Histogenesis of this tumour is controversial. The possibilities suggested for the cell of origin are endothelial, pericytic, bone marrow, osteoblastic, mesenchymal and neuroectodermal.

Treatment

Because almost all the patients with apparently localised disease at diagnosis have occult metastasis, multiple chemotherapy as well as local control with surgery and/or radiation is indicated in the treatment of all patients.

Behaviour: Most commonly, metastasis occurs in chest bone/or bone marrow. Less common sites include the central nervous system and lymph nodes.

SYNOVIAL SARCOMA

Common sites are shoulder, wrist, and knee.

Cause

Synovial sarcoma is characterised by specific chromosomal translocation t(x-18)(p11:q11) and the SSX10 or SSX2 gage on the chromosome (at Xp11) that is observed in more than 90% of cases.

Macroscopically

The mass tends to be sharply circumscribed, pink, fleshy mass with a heterogeneous appearance and has a glistening pseudocapsule.

Cut surface shows solid. haemorrhagic and cystic areas. Foci of calcification are occasionally noted. Heavy calcification tends to indicate less aggressive lesions and offers a more favourable prognosis.

Microscopically

The tumour consists of large polygonal cells (epitheloid) that secrete hyaluronic acid and show an organisation that is suggestive of microscopic joint spaces. These cells are surrounded by spindle cells that simulate subsynovial mesenchymal cells.

It can be monophasic or biphasic.

Biphasic variant consists of plump round cells, and fibroblasts alternating with gland-like areas that is lined by synovial-like cells and contain mucin.

Monomorphic: The monomorphic variant does not have glandular areas. Punctate areas of calcification may be present.

Spread: It can spread to other areas of body, particularly to involve regional lymph nodes. Metastases to distant body tissues occur in about half of all cases, usually months to years after the initial diagnosis is made.

VASCULAR TUMOURS

HAEMANGIOENDOTHELIOMA

The tumour is between the benign, well-differentiated haemangioma and the frankly anaplastic angiosarcoma.

Tumour appears as exophytic ulcerated painless masses of maxillary and mandibular gingival.

Microscopically, masses of plump and cuboidal endothelium having abundant lightly staining cytoplasm are seen lining and present in wall of vascular channel. The tumour cells are arranged in nests, cords and short strands.

HAEMANGIOPERICYTOMA

Clinical features

Early lesions may be small, discrete, painless, reddish, nodules, which may progress to large dark coloured ill-defined fresh tumour masses—often with extensive areas of haemorrhage and necrosis.

Microscopically

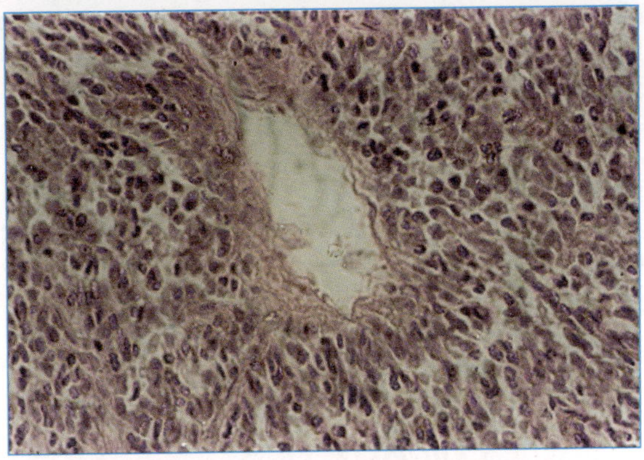

Fig.21.20: Shows microscopic appearance of haemangiopericytoma

The tumour consists of thin vascular channels surrounded by masses of spindle cells or polyhedral cells arranged in a radial fashion outside the basement membrane of the vascular channel. Areas with more spindle pericytes may show interlacing pattern of cells but usually there is a medullary tissue pattern, sometimes pallisading of cells, reminiscent of neural tumour. Reticulin staining will demonstrate lesional vessels lined by a single layer of endothelial cells, with pericytes outside the basal lamina, although they are often individually surrounded by reticulin and collagen fibre.

Lesional cells are immunoreactive for vimentin, factor XIIa antigen, HLA- DR antigen and QUE-BAND 10(CD34). Chromosomal translocations T(12, 19) and (13, 22) have been observed in lesional cells.

ANGIOSARCOMA

The angiosarcoma is a malignancy of vascular channels and half of the skin angiosarcomas occur in the head and neck regions, usually affecting the scalp of elderly men. It is very uncommon in oral cavity but when occurring there it usually involves the mandible or the maxilla.

Causes

The causes of angiosarcoma are unknown. Various predisposing factors have been found in association with angiosarcomas:

1. Chronic lymphedema, radiations and altered immune status. Chronic lymphedema occurring on a congenital, idiopathic, traumatic, or infectious basis also predisposes to angiosarcoma.
2. Angiosarcoma occurs with increased frequency in those with AIDS.
3. Less common cause is the high dose of ionising radiation like radiation therapy.
4. The usual ways a patient develops angiosarcoma are through exposure to vinyl chloride when working in vinyl chloride factories, beauty shops and other plastic industries.

Clinical features

Age: Angiosarcoma of the oral region is a disease of older individuals, averaging more than 65 years of age, but it has been reported in infancy.

Sites: Most cases have involved the mandible, but other less frequent sites of involvement have included the maxilla, parotid glands, lips, tongue, floor of mouth, cheek, palate and antrum.

It is seen as painful, spontaneously bleeding round or ovoid nodules that appear red to bluish in colour and firm on palpation. The lesions may be extensive and ulcerate rarely in form of bruise or a pyoderma.

Some tumours grow rapidly while others take many months to reach a size of 4.5 cm.

Microscopically

Angiosarcoma mainly consists of vascular channels, often overshadowed by the markedly cellular clumps of proliferating endothelial cells with mitosis. The cells are round, plump, polygonal and fusiform with hyperchromatic nuclei and project into the lumen as '*hobnails*'. Red blood cells are seen within the vascular channels.

CD 31, CD34 and factor VIII staining reveals its origin from endothelial cells.

Prognosis

Prognosis is generally poor and depends much on two factors: (i) clinical size of tumour (ii) degree of cellular differentiation. Overall survival is poor—only 10-15 percent after 5 years.

Treatment

Treatment of angiosarcoma includes chemotherapy, surgery (radical neck dissection), radiotherapy, anti-angiogenesis drugs—or a combination of these treatment modalities.

KAPOSI'S SARCOMA

In 1872, Moritz Kaposi described blood vessel tumour.

Kaposi's sarcoma is a multifocal vascular malignancy seen predominantly in HIV-infected individuals. The development of this tumour is diagnostic of AIDS prognosis.

Prior to the HIV epidemic, Kaposi's sarcoma was a rare tumour restricted to elderly males of Mediterranean or Jewish descent, immunosuppressed transplant recipients, and children, and young adults in sub-Saharan Africa.

There are four types of Kaposi's sarcoma:

- The classic type of Kaposi's sarcoma affects elderly men of Mediterranean or Jewish descent and middle European descent and in sub-Saharan Africa. Classic Kaposi's sarcoma is rare, and unassociated with HIV infection.
- HIV associated Kaposi's sarcoma mainly affects men who have sex with men. It occurs less frequently in intravenous drug users and rarely in women, haemophiliacs or their sexual partners. HIV associated Kaposi's sarcoma is more common in women in some parts of Africa. It is less common in the USA and Europe because of effective highly active retroviral therapy (HAART).
- Endemic African Kaposi's sarcoma arises in some parts of Africa (Uganada and Zambia) in children and young adults. It is becoming more prevalent with the rise of HIV infection.
- Iatrogenic Kaposi's sarcoma is a particular concern for organ transplantation patients, especially in geographic areas associated with high levels of infection with KSHV. Most have virus prior to transplantation but the drugs cause it to reactivate.

Cause

1. A human herpes virus (HHV-8)—also called Kaposi's sarcoma associated herpes virus—has been implicated as the cause.
2. Elevated degree of expression of numerous cytokines and angiogenic growth factors, including TNF-alpha, IL-6, bFGF, HIV-tatprotein and oncostatin M.
3. Genetic.
4. Hormonal.

Clinically

Cutaneous lesions include purple non-tender, non-pruritic papules over nose, genitalia, and lower limbs. Ulceration on feet shows crease line arrangement and often associated with edema and lymphadenopathy. As the disease progresses the skin lesions become more numerous and larger.

Early lesions appear as flat or slightly elevated brown to purple lesions that are often bilateral. Advanced lesions appear as dark red to purple plaques or nodules that may exhibit ulceration, bleeding and necrosis.

Pulmonary lesions: Pulmonary Kaposi's sarcomas occur in 10-15% of patients and presents with breathlessness, cough, haemoptysis, chest pain, and fever. Pleural effusion is present in 25% of cases.

Gastrointestinal lesions can occur anywhere within the gastrointestinal tract. The lesions are often asymptomatic and clinically indolent. Gastrointestinal disease is usually an indicator of more advanced HIV infection. Symptoms include dysphagia, nausea, haematemesis, haematochezia, melena, and bowel obstruction.

Lymph nodes: When lymph nodes are affected there may be swelling in the arm and legs, which can be very painful and uncomfortable. This is known as lymphedema and is caused by the Kaposi's sarcoma cells blocking the flow of fluid through the body tissues.

Oral manifestations

Oral cavity is involved in about 30% and is the initial site in 15% of AIDS related Kaposi's sarcoma.

Sites: Kaposi's sarcoma of mucosa most commonly affects the hard palate, gingiva, and tongue. Intraorally, Kaposi's sarcoma appears as brown, bluish, purple or red patches or papules on the hard palate mucosa and gingival. The initial lesions are flat macules or patches on the mucosal surface, but, over time, they become nodular and often ulcerate and bleed. Ulcerated and bulky tumour involvement may interfere with speech or mastication.

Microscopically

The tumour is composed of a proliferation of spindle tumour cells arranged in nests, cords, and short strands. Epitheloid cells exhibited abundant eosinophilic cytoplasm with nuclear and cellular pleomorphism and intracytoplasmic vacuoles. There are presence of fibroblasts, inflammatory cells, haemosiderin and extravasated erythrocytes.

Treatment

Prognosis of Kaposi's sarcoma depends upon the CD4 count and the extent of disease. Epithelial haemangioendothelioma is a rare vascular neoplasm, which exhibits the potential for malignancy and recurrence as well as the ability to metastasise.

Kaposi's sarcoma is usually a localised tumour that can be treated surgically, or by liquid nitrogen or laser therapy, through local irradiation and retinoic gel. Chemotherapy with drugs such as liposomal anthracyclines or paclitaxel may be used particularly for invasive disease.

MUSCLE

RHABDOMYOSARCOMA

Rhabdomyosarcoma is the sarcoma arising from a primitive rhabdomyoblast. It is a malignant tumour made up of cells that normally develop into skeletal muscles of body. It is a highly malignant tumour, which accounts for over half of the soft tissue sarcomas. In the oral cavity the common sites are tongue, palate and buccal mucosa.

Pleomorphic rhabdomyosarcoma

Macroscopically: Rhabdomyosarcomas present as one or more firm, white, well-circumscribed nodules.

Microscopically: Tumour is very pleomorphic, with numerous tumour giant cells. There are large and small spindle-shaped cells, mononucleated or multinucleated round giant cells with non-pyknotic nuclei, star-shaped cells and cells shaped like tennis rackets.

Histologically, embryonal rhabdomyosarcoma is being composed of small round and oval cells with primitive hyperchromatic nuclei, scanty cytoplasm and a high mitotic rate.

There is myxomatous tissue resembling embryonic mesenchyme as a prominent component.

Mutations in ras oncogene are common in embryonal rhabdomyosarcoma.

GIANT CELL TUMOUR (OSTEOCLASTOMA)

Osteoclastoma or giant cell tumour of bone is a specific type of primary neoplasm of bone and account for 5 percent of all primary bone tumours.

Age: The lesion arises chiefly in 20-40 years of age groups.

Site of occurrence: 50 percent of all the tumours arise around knee joint, lower end of femur, upper end of tibia and proximal end of fibula. Another common site is lower end of radius. Other bones involved are vertebral spines and jaw bones.

Clinical features

Giant cell tumour produces severe pain on movement. The tumour expands the bone asymmetrically. The tumour is soft grey tissue with areas of haemorrhages. The bone is markedly thinned out as to produce a crackling sound on pressure under the fingers like an egg shell. The tumour may be detected for the first time by a spontaneous pathological fracture.

X-ray: Giant cell tumour appears as large lobulated osteolytic lesion and shows characteristic honey mosaic or ***'soap bubble appearance'***.

PATHOLOGY

Macroscopically: These tumours are soft, cellular, often jelly-like reddish-brown and frequently undergo central lytic degeneration.

Cut surface shows soft friable reddish-brown tissue of variegated appearance. These are yellow areas of lipid deposition. When tumour has attained a larger size there remains a thin covering in the process of resorption and replacement of bone resulting in thinning of the cortex.

Microscopically

Stromal cells: The stroma consists especially of mononuclear spindle, ovoid or round cells with numerous mitotic figures.

Giant cells: Embedded in stroma are numerous large multinucleated giant cells. They measure from 20 to 100 nuclei that are often set centrally in a vacuolated cytoplasm. Giant cells are osteoclastic type (foreign body) and have very high acid phosphatase.

Other features: Tumour blood vessels are numerous and thin-walled; gives rise to haemorrhages and haemosiderin together. Stroma contains scanty collagen tissue.

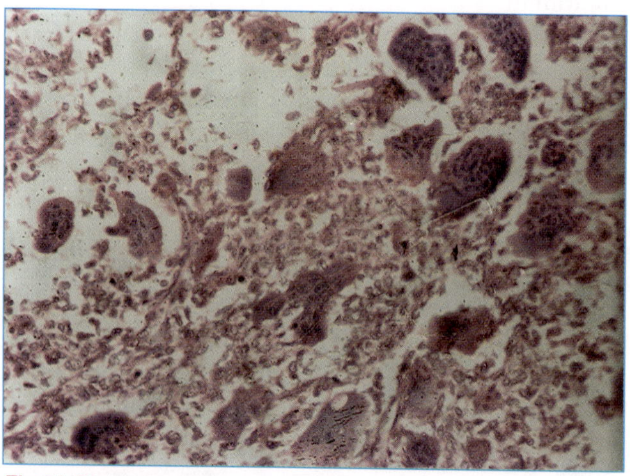

Fig.21.21: Tumour is mainly consists of osteoclastic Giant cells and spindle and round stromal cells osteoclastoma

Cell of origin: Osteoclastoma does not arise from osteoclast but possibly are mesenchymal in origin.

Biological behavior: Giant cell tumour is potentially malignant tumour. In 40 to 60% of them, following surgical treatment there may be recurrence, infiltration into surrounding tissue and even metastasis to lung—though the tumour is histologically benign. Most of osteoclastoma are cured by thorough removal; approximately 20 % recur; well under 5% are malignant or become malignant after radiotherapy and metastasise to lung.

MALIGNANT LYMPHOMA

Non-Hodgkin's lymphomas are a group of highly diverse malignancies and have great tendency to affect organs and tissues that do not ordinarily contain lymphoid tissue. 20-30% of non-Hodgkin's lymphoma arises from extranodal sites.

Non-Hodgkin's lymphomas are the third-most common of group of malignant lesions in the oral cavity and maxillary region.

Among various head and neck sites, Waldeyer's ring, which is an area encompassed by the nasopharynx, the tonsils, and base of the tongue is most often involved by malignant lymphoma. The nose and paranasal sinuses, orbits, and salivary glands are other sites in head and neck.

The oral cavity may be the primary site of non-Hodgkin's lymphoma. Usually the oral manifestations of non-Hodgkin's lymphoma are secondary to a more widespread involvement throughout the body. Non-Hodgkin's lymphoma arising within the oral cavity accounts for less than 5% of all malignancies. The estimated annual incidence is 1 : 1,000,000 population.

Cause

There is no known etiological factor for non-Hodgkin's lymphoma except the rare event of an underlying human immunodeficiency viral infection.

Clinical features

Age: It is a rare tumour, usually occurring before the age of 40 years but may be seen in younger age group.

Sex: There is no gender preference.

Sites: Involvement of various parts of the oral cavity is very uncommon. The gingival and hard palate are the most often involved intra oral sites. Involvement of buccal mucosa, tongue, floor of the mouth and lip has been reported quite frequently.

Symptoms and sign

In the oral cavity malignant lymphoma often appears in the form of pillow-like, soft, dark red, frequently ulcerated tumours on the palate, gingival and floor of mouth, or in the area of tonsils. The surface of the ulcer is irregular with inflammation at the periphery, the base of the ulcer and surrounding tissues. Bone is a relatively uncommon site of primary lymphoma. Most common presenting symptoms are local swelling, pain and discomfort. There is evidence of periodontal lesion, foetor, mucosal discolouration and mental nerve paraesthesia.

Non-Hodgkin's lymphoma can occur as a T-cell or B-cell lymphoma. In the oral cavity the B-cell lymphoma is more often observed.

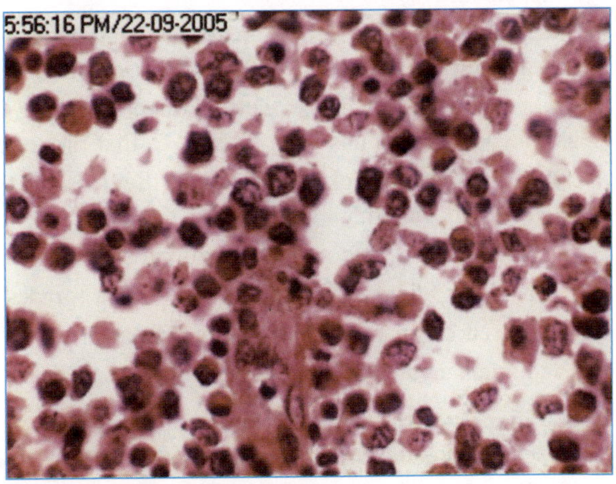

Fig.21.22: Section shows microscopic appearance of B cell lymphoma

HODGKIN'S LYMPHOMA

Incidence: In United States about 8,000 new cases of Hodgkin's disease occur every year.

Age: Median age is 31 years, first peak at 21-25 years and second at 50-70 years. The disease is rare under age of two years.

Sex: It is more common in men, except for the nodular sclerosis variant, which is more common in females.

There are important epidemiological observations that correlate socioeconomic factors and disease incidence. The disease is more common among individuals with few or no siblings, among those having higher education, and among urban than rural dwellers.

Thomas Hodgkin originally described the disease Hodgkin's lymphoma in 1832.

Macroscopically

Normal architecture of lymph node is completely lost.

Lymph nodes may be enlarged up to 10 cm. Consistency is rubbery. Cut surface is homogenous and fish flesh-like in lymphocytic predominance form of Hodgkin's disease.

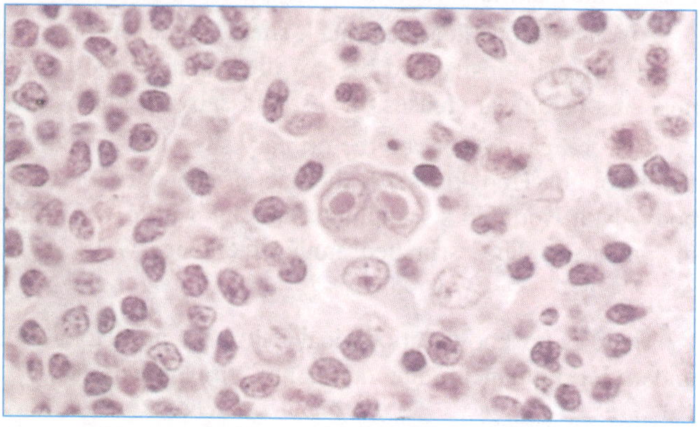

Fig.21.23: Mixed cellularity Hodgkin's lymphoma with characteristic Reed-Sternberg giant cells

Microscopically

The cellular infiltrate consists of lymphocytes, polymorphs, plasma cells and eosinophils. Noncaseating epitheloid cell granuloma occurs in the lymph node and spleen in some patients with Hodgkin's disease.

***Reed-Sternberg giant cell*:** The classic Reed-Sternberg cell is seen in all subtypes of classical Hodgkin's lymphoma. It is a large cell (20 to 50μm) in diameter or more with abundant weakly acidophilic or amphophilic cytoplasm, which may appear homogeneous or granular and which lacks a pale zone in the Golgi area. The nucleus is lobed or polylobed. The nuclear membrane is thick and sharply defined. The nuclear pattern is usually vesicular but with some coarse chromatin clumps scattered throughout. There is a very large, rounded, highly acidophilic central nucleolus surrounded by a clear halo. The two nuclear lobes face each other (mirror image) resulting in the oft-cited 'Owl eye' appearance.

Lacunar cells surrounded by an artefactual space in histological sections are characteristically seen in nodular sclerosing grade I Hodgkin's disease.

Popcorn cell: This is a variant of Reed-Sternberg cells. When multilobulation occurs in the nucleus, the appearance has been likened to that of 'egg basket cells or popcorn cells'.

Classification: Hodgkin's disease is divided into the four types defined at a conference held in Rye, New York in 1965:

- Lymphocyte predominant Hodgkin's lymphoma
- Nodular sclerosis Hodgkin's lymphoma (grades 1 and 2)
- Mixed cellular Hodgkin's lymphoma
- Lymphocyte depletion Hodgkin's lymphoma.

1. **Lymphocytic-predominant type:** Lymphocyte rich Hodgkin's disease is characterised by classical Reed-Sternberg cells set in a diffuse background of lymphoid cells.
2. **Nodular sclerosing type:** This accounts for about 40% of Hodgkin's disease and form 70% of the Hodgkin's cases in adolescent. In this type, the lymph node capsule is thickened and fine

or coarse bands of collagen subdivide the node into nodules of various size. The septa vary in thickness and sometimes they are so massive that they make up 50% of the volume of lymph node. Nodules in-between the septa consist predominantly of lymphocytes, histiocytes, eosinophils, neutrophils, and plasma cells.

3. **Mixed cellularity type:** There is occasional necrosis with moderate degree of fibrosis.
4. **Lymphocyte-depletion type:** This accounts for 15% of cases of Hodgkin's disease. Lymphocytes are sparse and other reactive cells, including eosinophils, are variable in number. It is seen in elderly adults. This subtype of Hodgkin's disease is rare and carries the worst prognosis. The infiltrate is composed of many pleomorphic Reed-Sternberg cells and shows few reactive lymphoid cells.

Oral manifestations

There may be inflammatory gingival overgrowth, premature root resorption of deciduous teeth, and alveolar bone loss.

Oral complications include xerostomia, radiation-induced caries, the risk of osteoradionecrosis in irradicated bone. Tooth mobility may be increased.

INVESTIGATIONS

I. **Changes in the blood**
   1. Anaemia with normal indices, with a normal or low reticulocyte count is seen in cases of Hodgkin's disease. Some patients develop an autoimmune haemolytic anaemia and rarely Coombs' test is positive.
   2. An eosinophila, neutrophilia, monocytosis, and leukopaenia may be present.
   3. Erythrocyte sedimentation rate is often elevated.
   4. Serum iron and TIBC are low but marrow iron stores are normal.
   5. There is hypergammaglobulinaemia and, occasionally, hypoalbuminaemia.
   6. Lactic dehydrogenase measurements, as raised levels are an adverse prognostic levels.

II. **Chest X-ray** may show a mediastinal mass.

III. **CT scans** of chest and abdomen to permit staging. Bulky disease (greater than 10 cm in a single node mass) is an adverse prognostic feature.

IV. **Lymph node biopsy** may be undertaken surgically or by percutaneous needle biopsy under radiological guidance.

Clinical features

1. The disease presents commonly with painless enlargement of superficial lymph nodes. Cervical lymph nodes and mediastinal lymph nodes are frequently involved. Sometimes other lymph node groups—like axillary, inguinal and mesenteric—are involved. Disease begins in a single lymph node, followed by spread to adjacent node and then to other organs. Often presents clinically as enlargement of accessible lymph nodes. Disease spreads to spleen, bone marrow, gastrointestinal tract and liver.
2. Spleen is enlarged in 75% of cases and liver in 50% of cases.
3. About 1/3rd of people with Hodgkin's disease may also notice some systemic symptoms such as low-grade fever, night sweats, weight loss, pruritis, hyperpigmentation of skin, and fatigue. Involved nodes are painful after alcohol consumption.
4. Recurrent fever persisting for a week with intervals of one or two weeks. This type of relapsing fever is known as Pel-Ebstein fever.

STAGING OF HODGKIN'S LYMPHOMA

I. Involvement of single lymph node region.

II. Disease in more than one site –all lesions above or below diaphragm.

III. Disease on both sides of diaphragm.

IV. Widespread involvement of extra lymphoid sites and lymphatic involvement.

Etiology

Viral theory: Viral theory of Hodgkin's lymphoma remains unknown, but there is considerable evidence to suggest that the EBV plays an important role. The EBV gene has been demonstrated in the nuclei of Reed-Sternberg cells. The incidence of Hodgkin's lymphoma is increased in patients with HIV infection.

Hodgkin's disease may be more prevalent in people who have contracted infectious mononucleosis. Also there is a link between Hodgkin's and the measles virus.

Neoplastic theory: Hodgkin's lymphoma is a neoplasm of lymphoid tissue that is defined histopathologically by the presence of malignant Reed-Sternberg cells. Surface-markers on the RS cells indicate that these cells are most probably the B cell origin. Markers of antigen presenting cells like MHC –2 antigens and co-stimulatory antigens B7 present on the surface of RS cells.

A defect in cell-mediated immunity has been recognized in patients with Hodgkin's disease.

Reed-Sternberg giant cells are capable of secreting many cytokines like IL-4, IL-5, TNF-alpha, GMCSF and TGF-b (an intensely fibrogenic cytokine). This is probably why there are broad bands of fibrosis in the nodular sclerosis subtype of Hodgkin's lymphoma.

Genetic theory: There is also evidence for a genetic susceptibility factor. It has also been noted that there is an increased susceptibility to these individuals who have HLA antigen belonging to 4C system.

BURKITT'S LYMPHOMA

Burkitt's lymphoma is a cancer of the lymphatic system (in particular; B lymphocytes). It is named after Denis Burkitt, who mapped its peculiar geographic distribution across Africa. It has three major forms—the endemic (African form), the non-endemic (sporadic) form, and the immunodeficiency form.

Endemic Burkitt's lymphoma refers to those cases occurring in African children usually 4-7 years old, with a male female ratio of 2 : 1, involving the bones of the jaw and other facial bones, as well as kidneys, gastrointestinal tract, ovaries, breast, and other extranodal sites. It is seen in equatorial strip of Africa.

Sporadic: Worldwide distribution. It is seen mainly in children and adolescents. There is greater tendency for involvement of abdominal cavity than endemic form.

Immunodeficiency associated: Primarily associated with HIV infection.

Sites: The African form most often involves the maxilla or mandible.

Histologically

The tumour cell exhibits a diffuse, almost coherent pattern, is a little larger than small lymphocytes (10-25 μm), round, nuclei with several prominent basophilic nucleoli and has a high nuclear/cytoplasmic ratio. Chromatin is coarse with thick nuclear membrane and numerous motoses. In most patients, non-neoplastic macrophages with abundant, pale cytoplasm are scattered among the tumours. Cytoplasm is amphophilic and strongly pyronophilic.Often they contain phagocytosed debris of tumour cells. The pale macrophages scattered among the dark tumour cells give the lesion a *starry sky appearance,* often striking in Burkitt's lymphoma.

Causes

1. **Chromosomal abnormality:** Examination of chromosomes from these tumour cells often shows translocation of the mYc and Ig genes (t, 8; 14).
2. **Epstein-Barr viruses** are closely associated with the African form of Burkitt's lymphoma. Some have postulated that, because of immunosuppression caused by coexistent malaria or another infection, the host is unable to generate an adequate T- lymphocyte response (e.g. EBV-specific cytotoxic T cells) against B cells that are infected latently with EBV. This subsequently results in excessive B cell proliferation.

METASTATIC TUMOURS

Malignant epithelial neoplasms have a tendency to metastasise to bone via the blood stream as well as via lymphatics. Metastatic tumours may present as primary intraoral masses, with or without oral involvement.

In jaws, particularly mandible may be a site of intraosseous metastases.

The lung is the most common site of the primary lesion.

In most site of origin of secondary jaw, tumours occur in the following order of frequency: breast, large intestine, prostate, kidney, thyroid gland, skin (melanoma), endometrium, mesothelioma and testis. Less common sites of origin include the ovary and liver. Chordoma of cervical vertebrae can protrude into the oral cavity.

Metastatic spread occurs more frequently to the mandible than to the maxilla.

X-ray: In more advanced cases, well-defined osteolytic areas with root destruction may be evident.

Clinically: There is swelling, pain, burning, paresthesia, and loosening of teeth.

Bibliography

James William, Berger Timothy, Elston Dirk: (2005) Andrew's Diseases of the Skin: Clinical Dermatology, Tenth Edition. Saunders.

K. Pavithran, D. Doval, G. Mukherjee. V. Kannan, S.V. Kumarswamy and P P Bapsy: Rhabdomyoma of the oral cavity. Report of eight cases, Acta Oncol 36 (1997). P819- 821.

Noorshin Mohtasham, Ali AH kharrazi, Shokoo Feh Jamshidi and Hamid Jafarzadeh: Journal of Oral Science Vol 50 (2008), no 2 June 219-223.

CHAPTER

22

SALIVARY GLAND

DEVELOPMENTAL DISTURBANCES OF SALIVARY GLANDS

APLASIA

Aplasia of one or more glands has been reported but is exceptionally rare. Even more rarely, it is complete and then results in total failure of secretion of saliva. Autosomal dominant aplasia of lacrimal and salivary gland is a rare condition caused by mutation in the gene encoding fibroblast growth factor-10 (FGF 10). Aplasia of parotid glands can be associated with mandibulofacial dystosis, aplasia of the lacrimal glands, and hemifacial microstomia, lacrimoauriculodentodigital syndrome (LADD), cleft palate and microstomia.

Clinical features

Salivary gland aplasia has been reported more frequently in males than in females by a 2 : 1 ratio. Parotid gland is more commonly affected than submandibular glands. Some individuals are affected by agenesis of all four of the largest glands (both parotids and submandibular glands).

Aplasia of salivary gland is characterised by irritable eyes, epiphora and xerostomia, which increases risk of dental erosion, dental caries, leathery tongue, periodontal disease, and oral infection. Other complications include soft tissue inflammation and disorders of smell, chewing, and swallowing.

Treatment

Salivary flow may also be stimulated via the use of sugarless gum or sour candy. Good oral hygiene to reduce dental caries and other complications.

HYPERPLASIA OF SALIVARY GLANDS

It is common in Caucasians and uncommon in Asians.

Clinical features

The lesion is predominant in male patients with a ratio of about 1.5 : 1. It is found in all ages but more frequently between the fourth and sixth decades.

The lesion presents as nodular swelling mimicking a salivary gland neoplasm or a fibroma.

Adenomatoid hyperplasia typically presents as a painless mass located on hard or soft palate in up to 90% of cases. Other intraoral sites are mandibular retromolar area, buccal mucosa, tongue, and lips.

Macroscopically

Grossly, these lesions range from 0.5 to 3 cm. They are usually non-ulcerated well-circumscribed masses. They are covered by normal-appearing mucosa and may represent developmental anomaly or a focal glandular hyperplasia.

Microscopically

Microscopic examination of excised tissue reveals that it is composed of lobules of mucinous salivary acini separated by fibrous septa.

Management

No treatment is required because this lesion does not recur.

ABERRANCY

Aberrant salivary glands are salivary tissue that develops at unusual anatomic sites. Aberrant salivary glands have been reported in a variety of locations including the middle ear cleft, external auditory canal, neck, posterior mandible, anterior mandible, pituitary and cerebellopontine angle.

Sometimes the salivary tissue may be present within the body of the mandible and, in such cases, the intraosseous gland maintains a communication with the extraosseous normal salivary gland with the help of a stalk, which has perforated through the lingual cortical plate of bone.

Pathological conditions like sialolithiasis, neoplasms and cysts etc., which commonly affect the normal salivary gland can also involve the ectopic salivary gland tissues. Ectopic salivary gland tissues may be found in gingival and these tissues may produce a tumour-like mass, which is known as gingival gland choristoma.

ACCESSORY SALIVARY DUCTS

An accessory salivary ducts is defined as an ectopic salivary gland tissue with duct system.

An accessory parotid lobe is the most common developmental anomaly. The most common example of accessory salivary gland tissue is accessory parotid gland tissue.

Accessory parotid tissue is seen in 21 to 56% of normal adults. The accessory parotid gland is typically found overlying the masseter, and accessory duct typically lies cranial to Stensen's duct.

Interestingly, 1 to 8% of parotid tumours arise from accessory tissue and higher percentage of these lesions are malignant.

Treatment

Accessory salivary ducts are common and do not require treatment.

DIVERTICULI OF SALIVARY DUCT

Diverticuli in the ducts of the major salivary glands often lead to pooling of saliva and recurrent sialadenitis.

POLYCYSTIC DISEASE OF PAROTID GLAND

This rare anomaly described by Seifert et al (1981) may be unilateral or bilateral.

Clinical features

It has been found almost exclusively in females. Overt clinical signs are usually delayed, even in adulthood. Usually disease is bilateral but unilateral disease has been documented.

Macroscopically

Grossly, these lesions present as spongy masses of the involved salivary glands.

Microscopically

The cysts vary in size and are lined by a single layer of flattened, cuboidal or columnar cells. At places, the cyst lining cells may be heaped up to give a pseudo-papillary appearance. Amorphous eosinophilic material is present in many of the cyst cavities and there are, also typically, rounded concretions with a concentric laminated or radial pattern or conglomerates of smaller bodies. These may be congophilic. Remnants of gland tissue with acini are recognised between the cysts, but inflammatory changes are absent.

Treatment

A history of fluctuating non-tender parotid gland swelling for several years is antecedent to surgical intervention.

SIALADENOSIS

Sialadenosis has been defined as a non-inflammatory, diffuse enlargement of salivary glands due to acinar hypertrophy and hyperplasia. It usually involves the parotid glands and, less commonly, the submandibular glands. Minor salivary gland involvement has also been reported.

TABLE 22.1 CAUSES OF SIALADENOSIS
❍ **Nutritional:** Vitamin deficiency, bulimia, alcohol, eating disorders, kwashiorkor, pellagra, beri beri.
❍ **Endocrinal:** Diabetes mellitus, gonadal dysfunction, hypothyroidism, hyperthyroidism, pancreatitis.
❍ **Metabolic:** Obesity, pregnancy, cirrhosis, malabsorption, kidney failure, drug induced e.g., thiourea.
❍ **Inflammatory autoimmune:** Sarcoidosis and Heerfordt syndrome.
❍ **Neurochemical:** Lead, mercury, iodine, thiouracil, isoprotenelol.

Clinical features

- Recurrent bilateral, symmetric, diffuse, soft and non-tender swelling of the parotid glands.
- The condition usually begins between the ages of 20 and 60 years.
- Disease may persist for more than 20 years.

Microscopically

Histological patterns of sialadenosis are recognised: Granular, honeycomb, or vascular transformation, and mixed. There is infiltration or lipomatosis and fibrosis of interlobular septae.

Treatment

A superficial parotidectomy must be performed because of the cosmetic deformity caused by swollen glands.

XEROSTOMIA

Definition: An abnormal dryness of the mouth, caused by lack of normal secretion of saliva. It is derived from new Latin word *xero* + Greek *stomas*, mouthed.

TABLE 22.2
CAUSES OF XEROSTOMIA

I. Water and metabolic loss
  a. Impaired water intake
    Loss of water through the skin (fever, burns, and excessive sweating)
    Blood loss
    Emesis
    Diarrhoea
  b. Renal water loss
    Polyuria: Diabetes insipidus
    Osmotic diuresis: Diabetes mellitus
  c. Protein calorie malnutrition
II. Damage to the salivary glands
  a. Therapeutic irradiation to head and neck region
  b. Autoimmune diseases:
    Sjogren's syndrome (SS)
    Graft-versus-host disease (GVHD)
    Systemic lupus erythematosus (SLE)
    Rheumatoid arthritis (RA)
  c. HIV-1 infection
  Aging.
III. Interference with neural transmission
  Medication/drugs
  Autonomic dysfunction, e.g., ganglionic neuropathy
  Conditions affecting the CNS, e.g., Alzheimer's disease
  Psychological disorders (depression, anxiety)
  Trauma
  Decrease in mastication
IV. Local causes
  Decreased mastication
  Smoking
  Mouth breathing
V. Idiopathic.

Clinical features

- Difficulty in chewing, swallowing, and speaking.
- A dry, burning feeling in the mouth and throat.
- A pasty and/or sticky feeling in the mouth.
- Bad breath (halitosis).
- Thirst: Frequent ingestion of fluids, especially while eating.
- Difficulty with eating dry foods, and difficulty with use of a denture.
- Oral fissuring, cracked lips, ulceration in oral cavity, and increased susceptibility to caries.
- Patient is more prone to candidiasis.

Complications of xerostomia include acute gingivitis, dysphagia, parotitis, abrasion and erosion of teeth.

Treatment

- Drinking water or sugarfree beverages with each meal to keep food particles from becoming trapped in mouth.
- Sugarfree gum and candy, especially one that has a sour taste, may increase saliva production.
- Don't use tobacco, alcohol that dries out the mouth.
- Systemic use of certain drugs, e.g., pilocarpine, salivary stimulants, bromhexine and vitamin supplements.

INFLAMMATION

ACUTE SUPPURATIVE SIALADENITIS

Acute inflammation of the salivary gland most frequently occurs in the parotid, but occasionally the other salivary glands may be involved. The infection can occur due to spread of organisms from mouth through their ducts. The organisms isolated are Staphylococcus, Streptococcus pneumoniae, Hemophilus influenzae, and Escherichia coli. The various predisposing factors that help in causation of acute sialadenitis are dehydration, debilitation, malnutrition, and chronic illness.

It typically presents with acute swelling of the gland, increased pain and swelling with meals, tenderness and erythema of the duct-opening. Pus often can be massaged from the duct.

There may be widespread cellulitis of the overlying skin, which looks dusky red.

Complications

Parotid abscess may form which can be single or multiple and these can coalesce to form a large abscess.

Treatment

Therapy is initially conservative with adequate hydration, sialogogues, heat, massage of the affected glands, and administration of an appropriate antibiotic, usually a penicillinase-resistant antistaphylococcal antibiotics.

Chronic sialadenitis

Chronic sialadenitis is unilateral swelling with mild pain. Chronic sialadentis form of the disease is associated with conditions linked to decreased salivary flow, rather than dehydration.

Chronic sialadenitis can occur in either the parotid or submandibular glands.

Chronic inflammation of a salivary gland is often associated with obstruction of the duct, usually by a calculus. Duct orifice is reddened and flow decreases.

Microscopically: There is follicular collection of small lymphocytes in a band of eosinophilic fairly dense fibrous tissue, which divides the affected gland into multiple lobes. There is extensive loss of acini. Remaining ducts have double lining. A single thin layer of flat epithelial cells surrounds the acini. The small ducts are markedly dilated and lined by a single thin layer of flat epithelial cells. The lumen of the dilated duct is filled with pus-like material, which consists largely of polymorph leukocytes. There is interstitial fibrosis.

TUBERCULOUS SIALADENITIS

Primary tubercular infection of the salivary gland is uncommon and more often consists of unilateral parotid gland involvement. Parotid and submandibular glands are involved in 63% and 37%, respectively. The infection is thought to arise in the teeth or tonsils and result in a chronic tumour-like lesion. Direct extension of salivary gland parenchyma by the bacillus may occur by way of glands ductular system.

Secondary tuberculosis more often involves the submandibular or sublingual gland and is accompanied by pulmonary disease.

Clinical features

Patient presents with swelling over side of the face, with multiple fistulae, irregular fever, pain during opening of the mouth, occasional dry cough, loss of appetite, and gradual loss of weight.

Microscopically

There is chronic granulomatous lesion consisting of caseation, epitheloid cells, Langhan's giant cells, lymphocytes and fibrosis.

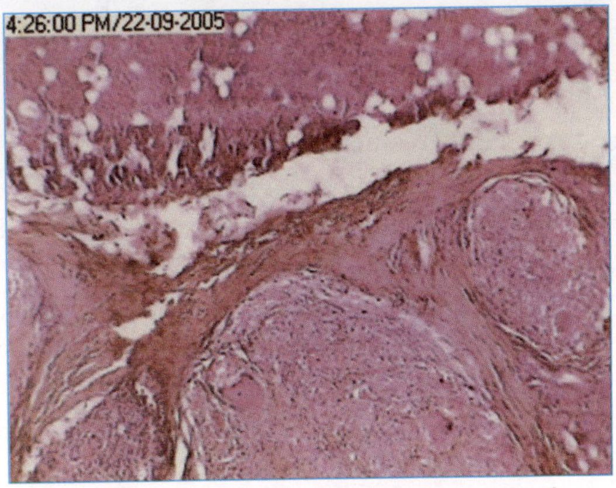

Fig.22.1: Shows microscopic appearance of tuberculosis of salivary gland

VIRAL INFECTION

Mumps

Mumps is a self-limiting benign viral infection of the salivary glands. This illness is caused by an RNA virus from a paramyxovirus group and typically involves parotid bilaterally.

Most patients are children, and the incidence is highest in spring. The incubation period is 14-21 days. Infectivity occurs via saliva and urine and precedes the symptoms by about 1 day and is maximal for 3 days but it may last a week.

Clinical features

The patient complains of pain near the lobe of ear and difficulty in chewing within 24 hours of onset. There is diffuse enlargement of parotid gland. The enlarged parotid obliterates the mandibular angle. The skin over the salivary gland is oedematous.

Complications

1. **Deafness**: It may cause unilateral irreversible sensory neural deafness.
2. **Viraemia**: It can lead to epididymoorchitis, pancreatitis, meningitis, encephalitis, or thyroiditis, myocarditis, pancreatitis, and oophoritis, which are more likely to occur in adults.

HIV associated salivary gland disease

HIV infected patients often develop bilateral painless parotid enlargement, much more often than women.

Microscopically

There are hyperplastic lymphoid follicles and a predominantly CD4 + cell population. The cells consisting the reactive follicles also include tangible body macrophages and follicular dendritic cells, all of them showing a positive staining for HIV p24 antigen.

Salivary gland involvement may be seen in a wide range of other viral illness including those caused by cytomegalovirus, lymphocytic choriomeningitis virus, coxsackie virus A, echo virus and parainfluenza virus.

SIALOLITHIASIS (salivary duct stones)

Salivary gland lithiasis accounts for approximately 30% of all salivary disorders and about 0.01-1.0% of population is held to be affected, with a higher incidence in males aged 30 to 60 years.

Salivary calculi are almost exclusively located in the major salivary glands.

They are common in submandibular gland (Wharton's duct), sublingual and minor salivary gland. It is uncommon in parotid gland (Stensen's duct). Sublingual gland is affected in 2% of cases and minor salivary glands in another 2%. High frequency of submandibular involvement is believed to be secondary to the tortuous course of Wharton's duct, high levels of calcium and phosphate, and the relative dependent position of the glands thus facilitating stasis and stone formation.

Etiology

Exact etiology of stone formation is unclear, but it appears to be related to the following conditions:

- **Higher mucin content** in the salivary gland secretion. Inspissated secretions due to salivary stagnation, dehydration, decreased food intake, and medications.
- **Epithelial injury along the duct** resulting in sialolith formation, which acts as a nidus for further stone formation.
- **Calcium and phosphate content** in the secretion is high. Precipitated calcium phosphate coalesces to inflammation or stasis. Hence, 80% of them are radio-opaque. Detected by plain X-ray.
- **Non-dependent drainage** of the secretions. Gland is in the neck and opening of the duct in oral cavity.
- **Kinking or hooking** of submandibular duct by lingual nerve.

Stones are primarily crystalline in nature composed of mostly hydroxyapatite (calcium phosphate and carbon with trace amounts of magnesium, potassium chloride and ammonium).

Clinically

Salivary gland stones are most common in adults; 25% of those with stones have more than one. Submandibular stone may be palpable or inspected in the floor of the mouth. Moreover, when the calculi are located in the distal parts of the ductal system, introducing a probe into the orifice of Wharton or Stensen's duct can often substantiate their presence:

1. **Salivary colic**: Partial obstruction causes enlargement and pain on eating, with return to normal as saliva drains. Salivary secretions are induced by a meal or lemon. As a result of blockage due to a stone, the tension within the gland increases, resulting in pain.
2. **Lingual colic**.
3. Total obstruction leads to **chronic enlargement** and often infection.

Complications of sialolith include fistula formation, acute sialadenitis, stricture, mucus retention cyst, ductal dilatation, recurrence of stones, and discomfort.

Treatment

The first diagnosis of sialolithiasis with a painful, swollen gland should initially be treated with secretory stimulants and massage of the affected glands. Dilatation of duct orifice, the narrowest part of the duct, can provide, in cases of small stones. In acute phase, antibiotics, and then surgical removal. Extracorporeal shock wave lithotripsy (ESWL) is proposed as an alternative therapeutic approach in the treatment of salivary stones.

CHEILITIS GLANDULARIS

Synonyms: Baelz' disease, myxadenitis labialis, Volkmann's cheilitis.

Cheilitis glandularis is a condition characterised by swelling and eversion of the lower lip.

The cause is unknown, although in some cases hereditary pattern is observed. Other causes include syphilis, bacterial infection, actininc damage, tobacco use, and poor oral hygiene.

Clinical features

Clinically, it consists of enlargement of the lip due to minor salivary gland hyperplasia and chronic inflammatory infiltration.

Three forms of cheilitis glandularis are recognised: A simple form, which is most common, a superficial suppurative form, and a deep suppurative form.

The condition most frequently occurs between the fourth and seventh decades of life, however, the range is wide. One report exists in a child. Cheilitis glandularis affects the lower lip almost exclusively although there are also purported cases involving the upper lip and palate.

It manifests as progressive, often multinodular enlargement, eversion, and induration. Salivary gland duct orifices are dilated and appear as red or black puncta. Viscous clear secretions initially exist the duct openings spontaneously. Crusting, erosions, and microabscesses may occur.

Cheilitis glandularis can be considered a potential predisposing factor for the development of actinic cheilitis and squamous cell carcinoma.

Microscopically

The microscopic findings of cheilitis glandularis are not specific and usually consist of chronic sialadenitis and ductal dilatation. Concomitant actinic, dysplastic changes and hyperkeratosis may be observed in the overlying surface epithelium in some cases. The subepithelial connective tissue shows minor mucus salivary gland with chronic inflammatory infiltrate.

Treatment

Tropical steroids are of limited value. In advanced cases, plastic surgery is indicated.

CHEILITIS GRANULOMATOSA

Granulomatous cheilitis is a chronic swelling of the lip due to granulomatous inflammation.

Clinical features

The condition is rare, and may occur in people of any race, age, sex, although onset is usually in early adulthood.

Cheilitis granulomatosa is episodic non-tender swelling and enlargement of one or both lips. In most cases, this first episode goes away completely within hours or days.

Melkersson-Rosenthal syndrome is associated with facial nerve palsy and cheilitis ganulomata.

Causes

Cause is unknown. A genetic predisposition may exist in Melkersson-Rosenthal syndrome. Siblings have been affected. Crohn's disease, sarcoidosis, and orofacial granulomatosis may present in a similar clinical fashion and with identical histologic findings.

Orofacial granulomatosa may result from reactions to some foods or medicaments, such as cinnamon aldehyde and benzoates.

Clinical features

The earliest manifestation is sudden diffuse or occasionally nodular swellings of the lip or the face involving the upper lip, the lower lip or both cheeks. The forehead, the eyelids, or one side of the scalp may be involved. Once chronicity is established, the enlarged lip appears cracked with reddish brown discolouration and scaling. Regional lymph nodes are enlarged in 50% of patients. Other symptoms that may occur include fever, headache, and visual disturbances. Fissured and plicated (pleat-like effect) tongue is present in 20-40% of cases.

Microscopically

The swelling is accounted for by the presence of granulomatous inflammation with infiltration and replacement of minor salivary glands. The granulomas are multinodular, composed of swirled collagen fascicles with interspersed multinucleated giant cells.

Treatment

1. Tropical corticosteroids
2. Long term anti-inflammatory antibiotics, e.g., a six to twelve month course of tetracycline and erythromycin.

NECROTISING SIALOMETAPLASIA

This lesion was first described in 1990 by Werning et al.

Necrotising sialometaplasia is a non-neoplastic inflammatory condition of the salivary glands.

Causes

The cause is unknown, however, predisposing factors are:

- Cases are reported in which vascular compression is caused by a necrotic mucocutaneous reconstruction flap, embolisation from carotid enarterectomy, sickle cell anaemia, Burger's disease, or Raynaud's phenomenon.
- Necrosis of minor salivary glands due to trauma caused during intubation.
- Sialometaplasia is associated with parotid tumours, vocal cord squamous carcinoma and carcinoma of maxillary antrum.
- Infiltration of palate by local anesthetics.
- Chemical injury.
- Infections.
- Tobacco use is suggested as a possible etiologic risk factor for necrotising sialometaplasia.
- Ill-fitting denture.
- Bulimia with chronic vomiting.
- Atherosclerosis.

Clinical features

Sites: 75% of all cases occur on the posterior palate. Reports of this entity in the minor salivary glands of the retromolar pad area; buccal mucosa, tongue, incisive canal, and labia mucosa are available. In addition, necrotising sialometaplasia is recognized in the parotid and submandibular salivary glands.

It is more common in men than women (male female ratio 2 : 1) and usually seen in the fourth to fifth decades of life.

Most of the lesions are unilateral, with one-third occurring in a mid-palatal location. Submucosal ulcerative, nodular, crater-like lesion characterises it. The lesion usually measures 3 cm in its greatest diameter.

Microscopically

The solitary lobules show a heavy, diffuse infiltrate of acute and chronic inflammatory cells and focal acinar necrosis. There is ductal and acinar squamous metaplasia, enlarged nuclei, prominent nucleoli, mitotic figures and apoptosis. There is pseudoepithelial hyperplasia of overlying epithelium. Histopathologically, it is important to differentiate necrotizing sialometaplasia from squamous cell carcinoma or mucoepidermoid carcinoma.

Treatment

The lesion gradually heals spontaneously without treatment within 4 to 10 weeks.

BENIGN LYMPHOEPITHELIAL LESION (MIKULICZ'S DISEASE)

It is characterized by the triad which includes (i) the parotid enlargement—may be accompanied by enlargement of minor salivary glands (e.g., salivary glands of the tongue and palate). (ii) Enlargement of lacrimal glands, which causes narrowing of lacrimal fissures, and (iii) dryness of mouth.

Clinical features

Benign lymphoepithelial lesion is most likely to occur in adults around 50 years of age. There is predilection for gender with 50-60 percent being female. The gland affected has a diffuse swelling.

The swelling can be asymptomatic, but mild pain can also be associated. There is preponderance of this disease in those who suffer from HIV infection.

Causes

Tuberculosis, leukaemia, lymphosarcoma, poisoning, sarcoidosis, syphilis, gout and idiopathic lymphoid hyperplasia may cause it.

Microscopically: The lymphoid tissue replaces the glandular parenchyma. There is also intraductal proliferation of the epithelial cells with formation of both epithelial and myoepithelial elements.

Complications: Rare complication of Mikulicz's disease is the development of malignant lymphoma in salivary glands.

TUMOURS OF SALIVARY GLANDS

Neoplasms of salivary glands have an incidence of about 1 to 2 per 100,000 per annum in England and Wales, with about 470 new cases diagnosed every year.

They are less than 1% of all cancers and 3 to 6% of all tumours of head and neck.

Salivary gland tumours represent 2-3% of head and neck neoplasms. They are more common in females than in men. Benign tumours are more common in women while malignant tumours have an equal sex distribution.

Tumours are most common in the sixth decade of life. Malignancy typically presents after the age of sixty.

About 85% of salivary tumours occur in the parotid glands, followed by submandibular and minor salivary glands, and about 1% occur in the sublingual glands. Palate is most common site of minor salivary gland tumours.

Etiology of salivary gland tumours

Predisposing factors for salivary gland neoplasms are:

1. **Increased alcohol consumption**
2. **Increased smoking:** Smoking is an important risk factor for the development of Warthin's tumours but its relationship to malignant parotid tumour is less clear. Warthin's tumours are eight times more common in smokers as compared to non-smokers.
3. **Exposure to aflatoxin:** Salivary gland cancers are common in workers working in life stock processing unit. This has been attributed to the presence of excessive amounts of aflatoxin B_1 present in the feed. Infact aflatoxin happens to be a contaminant in livestock feed.
4. **Exposure to radiation:** The risk of salivary gland cancer is increased in atomic bomb survivors and after radiotherapy. Radiation to the neck increases the risk of malignancy of salivary glands with 15 to 20 year latency.
5. **Virus infection:** There is also evidence that people infected with herpes viruses and Epstein-Barr virus may be at higher risk for salivary gland tumours. An individual infected with human immunodeficiency virus (HIV) has more salivary gland disease, in general, and may be at higher risk for salivary gland tumours.
6. **Diet and nutritional habits:** Intake of polysaturated fatty acids has a protective effect from these tumours.
7. **Occupations** associated with an increased risk for salivary gland cancers include rubber products manufacturing, asbestos mining, plumbing, and some types of woodworking. People who are exposed to mustard gas, isopropyl oils, volatile hydrocarbons, or metals-like nickel and chromium are more prone to carcinoma of salivary glands.

8. **Oncogenes:** Over-expression of TP53 has been identified in a high proportion of carcinomas arising from pleomorphic adenomas while few TP53 mutations has been described in other salivary gland tumours.

   Hepatocyte growth factor (HGF), a protein that causes morphogenesis and dispersion of epithelial cells, has been found to increase adenoid cystic carcinoma scattering and perhaps invasiveness.

   Expression of proliferating nuclear antigen (PCNA) was found in adenoid cystic carcinomas with higher expression in salivary gland malignancy.

   c-fos oncogene under expression in salivary gland tumours as measured by in situ hybridisation.

   Protein product of the c-erb B-2 proto-oncogene is frequently expressed in salivary gland tumours.
9. Some studies suggested an association between high use of mobile phones and an increased risk of benign and malignant parotid tumours although others found no evidence of such relationship.

Symptoms of benign tumours

- Painless swelling in one of the salivary glands, e.g., in front of ears, under the chin, or floor of the mouth. The size of the tumour gradually increases.
- Pain in the jaw or side of the face
- Difficulty in swallowing
- Difficulty in breathing
- Difficulty in speaking.

Symptoms of malignant tumours

Pain and neural involvement are common. Eventually, the overlying skin or mucosa becomes ulcerated or the adjacent tissues may become invaded.

Features suggestive of malignancy are hardness, fixation, tenderness, and infiltration into the surrounding tissue, e.g., facial nerve, and local lymph nodes.

Malignant tumours involving the salivary glands are challenging to treat because of following reasons:

1. Diversity of histological types
2. Anatomical constraints
3. Rarity of these tumours.

Theories of cellular origin

Two theories predominate in the study of cellular origin of salivary gland malignancy:

Bicellular theory: This theory postulates that tumours arise from one of the two undifferentiated stem cells, the excretory duct reserve cell or the intercalated duct reserve cells. Excretory stem cells give rise to squamous cell carcinoma and mucoepidermoid carcinomas, while intercalated stem cell give rise to pleomorphic adenomas, oncocytomas, adenoid carcinomas, and acinic cell carcinoma.

Multicellular theory: This theory assumes that each tumour type is associated with a specific differentiated cell of origin within the salivary gland unit. Squmous cell carcinomas arise from excretory duct cells, pleomorphic adenomas arise from the intercalated duct, oncocytomas from striated duct cells and acinic cell carcinomas arise from acinar cells.

INVESTIGATIONS

Biopsy

Fine needle aspiration cytology: It is useful for preoperative evaluation of salivary gland swelling and documenting of recurrent and metastatic disease. Accuracy is 90%.

CT scan and MRI of the major salivary gland can detect inflammatory disorders, obstruction, and tumours.

Sialography: Retrograde sialography is particularly useful when an inflammatory disorder or obstruction is suspected.

Gallium scan.

TABLE 22.3
SALIVARY GLAND NEOPLASM

A. Benign tumours
1. Adenomas
   i. Pleomorphic adenoma (mixed parotid tumour)
   ii. Adenolymphoma (Warthin's tumour)
   iii. Monomorphic adenoma
   iv. Oxyphil adenoma.
2. Mesenchymal tumour.

B. Malignant tumours
1. Adenocarcinoma
2. Mucoepidermoid carcinoma
3. Malignant mixed tumour
   i. Carcinoma ex-pleomorphic adenoma
   ii. Carcinosarcoma
   iii. Metastasizing mixed salivary gland tumours
4. Adenoid cystic carcinoma
5. Acinic cell carcinoma
6. Epidermoid carcinoma
7. Undifferentiated carcinoma
8. Miscellaneous

BENIGN TUMOURS

PLEOMORPHIC ADENOMA

Synonyms: Mixed parotid tumour, iceberg tumour, endothelioma, branchioma, or enchondroma, enclavaoma.

The term benign mixed tumour or pleomorphic adenomas was first proposed by Minssen in 1874 to describe the two components of tumour.

Pleomorphic adenoma is the most common parotid gland tumour. It accounts for 70 to 80 percent of all benign parotid tumours. Over 84% of pleomorphic adenomas occur in submandibular salivary glands. Intraoral minor salivary gland tumour constitutes approximately 8%. The palatal glands are the most affected in this group (65-65%). Other sites included in oral cavity are sublingual glands, cheek, and floor of the mouth.

Clinical features

They generally occur in adults between the ages of 30 and 60 years. More commonly, these occur in females with a ratio of M : F 1 : 4. It present as a painless slowly growing mass. Transformation to a malignant tumour is seen in only 2-5% of cases and is usually associated with tumours that have been present for 10-15 years.

Macroscopically

Pleomorphic adenomas vary in size from a small nodule to a bosselated mass weighing over a kilogram. Pleomorphic adenomas are typically smooth, well marginated tumours, though the nodularity along the outer surface is sometimes present. It is well-encapsulated to partially encapsulated or the tumour may even directly abut salivary gland parenchyma without an intervening capsule. The cut surface shows mucoid and cartilage-like areas and the greyish-white solid areas. Sometimes cystic degeneration may be seen.

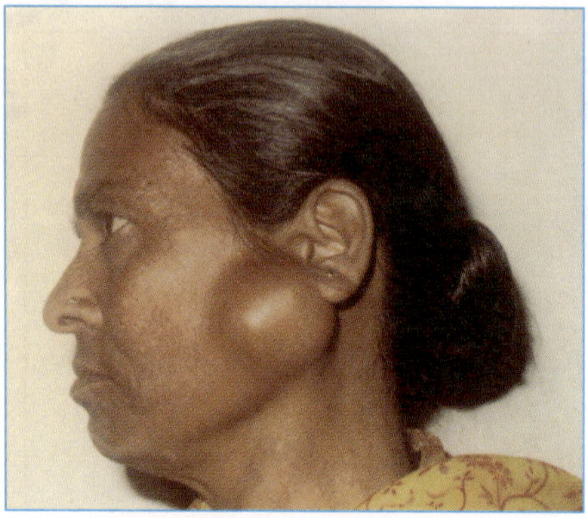

Fig.22.2: Photographs showing swelling below the ear lobule—Pleomorphic adenoma salivary gland

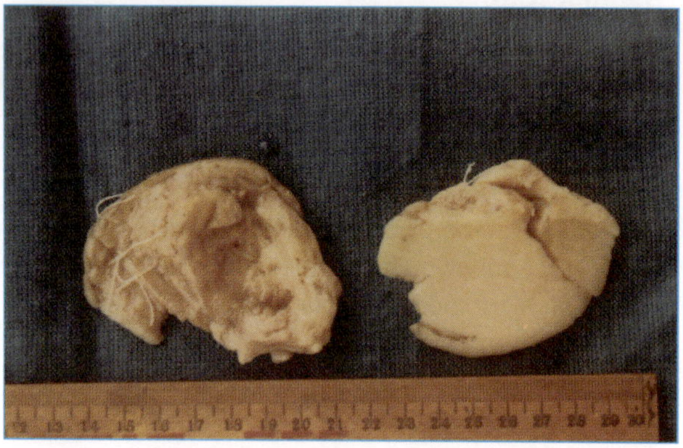

Fig.22.3: Resected specimen from a case of pleomorphic adenoma shows smooth mass with myxomatous element

Microscopically

Tumour composed of 2 subtypes of cells—epithelial and mesenchymal. Epithelial elements arranged in ducts, tubules, acini, single cell strands, sheets, or even single cells along with mesenchymal elements that resemble cartilage, or, rarely, bone. The myoepithelial cells form well-defined sheaths, cords or nests and often they are separated by a cellular ground substance, which resembles cartilaginous, myxoid or mucoid material and appears to be the product of the myoepithelial cells. Stroma consists of mucoid, fibroid, vascular and chondroid elements. The dilated and cystic ducts may contain eosinophilic and PAS positive material. Foci of squamous epithelium either in the form of solid clumps of prickle cells or cysts filled with laminated keratin are also seen. Haemorrhages, calcification, and necrosis are occasionally present.

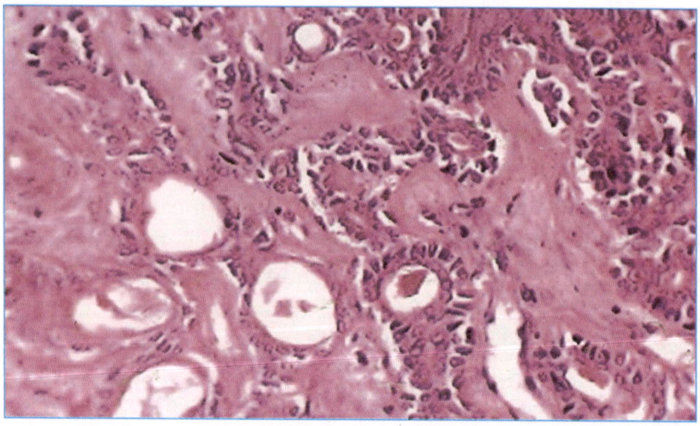

Fig.22.4: Pleomorphic adenoma salivary gland showing acini with epithelial mucin and pseudocartilage

Pleomorphic adenoma has a strong tendency to recur particularly when enucleated. This is largely due to the fact that small outgrowths of the tumour often protrude through the capsule and are left behind if close excision is done, while wide excision is made difficult by the facial nerve. Malignant transformation may occur in a mixed tumour after ten to fifteen years. It is characterized by sudden rapid growth and is accompanied by pain and paralysis of the facial nerve. There is a greater chance of malignancy in the submandibular and sublingual glands with 50% being benign.

Metastasis occurs to the regional lymph nodes and lung.

Treatment

Treatment of pleomorphic adenoma is complete surgical excision with a surrounding margin of normal tissue, e.g., superficial parotidectomy with facial nerve preservation, submandibular gland excision or wide local excision for minor salivary glands.

MONOMORPHIC ADENOMA

Monomorphic adenomas are slowly growing tumours less than 5% of all salivary gland tumours.

The term '*monomorphic adenoma*' refers to a group of rare salivary tumours that includes basal cell, canalicular, sebaceous, glycogen rich and clear cell adenoma.

Basal cell adenoma

Basal cell adenoma is a benign neoplasm composed of baseloid cells with peripheral palisading.

Clinical features

It is usually seen in adults with slightly predilection for females and usually between the fourth and ninth decades of life. The parotid gland is most common site involved. Basal cell adenomas usually arise on one side and bilateral occurrence is rare, accounting for 1-3% of all parotid tumours.

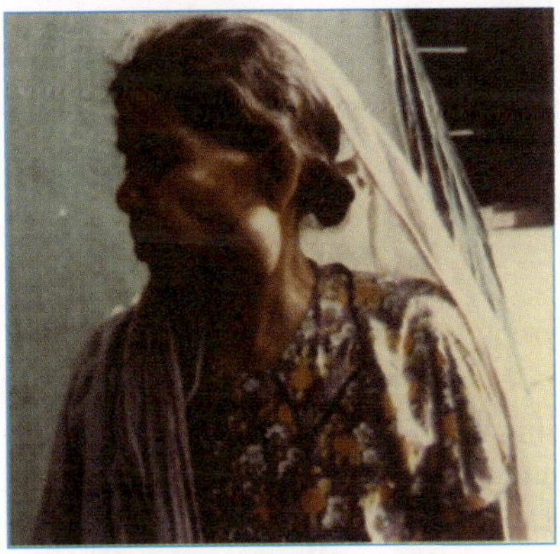

Fig.22.5: Shows monomorphic adenona salivary gland

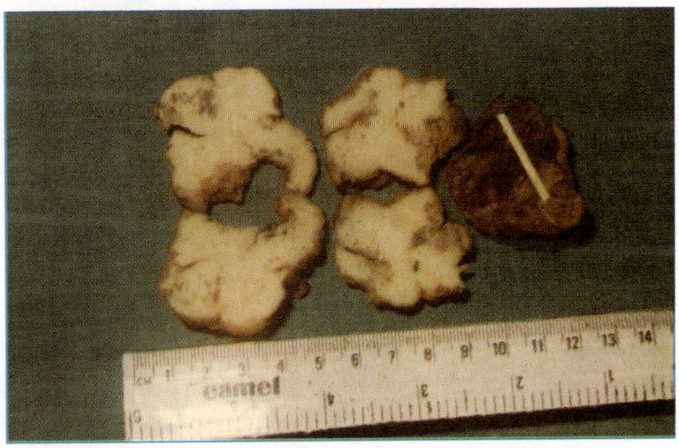

Fig.22.6: Shows gross appearance of monomorphic adenoma

Macroscopically

Basal cell adenomas are round to oval in shape. They tend to be smaller than pleomorphic adenomas; most measure 3 cm or less in diameter.

On cut section they are typically uniform and solid, without necrosis.

Microscopically

Basal cell adenomas are circumscribed capsulated by fibrous connective tissue.

Basal cell adenomas are benign tumours composed of relatively baseloid cells, a conspicuous basal cell layer, and dinstinctive basement membrane-like material. Basal cell adenoma lacks the characteristic myxochondroid matrix of pleomorphic adenoma.

Malignant transformation is seen as adenoid cystic carcinoma and basal cell adenocarcinoma.

Canalicular adenoma

The canalicular adenoma is a benign neoplasm that affects the minor salivary glands.

Canalicular adenomas tend to be multifocal and often occur in the upper lip mucosa (80% of cases) especially in the elderly around the 70 years of age. The next most common location is buccal mucosa. There is a predilection for gender with most cases being in females. The female-to-male preponderance is approximately 2 : 1.

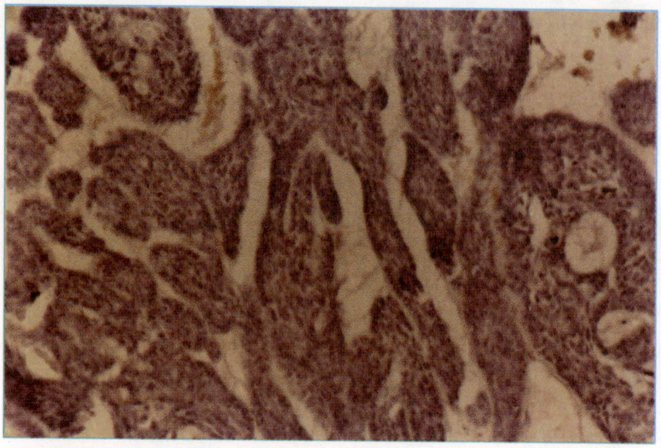

Fig.22.7: Showing microscopic appearance of baseloid type of monomorphic adenoma

Macroscopically

Canalicular adenomas are typically smaller than 2 cm. It is usually a single nodule. It may be multinodular of multifocal. The tumour is well-circumscribed with light tan to brown appearance.

Microscopically

The tumour is made up of columnar epithelial cells that form thin branching and intercommunating cords in a very loose but highly vascular and fibroblastic stroma. Double rows of cells alternately oppose and then separate from one another, producing a '*beads-on- a- string*' or '*canaliculi appearance*'. The cuboidal to tall columnar cells are with eosinophilic cytoplasm and round to elliptical nuclei. The chromatin is basophilic and stippled. There is lack of pleomorphism and mitosis. The epithelial cells have basal lamina with few microvilli and occasional secretory granules. Myoepithelial and basal cells are lacking.

The cells are reactive with keratin, vimentin and S-100 protein.

ADENOLYMPHOMA

Synonyms: ***Warthin's tumour***, benign papillary cystadenoma lymphomatosum and branchial cyst of parotid.

Warthin gave the name papillary cystadenoma lymphomatosum in 1929 in USA. Warthin's tumour is the second most common benign lesion in the parotid gland. It comprises 6 to 10% of cases of parotid tumour with rarely extraparotid. The tumour occurs in males predominantly with a male to female ratio of 5 : 1. They are present in 40-70 year old age group and are more common in whites than black.

The tumour is slow-growing, painless, and usually appears in the tail of the parotid gland near the angle of the mandible. It takes the form of an ovoid or round mass, often flattened and sometimes bilateral.

Macroscopically: On gross examination, the tumour is seen as well-defined oval or spherical mass with a smooth lobulated surface. The usual size of tumour is 1 to 8 cm. The tumour is well-capsulated, with pale grey homogeneous surface.

Cut surface: Characteristically, there are cleft-like spaces filled with mucin and showing papillary configuration in the wall. The solid areas are grey in colour with white nodules that represent the lymphoid follicles.

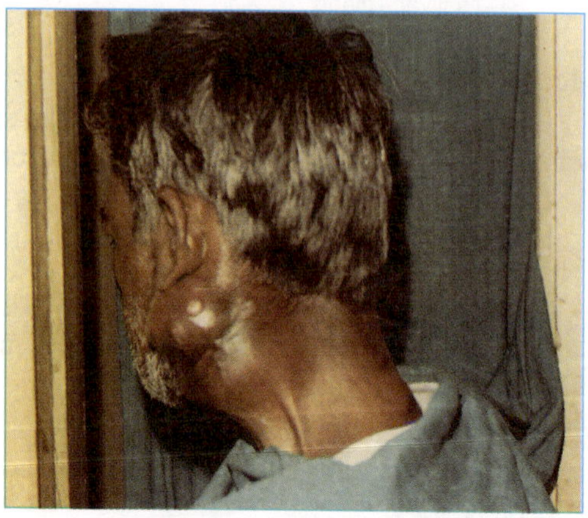

Fig.22.8: Photograph showing swelling below the ear lobule. Outer surface is nodular

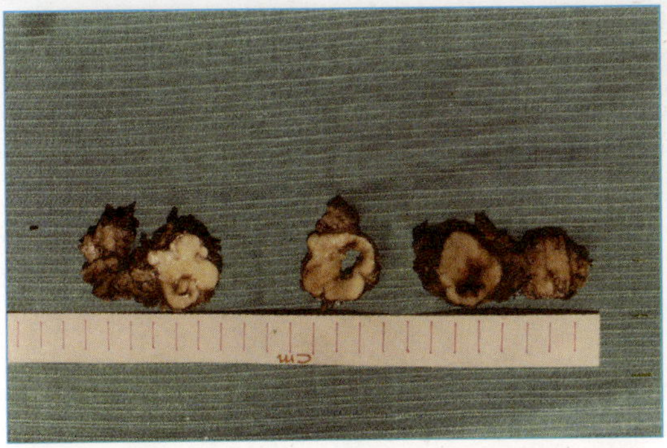

Fig.22.9: Showing cut surface of Warthin's tumour

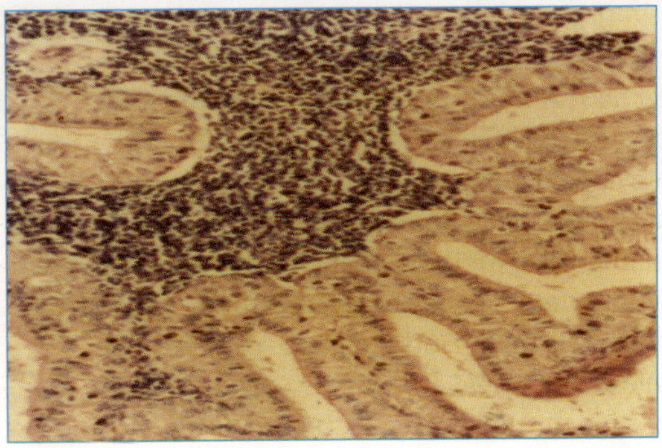

Fig.22.10: Shows lymphoid stroma and cystic spaces lined by papillary projections

Microscopically

The stroma contains a considerable amount of lymphoid tissue and there are many irregular cystic spaces into which papillary structures projects. The epithelium is two-layered; the inner tall columnar cells with eosinophilic granular cytoplasm with nuclei regularly arranged towards the lumen and outer small cuboid cells with eosinophilic cytoplasm. The nuclei of inner cells are vesicular and oriented towards the basement membrane. Sometimes piling up of epithelium or focal areas of squamous metaplasia may be seen.

Very rarely, malignant transformation to lymphoma or adenocarcinoma or squamous cell carcinoma can occur. It is thought that the tumour represents heterotopic salivary tissue trapped within a regional lymph node during embryogenesis.

Hypersensitivity theory: The lymphocytes being an immune reaction to the salivary ducts, which undergo oncocytic change.

There is some unique association of Warthin's tumour with cigarette smoking, but it is yet to be explained.

Treatment

Treatment of Warthin's tumour is surgical resection. Enucleation of the tumour may be adequate therapy but superficial parotidectomy with facial nerve preservation is the standard treatment. A recurrence rate of about 10% is attributed to incomplete excision, multicentricity, or a second primary tumour.

ONCOCYTOMA (OXYPHIL ADENOMA)

They arise from acidophilic cells called oncocytes and comprise less than 1% of all salivary gland tumours. Malignant oncocytomas are also seen.

Clinical features

Oncocytomas are common in parotid gland and then in submandibular glands. There is equal frequency in men and women. Patient presents with swelling and rarely pain. There is history of ionizing radiation. Pain is usually absent.

Mostly seen in the elderly, they usually do not grow larger than 5 cm and involve the superficial lobes of parotid.

Macroscopically

Tumour is well-circumscribed, single nodule and partially capsulated. Cut surface is red to brown. The tumour usually measures 3-5 cm in diameter.

Microscopically

Oncocytic cells are arranged in glandular and solid pattern. There are sheets, nests or cords of uniform oncocytes. These cells are large with distinct borders and filled with an acidophilic granular cytoplasm. The granularity of cytoplasm is due to the presence of large numbers of mitochondria they may constitute up to 60% of the volume. The nucleus is round with dispersed chromatin, prominent nucleoli with rare mitosis. Fine fibrovascular stroma may contain lymphoid infiltrate.

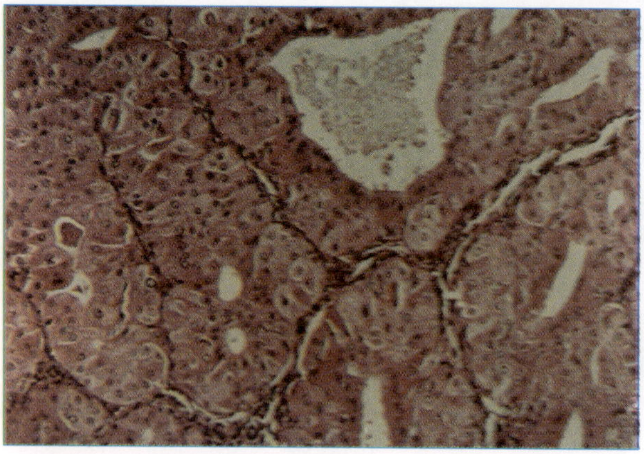

Fig.22.11: Oncocytoma: Oncocytic cells are arranged in glandular and solid pattern

Management

Surgical excision should be carried out.

MALIGNANT TUMOURS

MUCOEPIDERMOID TUMOUR

Stewart, Foote and Becker introduced the term mucoepidermoid tumour in 1945.

Mucoepidermoid carcinoma arises from the ductal epithelial cells and is composed of varying proportion of squamous cells, mucus secreting cells and intermediate cells.

Clinical features

It is the most common parotid salivary gland malignancy. It forms 3 or 4% of all tumours of major salivary glands. It occurs in parotid gland (60%), minor salivary glands (30%). It can occur deep within the bone such as in the wall of dentigerous cyst.

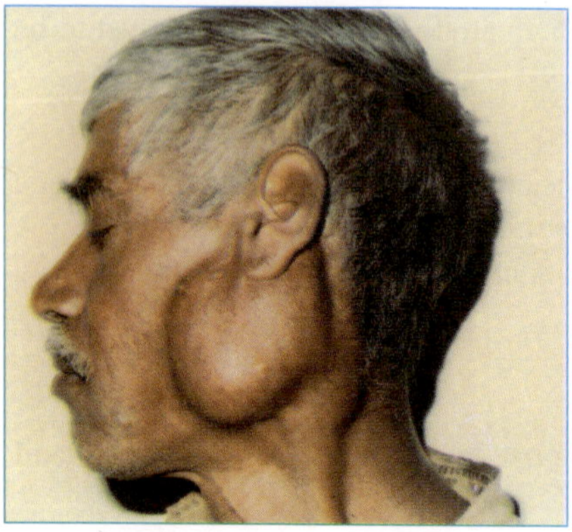

Fig.22.12: Mucoepidermoid carcinoma

In oral cavity it is seen in palate, buccal mucosa, tongue, and retromolar area.

There is history of ionising radiation. It occurs in adults and more often in women than men (1.5 : 1). It occurs as painless solitary nodule. Other clinical features include tenderness or pain, trismus, facial paralysis, discharge from ear, dysphagia, and numbness of teeth when tumours are situated close to teeth. There is ulceration or haemorrhage from minor salivary gland tumours.

Macroscopically

Tumour is uncapsulated or may be partially capsulated. Cut surface shows pink to tan coloured multiple cysts filled with mucoid material. Size varies from 1-12 cm.

Microscopically

It can be classified as low-grade, intermediate-grade and high-grade.

It consists of neoplastic mucus secreting cells organised into microcysts, malignant epithelial cells and intermediate cells (also known as transitional cells). Pleomorphism and mitoses are frequent in the high-grade mucoepidermoid tumours and indicate poor prognosis. Stroma is fibrous, infiltrated by abundant lymphocytes showing lymphoid follicles.

Recent increase in size, pain, facial palsy and local fixation suggest a higher grade of tumour.

Almost 95 to 98% 5-year survival have been reported in low-grade tumours. Five-year survival reported for high-grade variety is 50 to 55%.

More aggressive tumours metastasise to lymph nodes and may invade the blood vessel. Distant metastases to lungs, bones, brain and subcutaneous tissue are common.

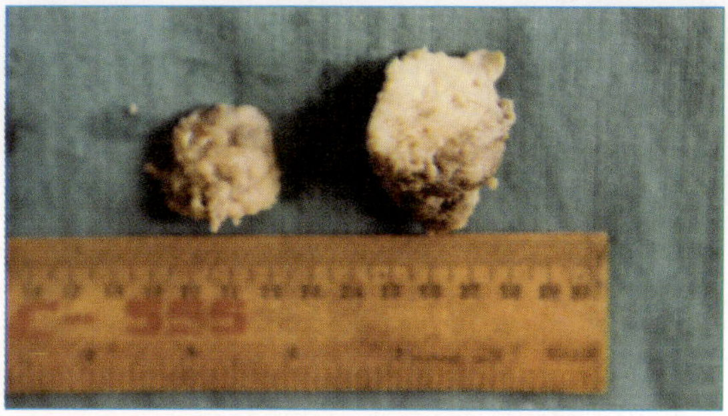

Fig.22.13: Showing gross appearance of mucoepidermoid carcinoma

Treatment

Treatment of mucoepidermoid carcinoma consists of wide excision and postoperative radiation. The 5-year survival rate is 95% with low grade type, primarily mucus cells and 50% with the high-grade type, primary affecting epidermoid cells.

ADENOID CYSTIC CARCINOMA

Adenoid cystic carcinoma is also known as cylindroma.

Adenoid cystic carcinoma is usually slow-growing and often appears to be a low-grade tumour. It constitutes 5% of all tumours of the major salivary glands and 20% of minor salivary glands. It represents 28% of malignant submandibular gland tumours.

Pathogenesis

Slow-growing tumour of salivary glands, thought to arise from intercalated mucus secreting ducts and myoepithelial cells.

Hepatocyte growth factor (HGF)—a protein that causes morphogenesis and dispersion of epithelial cells—has been found to increase adenoid cystic carcinoma scattering and, perhaps, invasiveness.

Expression of proliferating nuclear antigen (PCNA) was found in adenoid cystic carcinomas with higher expression in salivary gland malignancy.

Clinical features

Female to male ratio is 3 : 2. The peak age for the development of adenoid cystic carcinoma is between 50 and 60 years of age. The tumour seldom occurs in people under 30 years of age.

Most common glands involved are the parotid and submaxillary. The palate is the most common location in the oral cavity.

Early lesions of salivary glands present as painless masses of mouth or face, usually slow-growing. Advanced tumours may present with pain, tenderness and/or facial nerve paralysis.

Several factors have been considered indicative of a poor prognosis in patients with adenoid cystic carcinoma, including an advanced stage, a solid histologic type, the presence of nodal metastasis, and presence of positive margins and perineural lymphatics.

Microscopically

Adenoid cystic carcinomas can be graded as well-differentiated, moderately-differentiated and poorly-differentiated.

Well-differentiated adenoid cystic carcinoma shows **tubular pattern.** It is composed of ductal structures formed of outer myoepithelial cells and inner epithelial cells enclosed by hyaline material.

Moderately-differentiated adenoid cystic carcinoma: It is a malignant tumour, consisting of cords of darkly staining cells with cystic spaces containing mucin, which show a characteristic sieve-like or **cribriform pattern**. This pattern is also called honeycomb pattern.

Poorly differentiated adenoid cystic carcinoma: This tumour exhibits a **solid pattern** of growth and is composed of anaplastic tumour cells forming solid nests or sheets. Inside the solid nests, areas of comedo-like necrosis may be present.

Immnunohistochemically, tumour cells are positive for keratin, carcino-embryonic antigen (CEA), isozyme, lactoferrin, S-100 and CD117 (c-kit).

Adenoid cystic carcinoma tends to infiltrate the perineural spaces. These tumours have high incidence of distinct metastasis to lungs but, in general, they display indolent growth. Skin lesions are more common as it spreads along the nerve tissue, which leads to treatment failure. The tumour metastasises to lymph nodes.

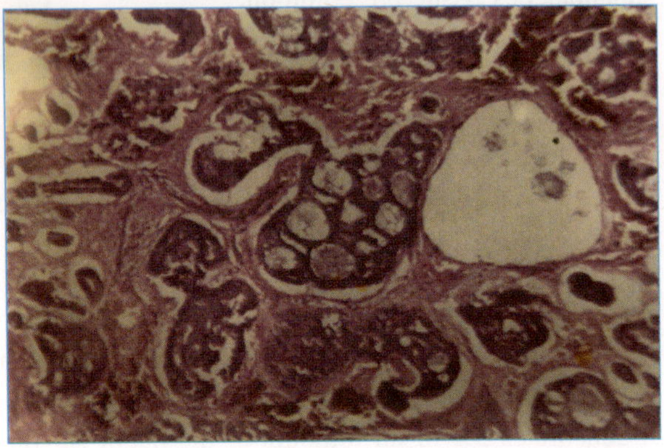

Fig.22.14: Shows microscopic appearance of adenoid cystic carcinoma

Adenoid cystic carcinoma is characterised by persistent local recurrences, perineural spread, and distant metastases to lung and liver; lymphatic spread is less common.

Treatment

Primary treatment of this tumour is surgical removal with clear margins. Adjuvant or palliative radiotherapy is commonly given following surgery. Neutron therapy has been shown to be superior for some types of cancer including adenoid cystic carcinoma of head and neck. Chemotherapy is used for metastatic disease.

ACINIC CELL TUMOUR

Acinic cell tumour is a neoplastic growth of epithelial cells showing serous acinar pattern. They arise from both acinar cells and intercalated ducts.

Clinical features

Acinic cell carcinoma accounts for 2.5 to 4% of all tumours of salivary gland and 15% of all malignant tumours of parotid glands.

The tumour occurs principally in young men between the ages of 20 and 30 years. The tumour is most common in whites than blacks.

Patient presents with slowly growing, mobile, or fixed mass of various duration. It is asymptomatic, may complain pain, tenderness and facial muscle weakness.

Acinic cell carcinoma has been reported to be the most likely of carcinomas which occurs bilaterally. The cancer affects women more commonly than men.

Macroscopically

It is seen as an encapsulated, round mass, usually smaller than 3 cm across, and is sometimes cystic. Cut surface is lobular, red to tan coloured, firm and cystic.

Microscopically

The tumour shows various histological patterns: Acinar, tubular, microcystic, follicular, papillary cystic, medullary, ductoglandular and primitive tubular.

Acinic type: The acinic cell carcinomas are composed of large round to polygonal cells with basophilic cytoplasm, similar to the secretory (acinic) cells of the normal salivary gland. Nuclei are vesicular, small, round and uniform. The cytoplasm contains granules stimulating the normal acinar cell. Lattice-like appearance may be seen due to accumulation of the fluid. In some tumours clear cells predominate having vacuolated cytoplasm (hypernephroid appearance). Clear cells do not contain fat or mucin but may be variable amounts of glycogen.

Follicular type is rare and comprises of cystic spaces lined by cuboidal to columnar cells.

In microcystic variety, multiple small cystic spaces are created that contain some mucinus or eosinophilic material.

Papillary acinic cell tumour shows features of acinic cell tumour with papillary areas. The cells of tumour seemed to follow a sequence from large cells with rounded nuclei with open chromatin and prominent nucleoli. Vacuolated cells have granular material, and, finally, cells undergo apoptosis. There are presence of concentrically laminated to polygonal, Congo-red positive, birefringent bodies that in areas accumulated and formed extensive areas with massive deposits. Some authors report that huge globular deposits are amyloid in nature.

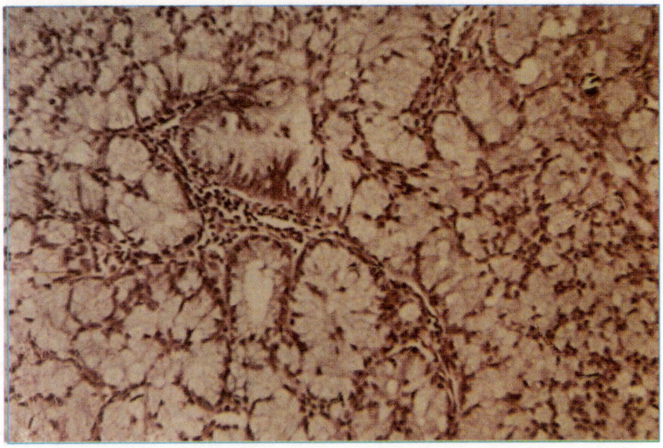

Fig.22.15: Basophilic tumour cells in acinar pattern with lymphoid tissue in the stoma

A lymphoid infiltrate sometimes with germinal center formation is not unusual.

Acinic cell carcinomas are generally associated with good prognosis. However, recurrences are known to occur.

The most sites of metastases are lymph nodes, lungs, bone, central nervous system, mediastinum, liver and brain.

MALIGNANT PLEOMORPHIC ADENOMA

It is mainly of three types: Carcinoma ex-pleomorphic adenoma, carcino sarcoma and metastasising mixed tumours.

CARCINOMA EX-PLEOMORPHIC ADENOMA

Carcinoma ex-pleomorphic adenoma is defined as a malignant transformation in a pre-existent mixed tumour.

Clinical features

It is most common in middle-aged and older adults with peak prevalence in the sixth decades of life. It accounts for 1% of all parotid tumours and 7% of all malignant tumours.

More than 85% of cases of carcinoma ex-pleomorphic adenomas are seen within the major glands, primarily the parotid gland. Nearly two-thirds of minor salivary gland cases occur on the palate.

Usually the patient will have a long-standing history of a salivary gland lesion, and may have undergone multiple operations for recurrent pleomorphic adenoma. There is sudden increase in growth, pain and facial paralysis. There is destruction of capsule, invasion of and adhesion of the surrounding tissue and the tumour metastasises to regional lymph nodes, lungs, bone, and abdominal organs.

Macroscopically

The tumours are firm with minimal encapsulation and widely infiltrative with areas of haemorrhage and necrosis. Neurovascular invasion and necrosis are frequent findings.

Microscopically

There is microscopic evidence of pre-existing benign tumour; sometimes represented by only a totally hyalinised round nodule surrounded by carcinoma, or benign or malignant tumour. Malignant neoplasm may be salivary duct carcinoma, undifferentiated carcinoma, myoepithelial carcinoma and unclassified carcinoma.

CARCINO SARCOMA (true malignant mixed tumours)

It is a exceeding rare tumour of the salivary gland, comprising 0.04% to 1.6% of all salivary gland neoplasms. Kirklin et al first described it in 1951.

Clinical features

There is no sex predominance. The mean age at presentation is 58 years with a range of 14-87 years.

True malignant mixed tumours of the oral minor salivary glands (e.g., situated within the hard and soft palates, cheeks, lips, tongue, and tonsillar crypts) are rare yet cases are reported in medical literature. Haematogenous metastases are more common in the lung, bone, and liver. Cervical and hilar lymph node metastases are common.

Pathogenesis

Pathogenesis and histogenesis of true malignant mixed tumours of the salivary glands are controversial. According to some authors, carcinosarcoma and pleomorphic adenoma of salivary gland share a common precursor, possibly myoepithelial cell.

Microscopically

Carcinosarcomas of the salivary glands are biphasic tumours that exhibit both carcinomatous and sarcomatous elements. These tumours are thought to develop de-novo in the salivary gland and contain malignant stromal and epithelial elements. The most common malignant epithelial element component is squamous cell carcinoma or adenocarcinoma, whereas the most common mesenchymal component is chondrosarcoma, followed by fibrosarcoma, leiomyosarcoma, osteosarcoma, liposarcoma and rhabdomyosarcoma.

Immunohistochemically, cytokeratin and EMA are epithelial markers whereas vimentin and S-100 are sarcomatous mesenchymal markers.

Treatment

Carcinosarcoma is an aggressive, high-grade neoplasm and require radical surgery, with and without radiation therapy and chemotherapy.

METASTASISING BENIGN MIXED TUMOURS

Metastasising mixed tumour is rare. As with other malignant tumours, most cases originate in the parotid gland, but the primary tumour may occur in the submandibular gland or minor salivary glands.

Metastasising benign mixed tumours are histologically benign but usually have a history of multiple local recurrences. Metastases occur several years after the initial diagnosis and may occur to the lungs, regional lymph nodes, skin and bone.

ADENOCARCINOMA

It is slightly more common in women.

Adenocarcinomas are most frequently found in minor salivary glands of nose and paranasal sinuses. Adenocarcinoma may arise from a pleomorphic adenoma. Adenocarcinoma develops from the secretory element of glands or excretory ducts. The tumour, which is generally firm and non-tender, tends to infiltrate blood vessels, lymphatic channel and perineural spaces. The lesion is seen on the soft and hard palate, cheek, and upper lip.

Macroscopically

Size varies from 2-3 cm. Cut surface is yellowish-white with areas of haemorrhage and necrosis.

Microscopically

Malignant tumour cells are arranged in solid cords, sheets, nests, tubular, islands and cystic pattern with papillae. Ductal glandular differentiation is present in all cases. There are presence of clear cells or oncocytic cells.

This is an aggressive lesion with potential for both local and distant metastasis. Approximately 33% of patients have nodal or distant metastasis present at the time of initial diagnosis. Overall, 5-year survival is 19-75% as it is highly variable and related to grade and stage of presentation.

METASTATIC CARCINOMA

Metastatic tumours in salivary glands account for 5 to 20% of salivary swellings.

Melanomas (46%), squamous cell carcinoma (37%), and other tumours (17%) comprise the overwhelming majority of head and neck malignant neoplasms that metastasise to the parotid gland. There have been few reported cases of renal cell carcinoma in submandibular glands. Other tumours, which metastasise to salivary glands, include olfactory neuroblastoma, retinoblastoma, thyroid tumours, Merkle cell carcinoma, eccrine carcinoma, nasopharyngeal carcinoma, hepatocellular carcinoma, adenocarcinoma of ampulla of Vater, carcinoma breast, and small cell carcinoma of lung.

Bibliography

Sousa J De, Sao O: 2001 Salivary gland tumours: Indian J Cancer March: 38 (1): 38-45.

Bhargawa S, Sant MS and Arora, MM: Histomorphological spectrum of minor salivary glands. Indian J. Cancer: 19: 134-140, 1982.

Das S: A Concise Textbook of Surgery. 4th edition, Dr S Das Publication, 2006.

James William D, Berger Timothy G, et al: (2006) Andrew's diseases of the Skin: Clinical Dermatology. Saunders Elsevier.

Joshi SW, Pawar A, Lakhka Dr: Unusual metastatic tumours of parotid—report of two cases. Indian Journal of Radiology and Imaging: 2005; 15: 205-207.

Kahn, Michael A: Basic Oral and Maxillofacial Pathology, Volume 1. 2001.

Kernohan NM, Blessing K, King G, Miller ID: 2005. The Journal of Pathology, Volume 163 (1) 77-80.

Mashberg A, Bofetta et al: Tobacco smoking, alcohol drinking and cancer of the oral cavity and oropharynx among US Veterans. Cancer 72:1369-75, 1993

Sadetzki S, Chetrit A, Jarus-Hakak A, et al; Cellular phone use and risk: Benign and malignant parotid gland tumours—a nationwide case-control study. American J Epidemiol. 2008 feb 15; 167 (4): 457-67.

Nevelle, Brad W: (2002). Oral and Maxillofacial Pathology: Second Edition, Philadelphia, W B Saunders.

Verma S: Cheilitis glandularis: a rare entity. British J Dermatol 2003 148: 362

Y. Danshbal, S. Negahban, and B. Khademi: Acinic cell carcinoma of salivary gland with massive deposits of globular amyloid. International Journal of Surgical Pathology, June 1, 2009: 17(3): 276-278.

CHAPTER

23

ODONTOGENIC TUMOURS

ODONTOGENIC TUMOURS

TABLE 23.1
CLASSIFICATION OF ODONTOGENIC TUMOURS

A. Benign epithelial odontogenic tumours
   1. Tumours producing minimal inductive change in connective tissue
      a. Ameloblastoma
      b. Calcifying epithelial odontogenic tumour
      c. Odontogenic adenomatoid tumour
      d. Squamous odontogenic tumour.
   2. Tumours producing extensive inductive change in connective tissue
      a. Ameloblastic fibroma
      b. Ameloblastic fibroodontoma
      c. Odontoma
      1. Compound odontoma
      2. Complex odontoma.

B. Mesenchymal odontogenic tumours
   1. Odontogenic fibroma
   2. Odontogenic myxoma
   3. Cementoma
      a. Periapical cemental dysplasia
      b. Cementifying fibroma
      c. Benign cementoblastoma

Contd.

Contd.

4. Dentinoma.

C. Tumours of unknown origin

1. Melanotic neuroectodermal tumour of infancy.

D. Malignant odontogenic tumours

1. Ameloblastic carcinoma
2. Primary intraosseous carcinoma
3. Ameloblastic fibrosarcoma
4. Clear cell odontogenic sarcoma
5. Ameloblastic dentosarcoma.

AMELOBLASTOMA (ADMANTINOMA)

Ameloblastoma is the most common of the epithelial odontogenic tumours. The tumour is seen commonly in the fourth to the fifth decade of life.

Origin: It may arise from the epithelial lining of dentigerous cyst, Hertwig sheath, from the remnants of the dental lamina and enamel organ, or from basal layer of the oral mucosa.

Ameloblastomas have been classified as:

- Peripheral (extraosseous)
- Central (intraosseous)
- Unicystic
  - Intraluminal
  - Mural
  - Intramural
- Plexiform unicystic
- Muilticystic or solid.

Peripheral ameloblastoma: It occurs in soft tissue outside and overlying alveolar bone. This neoplasm arises from the basal layer of the surface epithelium or remnants of dental lamina. It occurs most frequently in the fourth to sixth decade of life and has a slight male predilection. Mandible is affected twice as frequently as the maxilla.

Central ameloblastoma

Clinical features

The lesion occurs in both the maxilla and mandible, but the posterior mandible is the most common location, only 20% of the lesions are found in the maxilla. It is uncapsulated and infiltrates surrounding bone marrow. Even though they are infiltrative, they do not metastasise.

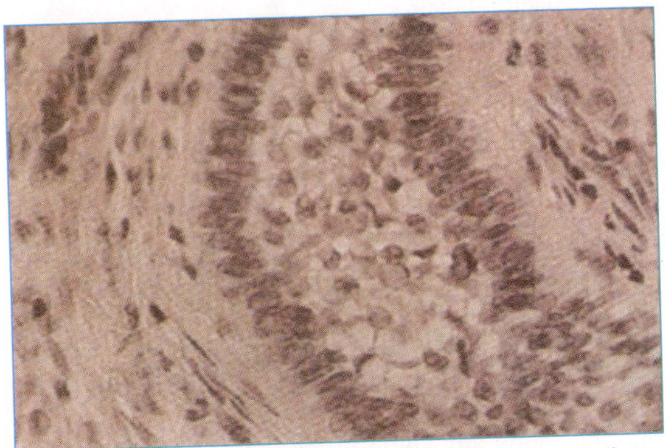

Fig.23.1: Microphotograph shows ameloblastic epithelium in a loose fibrous stroma. There is palisading at the periphery

Microscopically

The tumour consists of numerous solid and cystic epithelial masses embedded in fibrous tissue. The solid portions are mostly of small size and round, oval or irregular contour and supported by a delicate basement membrane. Marginal cells are constantly columnar, and palisaded, with oval nuclei, away from the base. The core is invariably made up of prickle epithelium are flattened, oval, round, or polyhedral with central nuclei and joined across, narrow canals by numerous delicate processes.

Several histological patterns are recognised

Granular cell pattern

Tumour consists of abundant coarsely granular eosinophilic cytoplasm in the stellate cells. These granular cells may be cuboidal, columnar, or rounded. Electron microscopy shows these granules to be lysosome.

Basal cell pattern

The least common type; shows a strong resemblance to epidermal basal cells. These lesions are composed of nests of uniform baseloid cells, and they are very similar to basal cell carcinoma of skin. No stellate reticulum is present in the central portions of the nests. The peripheral cells of the nests tend to be cuboidal rather than columnar.

Acanthomatous type: The central core of loosely epithelial cells in follicular pattern may undergo squamous metaplasia. They lose their star-shape and become polygonal.

Plexiform pattern

The cords or sheets are bounded by columnar or cuboidal 'ameloblastic-like' cells and surround loosely arranged angular 'stellate reticulum cells'. Fibrous stroma is loosely arranged, are vascular and undergoes cystic degeneration.

Desmoplastic pattern

Desmoplastic ameloblastoma is a rare variant, initially described in 1984 by Eversole et al. It presents accentuated predilection for the anterior region of the maxilla and the mandible, preferably for the maxilla. The tumour usually occurs between the third and fifth decades of life, with equal prevalence between male and females. It represents 4-5% of all ameloblastomas.

Microscopically

The desmoplastic ameloblastoma is characterised by a stroma with intense desmoplasia, densely collagenised, comprising little odontogenic epithelium islands and cords of various sizes.

Immunohistochemical studies have shown increased production of the cytokeratin known as transforming growth factor (TGF-β) in association with this lesion, suggesting that this may be responsible for the desmoplasia.

Follicular pattern

The peripheral cells are tall and columnar. The central cells of the follicle resembling stellate reticulum undergo cystic degeneration.

X-ray of the jaw shows a multilocular or unilocular cystic lesion of the jaw. Ameloblastoma typically appear as an expansile multilocular radiolucency in the area of the lower third molar, but they may be found anywhere in the jaw.

Treatment

The treatment of ameloblastoma is surgical excision with wide free margins.

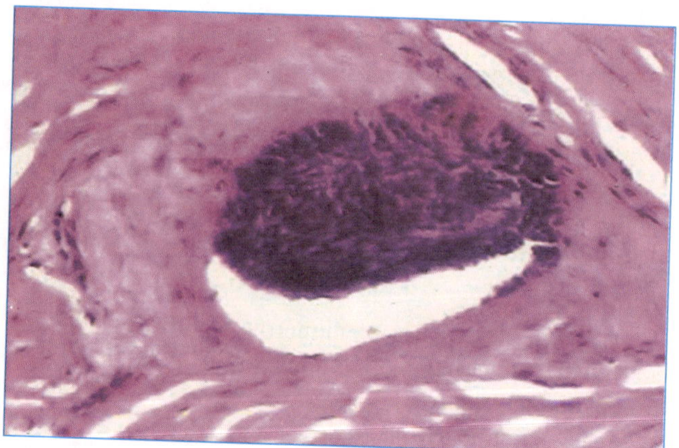

Fig.23.2: Microphotograph showing ameloblastic epithelium. Peripheral cells are columnar

ADENOMATOID ODONTOGENIC TUMOUR

Adenomatoid odontogenic tumour is a benign capsulated odontogenic tumour that probably arises from the odontogenic epithelium of the dental lamina complex or its remnants.

It occurs in the middle and anterior portions of the jaws. It is more common in females. Adenomatoid odontogenic tumour is usually seen between the ages of 5 and 30 years. This is a tumour mostly of teenagers.

Two-third of the cases occur in the anterior maxilla, one-third occur in the anterior mandible, and are never found posterior to the premolars. The lesion usually presents as asymptomatic swelling, slowly growing and often associated with an unerupted tooth. Facial asymmetry is one of the first signs to be noticed by the patient as the tumour increases in size.

Macroscopically: The tumour is encapsulated, somewhat cystic. Cut surfaces feel gritty and the cystic cavity is partially or completely filled with a solid tumour mass. The crown of the tooth is usually found projecting into the cystic cavity.

Microscopically

On microscopic examination, at low magnification, the tumour exhibits distinctive histomorphic features. There is thick fibrous capsule encompassing ameloblastic epithelium that may be arranged in sheets or whorled pattern. The tumour fills the central cavity. The lumen of the duct-like spaces may be empty or contain a variable amount of cell debris. The trabeculae of the epithelium may be noted toward the periphery of the lesions. There is little stroma. The tumour cells frequently form ball-like structures referred to as rosettes. Calcified material may be noted throughout the epithelial tissue and stroma. Melanin may be present.

At high magnification, the epithelial component usually shows a duct cell population consisting of polyhedral spindle-shaped to columnar and cuboidal cells. The first type of epithelial cell forms large aggregates with a surviving pattern exhibiting the overall nodular pattern. The second cell type, which is more cuboidal to columnar in nature, forms duct-like spaces, producing a characteristic glandular pattern, as well as convoluted cords in complicated patterns.

Radiological findings

This lesion generally appears as a well-demarcated radiolucency. In 75% of cases, it is associated with unerupted tooth, usually the canines. Small calcifications may be found in the tumour. If they are present in sufficient size and number, they may show a radiograph as a ***'snow-flake pattern'***.

Treatment

Complete removal of tumour is necessary and the prognosis is excellent without any recurrences.

CALCIFYING EPITHELIAL ODONTOGENIC TUMOUR (PINDBORG TUMOUR)

The calcifying epithelial odontogenic tumour—also known as Pindborg tumour or calcifying epithelial tumour—was first recognised by the Dutch pathologist Jens Jerger Pindborg in 1955. Calcifying odontogenic tumour (CEOT) is a rare benign odontogenic neoplasm, forming only 3-4% of all intraosseous odontogenic tumour.

It is a odontogenic tumour and thought to arise from the epithelial element of enamel origin. But the exact part from which it originates is not known. However, it has been postulated that it may arise from either the external enamel, stratum intermedium of the enamel organ or from the cellular remnants of the basal sheet or basal stratum of gingival epithelium.

Clinical features

The age range is wide—8-92 years—although it is most commonly seen in the fourth and fifth decades of life. Intraosseous tumours are more likely 94% versus extraosseous tumours 6%. Introsseous

CEOT shows a maxilla-to-mandible site ratio of 1 : 2 and is mainly located in mandibular premolar/molar area associated with embedded tooth. Clinically, it has two types, the central and peripheral. In few cases it is located peripherally in gingival. It is a typically slow-growing, but invasive, neoplasm. There is no sex predilection.

Clinically, it presents as a slowly growing expansile jaw lesion, which may be associated with pain, nasal obstruction, epistaxis, and headache. Maxillary tumours may be present with facial alteration.

Painless swellings—often along with an unerupted tooth—are the common presentation. They behave like ameloblastomas, tending to be invasive and recur locally after removal, but they do not metastasise.

Microscopically

It is composed of strands and buds of polyhedral epithelial cells embedded in a cellular connective tissue stroma. This tumour forms an amorphous material that is said to be amyloid or amyloid-like material, it calcifies in a concentrically lamellated tree-ring pattern, known as **Leisegang** calcifications. There is frequently polymorphism.

Immunohistochemical studies with antibodies against basement membrane proteins (laminin 1 and 5) fibronectin, cytokeratins and vimentin.

Radiographic findings

These lesions can be radiolucent, but they are more characteristically mixed lucent and opaque masses, exhibiting a 'snow-driven' appearance. Small intramural calcification starts appearing in the second phase, which is characteristic but not diagnostic. The final stages are associated with osseous destruction and tumoral calcification giving a honeycomb appearance. In intraosseous lesions they are large and generally multilobulated, and can simulate ameloblastoma radiologically.

Treatment

Treatment of this lesion is complete surgical excision varying from simple enucleation to partial resection of the affected bone. The tumour can be locally aggressive, but malignant transformation and metastasis is rare. The local recurrence rate is 10-15%.

SQUAMOUS ODONTOGENIC TUMOUR

Squamous odontogenic tumour is a hamartomatous proliferation of odontogenic epithelium, probably arising from the rests of Malassez.

The maxillary incisor-canine area and mandibular molar area are most commonly involved.

Clinical features

It is a benign tumour having predilection for posterior mandible and anterior maxilla. Males are more commonly affected than females (M : F ratio 1.4 : 1). Age range is 8-74 years with a mean age of 38.7 years. Most cases are unifocal and tooth mobility is the usual chief complaint. Local pain, swelling of the gingival, osseous expansion or mild gingival erythema may be observed.

Microscopically

It is composed of nests and islands of a well-differentiated squamous epithelium, surrounded by collagenous stroma. Part of the tumour may show the characteristic ameloblast-like cells, which resemble stellate epithelium. Individual tumour islands reveal a peripheral layer of low cuboidal or flat epithelial cells. Epithelial islands may undergo microcystic degeneration. Recurrences are rare and probably due to incomplete removal.

Radiologically

It is well-circumscribed, semicircular, radiolucent, and surrounded by a sclerotic border. Extensive squamous odontogenic tumours may present as multilocular pattern. The peripheral variant may produce some 'saucerization' of the underlying bone—a result of pressure from tumour expansion rather than neoplastic infiltration.

Treatment

Complete excision of the tumour is necessary to prevent recurrence.

AMELOBLASTIC FIBROMA

This is a tumour of childhood; the typical patient is about 12-14 years old, seldom beyond age 20. The posterior segment of the mandible is the most common location.

Microscopically

It is composed of a diffused mass of embryonic mesenchyme, which is traversed by elongated cords of cuboidal or columnar odontogenic epithelial cells that resemble the dental lamina. These cords terminate in bulbous projections that contain a central stellate reticulum.

In the larger islands, peripheral palisading of columnar cells with reverse nuclear polarity may be seen. The tissue surrounding the epithelium is cellular connective tissue that bears some resemblance to dental pulp.

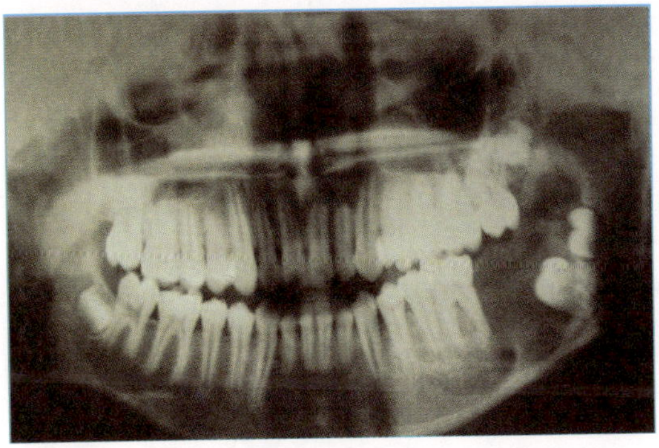

Fig.23.3: X-ray of jaw from a case of ameloblastic fibroma showing unerupted teeth

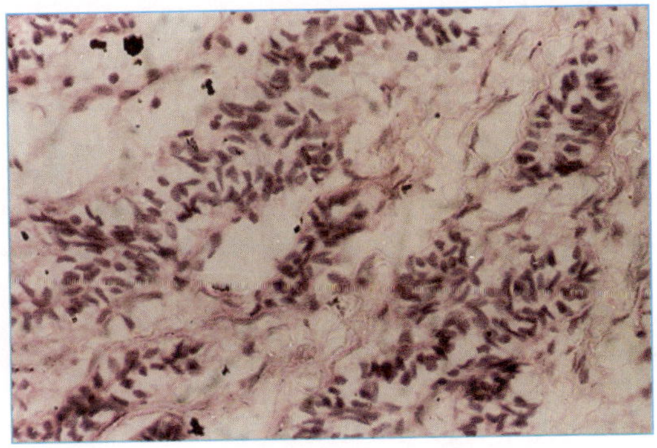

Fig.23.4: Histological picture from a case of ameloblastic fibroma showing strands of odontogenic epithelium lying in loose fibrous stroma

Radiographic findings

This lesion appears as a unilocular or binocular radiolucency, most often in the posterior mandible.

Proliferating cell nuclear antigen (PCNA) and MIB-1 are recently recognised proteins that bear a relationship with the cell proliferation.

AMELOBLASTIC FIBRO-ODONTOMA

Ameloblastic fibro-odontoma is a relatively rare, slow-growing expansile epithelial odontogenic mesenchyme. The incidence of ameloblastic fibro-odontoma is between 1 to 3% of odontogenic tumour.

Clinical features

It may inhibit tooth eruption or displace involved teeth, although the teeth in the affected area are vital, occurs with equal frequency in the maxilla and mandible, its usual location is in the posterior pre-molar-molar region.

Average at diagnosis is nine year old, only one reported case in a patient beyond the age of 20 year old.

Fibro-odontoma, involving canine area of maxilla, was reported in one-year-old child.

Microscopically

Histological examination reveals a fibrous soft tissue, islands of odontogenic epithelium and a disordered mixture of dental tissues. The tumour produces enamel or enamel matrix, dentin, and cementum.

X-ray findings

Ameloblastic fibro-odontoma appears as a well-demarcated radiolucency with a large central opacity. These lesions are always found in association with a tooth.

Treatment

The treatment of ameloblastic fibro-odontomas usually consists of enucleation or surgical curettage, which is possible due to their benign biological behaviour. The lesion does not often recur. Medical literature contains some support for sarcomatous change with recurrence.

ODONTOGENIC MYXOMA

Odontogenic myxoma is a locally aggressive tumour, only occurring in the jaw. It is commonly associated with an unerupted or congenitally missing tooth. Myxomas are seen equally in the maxilla and mandible.

The tumour is believed to originate from the dental papilla or follicular mesenchyme. Root resorption and displacement may be seen in some cases.

Clinical features

Odontogenic myxomas are asymptomatic and are found when a cause for loose teeth malocclusion secondary to tooth migration, or unerupted teeth, is investigated.

Odontogenic myxoma is a tumour that occurs over a wide age range but is more common in the second and third decades of life. It is rare in over 50-year old age groups. There is no gender preference for this lesion.

Microscopic appearance

Microscopically, spindle and stellate fibroblasts are associated with basophilic ground substance and myxomatous tissue.

Radiographically, the tumour appears as unilocular or multilocular lucency, often with honeycombing and may have scalloped appearance. The margins may be well-defined or diffuse. These lesions may be extensive and involve expansion of a condyle, an entire ramus, or, perhaps, half of the mandible or maxilla.

MELANOTIC NEUROECTODERMAL TUMOUR OF INFANCY

Synonyms: Melanoameloblastoma, congenital melanocarcinoma, melanotic epithelial odontoma, melanotic progonoma, and retinal analage tumour.

In 1918, Kropechar reported first case in a 2-month-old child in the maxilla. The tumour constitutes about 0.7% of all odontogenic tumours of the jaws. The tumour arises from neuroectoderm, the precursor of the retina, or it is odontogenic.

Clinical features

They are commonly seen in maxilla, however, they may occur in mandible, skull, mediastinum, soft tissues of thigh, forearm and cheek. The tumour is more common in females.

Melanotic neuroectodermal tumour of infancy appears as soft or hard and rapidly growing pigmented swellings, which are blue or black in colour. They may destroy the underlying bone and may be associated with displacement of developing teeth. The tumour ranges from 1.0 to 10.0 cm.

Melanotic neuroectodermal tumour of infancy may rarely be associated with elevated levels of α-fetoprotein. High levels of vanillymandelic acid (VMA) often are found in patients with melanotic neuroectodermal tumour of infancy.

Microscopically

Tumour consists of numerous tubules of varying sizes in a fibrovascular stroma. The tubules are lined by cuboidal to flattened cells with abundant intracytoplasmic melanin pigment, the lumina of the tubules contain groups of dark staining neuroblast-like cells with scanty cytoplasm. In some of the tubules, these cells are enmeshed in fibrillary matrix. There are presence of clusters of round, small basophilic cells, which have round hyperchromatic nuclei and a scanty rim of cytoplasm.

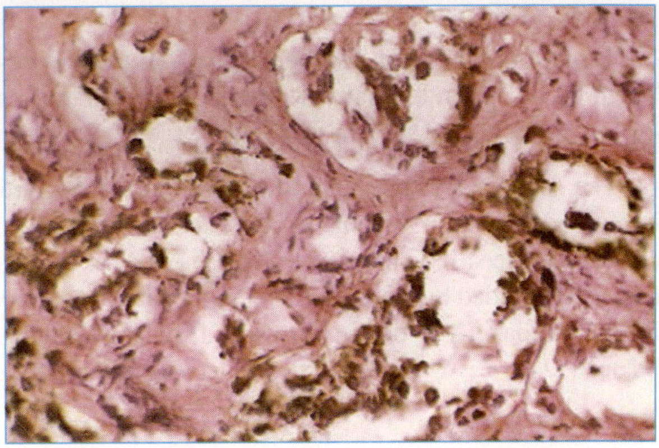

Fig.23.5: Microphotograph showing pigmented melanotic cells arranged in adenomatous pattern and small basophilic cells. (Neuroectodermal tumour of infancy)

Immunohistochemistry: The small darkly staining cells comprising the first population stain positively for synaptophysin, showing them to be neuroblasts and large epitheloid cells comprising of the second population stain positively with the antibodies HMB-45 (melanoma associated antigen) and NKI-Beteb, showing them to be melanocytes. They are less reactive for vimentin and neuron specific enolase (NSE).

Radiological findings

In some instances, there may be associated osteogenic reaction, which exhibits a 'sunray' radiographic pattern that can be mistaken for osteogenic sarcoma.

Differential diagnosis

Primary malignant melanoma: It is especially mucosal and rare in this age group.

Neuroblastomas are rarely pigmented, but usually show diffused reactivity for neuroendocrine markers.

Treatment

Malignant transformation has been reported to be rare. Because of its locally aggressive behaviour the melanotic neuroectodermal tumour of infancy is treated by wide surgical excision. When bone is involved, 0.5 cm margin of radiographically normal bone should also be involved.

ODONTOMA

Odontoma may develop from the enamel organ or the dental lamina, either in place of a normal tooth or a supernumerary lamina, or even in association with the follicle of an unerupted tooth.

COMPOUND ODONTOMA

Compound odontoma is more common in the anterior jaw segment.

Etiology

Though exact etiology of odontoma formation is unknown, a number of factors including prior trauma, genetic factors and infection seem to be involved.

Clinical features

Odontoma compound type are painless, slowly-growing lesions. When fully-matured, development ceases. The size varies from 1 to 2 cm in diameter, up to 6 cm has been reported.

Macroscopically

Tumour consists of a number of tooth-like structures enclosed in a fibrous capsule, which is thin. Teeth do not resemble normal teeth but are usually cone shaped.

Microscopically

The section shows both a tooth-like and haphazard arrangement of dental hard and soft tissue including cementum, dentin, enamel matrix, pulp and periodontal tissue. Reduced enamel epithelium can also be seen in some areas. There is normal arrangement of centrally placed fibrovascular pulp tissue surrounded by dentin with an outer surface covered by enamel in the crown area and cementum in the root part. The dentin is mainly tubular in type but extensive areas of atubular dentin can also be seen. There is no inflammation or evidence of malignancy.

Radiological features

Multiple tiny teeth-like structures are contained within a fine radiolucent rim give a characteristic 'bag of marbles' radiographic appearance.

COMPLEX ODONTOMA

Complex odontomas appear as an amorphous and disorderly pattern of calcified dental tissues.

Complex odontoma is more commonly in posterior jaws. It is more frequent in molar areas of mandibular premolar-molar area than in maxilla.

The etiology is unknown but there is some evidence in favour of a genetic basis for odontomas.

Clinical features

Complex odontomas most commonly occur in the second to third decades of life but have been known to occur at any age. There is no sex predilection.

Complex odontomas are usually small, produce few clinical sign and symptoms, and are usually discovered on routine dental radiographs. They could be suspected because of failure of a tooth to erupt. When they occur in the maxilla they tend to push the antrum upwards and bulge into antral cavity. Occasionally, they may expand and thin out cortical bone, resulting in facial asymmetry.

Complex odontomas may reveal their existence by disturbances in tooth eruption, missing teeth or jaw expansion.

Radiological findings

These lesions are generally described as sunburst radiopacities surrounded by a thin, uniform, radiolucent rim.

Treatment consists of conservative removal. Recurrences are not seen.

CEMENTOBLASTOMA

Cementoblastoma is a rare lesion first described by Norberg in 1930.

Cementoblastoma is a rare odontogenic tumour of mesenchymal origin. The benign cementoblastoma or true cementoma is a slowly-growing benign odontogenic tumour arising from cementoblasts. It accounts for less than 1 % of all odontogenic tumours.

Clinical features

Cementoblastoma usually occurs in people under the age of 25, often involving mandibular molars or premolars. The male-to-female ratio of prevalence of benign cementoblastoma has been reported to be 2.1 : 1, with a mean age of 20.7 years. The involved tooth usually has a vital pulp. Most patients initially present with mild pain and bony swelling in the area of the lesion. The pain and swelling is due to bony expansion of the buccal and lingual aspects of the alveolar ridges.

This tumour typically occurs around the roots of the lower posterior teeth.

Macroscopically

Cementoblastoma is round to ovoid, well-circumscribed mass of hard, calcified tan-coloured tissue surrounding the root of the affected tooth.

Microscopic appearance

The tumour consists of radially oriented trabeculae from the attached root cementum with a rim of osteoblasts and fibrous marrow is apparent. The cementum displays prominent basophilic reversal lines and cementoblastic rimming. The cementoblasts were plump with moderate amounts of cytoplasm, hyperchromatic nuclei, and conspicuous nucleoli. The intervening stroma consisted of loose fibrovascular tissue with scattered multinucleated osteoclast-like giant cells at the periphery of the lesion.

Radiological features

A cementoblastoma in a radiograph appears as a well-defined, markedly radiopaque mass, with a radiolucent '*peripheral line*' which overlies and obliterates the tooth. There is usually external resorption of the root where the tumour and the root join.

Differential diagnosis

Osteoclastoma: Osteoclastomas arises in the medullary cavity of many bones including the long bones, vertebrae and jaws, whereas cementoblastoma are in intimate association with a tooth root.

Odontome: The odontome is usually not fused to the adjacent tooth and appears as a more heterogeneous radioopacity, reflecting the presence of multiple hard tissues.

Peripheral cemental dysplasia: It usually produces a smaller lesion than cementoblastoma and shows a progressive change in radiographic appearance. Over time-change from radiolucent to mixed radiopaque.

Treatment

Treatment of cementoblastoma consists of surgical extraction of the tooth together with the attached calcified mass. Surgical excision of the mass with root amputation and endodontic treatment of the involved tooth may be considered.

MALIGNANT TUMOURS

MALIGNANT AMELOBLASTOMA

AMELOBLASTIC CARCINOMA

Odontogenic carcinomas that can emanate from any of four sources:

a. De novo from remnants of odontogenic epithelium—that is, primary intraosseous carcinoma.

b. Malignant variants of other odontogenic tumours.

c. Malignant transformation of preexisting ameloblastoma.

d. Malignant conversion of epithelial lining of osteogenic cysts.

Clinical features

The tumour more frequently involves the mandible and presents as a painful rapidly growing swelling. The tumour usually perforates the cortical plates of jaws and presents intraorally as ulcerated exophytic mass. Root resorption is common.

Metastasis to regional lymph nodes, lungs, and other sites has been documented.

Microscopically

The tumour shows irregular masses of and interdigitating cords of epithelial cells with palisading around the periphery of the epithelial islands. The tissue in the centre of the cellular islands is composed of stellate reticulum. Other areas show islands of keratinising well-differentiated carcinoma infiltrating the adjacent bone.

Radiologically

It presents as an ill-defined radiolucency.

Management

Surgery is mainstay of treatment for ameloblastic carcinomas. The optimal treatment for ameloblastic carcinomas is resection with wide margins.

PRIMARY INTRAOSSEOUS CARCINOMA

Primary intraosseous carcinoma is an uncommon neoplasm. It was first described by Loos in 1913, and named intra-alveolar epidermoid carcinoma by Willis in 1948. The term intraosseous carcinoma (PIOC) was suggested by Pindborg et al in 1972. According to World Health Organization (WHO) classification, PIOC is an odontogenic carcinoma defined as squamous cell carcinoma arising within the jaw, having no initial connection with the oral mucosa.

Origin: These tumours are thought to originate from residues of the odontogenic epithelium and known as odontogenic carcinomas. There are two possible pathogenesis origins: either by malignant transformation of the epithelial lining of the odontogenic cysts or the remnants of odontogenic tissue.

Clinical features

Primary intraosseous carcinoma occurs only in the jaw bones and predominantly in the posterior mandible (90%). It affects men more than women with the ratio about 1.2 : 1, and mostly in the elderly patients aged above sixty. Symptoms are non-specific while pain swelling and sensory disturbances presented in most of the patients. There is no ulceration of oral mucosa, except when caused by other factors, such as trauma or tooth extraction. Unexplained loosening of teeth occurs. The tumour may metastasise to regional lymph nodes as well as lungs.

Radiologically

It appears as a non-specific osteolytic lesion generally with diffuse irregular or ill-defined margins. Root resorption is seen only in few cases.

Microscopically

Microscopically, intraosseous carcinoma shows sheets and islands of neoplastic epithelium manifesting the cardinal signs of malignancy—hyperchromatism, pleomorphism and mitoses. Most lesions are moderately differentiated without prominent keratinisation. The stroma may or may not exhibit an inflammatory infiltrate.

There is cytological atypia, increased cellularity and diminution or absence of epithelial component. Expansion or cortical perforation is encountered.

Management

Radical surgery with/without post-operative radiotherapy is recommended for management of de novo primary intraosseous carcinoma. Other modalities such as radiotherapy or chemotherapy, should be considered only for lesions that cannot be surgically controlled.

CLEAR CELL ODONTOGENIC TUMOUR OR CARCINOMA

In 1945, Hansen et al reported a locally aggressive odontogenic neoplasm, and named it clear cell odontogenic carcinoma.

Clinical features

Clear cell odontogenic carcinoma is a rare odontogenic tumour occurring in the anterior region of the mandible in 5th-7th decades of life and shows a female preponderance. It is potentially aggressive, uncapsulated and metastases are found in lymph nodes as well as in the lungs and skeleton.

Microscopically

Microscopic examination of tissue shows a neoplasm composed of epithelial cells arranged in irregular nests separated by fibrovascular septa. The cells adjacent to the fibrovascular septa are cuboidal to columnar with high nuclear-cytoplasmic ratio and eosinophilic cytoplasm, while those in the centre of the nests are larger and polygonal, with abundant clear cytoplasm. Each cell had a single nucleus and prominent eosinophilic nucleolus. The cells at the periphery of the nests occasionally demonstrate nuclear palisading away from the basement membrane, e.g., reverse nuclear polarity. These peripheral cells also show occasional mitoses. The central areas of the nests and fibrous septae showed infiltration by neutrophils.

Immunohistochemistry: The cells are immunoreactive for pan-cytokeratin, epithelial membrane antigen, and S-100 protein; they did not stain for vimentin, smooth muscle actin, and HMB-45.

AMELOBLASTIC FIBROSARCOMA

It is also known as odontogenic carcinosarcoma.

Ameloblastic fibrosarcoma an odontogenic tumour that is the malignant counterpart of an ameloblastic fibroma, within which it usually arises. The tumour can occur de novo but can be associated with recurrent ameloblastic fibroma or ameloblastic fibroodontoma.

Clinical features

Approximately 80% of cases occur in mandible predominantly posterior segment, 60% occur in men.

Pain and swelling are most common symptoms, in with most other odontogenic tumours. Ulceration, bleeding and paresthesia may be additional local findings.

Death follows after extensive local recurrence and extension.

Macroscopically

Surface of the bone is destructed. The cut surface is pinkish grey with central small areas of bleeding and cystic degeneration.

Microscopically

There are numerous islands and cords of odontogenic epithelium, often resembling the dental lamina of early tooth development. The islands are lined with cuboidal cells intermingled with keratinised epidermoid cells. A few islands had central cystic degeneration. The mesenchymal component mainly consists of myxomatous tissue very poor in intercellular collagenous matrixial elements. The mesenchymal cells have round or ovoid pale-staining nuclei. Besides all these features resembling a typical ameloblastic fibroma, in a few cases there is cytological atypia, increased cellularity and diminution or absence of epithelial component.

Immunohistochemically, the sarcomatous mesenchymal component of ameloblastic fibrosarcoma is positive to K167, PCNA, and TP53, in front of the negativity of ameloblastic fibroma.

Radiologically

Varying radiographic patterns can be seen that include destructive/permeative, uniocular, or multilocular.

Management

Ameloblastic fibrosarcomas are aggressive and commonly recur after curettage, therefore en bloc resection is recommended for these tumours.

ODONTOGENIC FIBROSARCOMA

First documented case of odontogenic fibrosarcoma was reported by Thoma in 1940.

Odontogenic fibrosarcoma is a malignant tumour of jaws that develops in a mesenchymal component of a tooth or tooth germ.

Clinical features

Pain and swelling are two most common clinical symptoms of this neoplasm.

Histopathological features

Microscopically, the tumour shows an intense proliferation of spindle shaped-cells, varying little in size and shape and arranged in parallel bands, partly crossing each other, the mitotic activity is increased and there is nuclear pleomorphism. Islands of odontogenic epithelium with a surrounding malignant mesenchymal proliferation are seen.

Immunohistochemically, the cells only showed immunoreactivity for vimentin and alpha smooth muscle actin.

Radiologically

A large radiolucent lesion with ill-defined margins.

Management

Treatment of choice is radical surgery with mandibular reconstruction. Radiation therapy and chemotherapy can be used as adjuvant treatment.

Bibliography

Aoron R, Huber and Gretchen S Folk: Cementoblastoma Head and neck Patholo. 2009 June; 3 (2) 133-135

Eversole LR, Leiden AS, Hansen LS: Ameloblastoma with pronounced desmoplasia. J Oral Maxillofac Surgery: 42 (11): 135-40. 1984.

Hansen LS, Eversole LR, Green TL, Powell NB: clear cell odontogenic tumour—a new histologic variant with aggressive potential. Head and neck Surgery1985, 8 115-123.

Kramer JR, Pindborg JJ, Shear M: Histological typing of odontogenic tumours, cysts, and allied lesions. In: International histological classification of tumours. Geneva; World Health organization: 1992 p. 23-40

Sharmana Mandal, Kachnar Varma, Nita Khurana, Mandal AK: Calcifying epithelial odontogenic tumour: Report of a two cases. Indian Journal of Pathology and Microbiology—51(3) 2008 397-398.

CHAPTER

24

CYTOLOGY

INTRODUCTION

Definition: Cytology is the scientific study of the morphology of cells.

Exfoliative cytology

Exfoliative cytology can be powerful tool for early detection of malignant and premalignant lesions as well as for some viral and fungal lesions of oral cavity.

Advantages

1. Simplicity of procedure.
2. Material can be collected without surgical operation.
3. Results are available in few hours.
4. It is inexpensive, non-invasive and least disturbing to the biology of the lesion.

Disadvantages

1. Since it depends upon 'Nature' for desquamation of abnormal cells from the lesion the chance of getting a positive finding is less than that of a surgical biopsy or an interventional cytology.
2. Sometimes it is not possible to ascertain the specific area/organ from which the abnormal cells have come.

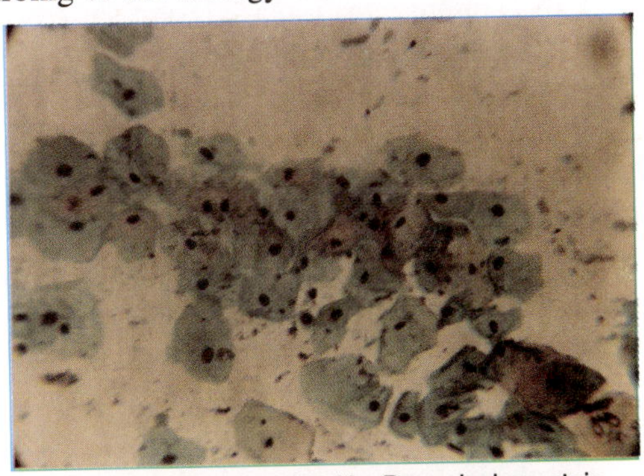

Fig.24.1: Smear stained by Papanicolaou stain shows superficial epithelial cells

Superficial cell: Superficial cells in the smear occur usually singly, polyhedral in shape, translucent cytoplasm usually acidophilic (yellow to orange to pale pink to blue). The nucleus is pyknotic, stains uniformly dark without a recognisable structure.

Intermediate cells: The size of intermediate cells varies from 30-60 μm depending on the degree of maturation; those from the lower rows are smaller in size and stain bluish-green, whereas those nearer the surface are larger and may take up the eosinophilic stain.

Parabasal cells: Small round or oval cells with opaque usually basophilic vacuolated cytoplasm, 15 to 30 μm in diameter with a large vesicular nucleus, which is similar in size to the nucleus of an intermediate cells.

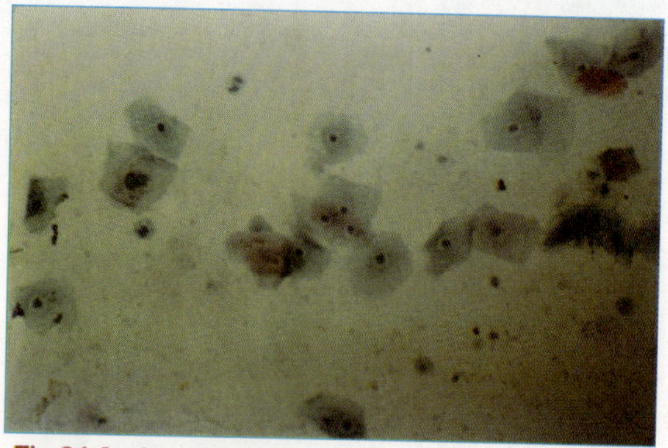

Fig.24.2: Shows intermediate cells in the smear stained by Papanicolaou stain

Basal cells: Basal cells are smallest cells (10-12 μm diameter) of squamous epithelium and are round or oval. Cytoplasm is scanty, stain dark to deep blue with Papanicolaou stain.

Role of exfoliative cytology in diagnosis of oral cancer

1. For screening large areas of abnormal appearing mucosa , in order to choose the site for a biopsy in an area from which the most suspicious cells are found.
2. As a preliminary investigation for oral cancer in a patient too nervous to allow biopsy.
3. For preliminary investigation of lesions forming on the site of a treated cancer, to exclude a recurrence or a new primary.

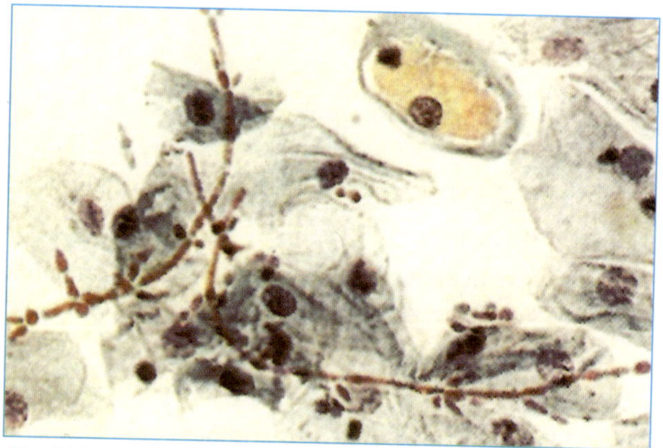

Fig.24.3: Candidiasis with budding yeast cells and pseudohyphae

CIN I (Mild dysplasia): The cells have plentiful clear cytoplasm translucent cytoplasm with well -defined borders. Cells resembled superficial and intermediate squamous cells having enlarged nucleus, high N : C ratio and finely granular, evenly distributed slightly hyperchromatic nuclear chromatin.

CIN II (moderate dysplasia) Cytology from CIN II: lesions revealed round to polygonal cells having cyanophilic cytoplasm, distinct cell borders, enlarged nucleus and high nuclear cytoplasmic ratio. Nuclear chromatin was coarsely granular and evenly distributed.

Lesions revealed round to polygonal cells having cyanophilic cytoplasm, distinct cell borders, enlarged nucleus and high nuclear cytoplasmic ratio. Nuclear chromatin was coarsely granular and evenly distributed.

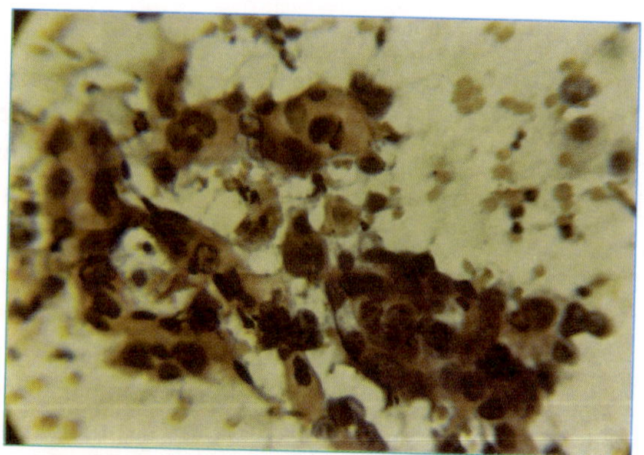

Fig.24.4: Shows features of moderate dysplasia

Cytological smear from keratinising squamous cell carcinoma shows loosely cohesive

and singly lying cells having marked anisocytosis, moderate to abundant amount of dense waxy cytoplasm, pleomorphic hyperchromatic nuclei and coarsely granular unevenly distributed chromatin. Bizarre cells are also seen.

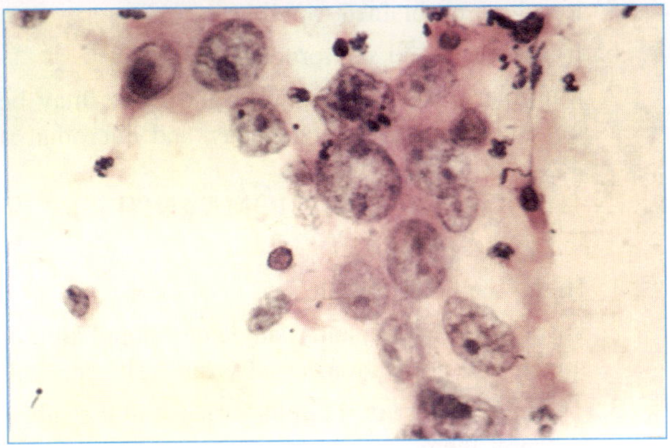

Fig.24.5: Shows smear from malignant squamous cells with hyperchromatic nuclei, macronucleolus and mitosis

Fine needle aspiration cytology is a simple, rapid, and minimally invasive technique of obtaining cells for diagnosis, with an accuracy more than 90%, by using 23 or 24 gauze needles attached to 20 ml disposable plastic syringe. The main purpose of FNAC is to confirm malignancy preoperatively and to avoid unnecessary surgery in specific benign conditions. Even though specific diagnosis may not be possible in all cases, FNAC provides valuable information for making a proper therapeutic decision. However, it requires considerable experience and skill before expertise is achieved. The aspirated material can also be used for immunohistochemistry and cytogenetic studies.

Technique

1. The patient was examined with review of clinical history. Utility of FNAC and its procedure should be explained to the patients.
2. Skin over the site is thoroughly cleaned with spirit. No local anesthesia is used.
3. A 23 or 24 gauge needle attached to a 10 cc disposable plastic syringe is introduced into the lesion with the plunger in the resting state. Then, the plunger of the syringe is retracted maximally, thus creating vacuum in the system. The needle is then moved back and forth in different directions under constant suction to detach the tissue fragments.
4. When the aspiration is complete, the plunger is released to eliminate the vacuum in order to reach pressure equilibrium in the system. Only then the needle is withdrawn from the lesion, thus avoiding aspiration of the material into the syringe.
5. The contents of the needle are carefully expelled on to the glass slides. After that the syringe is disconnected from the needle, filled with air, and reconnected. The needle content is then blown out on the slide by pushing down the plunger, as the needle top touches the glass.
6. If the specimen is semisolid droplet, it is gently squeezed with other slide by exerting slight pressure. If the aspirate is fluid from a cystic lesion, as much of the fluid as possible is aspirated and spread directly or after centrifugation.
7. Smears were immediately fixed in 95% ethanol for Haematoxylin and Eosin staining.

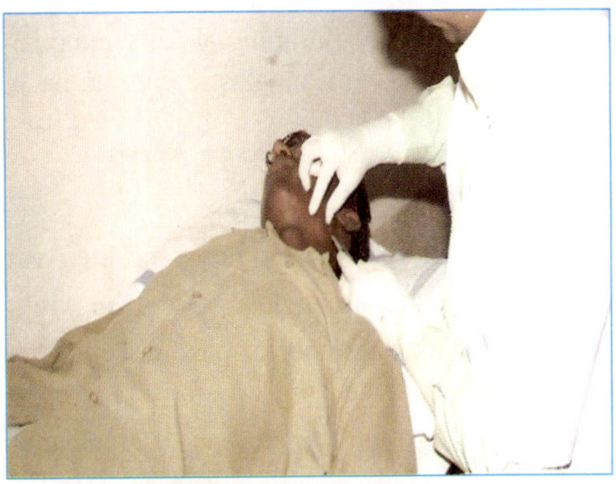

Fig.24.6: Procedure for fine needle aspiration from swelling salivary gland

Advantages of FNAC over biopsy

1. It is a non-invasive simple procedure that can be performed on any swelling or localised lesion.
2. It is OPD procedure, no hospitalisation and anesthesia required.
3. Less traumatic than usual knife biopsy.

4. Low cost procedure which is cost effective.
5. Results are obtained rapidly.
6. It is a cheap and safe procedure.
7. Multiple passes can be made and tissue may be obtained even for special studies such as immunochemistry, cytogenetics, and microbial studies.

NON-HODGKIN'S LYMPHOMA (NHL)

General features of NHL

1. Highly cellular aspirate.
2. Display a predominantly single cell population of discretely arranged cells. Even in cases of mixed cell population, usually one cell type will predominate.
3. The morphology of the cells varies with the subtype and requires great experience to correctly interpret them.
4. Based on the size and nuclear characteristics, it can be further classified into small, large, or mixed small and large cell types; anaplastic large cell (Ki-1) and, to some extent, lymphoblastic and immunoblastic.
5. Presence of small cytoplasmic fragments called lymphoglandular bodies indicates lymphoid origin of the neoplasm.

MALIGNANT LYMPHOMA—SMALL CELL TYPE

A monotonus population of small cells resembling small lymphocytes with round nuclei characterises it. The cells are slightly larger (1.5-2 times the size of a small lymphocyte) and the chromatin paler and more granular with varying degrees of clumping.

LARGE B-CELL TYPE

This high-grade lymphoma is characterised by

1. A monotonus population of large cells with the nucleus 3-4 times the size of normal small lymphocytes.
2. Large hyperchromatic or vesicular nuclei with large and multiple nucleoli. The nucleus may be cleaved or non-cleaved.
3. Varying amounts of cytoplasm from rim to moderate.
4. The cells are usually seen discretely with minimal overlap.
5. Occasionally clumping of cells and phagocytosis of malignant cells by macrophages may cause confusion with anaplastic carcinoma.

HODGKIN'S LYMPHOMA (HL)

Characteristic features

1. Reed-Sternberg (RS) cells and their variants.
2. Atypical mononuclear cells–Hodgkin's cells.
3. A variable number of plasma cells, eosinophils, neutrophils, and histiocytes often epitheloid in appearance.
4. A background population of small mature lymphocytes.
5. Occasionally resetting of the neoplastic cells by T cells is seen and, if present, it is very characteristic.

SALIVARY GLAND

Mixed tumour of salivary glands: This is the commonest tumour of the major salivary glands. It has characteristic cytological features and can be diagnosed easily by FNAC.

Aspirate is characterised by

1. A mixture of epithelial and mesenchymal elements.
2. Epithelial cells which are small and uniform with round or oval eccentric nuclei with bland chromatin and moderate amount of granular densely staining cytoplasm, arranged in cohesive sheets, branching cords, ductal structures or singly.
3. Fibrillary chondromyxoid matrix staining bright red or purple with Giemsa stain and grey or greenish-blue with pap stain.
4. Spindle-shaped mesenchymal cells seen in stromal matrix.

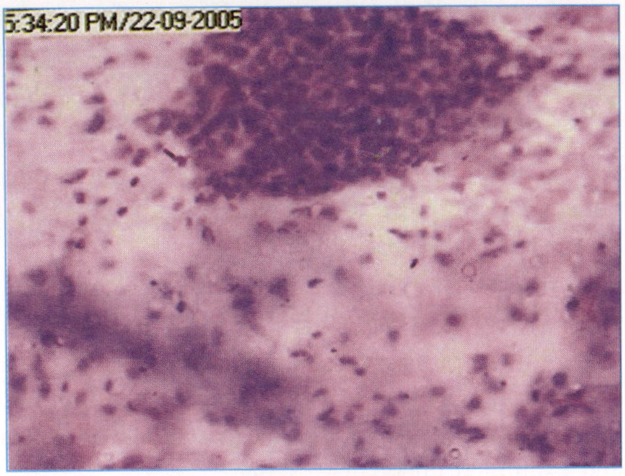

Fig.24.7: Cytological smear showing sheets of acinic cell and abundant mucin (Pleomorphic adenoma)

WARTHIN'S TUMOUR

Characteristic features

1. Oncocytic cells in cohesive monolayered sheets with irregular outline. These cells have abundant pink granular cytoplasm in pap stained smears. The nuclei are central, small, round, and irregular with blunt chromatin and small inconspicuous nuclei.
2. Many lymphoid cells in the background.
3. Amorphous or granular debris representing cyst contents.

ONCOCYTOMA

The characteristic features are oncocytic cells with small, regular nuclei arranged in cohesive, multilayered clumps with absence of debris and lymphoid cells in the background.

ACINIC CELL CARCINOMA

Diagnostic features

1. Cellular aspirate in a clean background.
2. Cohesive clusters of cells often with central fibrovascular core. The cells have abundant finely vacuolated or dense oncocyte-like cytoplasm and mildly pleomorphic medium-sized nuclei.
3. Scattered bare nuclei resembling lymphocytes are seen amongst the cells.

ADENOID CYSTIC CARCINOMA

Diagnostic features

1. Close packed cohesive cells with hyperchromatic, uniform, round or oval nuclei, coarse nuclear chromatin, small nucleoli and scanty cytoplasm.
2. Hyaline spherical globules of varying size (basement membrane material) surrounded by tumour cells most distinctive features of the neoplasm. In Pap-stained smears these are pale and translucent and in Giemsa stain these appear red and purple and dense.
3. Rounded or finger-like stromal structures may be seen between cell clusters.

MUCOEPIDERMOID TUMOURS

This neoplasm is one of the most difficult to diagnose cytologically.

Diagnostic features of low-grade mucoepidermoid tumours

1. Cohesive sheets and clump of cells in a dirty background of mucus and debris. Small streams of cells are seen within mucus also. Coexistence of cells with squamous and glandular differentiation helps in a definite diagnosis.

Variation in cell types: Squamous, intermediate and mucin secreting. Most of the cells have abundant cytoplasm, some having vacuolated or foamy appearance. The cells have regular nuclei and prominent nucleoli in some cells.

IMPRINT CYTOLOGY

In this form of cytology, tissue is collected by surgical resection, cut by a sharp knife to have an even surface, which is then pressed on an albuminised slide or dry slide to obtain an impression of the cut surface of the tissue on the slide. The smear is fixed or air-dried, stained by a suitable stain and examined under microscope.

Advantages of imprint cytology

1. It is extremely useful in the typing of lymphomas, as nuclear details with grooves etc. are well-seen on imprint smears which are air-dried and stained with Rominowsky's stains.
2. As a supplement to a biopsy—particularly small endoscopic biopsy.
3. As a supplement of frozen section.

Bibliography

Atkinson/Silverman: 1998 Atlas of difficult diagnosis in Cytopathology: Saunders

Bizjak-Schwarzbartl M: Cytomorphologic characteristics of non-Hodgkin's lymphoma. Acta Cytol 32:216, 1988

Cohen MB, Reznicek MJ, and Miller TR: Fine needle aspiration cytology of salivary glands. Pathology Annual 27:213, 1992

Masayoshi Takahashi: 2000: Colour atlas of cancer cytology: 3rd edition, Ikaku-Shon Tokyo.

CHAPTER

25

SPREAD OF ORAL INFECTION

INTRODUCTION

A major portion of human diseases—especially in the tropical and underdeveloped countries—are caused by biological infective agents, namely, bacteria, fungi, viruses and parasites.

FACTORS RELATING TO INFECTIOUS AGENTS

A. MODES OF ENTRY. Pathogenic organisms can spread from one host to another by a variety of mechanisms. These include:

1. **Inhalation, (Respiration)** dust and droplets, e.g., influenza, tuberculosis, measles, and mumps.
2. **Ingestion:** Contaminated food and water, e.g., enteric fever, hepatitis A, poliomyelitis, cholera, parasitic infestations.
3. **Contact, (contagious):** The organisms enter inside the body by direct close contact, e.g., venereal diseases, syphilis, gonorrhoea, infectious mononucleosis and AIDS.
4. **Inoculation:** e.g., insect bite—yellow fever and malaria. Infected needles- hepatitis B and C, AIDS, soil—tetanus.
5. Contamination of wounds and abrasions e.g., wound infection and rabies.
6. **Iatrogenic and laboratory infections:** Infection may be transmitted during procedures like injections, lumbar punctures, catheterisation and in laboratory technicians if proper care is not taken.
7. **Congenital (perinatal):** Congenital syphilis, rubella, Listeria monocytogens, toxoplasma, cytomegalic inclusion disease, AIDS, hepatitis, and herpes.
8. **Animals (Zoonotic infections):** The organisms are transmitted from animals to human beings e.g., rabies, mad cow disease, hydatid cyst.

B. Virulence of organisms, for example different strains of E. coli cause several distinct gastrointestinal diseases, urinary tract infections, septicemia, meningitis and a range of other minor infections.

C. Production of toxins: These are the substances produced by or present in bacteria, which have a direct toxic action on tissue cells.

D. Product of organisms

E. Spread of infection can be by several routes. Once an infective organism has gained entry to the body, it seldom remains localised but spreads to other tissues via several possible routes:

1. **Local spread.**
2. **Lymphatic spread:** Microorganisms are often carried in the lymph to the regional lymph nodes.
3. **Haematogenous spread:** Microorganisms can be carried in the blood, and, because of their small size, circulate throughout the body.
4. **Spread in tissue fluid:** Widespread peritonitis can result from the rupture of an appendiceal abscess, which releases great numbers of bacteria into the peritoneal cavity.
5. **Neural spread:** The rabies virus and the varicella zoster virus produce infection by travelling along nerves.

Oral microflora

Oral cavity is the sites of many infectious and inflammatory diseases, which has recently been associated with systemic diseases such as diabetes, cardiovascular disease, bacterial pneumonia and preterm low births. Three mechanisms or pathways linking oral infections to secondary systemic effects have been proposed.

(i) Metastatic spread of infection from the oral cavity as a result of transient bacteraemia.
(ii) Metastatic injury from the effect of circulating microbial toxins.
(iii) Metastatic inflammation caused by immunological injury induced by oral microorganisms.

CELLULITIS

Cellulitis is a bacterial infection of the deeper layers of the skin, the dermis, and the subcutaneous tissue. In adults and children, cellulitis is most often caused by streptococcus, and staphylococcus aureus bacteria. Cellulitis due to hemophilus influenzae type B occurs commonly in the buccal soft tissues of infants. Facial cellulitis may result after a dental infection.

Clinical features

Before skin changes occur, someone with cellulitis has fever, chills, and fatigue. The skin infection is usually red, diffuse, swollen, warm to touch and painful. Overlying skin shows a deep purplish discolouration.

INFECTIONS OF SPECIFIC TISSUE SPACES

Most infections of odontogenic origin do not spread beyond the confines of the root space of the tooth; however, spread to distant sites of the body may occur. Direct spread is the major patch of dissemination of infection. Once the infection is outside the maxilla and mandible, further spread is to a large degree governed by the facial planes of the floor of the mouth, neck and mediastinum.

Infratemporal space

Infratemporal and temporal fossa together is called the masticator space.

Boundaries enclosed by the splitting of the investing fascia in the head.

Lateral: Outer border of masseter muscle, zygomatic arch, and temporalis muscle.

Medial: Medial border of the medial pterygoid muscle.

Mastigatory space infection is created iatrogenically when dentists inject needles into infratemporal fossa and carry infection into that place. Dental infections of the maxillary molar teeth may spread to infratemporal space.

Clinical sign and symptoms include trismus, pain, dysphagia, swelling in floor of mouth, pharyngeal wall and pushes palatine tonsil towards the midline.

Retropharyngeal space

Retropharyngeal space bounded anteriorly by posterior wall of pharynx, posteriorly by prevertebral fascia, superiorly by base of skull, and, inferiorly, it communicates with superior mediastinum.

Infection reaches from lateral pharyngeal space and an abscess may form.

The clinical presentation of retropharyngeal space infection includes difficulty in swallowing or breathing, anterolateral neck swelling, cervical lordosis, and unilateral cervical lymphadenopathy. Examination of the posterior pharynx reveals a tender, asymmetric swelling and, sometimes, the presence of gas. Infection may spread down to the mediastinum.

Parapharyngeal space

It is also known as lateral pharyngeal space, peripharyngeal space, pharyngomaxillary space.

These lie immediately posterior and lateral to the pharynx, and extend forwards into the sublingual region, so that together they actually form a ring around the pharynx. They lie entirely deep to the superficial or anterior layer of the deep fascia, and communicate more or less freely with each other around the muscles and vessels, which traverse them.

Parapharyngeal space is more subject to infection than any other spaces. It may receive infection from teeth, submandibular gland, masticator space, pharyngeal space, parotid space and paratonsillar space. From this space infection can pass to retropharyngeal space and then to superior mediastinum.

Extension from peritonsillar abscesses can occur by dissection through the pharyngeal wall, lymphatic spread, perivascular extension, or septic thrombosis of the peritonsillar veins.

Symptoms differ according to whether the pre-or-post styloid space is involved. Common features include fever, otalgia (ear pain), and odynophagia (pain on swallowing).

The cardinal signs of pre-styloid involvement are trismus, lateral wall fullness, induration, swelling and tenderness at the angle of mandible, and systemic toxicity.

Post-styloid involvement usually accompanied by marked sepsis, little or no trismus, and, sometimes, cranial nerve palsy and Horner's syndrome.

Complications include airway obstruction, jugular thrombophlebitis, descending suppurative mediastinitis, septic pulmonary foci, carotid rupture, aspiration pneumonia, and extension to adjacent neck space.

Parotid space

The parotid gland is completely enclosed in a well-defined compartment of deep fascia derived from superficial layer of deep cervical fascia. It becomes very thin on its deep aspect antero-superior to the thickened stylomandibular ligament where it can readily rupture.

Contents of parotid compartment include parotid gland with its substance—superficial parotid lymph nodes or lateral aspect of the gland, deep parotid lymph nodes within the gland.

Infection from the lateral pharyngeal space reaches the parotid space or retrograde extension through the parotid duct. Complications of parotid space infection include extension of infection into the temporal fossa and lateral pharyngeal space.

Space of the body of the mandible

It is bounded anteriorly by attachment of anterior belly of diagastric, posteriorly, attachment of medial pterygoid to jaw, inferiorly it is closed by continuity of fascial layers and superiorly closed by attachment of layers of mandible and myelohyoid line.

Infection in space of body of mandible can occur from osteomyelitis, secondary to dental infection. It may discharge into the mouth or may spread to masticator space.

Submandibular space

The investing layer splitting above the hyoid bone to enclose the submandibular gland forms the submandibular fascial space; superiorly, this layer of fascia is attached to the mentum and anterior body of mandible.

Involvement of submandibular space causes severe symptoms, such as neck rigidity, trismus, dysphagia, respiratory distress, sialorrhea, and pyrexia.

Submasseteric space

The submasseteric space is situated between the masseter muscle and the lateral surface of the mandibular ramus. Patient complains of trismus, pain and swelling. The infection from a mandibular third molar passes through the retromolar fossa to the submasseteric space.

Submaxillary space

The submaxillary space is located medial to the mandible and below the posterior portion of the mylohyoid muscle.

It is bordered by:

Medially: Hypoglossus and diagastric muscle.

Laterally: Superficial fascia and skin.

Sublingual space

Sublingual space is located between the mylohyoid muscles inferiorly and laterally, and the genioglossus and hypoglossus muscle complexes medially. Major components of sublingual space include the geniohyoid and genioglossus muscle, the hypoglossus-styloglossus muscle complex, the sublingual gland, deep portions of the submandibular gland and duct, the lingual nerve, and artery, and the twelfth nerve.

Clinically, there is swelling in the floor of the mouth. It gives rise to dyspnea and dysphagia.

Submental space

Early manifestations are pain in any involved teeth, with severe tender localised submental and sublingual induration. Boardlike firmness of the floor of the mouth and brawny induration of the suprahyoid soft tissues may develop rapidly. Drooling, trismus, dysphagia, stridor from laryngeal edema, and elevation of the posterior tongue against the palate may be present. Fever, chills, and tachycardia are usually present as well. The condition can cause airway obstruction.

LUDWIG'S ANGINA

It is named after the German physician, Wilhelm Friedrich von Ludwig, who first described this condition in 1836. Other names include '*angina maliga*' and '*Morbus strangularis*'.

Ludwig's angina is characterised as rapidly progressive gangrenous cellulitis of soft tissues of the neck, and floor of the mouth.

Causes

It is usually a bacterial infection, most often streptococcus supp, staphylococcus and bacteriodes. The route of infection in most cases is from infected lower third molars or from pericorontitis, which is an infection of the gums surrounding the partially erupted lower third molars. Addition etiologies include mandible fracture, neck trauma, tongue piercing, sialadenitis, neoplasm, and other parapharyngeal infections.

Clinical features

Symptoms include fever, neck pain, neck swelling, dysphagia, redness of neck, weakness, fatigue, excessive tiredness and breathing difficulty. Many patients of Ludwig's angina demonstrate a *'bull neck'* appearance as the inflammation spreads to submandibular region, giving the appearance of a large double chin. Trismus is often present and suggests irritation of the masticator muscles. Dyspnea, tachypnea, inspiratory stridor, and cyanosis are signs of impending airway obstruction related to progressive supraglottic edema.

BACTERAEMIA

The oral cavity, and particularly teeth with deep periodontal pockets, is an ideal habitat for hundreds of microbial species. Dentogenic bacteraemia can result even after a minimum trauma in the mouth. Oral microorganisms spread easily into the blood stream through inflamed gingival tissue, deep caries cavities, or ulcers of the mucosa.

The incidence of bacteraemia following dental procedures as tooth extraction, endodontic treatment, periodontal surgery, root scaling, and root planing has been well-documented. Even routine oral hygiene procedures such as daily tooth brushings, subgingival irrigation, and flossing may cause bacterloemia. Oral microorganisms and cytotoxic by-products associated with local infections can enter the blood stream or lymphatic system and cause damage or potentites an inappropriate immune response elsewhere in the body.

SEPTICAEMIA

It is the condition where bacteria circulate and multiply in the blood, form toxic products, and cause fever. Causative organisms of septicaemia are staphylococcus, streptococcus pyogens and streptococcus pneumoniae.

INFECTIVE ENDOCARDITIS

Infective endocarditis is a serious and often fatal systemic disease that has been associated with dental diseases and treatment. Bacteria that adhere to damaged or otherwise receptive surfaces of the tissue that lines heart valves cause endocarditis. Dental and other surgical procedures may predispose to susceptible patients to infective endocarditis by inducing bacteraemia. However, bacteraemia from oral infections that occur frequently during normal daily activities—coincidental even with chewing food, tooth brushing, and flossing—contribute more substantially to the risk of infective endocarditis.

Oral microorganisms: Microorganisms are common etiologic agents of infective endocarditis. For example, strains of S. sanguis, as well as Gram-negative oral bacteria including haemophilus aphrophilus, A. actinomycetemcomitans, E. corrotens, Capnocytophaga spp, and Fusobacterium nucleatum—have been associated with bacterial endocarditis.

BACTERIAL PNEUMONIA

Pneumonia can result from infection by anaerobic bacteria. Dental plaque would seem to be the logical source of these bacteria, especially in patients with periodontal disease. Such patients harbour a large number of subgingival bacteria, particularly anaerobic species. Among the oral bacterial species implicated in pneumonia are Actinomycetemcomitans, Actinomyces israeli, Capnocytophaga spp, Eikenella corrodens, Prevotella intermedia and Streptococcus consellatus.

Route of infection: A more likely and common route of systemic infection by oral microorganisms is through aspiration of oropharyngeal fluids containing oral pathogenic microorganisms, which colonize the lower respiratory tract and cause pneumonia.

LOW BIRTH WEIGHT

Pregnancy can influence gingival health; changes in hormone levels during pregnancy promote an inflammation termed pregnancy gingivitis.

Oral infections also seem to increase the risk for or contribute to low birth weight in newborns. A Gram-negative infection, periodontal disease, may have the potential to effect pregnancy outcome. During pregnancy, the ratio of anerobic bacteria increases in dental plaque in the second trimester. The Gram-negative bacteria associated with progressive disease produce a variety of bioactive molecules that can directly affect the host. One microbial component, LPS (lipopolysaccharide), can activate macrophages and other cells to synthesise and secrete a wide array of molecules, including cytokines, TNF-II-1, and PGE2. If they escape into the general circulation and cross the placental barrier, they could augment the physiologic levels of PGE2 and TNF in amniotic fluid and induce premature labour.

DIABETES MELLITUS

Periodontal disease can coexists with severe diabetes mellitus. Severe periodontal disease increases the severity of diabetes mellitus and complicates metabolic control. An infection mediated upregulation of cytokine. Synthesis and secretion by chronic stimulus from LPS and products of periodontophilic organisms may amply the magnitude of advanced glycation end products mediated cytokine response in diabetes mellitus. Cytokine upregulation explains the increase in tissue destruction seen in diabetes periodontitis and how periodontal infection complicates the severity of diabetes and degree of metabolic control.

CAVERNOUS SINUS THROMBOSIS

Cavernous sinus is most likely to be involved in the potentially fatal of dental infections. Cavernous sinus thrombosis is relatively uncommon, and orodental infections are responsible in approximately 10% of the cases.

Cavernous sinus thrombosis can also develop from an infection of the maxillary third molars that haematogenously spreads through the pterygoid plexus of veins to the angular vein, ophthalmic vein, and cavernous sinus.

MAXILLARY SINUSITIS

Maxillary sinusitis could result from infection and the percentage varies considerably between 4.6 and 4.7%.

Etiology

Maxillary sinusitis is usually caused by nasal infection due to viral influenza or common cold but sinus infection may be of dental origin.

Usually, periapical abscess in the upper premolar or molar teeth may spread to the maxillary sinus. A contaminated tooth or root fragment can also be displaced into maxillary sinus during an extraction, stimulating infection.

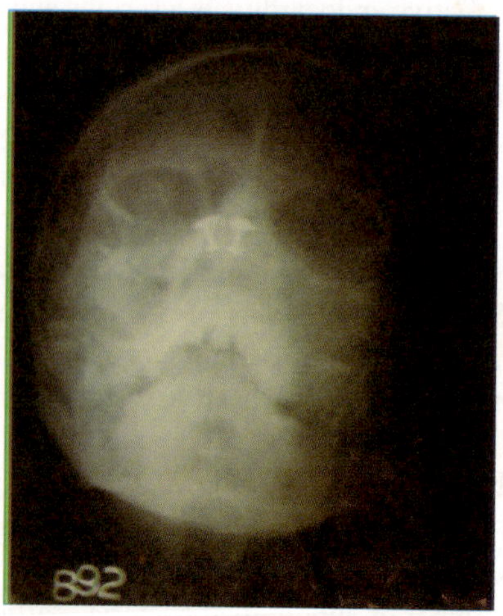

Fig.25.1: Showing haziness of both maxillary sinuses in a case of maxillary sinusitis

Signs and symptoms of maxillary sinusitis include tenderness over sinuses, nasal congestion, headache, foul odour, discharge down the back of the throat, nasal discharges, fever, and dental pain.

Chronic maxillary sinusitis

Chronic sinusitis is a complicated spectrum of disease that share chronic inflammation of the sinuses is common. It is divided into cases with polyps and cases without polyps, and the former is sometimes called chronic hyperplastic sinusitis.

Very rarely, the spreading of bacteria from a dental infection can also bring on chronic maxillary sinusitis.

Symptoms include nasal congestion, facial pain, headache, fever, general malaise, thick green or yellow discharge, vertigo, or lightheadedness, blurred vision, feeling official fullness or tightness which worsens on bending over, aching teeth and halitosis, and, occasionally, diarrhoea with mucus-like substance in it.

Microscopically

Histological findings in chronic sinusitis include basement membrane thickening, atypical gland formation, goblet cell hyperplasia, mononuclear inflammatory cell infiltration and subepithelial edema. There is thickening of sinus lining with squamous metaplasia of the mucosal lining and haemorrhage.

BRAIN ABSCESS

Definition: Brain abscess is a mass of immune cells, pus, and other material due to a bacterial or fungal infection.

Brain abscess usually occurs secondary to a focus of infection outside the central nervous system. Infected brain cells, white blood cells, and live or dead microorganisms collect in a limited area of the brain. An abscess begins as cerebral inflammation and progresses from focal necrosis to form encapsulated lesions.

The most common organism recovered form cultures is the bacterium Streptococcus. However, a wide variety of other bacteria (Proteus, Pseudomonas, Pneumococcus, Meningococcus, Haemophilus), fungi, and parasites may also cause the disease. Organisms that are most frequently associated with brain abscess in patients with AIDS are Mycobacterium tuberculosis, Toxoplasma gondii, and Cryptococcus neoformans.

Predisposing factors

1. Ear sepsis, e.g. chronic suppurative otitis media (CSOM) and mastoiditis.
2. Congenital cyanotic heart disease.
3. Sinusitis.
4. Bronchiectasis, subacute bacterial endocarditis.
5. Head injury, meningitis, and previous neurosurgical procedures.
6. Any major septic focus elsewhere in the body.

Complications: The swelling inside the brain can put pressure on the delicate brain tissue and the mass of pus itself can block blood vessels that are supplying essential blood to parts of the brain.

Clinical features

The symptoms of brain abscess are caused by a combination of increased intracranial pressure due to a space occupying lesion (headache, vomiting, confusion, coma), infection (fever, fatigue, etc.), and focal neurologic brain tissue damage (hemiparesis, aphagia etc.), The symptoms and findings depend largely on the specific location of the abscess in the brain. An abscess in the cerebellum may cause brain stem compression and hydrocephalus.

Brain abscesses are life-threatening infections. Recent progress in microbiological classification and identification has indicated that they are sometimes caused by oral infection and dental treatment.

It has been postulated that oral microorganisms may enter the cranium by several pathways:

1. By direct extension.
2. Oral infections spread along the facial planes.
3. Haematogenous spreading occurs along the facial, angular, ophthalmic, or other veins which lack valves, through the cavernous sinus, and into the cranium.
4. Through the general circulation.
5. Oral bacteria may cause systemic infections, e.g., endocarditis, and, then, indirectly initiate brain abscess.

MENINGITIS

It is the most common neurologic complication resulting from oral and maxillofacial infections. In this condition bacteria infect arachnoid mater and cerebrospinal fluid. As the brain abscess increases in size, it may rupture into the ventricular system and the result is usually fatal—if it extends into subarachnoid space, meningitis may develop.

Clinical features

Clinical features include fever, nausea and vomiting, headache, neck stiffness, seizures, and tachycardia.

Pathology

Macroscopically: Rosy red colouration of the meninges due to distention of the surface vessels. There may be a few petechial or longer haemorrhagic areas. The pia-arachnoid is congested; a turbid inflammatory exudate covers the surface of the brain.

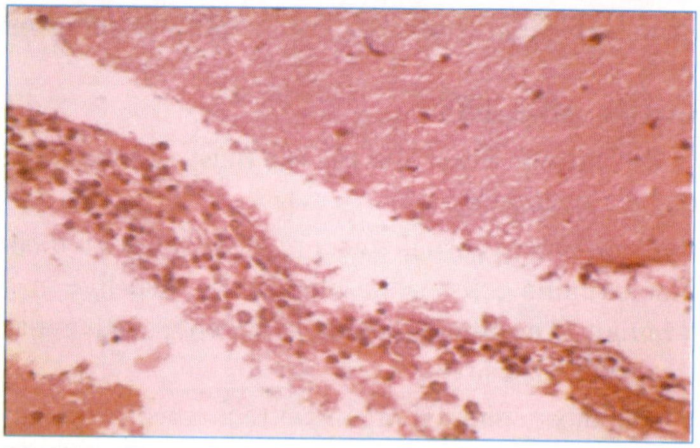

Fig.25.2: Shows brain tissue and acute inflammatory cells

Microscopically: The exudate consists principally of neutrophils mixed with a few lymphocytes.

Complications

1. A thin layer of pus forms and this may later organise to form adhesions. These may cause obstruction to the free flow of CSF leading to hydrocephalus or they may damage the cranial nerves at the base of the brain.
2. An obliterative endarteritis of the leptomeningeal arteries passing through the meningeal exudates may produce secondary cerebral infarction.

ATHEROSCLEROSIS AND MYOCARDIAL INFARCTION

Recent studies point to an increased incidence of heart disease and stroke in people with gum infections; the risk increases with the severity of the oral infection. Yet there is enough evidence to establish oral infection as an independent risk factor for heart disease or stroke.

ODONTOGENIC INFECTION OF ORBIT

Maxillary odontogenic infections can spread to the orbit by extension into infratemporal and pterygopalatine fossae and communicate with the inferior ophthalmic vein through the pterygoid plexus of veins. Anteriorly, infections of the incisors—especially the canine teeth—can spread directly or via communication of the non-valved angular fascial veins in the medial aspects of the orbit.

MEDIASTINITIS

Acute purulent mediastinitis caused by oropharyngeal infection is termed descending necrotising mediastinitis. Such infections usually have a fulminate course, leading to sepsis and frequently to death.

Mediastinitis occurring from a descending odontogenic infection occurs rarely.

Descending necrotising mediastinitis is caused by downward spread of neck and has a high fatality rate of 31%.

NECROTISING FASCITIS

Necrotising fasciitis of head and neck is a fulminant infection associated with necrosis of connective tissue, which spreads along the fascial planes with high mortality rate. It is a rapidly progressing condition, with a high morbidity and mortality rate.

The etiology in most of the cases reports being radicular abscess due to extensive caries, periodontal diseases, peritonsillar and pharyngeal abscesses, trauma, periodontitis, pericoronitis and osteonecrosis.

Although many underlying disease processes predispose patients to necrotising fasciitis, four common factors are invariably present:

(i) Impairment of immune system, e.g., diabetes mellitus, malignancy, and alcoholism.
(ii) Compromise of the facial blood vessels.
(iii) The presence of microorganisms that are able to proliferate within this area.
(iv) The disease is caused by a polymicrobial or mixed aerobic infection.

Face and neck is involved

The pathological changes of necrotising fasciitis include thrombosis of blood vessels, suppuration and necrosis of the superficial fascia with subcutaneous fat.

The characteristic features of necrotising fascitis are accumulation of gas in the tissues, odontogenic infection spreading to the neck, and anterior chest and an orange-peel appearance of the skin involved, which may change to a dusky discolouration. Skin is smooth, tense, and shiny with no sharp demarcation and poorly defined borders. There is necrosis of skin, which is secondary to thrombosis of nutrient blood vessels as they pass through the zone of involved fascia. If untreated, this will progress to frank cutaneous gangrene.

Focal infection

ARTHRITIS

There are evidences, which suggest that there is strong association between rheumatoid arthritis (RA) and periodontopathic bacteria. Clinical studies of rheumatoid arthritis and periodontal disease have provided evidence for a significant association between the two disorders. Patients with long standing active RA have a substantially increased frequency of periodontal disease compared with that among healthy subjects. High levels of oral anaerobic bacterial antibodies have been found in the serum of synovial fluid of RA patients.

OCULAR DISEASES

Inflammatory and infectious processes seen by those who perform facial surgery frequently affect the eye and orbit. The anatomical proximity and the common blood supply and drainage system make the orbit susceptible to infectious processes in the soft tissue of the face, paranasal sinuses, nose, teeth, gingival, and nasopharynx. Bacterial, viral, or fungal infections can affect the eye and orbit by direct spread of pathogen or alteration of blood supply and venous or lymphatic drainage.

Skin diseases

An abscessed or decayed tooth may contribute to acne, fungus infections of skin, eczema, dermatitis, venenata, impetigo, scabies, urticaria, psoriasis, and pityriasis rosea.

Other oral infections associated with skin lesions include erythema multiforme, pustular dermatitis, lichen planus, lupus erythematosus, and pustular acrodermatitis.

Renal diseases

The organisms such as streptococcus and staphylococcus from oral cavity reach to the urinary system via blood stream. It causes urinary tract infection and pyelonephritis.

INDEX

Abberancy 357
Abrasion 42, 43
Acanthomatous ameloblastoma 380
Acanthosis nigricans 192
Accessory duct 357
Accessory tongue 27
Achondroplasia 220
Acinic cell carcinoma 374, 395
Acquired myotonia 272
Acquired nevi 293
Acral lentiginous melanoma 340
Acrodermatitis enteropathica 245
Acrodynia 97
Acromegaly 210
Acrylic resin burn 95
Actinic cheilitis 318
Actinic keratosis 312
Acute atrophic candidiasis 127
Acute bacterial sialadenitis 360
Acute leukaemia 161
Acute lymphoblastic leukaemia 163
Acute periapical abscess 67
Acute pulpitis 67, 67
Acute suppurative osteomyelitis 139
Acute suppurative sialadenitis 360
Admantinoma 379
Addisonian pernicious anaemia 150
Addison's disease 202, 203, 204
Adenocarcinoma salivary gland 376, 377,
Adenoid cystic carcinoma 373, 374, 395
Adenoid basal cell carcinoma 341
Adenomatoid odontogenic tumour 381
Adrenal insufficiency 203
Aggressive periodonitis 84
Aglossia 27
Agnathia 16
Agranulocytosis 160
AIDS 116
AIDS related complex 119
Alberes-Schonberg disease 216
Alcohol injury 94
Alpha thalassaemia 155
Alveolar osteitis 140
Amalgam tattoo 94
Ameloblastic carcinoma 387
Ameloblastic fibroma 383
Ameloblastic fibroodontoma 383
Ameloblastic fibrosarcoma 389
Ameloblastoma 379
Amelogenesis imperfecta 38
Amyloidosis 225, 226
Amylotrophic lateral sclerosis 263
Anatomy of tongue 5
Anaemia 147
Aneurysmal bone cyst 284
Angioneurotic edema 238
Angiosarcoma 347
Angular cheilitis 127, 148
Ankylosis 36
Anodontia 33
Anular lichen planus 320
Aplasia of salivary gland 356
Aplastic anaemia 158
Arthritis 405
Aspergillosis 130
Arsenic intoxication 96
Aspirin burn 93
Atrophic lichen planus 320
Atherosclerosis 404
Attrition 42
Atrophy of muscle 274

B cell defects 225
Bacteraemia 401
Bacterial meningitis 404
Bacterial pneumonia 401
Bamboo spine 223
Basal cell ameloblastoma 380
Basal cell carcinoma 340
Basal cell nevus syndrome 281, 282, 283
Baseloid squamous cell carcinoma 332
Behcet's syndrome 238, 239
Bell's palsy 261
Benign lymphoepithelial lesion 364
Benign metastasizing mixed tumour 355

Beri beri 252
Beta thalassaemia 155
Bismuthism 96
Bitot's spots 247
Blastomycosis 132
Blue nevus 299
Bohn's nodule 279
Branchial cleft cyst 289, 290
Brain abscess 403
Brazilian pemphigus 182
Brown tumour of hyperparathyroidism 206
Brushfield's spots 216
Bruxism 88
Buccal caries 60
Bullous pemphigoid 183
Burkitt's lymphoma 354
Burning mouth syndrome 265

Caffey-Silverman syndrome 222
Calcifying epithelial odontogenic tumour 381
Calculus 75
Callus formation 54
Canalicular adenoma 369, 370
Cancrum oris 111
Candidial leukoplakia 313, 315
Candidiasis 122, 127
Cannon's disease 194
Capillary haemangioma 301
Carcinomatous epulis 331
Carcinoma ex pleomorphic adenoma 375
Carcinoma buccal mucosa 335
Carcinoma of floor of mouth 337
Carcinoma lip 334
Carcinoma of maxillary antrum 337
Carcinoma of palate 335
Carcinosarcoma 376
Castleman's disease 31
Cat scratch disease 112
Causes of pulpal inflammation 66
Cavernous haemangioma 302
Cavernous sinus thrombosis 402
Cellulitis 398
Cementoblastoma 386
Cementum 4
Cementicles 47
Cementum caries 63
Cervicofacial actinomycosis 109
Cervicofacial emphysema 91
Characteristics of benign tumours 291
Characteristics of malignant tumours 325
Cheilitis glandularis 362
Cheilitis granulomatosa 363
Chemical burn 93
Chemical injury 93
Cherubism 220
Chip munk facies 155
Chondroblastoma 309
Chondroma 308
Chondromyxoid fibroma 309
Chondrosarcoma 344
Choristoma 357
Christmas disease 173
Chronic atrophic candidiasis 127
Chronic bacterial sialadenitis 360
Chronic focal sclerosing osteomyelitis 141
Chronic hyperplastic candidiasis 127, 315
Chronic hyperplastic candidiasis 72
Chronic inflammatory gingival enlargement 77
Chronic lymphatic leukaemia 165
Chronic myeloid leukaemia 165
Chronic pulpitis 71
Chronic proliferative osteomyelitis 143
Chronic diffuse sclerosing osteomyelitis 142
Chronic suppurative osteomyelitis 142
Cicatrial pemphigoid 184, 185
Classification of benign tumours 191, 292
Clear cell odontogenic carcinoma 388
Cleft lip 20, 21
Cleft tongue 28
Cleidocranial dysostosis 214, 215
Cleidocranial dysplasia 214
Cocaine injury 95
Cocccidioidomycosis 131
Codman's tumour
Collagen 49
Comedonecrosis 332, 374
Commussural lip pits 20
Complex odontoma 386
Compound nevus 299
Condyloma accuminata 115
Congenital epulis of newborn 295
Congenital erythropoietic porphyria 156
Congenital fistulas 20

Congenital myotonia 271
Congenital syphilis 111
Contact dermatitis 227
Contact stomatitis 227
Counter current immunoelectrophoresis 11
CREST syndrome 188
Cretinism 207
Crouzon syndrome 204, 205
Crohn's disease 233
Cyclic neutropaenia 161
Cystic hygroma 302
Cysticercus cellulosae 135
Cytology basal cells 392
Cytology intermediate cells 392
Cytology dysplasia 392
Cytology superficial cells 391
Cytology parabasal cells 391
Cytology salivary gland tumours 395

Darier's disease 197
Darkground microscopy 8
Delayed eruption 34
Dens evaginatus 38
Dens invaginatous 38
Dens in dente 37
Dental caries 57, 62
Dental fluorosis 97, 98
Dentigerous cyst 278
Dentin dysplasia 41
Dentinogenesis imperfecta 40
Denture stomatitis 91
Dermatitis herpetiformis 190
Dermatitis venenata 227
Dermatomyositis 191
Dermoid cyst 287
Desmoplastic ameloblastoma 380
Development of tooth 4
Di George syndrome 225
Diabetes mellitus 199, 200, 201, 202, 402
Dilaceration 37
Dilatin 93
Diphtheria 104
Discoid lupus erythematosus 322
Diverticuli of salivary gland 357
Donovanosis 113
Dot and blot hybridization 13
Double lip 23
Doubling-Meara type epidermolysis bullosa 186
Down's syndrome 214, 215
Dry beri beri 252
Dyskeratosis congenital 323
Dystrophic myotonia 270, 271

Echinococcosis 136
Ectodermal dysplasia 195
Ehler's Danlos syndrome 194
Electrical burns 98
Electron microscope 9
Embedded teeth 34
Enamel caries 63
Enamel hypoplasia 39
Enamel pearl 38
Entamoeba gingivitis 132
Eosinophilic granuloma 90, 169
Epidermal growth factor 48
Epidermoid cyst 287
Epidermolysis bullosa 185
Epidermolysis bullosa dystrophic dominent 186
Epidermolysis bullosa dystrophic recessive 186
Epidermolysis bullosa simplex 185
Epidermolysis bullosa acquisita 187, 188
Epithelial dysplasia 319
Epulis fissuratum 92
Erosion 43, 44
Erosive lichen planus 320
Eruption cyst 279
Erysipelas 102
Erythema multiformae 176
Erythematous candidiasis 122, 127
Erythroblastosis fetalis 157
Erythrodermic psoriasis 178
Erythroleukoplakia 314
Erythroplakia 314
Etiology of salivary gland tumours 365
Eugenol burn 95
Ewing's sarcoma 345
Exfoliative cytology 391
Exostosis 307
External resorption 46

Facial hemiatrophy 19
Facial hemihypertrophy 18

Facial space infection 398
Factors affecting healing 48
Fat soluble vitamins 246
Fibroblastic growth factors 48
Fibroma 300
Fibromatous gingivae 25
Fibronectin 49
Fibrosarcoma 342
Fibrous dysplasia 218
Fibrous epulis 292
Fibrous histiocytoma 300
Fine needle aspiration cytology 393
Fissured tongue 28
Flow cytometry 12
Fluorescence microscopy 9
Fluorescent in situ hybridization 12
Fluorosis 97
Focal epithelial hyperplasia 24, 25
Focal myositis 269
Focal reversible pulpitis 66
Follicular ameloblastoma 380
Fordyce's granules 24
Fracture of mandible and maxilla 87
Fracture of teeth 86
Frey's syndrome 262
Frictional keratosis 89
Fusion 37

Garre's osteomyelitis 143
Gaucher's disease 241
Generalized cortical hyperostosis 222
Geniculate neuralgia 261
Geographic tongue 29
Germination 37
Giant cell epulis 293
Ginat cell reparative granuloma 293
Ginat cell tumour 350
Gigantism 209, 210
Gingival cyst of adults 280
Gingival cyst of newborn 279
Gingival enlargement due to drugs 77
Gingival enlargement with leukaemia 77, 79
Gingival enlargement 78
Gingivitis 75
Glandular odontogenic cyst 283
Glanzmann's disease 173
Globulomaxillary cyst 285
Glossopharyngeal neuralgia 260, 261
Glucose 6 phosphate deficiency anaemia 157
Gonorrhoea 103
Gorlin cyst 281
Granular cell myoblastoma 303
Granulomatous epulis 293
Granuloma inguinale 113
Granuloma venereum 113
Gums 6
Gumma 110
Gutta percha 94

Haemangioma 301
Haemangioendothelioma 346, 347
Haemangiopericytoma 347
Haemoglobin Bart disease 155
Haemoglobin electrophoresis 11
Haemolytic anaemia 151
Haemolytic disease of newborn 157
Haemophilia A 173
Haemophilia B 173, 174
Haemophilia C 174
Hairy leukoplakia 122
Hallopeau type of pemphigus 182
Hand-Schuller-Christian disease 169
Hand foot and mouth syndrome 125
Hansen's disease 106
Hard palate 6
Harrison's groove 249
Healing of wounds 48
Healing of fracture 54
Healing by first intention 51
Healing by second intention 53
Healing by third intention 54
Heck's disease 24
Hemifacial spasm 272
Hereditary benign intraepithelial dyskeratosis 197
Hereditary elliptocytosis 157
Hereditary gingival fibromatosis 77
Hereditary haemorrhagic telangiectasia 192
Hereditary spherocytosis 151
Herlitz's disease 187
Herpangina 116
Herpes simplex virus 114
Herpes zoster 115

Herpetiform ulcer 229
Herpetic gingivostomatitis 114
Histiocytosis X 168
Histiocytosis Y 297
Histoplasmosis 130
HIV virus 117
Hodgkin's lymphoma 352, 353, 394
Homogenous leukoplakia 313
Homozygous β-thalassaemia 155
Homozygous sickle cell anaemia 153
Howell-Jolly bodies 150
Human bite 90
Hunter's syndrome 244
Hutchinson's freckle 399
Hydatid cyst 136
Hydrogen peroxide burn 95
Hypercementosis 46
Hyperparathyroidism 205
Hyperpituitarism 209, 210
Hyperplastic candidiasis 122, 127
Hypertrophy of muscle 274, 275
Hyperthyroidism 208, 209
Hypertrophic lichen planus 313
Hypervitaminosis A 248
Hypoparathyroidism 205, 206
Hypopituitarism 210
Hypoplasia of salivary glands 356
Hypothyroidism 207

Idiopathic thrombocytopaenic purpura 171
Immunoelectrophoresis 10
Impacted teeth 34
Impetigo contagiosa 101
Imprint cytology 296
Incontinenta pigmenti 195
Infantile beri beri 252
Infectious mononucleosis 126
Infective endocarditis 401
Infratemporal space 398
Inflammatory papillary hyperplasia 92
Internal resorption 45
Intramucosal nevus 299
Iron deficiency anaemia 148
Ionizing radiation 99
Iodine burn 95
Irreversible pulpitis 66

Junctional epidermolysis bullosa 187
Junctional nevus 299
Juvenile periodontitis 83

Kaposi's sarcoma 123, 348, 349
Keratinizing calcifying odontogenic cyst 280
Keratinocyte growth factor 49
Keratoacanthoma 327
Keratomalacia 247
Keratosis follicularis 197
Koeber type epidermolysis bullosa 186
Koplick's spots 126
Korsakoff's psychosis 252
Kwashiorkor disease 241

Laboratory diagnosis of AIDS 123, 124
Laminin 49
Lateral periodontal cyst 278
Lead poisoning 96
Leiomyoma 306
Leishmaniasis 133
Lentigo maligna melanoma 339
Lepromas 107
Lepromatous leprosy 107
Leprosy 106
Letterer-Siwe disease 169
Leukaemia 161
Leukoplakia 312
Leukoplakia erosive 313
Leukoplakia simplex 313
Leukoplakia verrucosa 313
Lichen planus 319
Light microscope 8
Life cycle of HIV virus 119
Linear IgA dermatosis 198
Lingual caries 62
Lingual thyroid nodule 30, 31
Lingual varicosities 30
Lipoma 305
Liposarcoma 343
Localized myositis ossificans 267
Low birth weight 402
Ludwig angina 400
Lupus erythematosus 322
Lymphangioma 302

Lymphoepithelial cyst 32
Lymphogranuloma venereum 113
Lymphoid patches 31
Lymphoma B cell type 123, 394

Macrocheilia 22
Macrodontia 36
Macroglossia 26, 27
Macrognathia 17
McCune-Albright's syndrome 220
Malignant ameloblastoma 387
Malignant fibrous histiocytoma 342
Malignant lymphoma 351
Malignant melanoma 338
Malignant pleomorphic adenoma 375
Management of AIDS 124
Mandible 1
Mandibular tori 296
Mandibulofacial dysostosis 32, 33
Marasmus 240
Marble bone disease 216
Marfan's syndrome 214
Massive osteolysis 222
Maxilla 3
Maxillary sinusitis 402
Measles 125, 126
Median rhomboid glossitis 28, 39
Mediterranian anemia 154
Mediastinitis 405
Melanotic ectodermal tumour of infancy 384
Mercurialism 97
Mesenchymal chondrosarcoma 344
Meniere's disease 265
Mesiodens 34
Metallic stains 74
Metastatic carcinoma salivary gland 377
Microbiology of dental caries 59
Microdontia 36
Microglossia 27
Micrognathia 16
Microscopy 3
Midline lethal granuloma 231
Mikulicz disease 364
Mikulicz cells 111
Mild restricted muscular dystrophy 270
Minor aphthae 229
Mobius syndrome 274
Mixed salivary gland tumour cytology 395
Molluscum sebaceum 327
Monomorphic adenoma 369
Monostotic fibrous dysplasia 218
Morulla cells 168
Motor neuron disease 262
Mucocele 286
Mucoepidermoid carcinoma 372, 373
Mucormycosis 128
Mulberry molar 111
Multiple myeloma 166
Mumps 361
Munro's abscess 179
Muscular dystrophy 269
Myasthenia gravis 273, 274
Myiasis 132
Myocardial infarction 404
Myositis ossificans 267
Myotonias 270
Myxedema 207
Myxoma 301

Nasoalveolar cyst 284
Nasolabial cyst 284
Nasopalatine cyst 283
Natto classification of dental stain 74
Necrosis of pulp 72, 153
Necrotizing sialometaplasia 364
Niemann-Pick disease 242
Neumann type of pemphigus 182
Neurilemmoma 304
Neurofibroma 303
Neurofibromatosis 304
Neurotoxoplasmosis 134
Neutropaenia 160
Nevi 298
Naevoid basal cell carcinoma 281
Niacin 253
Nicotine stomatitis 89
Nicotine reverse smoker's palate 317
Night blindness 247
Nocternal parafunctioning habits 87
Nodular leukoplakia 313
Nodular melanoma 339
Noma 111

Non-Hodgkin's lymphoma 351, 394
Nursing bottle caries 60
Northern blot 13

Ocular diseases 405
Occlusal caries 61
Odontogenic caries 61
Odontogenic dysplasia 42
Odontogenic fibrosarcoma 390
Odontogenic infection of orbit 404
Odontogenic keratocyst 281
Odontogenic myxoma 384
Odontogenic tumours 378
Odontoma 385
Oncocytoma 371, 395
Oral melanotic macule 23
Osler-Weber-Rendu disease 192
Osteoblastoma 307
Osteochondroma 307
Osteoclastoma 350
Osteogenesis imperfecta 213
Osteogenic sarcoma 344
Osteoid osteoma 307
Osteoma 306
Osteomalacia 250
Osteomyelitis 70, 138
Osteoporosis 212
Osteoradionecrosis 145

Paget's disease 217
Palatal caries 62
Palatine torus 296
Papillary cystadenoma lymphomatosum 370, 395
Papillion-Lefevre syndrome 85
Papilloma 297
Popular lichen planus 320
Paracoccidioidomycosis 131
Paramyotonia 273
Paraneoplastic pemphigus 183
Parapharyngeal space 399
Parotid space 399
Parry-Romberg syndrome 19
PCR 14
Pellagra 254
Pellicle 58, 73
Pemphigus 180
Pemphigus erythematosus 183
Pemphigus foliacious 181
Pemphigus vegetans 182
Pemphigus vulgaris 181
Periapical abscess 64, 67
Periapical granuloma 64, 68
Periodontitis 80, 83
Peripheral ameloblastoma 379
Peripheral giant cell reparative granuloma 294
Pernicious anaemia 150
Pharyngeal gonorrhoea 103
Phenol burn 95
Pigeon chest 249
Pierre-Robin sequence 221
Pindborg tumour 381
Pityriasis rosea 193
Pizza burn 98
Plaque lichen planus 320
Plasmacytoma 310
Platelet derived growth factor 48
Plexiform ameloblastoma 380
Pleomorphic adenoma salivary gland 367, 368
Plummer Vinson's syndrome 149, 319,
Plunging ranula 287
Polyarteritis nodosa 232
Polycystic disease parotid gland 357
Polycythaemia 159
Polymerase chain reaction 14
Polyostotic fibrous dysplasia 219
Porokeratosis Miebelli 196
Precancerous conditions 311
Pregnancy tumour 80, 295
Primary healing 51
Primary intraosseous carcinoma 388
Primary syphilis 110
Primary systemic generalized amyloidosis 226
Primordial cyst 281
Prion disease 137
Progeria 211
Progressive bulbar palsy 264
Progressive muscular atrophy 262, 263
Progressive myositis ossificans 268
Proliferative myositis 268
Proliferative verrucous leukoplakia 313
Protein deficiency 240
Psoriasis 178

Psoriatic arthritis 178
Pulp calcification 44
Pulp necrosis 72, 153
Pulpitis 66
Pulse granuloma 69
Pustular psoriasis 178
Pyogenic granuloma 295

Radiation injury 99
Radiation osteomyelitis 145
Radicular cyst 277
Rampant caries 61
Recurrent aphthous stomatitis 228
Reiter's syndrome 229
Rendu-Osler-Weber syndrome 193
Residual cyst 277
Reticular lichen planus 320
Retrocuspid papilla 26
Retropharyngeal space 399
Reversible pulpitis 66
Rhabdomyoma 306
Rhabdomyosarcoma 349
Rheumatoid arthritis 235
Rhinoscleroma 111
Rhinosporidiosis 128, 129
Rickets 248
Riboflavin 253
Rickety rosary 249
Riga Fede disease 88, 89, 91
Rodent ulcer 340
Root caries 63
Rootless teeth 41
Root resorption 46

Salivary gland 6
Salivary gland calculus 361
Sarcoidosis 229, 230
Seborrheic dermatitis 253
Scanning electron microscope 10
Scarlet fever 102
Schmorl's node 213
Schaumann bodies 230
Schwannoma 304
Scleroderma 188
Scrotal tongue 28
Secondary syphilis 110
Secondary systemic generalized amyloidosis 266
Septicaemia 401
Severe generalized muscular dystrophy 269
Sexual abuse 90
Shingles 115
Sialoadenosis 358
Sialolithiasis 361, 362
Sickle cell anaemia 153
Sickle cell crisis 153
Simple microscope 8
Sjogren's syndrome 225
Skeletal fluorosis 223
Smokeless tobacco keratosis 323
Smooth surface caries 60, 61
Snail track ulcer 110
Soft palate 6
Southern blot 13
Space of body of mandible 400
Spasmophilia 249
Sphingomyelin lipidosis 242
Spindle cell carcinoma 331
Spread of infection 397
Squamous cell carcinoma cytology 393
Squamous cell carcinoma tongue 332
Squamous odontogenic tumour 382
Squamous cell papilloma 297
Stafne's bone cyst 285
Steven's Johnson syndrome 177
Stomatitis venenata 227
Sublingual ulceration 88
Submandibular space 400
Submucus fibrosis 315, 316, 317
Sulphur granules 109
Superficial spreading melanoma 339
Supernumerary teeth 34
Synovial sarcoma 346
Syphilis 110
Syphilitic glossitis 319
Syphilitic osteomyelitis 145
Systemic lupus erythematosus 322

T- and B-cell defects 224
T-cell defects 225
Talon cusp 37
Tay-Sachs disease 243

Temporal arteritis 264
Tertiary syphilis 110
Tetracycline stains 93
Thalassaemia intermedia 155
Thalassaemia 154
Thermal burns 98
Thiamine 251
Thistle pulp tube 41
Thrombotic thrombocytopaenic purpura 172
Thrombocytopaenia 169, 170
Thrush 127
Thyroglosssal duct cyst 288
Thyroid storm 209
Thyrotoxicosis 208
Tic douloureux 259
Tobacco stain 74
Tongue tie 28
Tongue anatomy 4
Tooth anatomy 5
Torus mandibularis 296
Torus palatinus
Toxic epidermal necrolysis 178
Transitional cell carcinoma 342
Transmission electron microscope 10
Transforming growth factor 49
Traumatic bone cyst 90
Traumatic lesions due to sexual habits 90
Traumatic neuroma 304
Traumatic ulcer 88
Treacher-Collins syndrome 32, 33
Trench mouth 82
Trichinosis 136
Trichloroacetic acid burn 95
Trichomoniasis 135
Trigeminal neuralgia 259
Trisomy 21 syndrome 215
Trypanosomiasis 133
Tuberculosis 105
Tubercular osteomyelitis 144
Tuberculosis of salivary glands 360
Tuberculoid leprosy 107, 108
Tumour forming localized amyloidosis 226
Tumours of salivary gland 365, 366
Type I diabetes mellitus 200
Type II diabetes 200

Ulcerative lichen planus 320

Vascular endothelial growth factor 49
Verrucous carcinoma 331
Verrucous leukoplakia 313
Vitamin A 246
Vitamin B_1 251
Vitamin B_2 253
Vitamin B_3 253
Vitamin B_6 255
Vitamin B_9 255
Vitamin B_{12} 149
Vitamin C 256, 257
Vitamin D 248
Vitamin D resistant rickets 248
Vitamin E 250, 251
Vitamin K 250,
Von-Ricklinhghausen's neurofibromatosis 303

Waldeyer's ring 5
Warthin's tumour 370, 395
Water soluble vitamins 252
Waterhouse Friderichsen syndrome 204
Weber-Cockayne syndrome 186
Wegner granulomatosis 232
Wernicke's encephalopathy 252
Western blot method 13
Wet beri beri 252
White sponge nevus 194
Witkop-von-Salman syndrome 197
Wound healing 48

Xerostomia 358, 359, 360
Xerophthalmia 247

Zinc phosphate injury 94
Zinser-Engman-Cole syndrome 323